IMMUNE REACTIVITY
OF LYMPHOCYTES

Development, Expression, and Control

ADVANCES IN EXPERIMENTAL MEDICINE AND BIOLOGY

IMMUNE REACTIVITY OF LYMPHOCYTES

Development, Expression, and Control

Edited by

Michael Feldman and
Amiela Globerson
The Weizmann Institute of Science

PLENUM PRESS • NEW YORK AND LONDON

Library of Congress Cataloging in Publication Data

International Conference on Lymphatic Tissue and Germinal Centers in Immune
Reactions, 5th, Teverya, Israel, 1975.
Immune reactivity of lymphocytes.

(Advances in experimental medicine and biology; v. 66)
Includes bibliographical references and index.
1. Lymphocytes—Congresses. 2. Immune response—Congresses. I. Feldman, Michael.
II. Globerson, Amiela. III. Title. IV. Series. [DNLM: 1. Lymphocytes—Immunology—
Congresses. W1 AD559 v. 66/WH700 I604 1975i]
QR185.8.L9I55 1975   616.07'9   75-42123
ISBN-13:978-1-4613-4357-8   e-ISBN-13:978-1-4613-4355-4
DOI: 10.1007/978-1-4613-4355-4

Proceedings of the Fifth International Conference on Lymphatic
Tissue and Germinal Centers in Immune Reactions held in Tiberias,
Israel, June 24-30, 1975

©1976 Plenum Press, New York
Softcover reprint of the hardcover 1st edition 1976

A Division of Plenum Publishing Corporation
227 West 17th Street, New York, N.Y. 10011

United Kingdom edition published by Plenum Press, London
A Division of Plenum Publishing Company, Ltd.
Davis House (4th Floor), 8 Scrubs Lane, Harlesden, London, NW10 6SE, England

Foreword

The area of the Lake of Galilee, which is the site of the Fifth Conference on Lymphatic Tissues and Germinal Centers, has been a germinal center of dramatic events in human history. Thus, some two million years ago, it seems to have harbored an important phase of human evolution, when the descendants of the African Australopithecus migrated northwards, attempting to become Homo sapiens. Two thousand years ago, this very place was a germinal center for a new religion which determined some of the most important components of the history of western civilization. This may have been the first significant contribution of the people of the Lake of Galilee area to the world of ideas and values. More recently, some 70 years ago, this very place was a germinal center for a great experiment aimed at the translation into actual reality of ethical and social values, by the establishment of the first kibbutz in Israel on this shore. We, therefore, hoped that by selecting this place for the Fifth Germinal Centers Meeting we could expect the inspiration of the site to generate new concepts and views.

We should admit, however, that the lymphoid germinal center in senso stricto was not the subject of many of the contributions that were presented at the conference. However, this seems justified in view of the present state of the art, for it is realized that, in aiming at the understanding of the relations of cellular tissue structures to immunological function, a deeper insight ought to be obtained into more basic systems. Hence, the symposium opened with a discussion of the ontogeny of lymphoid cells which was followed by a series of presentations on surface properties of lymphocytes and their relation to processes associated with the immunological activation of these cells. This furnished the basis for an approach to an area intimately connected with germinal center formation and function, i.e., problems of microenvironment, lymphocyte migration and induction. The specificity of the immune response is obviously determined by the recognition of antigens by cells; hence, problems of cell receptors and the control of immune reactions constituted a significant

part of the conference.   Tumor immunity and immunopathology were the
natural extensions towards aspects of applied immunology and human biology.

In view of the wide spectrum of subjects covered, it seems unneces-
sary to explain the reasons for Dr. J. H. Humphrey's being the
invited speaker of the symposium.   He brought us all back to the focal
questions of the interrelation between morphological manifestations and
immunological reactions, i. e. , to the question of the significance of germinal centers.   And he did so in a most inspiring way.

                              Michael Feldman and Amiela Globerson

Contents

SESSION 2

SURFACE PROPERTIES AND ACTIVATION
OF LYMPHOID CELLS

Chairpersons: G. Möller and M. Schlesinger

SESSION 4

CELL INTERACTIONS IN IMMUNE RESPONSES

Chairpersons: J. F. A. P. Miller and A. J. S. Davies

SESSION 5

LYMPHOID CELL RECEPTORS AND ANTIGEN RECOGNITION

Chairpersons: G. L. Ada and G. E. Roelants

SESSION 6

TUMOR IMMUNOLOGY: INTERACTIONS BETWEEN
LYMPHOCYTES, ANTIBODIES AND NEOPLASTIC CELLS

Chairpersons: G. Klein and M. G. Hanna, Jr.

SESSION 7

ROUND-TABLE DISCUSSION: DEFINITION AND FUNCTIONS
OF IR GENES

Chairperson: M. Sela

SESSION 8

REGULATION OF IMMUNE RESPONSES: SUPPRESSOR CELLS, THEIR NATURE AND FUNCTION.   ENHANCING FACTORS

Chairpersons: R. K. Gershon and G. A. Voisin

SESSION 9

IMMUNOPATHOLOGY

Chairpersons: J. D. Feldman and H. Cottier

Ontogeny of Lymphoid Cells

DIFFERENTIATION AND ONTOGENY OF LYMPHOID CELLS

N.L. Warner

Genetics Unit, The Walter & Eliza Hall Institute

Royal Melbourne Hospital, Victoria, Australia

For many years it has been recognised that lymphocytes play a central role in the initiation and development of both cellular and humoral immunity. In considering the heterogeneous nature of specific immune responses it was proposed from studies in birds[1] that there were two distinct lymphoid cell differentiation pathways, in that the bursa of Fabricius controlled the development of cells of the antibody forming series, whereas the thymus controlled the differentiation of lymphoid cells involved in cellular immunity. With the subsequent development of the concept of cell interactions in immune responses[2,3], the specific roles of bone marrow derived cells, (termed B cells, implying either bursal equivalent derivation) and T cells, in production of antibody were clearly defined. The subsequent application of a variety of cell surface markers and receptors to the analysis of distinct populations of lymphoid cells has even further validated the concept of two broad streams of lymphocyte differentiation represented under the general groupings of T and B lymphocytes. In this presentation I would like to concentrate on several of the current problems relating to the differentiation and ontogeny of T and B lymphocytes.

The basic premise taken in this discussion, is that T and B cells represent independent lines of differentiation that are relatively fixed, cells of one line do not differentiate into the alternative pathway. However, both lines ultimately trace back to a common precursor cell termed the hematopoietic stem cell. In order to attempt to delineate some of the specific problems concerned with lymphoid cell ontogeny, reference will be made to the accompanying

3

figure, the numbers referring to the following ten topics. One general point to be noted is the contrast between the relatively simple concept of differentiation originally proposed from studies in the chicken, and the more elaborate scheme of lymphocyte differentiation currently envisaged. The original concept basically proposed that a hematopoietic stem cell encountered either bursal or thymic inductive influences and was there induced into differentiation of T and B lymphocytes. More recent studies however, suggest that there may be several distinct stages of differentiation both pre and post primary lymphoid organ involvement, and lymphoid ontogeny or differentiation might be considered in three areas: preceding primary lymphoid organ involvement, events occurring within or induced by primary lymphoid organ function, and post primary lymphoid organ differentiation, (the latter process being principally antigen induced.) In the following brief discussion, I will deal with several of the current topical questions in immunocyte differentiation. In dividing the following discussion into ten points, it is perhaps relevant to note that there is controversy over the question of whether lymphoid differentiation is a continuous process or can be divided into distinct stages. The general approach to be used in this discussion, is to consider lymphoid differentiation in terms of stages, where different inductive stimuli are required for the process of differentiation from one stage to another.

1. Existence of Lymphoid Stem Cells

It is generally accepted that both T and B cell lineages ultimately trace back to a common precursor cell termed the hematopoietic stem cell, which has itself originally derived in the yolk sac from precursor hemangeoblasts and during foetal to post natal life this pool progressively moves from the yolk sac to foetal liver to the adult bone marrow. Such stem cells are capable of self-renewal and under specific inductive influences (possibly from local micro environments), these cells progressively differentiate into the mature elements of the hematopoietic system[4]. Marker studies have formally shown that hematopoietic stem cells will give rise to all hematopoietic elements including lymphoid, erythroid and myeloid series. The unresolved problem in this area is to determine at what point the two pathways of B and T cell differentiation irrevocably diverge. The original concept that the pluripotential stem cell itself moves into the thymus or bursa and is therein separately induced into T or B cell differentiation must be still questioned. The first arrow on the proposed diagram indicates that there may be a specific inductive event that induces the differentiation of the pluripotential stem cell into a cellular element which is now specifically committed to lymphoid differentiation, i.e. what might be termed a <u>lymphoid</u> stem cell. The lymphoid stem cell can now no longer be induced into either erythroid or myeloid differentiation, but can still be induced into <u>either</u> T or B cell pathways. As will be discussed below, although pre-T or pre-B cells have been defined, it is not yet clear whether these are one and the same cell type, i.e. themselves to be termed lymphoid stem cells, or are the progeny of such a hypothetical cell as indicated in the diagram.

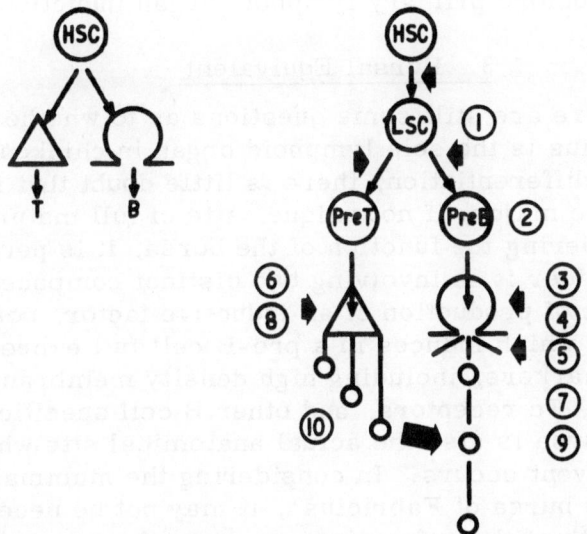

Fig. 1. Schemes of lymphoid cell differentiation. The simpler model proposes direct induction of hematopoietic stem cells (HSC) by thymus or bursa, whereas the complex model envisages multiple pre- and post- primary lymphoid organ stages. Solid arrows indicate possible induction stages and numbers refer to text sub-headings.

2. Pre T - Pre B Stages

In distinction to the concept that the pluripotential hematopoietic stem cell itself migrates into the primary lymphoid organs and is there induced to T or B cell differentiation, several recent studies[5, 6], have suggested that there are distinct precursor cell stages for both the T and B cell lineages, that are not pluripotential stem cells. The associated diagram suggests two possible stages; as noted above, the initial commitment of stem cells into the lymphoid differentiation pathway, followed by induction into a pre-T and pre-B cell stage. This model proposes that there is at least one definable stage prior to primary organ control, which has already involved commitment to the T or B cell pathway of differentiation. As will be discussed in this session by Dr. Roelants, some marker studies suggest that cells either in bone marrow or recirculating through blood are committed to the T cell pathway, as indicated by the minimal expression of several T cell specific markers, at a stage prior to thymic induction. The evidence for this is still preliminary, but is sufficient to warrant consideration as to whether the initial commitment to T or B cell pathways of differentiation is made within or before primary lymphoid organ induction.

3. Bursal Equivalent

Although there are still some questions as to whether the avian bursa of Fabricius is the sole lymphoid organ in chickens capable of inducing B cell differentiation, there is little doubt that in the normal situation it is the major, if not unique, site of full maturation of B cells[1]. In considering the function of the bursa, it is perhaps relevant to consider it as involving two distinct components. Firstly, the site of production of an inductive factor, possibly by epithelial cells, which induces in a pre-B cell full expression of mature B cell markers, including high density membrane immunoglobulin, Fc receptors, and other B cell specific markers. Secondly, the bursa is also the actual anatomical site where this differentiation event occurs. In considering the mammalian equivalent of the bursa of Fabricius[7], it may not be necessary to consider that both of these functions occur in the same site, i.e. there may be a bursal equivalent hormone, produced by an epithelial cell analogous to that in the avian bursa, but this may be a true hormone in inducing its action of differentiation in a distinct site. There is much evidence to suggest that the mammalian foetal liver is the primary site of B cell differentiation in ontogeny[8]. Whether the bone marrow also has this function[9] has not been fully clarified, as an alternative explanation is that the bone marrow contains a stem cell lineage of B cells perhaps in a somewhat early stage of differentiation, expressing some B cell markers such as MBLA[10], but not yet fully differentiated into mature B cells with high density membrane immunoglobulin. Further work is still required to determine whether the foetal liver is the site where the pre B cell encounters its inductive stimulus, or whether it is actually the site of formation of an as yet unidentified bursal type hormone.

4. Regulation of Isotype Expression

In considering B cell differentiation, it is particularly relevant to consider the expression of different constant region heavy chain genes. One view[7] proposes that sequential expression of IgM to IgG to IgA occurs only in foetal life and the respective precursor cells seed out during this period. An alternative[11] is that in the adult animal virgin precursor immuno-competent cells bear IgM type receptors, and on antigenic stimulation differentiation is initiated that results in expression of the other heavy chain classes. This second view basically proposes that a switch mechanism can operate following post antigen induced differentiation[11]. A variety of experimental models, particularly using purified cell preparations[12], are currently under analysis in attempts to resolve this situation.

5. IgD

A recently introduced aspect into the question of isotype expression concerns IgD immunoglobulin. It has been clearly shown that in man[13], IgD is expressed by B lymphocytes in the foetal and neonatal period, although relatively little secretion of IgD is occurring at this time. The exact sequence of expression of IgM and IgD in foetal life is still to be precisely determined. A series of recent studies (discussed in[14]) have suggested that in mice as in man, there is a second heavy chain type expressed by a large proportion of B lymphocytes. This second immunoglobulin type has been mainly detected by radioactive labelling of cell surface immunoglobulin. At present there is no distinct antigenic identification of this molecule although in some respects it appears to parallel human IgD. As it has been shown in mice, that the second heavy chain type is not detectable at the membrane level until after two weeks of life, it is perhaps unlikely that it plays an essential role in antigen induced lymphocyte activation. As several studies[14] with human chronic lymphatic leukemia cells (B cell neoplasms) have shown that cell lines express both IgM and IgD with the same variable region, the analysis of intracellular control of immunoglobulin gene synthesis in this regard is one of the most interesting current problems of control of immunoglobulin gene expression.

6.   Ontogeny of V Region Expression

In a somewhat analogous fashion to the problem of sequential or simultaneous expression of C region genes, is the question of expression of different V region genes, in both T and B cell lineages. For the purposes of this discussion, the thesis that the antigen specific receptor of T and B cells both involve V region genes will be held[11]. Several recent experimental models[15, 16] have been devised to study whether the ability to produce specific V region genes occurs simultaneously or sequentially during ontogenic development. In general these studies are suggesting that the cellular origin of different V region gene expression may be clonal in nature and occurs at different time intervals in development for different V region gene patterns. Alternatively, some studies[17] on antigen binding cells have suggested that particularly in sites representative of early B cell differentiation, the frequency of multiple antigen binding cells is considerable, suggesting that with B cell differentiation, restriction of V region gene expression in a given cell lineage occurs. Further analysis of this problem with particular reference to comparisons of the timing of expression of different V region gene activities in T and B cell lineages, will be valuable in comparing the nature of the antigen specific receptor in cells of these two types.

7.   B Cell Differentiation Markers

Analysis of distinct stages of B cell differentiation will be considerably aided by elucidation of the sequence of expression of various B cell markers. It has been shown that cell surface expression of high density membrane immunoglobulin increases from the pre-B cell stage through B cell maturation and then decreases with differentiation to the mature plasma cell[11]. Several studies also suggest that the surface expression of the Fc receptor parallels that of membrane immunoglobulin i.e. rises and then falls[11]. Studies on the ontogenic expression of the C3 receptor suggest a later expression of this marker[18]. Few studies in this regard have yet been performed on B cell hetero- or allo-antigens. By determining the sequence of expression of these various B cell specific markers, it may be possible to devise distinct phenotypes for characterising a given cell type e.g.(a neoplastic B cell line) at a particular stage of differentiation. Such a provisional scheme has recently been proposed by a UICC committee in considering immunoglobulin producing neoplasms in man and other animals[19]

8. Intrathymic Pathways

In considering T cell differentiation, it is perhaps convenient to divide the problem into prethymic, intrathymic and postthymic differentiation. Problems of prethymic differentiation have been discussed above. It should be noted however, that there are still several current alternative considerations regarding intrathymic differentiation. Although it is tempting to consider that a cell of phenotype low Thy-1, low Tl differentiates into a cell with high Thy-1, high Tl, and then further differentiates and peripheralises as a low Thy-1 negative Tl cell, an alternative scheme has been proposed [20] that suggests there are two pathways of T cell differentiation within the thymus. Firstly a terminal differentiation to a high Thy-1, high Tl positive cell which dies within the thymus, and a second pathway which represents the peripheralised T cell.

9. T Cell Control of Plasma Cell Differentiation

Although the majority of studies on cell collaboration between T and B cell lineages concern antigen specific collaboration, there are sufficient studies to recognise the concept that T cell factors of a non-antigen specific nature may be involved as true inductive stimuli for terminal plasma cell maturation from B cells. This concept may be particularly relevant in considering several clinical situations[21] wherein "suppressor T cells" appear to act to prevent terminal plasma cell differentiation. This may involve complex interactions where the so called suppressor T cell function acts to control a T cell inductive function, i.e. increasing suppressor activity negates T cell induction of terminal plasma cell differentiation. A variety of experimental models[22] are currently being used to analyse this concept that non-antigen specific T cell factors control terminal maturation of plasma cells.

10. T Cell Heterogeneity

A considerably active area of contemporary immunobiology concerns the nature of subpopulations of T cells, as defined by functional studies. In particular this concerns helper T cell function, cytotoxic T cells capable of direct target cell killing, suppressor type T cells, and T cell lineages involved in delayed type hypersensitivity. On the associated figure these have been represented as alternative pathways of differentiation at a postthymic stage. However, this diagramatic representation contrasts to the B

cell lineage in which different stages of differentiation are shown in
a sequential fashion. This raises the question as to whether the
various T cell functions represent distinctly different postthymic
differentiation pathways, rather than different functional activities
being associated with distinct stages of the one continuing and
sequential T cell differentiation pathway, as proposed for the B cell
lineage. The reciprocal argument is to propose that B cell
differentiation in a postbursal state, represents as for T cells,
alternative pathways of B cell differentiation, perhaps represented
by the terminal maturation of plasma cell lineages producing the
different isotypes of immunoglobulins.

In this discussion I have not attempted to propose answers to
these problems, but rather to indicate that the general area of the
differentiation and ontogeny of lymphoid cells still contain a large
number of unanswered questions for immunobiologists. Although
considerable progress has been made in recent years in further
defining possible stages in lymphoid cell differentiation,
particularly in regard to cell surface markers and analysis of T cell
inductive factors, considerably further research may not only
provide fascinating answers of interest to immunobiologists, but may
further reinforce the value of the lymphoid system as a general
model for cellular differentiation.

References

1.   Warner, N.L., Szenberg, A. and Burnet, F.M., Aust.J.Exp.
        Biol., 40, 373, 1962.
2.   Claman, H.N. and Chaperon, E.A., Transpl. Rev., 1, 92, 1969
3.   Miller, J.F.A.P. and Mitchell, G.F., Transpl. Rev., 1, 3,
        1969.
4.   Metcalf, D. and Moore, M.A.S., "Hemopoietic cells: Their
        origin, migration and differentiation". North-Holland, 1971
5.   El-Arini, M.O. and Osoba, D., J.Exp.Med., 137, 821, 1973.
6.   Lafleur, L., Miller, R.G. and Phillips, R.A., J.Exp.Med.,
        137, 1363, 1972.
7.   Lawton, A.R., Kincade, P.W. and Cooper, M.D., Fed.Proc.
        34, 33, 1975.
8.   Owen, J.J.T., Cooper, M.D. and Raff, M.C., Nature, 249,
        361, 1974.
9.   Osmond, D.G. and Nossal, G.J.V., Cell Immunol., 13, 117,
        1974.
10. Ryser, J.E. and Vassalli, P., J.Immunol., 113, 719, 1974.
11. Warner, N.L., Advances Immunol., 19, 67, 1974.

12. Jones, P.P., Craig, S.W., Cebra, J.J. and Herzenberg, C.A. J.Exp.Med., 140, 452, 1974.
13. Rowe, D.S., Hug, K., Forni, L. and Pernis, B., J.Exp.Med., 138, 965, 1973.
14. Seligmann, M., Preud'homme, J.L. and Kourilsky, F.M. (Editors) Membrane receptors of lymphocytes, in press, 1975.
15. Klinman, N.R. and Press, J.L., Fed.Proc., 34, 47, 1975.
16. Silverstein, A.M. and Segal, S. this volume.
17. Miller, A., DeLuca, D., Celada, F. and Sercarz, E. this volume.
18. Nussenzweig, V., Advances Immunol., 19, 217, 1974.
19. Warner, N.L., Potter, M. and Metcalf, D. (Eds) U.I.C.C. Technical report series, Vol 13, 1974.
20. Shortman, K. and Jackson, H., Cell Immunol., 12, 230, 1974.
21. Broder, S., Humphrey, R., Durm, M., Blackman, M., Meade, B. and Waldmann, T., Fed.Proc., 34, 1003, 1975.
22. Warner, N.L. and Anderson, R.E., Nature, 254, 604, 1975.

THE ONTOGENY OF BURSA- AND THYMUS-SPECIFIC CELL SURFACE ANTIGENS

IN THE CHICKEN

G. Wick and B. Albini

Institute for General and Experimental Pathology of the
University
Vienna, Austria

Antisera specific for the chicken bursa of Fabricius (ABS)
and for thymus (ATS) cells have been produced in turkeys (1) and
characterized in _in vitro_ (2) and _in vivo_ (3) experiments. Using
these antisera, the B-and T-cell populations of lymphoid organs of
chickens at different times after hatching have been delineated
(4). The present report summarizes experimental results on the
appearance and frequency of cells bearing antigenic determinants
defined by anti-bursa cell and anti-thymus cell sera during embryonal life of the chicken.

Materials and Methods

Normal White Leghorn eggs obtained from a local breeder were
incubated at standard conditions. Groups of 4-24 embryos were
sacrificed beginning with the 5th day of incubation until hatching.
The procedures for the preparation of cell suspensions from the
bursa of Fabricius, thymus, spleen and yolk sac have been described
elsewhere (5). Briefly, minced tissue from these organs was passed
through steel screens, the cells were washed in phosphate buffered
saline (PBS;pH 7.2;0.01 M) and the cell suspension was adjusted
to 10 - 15 X 10^6 cells/ml. Yolk sac cell preparations were subjected to collagenase treatment. Lymphocyte suspensions from the
spleen were obtained by sedimentation with 4% polyvinylpyrrolidone
(4). Antigenic determinants defined by specific ABS and ATS were
detected in an indirect immunofluorescent staining procedure on
viable cells (4-6). An anti-turkey γ-globulin serum raised in
rabbits and absorbed with chicken γ-globulin was coupled to FITC.
After conjugation, it had 16 standard precipitation units and a
molar F/P ratio of 5.3. The working dilution was determined

13

following the guidelines of Beutner et al (7), and found to be
1:32. The percentage of positive cells was determined using
either counterstaining with Evans blue (4,5) or dark-field illum-
ination with visible light. All readings were done with a
Reichert Zetopan microscope equipped with a "FITC 3" exciter
filter (Balzers) and a KV 418 barrier filter (Schott). A vertical illuminator with a dichroic mirror was used. Per preparation,
1 to 3 slides were examined and 20 to 60 visual fields were screened
per slide using a 63 x objective and a 10 x ocular. Control experiments were performed as described elsewhere (2,4,5), including
incubation of chicken lymphoid cells with the FITC-conjugate alone,
incubation of human and rat erythrocytes and rat liver cells, and
embryonal chicken brain, liver and red blood cells with ABS or
ATS and conjugate.

Results

ABS-reactive surface determinants. A low number of yolk sac cells
from 7 day old embryos reacted with ABS (Table I). The percentage
of such cells increased during the observation period constantly.
Cells reacting with ABS were found in the bursa on the 10th, in
the thymus on the 9th and in the spleen on the 11th day of incubation. The percentage of ABS-reactive cells increased in the bursa
sharply on day 12, and reached values of 70-80% on days 18 to 21
of embryonal life. In the thymus, ABS positive cells reached a
peak on the 13th day of incubation, to decline to values below 5%
at hatching. In the spleen, the percentage of cells reacting with
ABS increased from 1.1% on the 10th embryonal day to 29% on the
11th day of incubation, but the percentage of these cells remained
in the range of 10 to 30% until the time of hatching. No ABS-
positive cells were found in embryonal brain, liver or red blood
cell preparations.

ATS-reactive surface determinants. The first ATS-reactive cells
were found in the yolk sac of 7 day old embryos (Table II). The
number of these cells was 5 to 10 times lower than the number of
ABS positive cells. In the thymus of 9 day old embryos the first
cells reacting with ATS appeared. ATS-positive cells were present
in the bursa and spleen of 10 day old embryos. In the thymus,
the values for ATS positive cells reached a plateau of 80% to 90%
on the 14th day of incubation. In the bursa, the value for ATS
reactive cells reached 41% on day 15 of embryonal life. It then
declined rapidly until hatching. In the spleen, cells reacting
with ATS increased in number until three days before hatching.
There were no ATS-positive cells in preparations of embryonal
brain, liver or red blood cells.

TABLE I

PERCENTAGE OF CELLS REACTING WITH ABS IN INDIRECT IMMUNOFLUORESCENT STAINING

Embryonal Day	Yolk Sac	Bursa	Thymus	Spleen
5	0	ND	ND	ND
7	0.1	ND	ND	ND
8	0.3	ND	0	ND
9	0.4	0	1.2	ND
10	0.2	0.1	1.0	0.0
11	0.3	0.05	1.5	1.1
12	0.5	0.6	12.4	29.3
13	1.2	15.3	45.9	ND
14	0.7	33.2	27.0	12.4
15	ND	52.6	ND	ND
16	ND	48.4	ND	ND
17	ND	55.6	20.0	ND
18	ND	66.0	ND	23.1
19	ND	82.9	13.3	23.8
20	ND	73.5	ND	26.1
21	ND	78.2	7.4	11.7
Weeks after hatching				
2	ND	85.6	9.2	22.1
9	ND	86.2	ND	ND

ND   not done

TABLE II

PERCENTAGE OF CELLS REACTING WITH ATS IN INDIRECT IMMUNOFLUORESCENT STAINING

Embryonal Day	Yolk Sac	Bursa	Thymus	Spleen
5	0.0	ND	ND	ND
7	0.02	ND	ND	ND
8	0.02	ND	0.0	ND
9	0.02	0.0	0.6	ND
10	0.03#	0.1	3.7	0.02
11	0.01#	0.05	6.4	3.3
12	0.3	0.6	19.0	20.9
13	0.1	6.7	62.3	ND
14	0.5	33.5	84.1	46.3
15	ND	40.9	ND	ND
16	ND	26.1	ND	ND
17	ND	8.7	80.0	ND
18	ND	ND	ND	42.6
19	ND	2.5	95.4	67.2
20	ND	1.5	ND	56.3
21	ND	0.0	87.7	46.0

Weeks after hatching				
2	ND	5.4	91.2	48.5
9	ND	8.2	ND	ND

ND not done

\# only one cell stained in whole preparation

Discussion

The demonstration of cells bearing antigenic determinants reacting with ABS and ATS in yolk sac cell suspensions of chicken embryos beginning with the 7th day of incubation at a time, when no other of the lymphoid organs may be suspected to harbor or seed lymphoid cells, strongly supports the hypothesis of a yolk sac origin of lymphoid stem cells as proposed by Moore and Metcalf (8). As these yolk sac cells carry ABS and ATS reactive determinants, which are not found on cells in other than lymphoid embryonal and adult tissues, it may be suggested that in the embryonal yolk sac there are already stem cells present, which are predetermined to give rise only to lymphoid cell lines during maturation. Alternatively, it is possible that ABS and ATS reactive surface determinants present at certain times of otogeny on pluripotent hemopoietic stem cell are lost under the influence of an environment inducing non-lymphoid differentiation.

The presence of cells reacting with ATS in the bursa and of cells reacting with ABS in the thymus during early ontogeny may indicate the presence of both determinants on stem cells, with a subsequent loss or hiding of determinants accomplished during the maturation process. Alternatively, the thymus and bursa microenvironment at this early stage may not discriminate yet B- and T-cell specific determinants on different lymphoid stem cells. Double staining experiments are under way to establish, if both determinants occur on single embryonal cells or not. A disappearance of antigenic determinants during maturation has been described also for mammalian blood cells (9).

The spleen is populated by cells reacting with ABS and ATS almost at the same time as the bursa. ATS reactive cells in the spleen may either come from the yolk sac or from the thymus. However, cells reacting with ABS increase only slowly in number. As found earlier, the number of cells carrying immunoglobulin surface determinant increases also only slowly until hatching in this organ (5,10,11). Despite the much lesser percentage of B cells present in the spleen if compared to the number of B cells present in the bursa, the spleen could become a main source of B cells in bursectomized chickens. Indeed, bursectomies performed at certain times of embryonal life do not deplete the B cell population of the chicken significantly (11,12), and even after surgical bursectomy in ovo and subsequent x-ray irradiation, a low number of B cells is present in the spleen and blood (3). Tao-Wiedmann et al (13), however, did not find any increase of cells with immunoglobulin surface determinants in the spleens of bursectomized birds, if compared to untreated ones.

Acknowledgment

We thank Miss Renate Steiner for her competent and reliable technical assistance. This study was supported by grants from the Austrian Research Council (project 1997) and the Fund of the Austrian Cancer Society.

References

1. Wick, G. & Witebsky, E.   Fed. Proc. 29: 2, 1970.
2. Wick, G., Albini, B. & Milgrom, F.   Clin. Exp. Immunol. 15: 237, 1973.
3. Wick, G., Albini, B. & Johnson, W.   Immunology 28: 305, 1975.
4. Albini, B. & Wick, G.   J. Immunol. 112: 444, 1974.
5. Albini, B. & Wick, G.   Int. Arch. Allergy 44: 804, 1973.
6. Moller, G.   J. Exp. Med. 114: 415, 1961.
7. Beutner, E.H., Sepulveda, M.R. & Barnett, E.V.   Bull. WHO 39: 587, 1968.
8. Moore, M.A.S. & Metcalf, H.   Brit. J. Haemat. 18: 279, 1970.
9. Van den Engh, G.J. & Golub, E.S. submitted for publication.
10. Hudson, L. & Roitt, I.M.   Europ. J. Immunol. 3: 63, 1973.
11. Tao-Wiedmann, T. W., Loor, F. & Hagg. L.B.   Immunology 28: 821, 1975.
12. Pierce, A.E., Chubb, R.C. & Long, P.L.   Immunology 10: 321, 1966.

IGA SURFACE DETERMINANTS ON CELLS FROM THE CHICKEN EMBRYO

B. Albini and G. Wick

Institute for General and Experimental Pathology   of
the University
Vienna, Austria

Reports on chicken IgA were published almost simultaneously
in 1972 by three different groups of investigators (1-3). Antisera
to chicken IgA have been produced using serum, bile or oviduct
washings as antigen source in rabbits (1-3) or pheasants (4). IgA
is present in chicken serum and secretions in a variety of polymer
molecules (5). The distribution of cells with IgA surface determinants has been studied in different organs of the chicken (6,7).
Recently it has been suggested that IgA appears very early in
phylogenesis (8). In continuation of work on the distrubtion of
lyphoid cells bearing immunoglobulin surface determinants in
hatched chickens (9), cells from the yolk sac, bursa of Fabricius,
thymus and spleen of embryonal chickens have been tested in an
indirect immunofluorescence test for surface determinants reacting
with anti chicken IgA sera.

Materials and Methods

Normal White Leghorn eggs were obtained from a local breeder,
and incubated in our own facilities. Embryos were sacrificed from
the 5th day of incubation until hatching, and organs of embryos of
the same age group (4-24 embryos) were pooled to prepare cell suspensions as described elsewhere (10).

An anti-chicken IgA serum (AA1) produced in rabbits was kindly
donated by Drs. Orlans and Rose (3), and two other preparations of
anti-chicken IgA sera were given to us by Drs. Parry and Aitkens
(4), of which one was produced in rabbits (AA2) and the other in
pheasants (AA3). A commercial anti-rabbit γ-globulin-FITC conjugate produced in goats was obtained from Behringwerke, Marburg,
Germany, and found to have 16 standard precipitation units and a

molar F/P ratio of 3.0. It was used in a working dilution of 1:16 in an indirect immunofluorescent staining procedure on viable cells (11).

All readings were done on a Reichert Zetopan microscope with a vertical illuminator and "FITC 3" (Balzers) exciter and KV 418 (Schott) barrier filters. Per slide, 2000-6000 cells were counted using Evans blue (1:10 000) as counterstaining, and two to three slides were prepared per cell preparation.

Controls were performed as described elsewhere (10, 12). The specificity of the staining of embryonal bursal cells with AA1 and anti-rabbit γ-globulin conjugate was tested using AA3 to inhibit the staining.

Results

The percentage of cells from the yolk sac, bursa, thymus and spleen reacting with AA1 are summarized in Table I.

A low number of yolk sac cells reacted with AA1 already on the 5th day of incubation (Table I). At this time, no other anti-chicken immunoglobulin serum reacted with the cells. On the 9th day of embryonal life, AA2 reacted with 2.6% of yolk sac cells, and on day 14 after incubation with 6.8%.

In the bursa of Fabricius, 1.5% of cells reacted with AA1 on the 10th embryonal day, and the number of reactive cells increased to 43% three days before hatching (Table I). The first appearance of AAI-reactive cells in the bursa was simultaneous with the appearance of cells reacting with anti-chicken IgM serum in this organ. However, cells with IgM determinants on their surface were present only in minimal numbers (0.1%). On the other hand, cells reacting with anti-chicken IgG sera appeared for the first time on the 16th day of incubation. The percentage of cells reacting with AA1 reached a low of 3% after hatching and increased again at 9 weeks of age. AA2 reacted with 14.3% of bursa cells on the 14th day of incubation, with 11.9% of cells on the 15th day of incubation, and with 38.7% of the cells on the day of hatching.

On the 9th embryonal day, a low number of thymus cells reacted with AA1 (Table I). The percentage of AA1-positive cells increased significantly on the 12th day of incubation and reached a maximum of over 50% on the 17th day of embryonal life. It declined to values lower than 1% 2 weeks after hatching. There were 46.2% of thymus cells reacting with AA2 on the 14th embryonal day, 60.8% reacting with AA2 on the 17th embryonal day, and 27.9% reacting with AA2 2 days before hatching.

TABLE I

PERCENTAGE OF CELLS REACTING WITH AAI IN INDIRECT IMMUNOFLUORESCENT STAINING

Embryonal Day	Yolk Sac	Bursa	Thymus	Spleen
5	0.2	ND	ND	ND
7	0.6	ND	ND	ND
8	0.5	ND	0	ND
9	2.6	0	1.1	0
10	6.1	1.5	0.6	0.3
11	3.4	4.6	1.5	1.6
12	2.0	8.0	26.2	36.3
13	4.7	13.6	36.7	ND
14	8.2	17.1	52.6	56.6
15	ND	8.4	ND	ND
16	ND	23.3	ND	ND
17	ND	21.6	61.1	38.5
18	ND	35.6	ND	25.9
19	ND	43.7	39.3	23.6
20	ND	40.1	ND	21.9
21	ND	28.2	23.4	38.2

Weeks after Hatching				
2	ND	3.0	0.9	4.0
9	ND	13.7	ND	8.5

ND not done

In the spleen, low numbers of cells carrying IgA-surface determinants were detected on days 10 and 11 of embryonal life (Table I). The percentage of such cells increased on the 12th embryonal day to 36%, and reached a maximum of 47% on the 14th day of incubation. The percentage of IgA positive cells in this organ remained in the range of 20-40% in the late embryonal period.

There was no reactivity of embryonal chicken erythrocytes, brain or liver cells with AA1 or AA2, with exception of one brain cell preparation from a 9 day old embryo, in which one cell reacted with AA1. The immunofluorescent staining of bursa cells from a 14 day old embryo with AA1 could be blocked through prior incubation with AA3. There was no staining of any cells with conjugate alone.

Discussion

The anti chicken IgA sera used in these experiments were monospecific as judged from immunodiffusion and immunoelectrophoresis (7). The appearance of cells with AA1 reactive antigenic determinants in the yolk sac on the fifth day after incubation, when no cells reacting with antisera to any of the other immunoglobulins classes of the chicken were detectable suggests that the IgA like receptors may represent the earliest surface determinant of immunoglobulin-like specificity in the chicken. Much higher percentages of cells from the bursa of Fabricius and the spleen react with AA1 and AA2 during embryonal life than after hatching. Most notably, the embryonal thymus harbors high numbers of cells reacting with AA1 and AA2, whereas no such reactivity is found with thymus cells after hatching. This result indicates that the IgA determinant of embryonal cell membrane disappears or becomes undetectable in most of the cells of the thymus, bursa, and spleen in the course of maturation and differentiation. Recently, comparable decreases of cells reactive with rabbit erythrocyte antigens have been described in the bursa (13). As the cells reactive with AA1 or AA2 increase again in percentage several weeks after hatching in the bursa and the spleen, showing thus a biphasic behavior, these sera may detect different specificities of antigenic determinant in the embryo and in the hatched chicken: rudimentary or primitive immunoglobulin of the embryonal lymphoid or hematopoietic stem cell, and the classic IgA surface determinant of mature lymphoid cells. Absorption studies with IgA-positive lymphoid cells from adult and embryonal chicken bursa and thymus are under way in this laboratory. In agreement with our findings where recent reports showing that anti-IgA sera given during the embryonal period decreased the IgM, IgA and IgG serum levels in chickens after hatching (14) in a similar manner as anti IgM sera.

Acknowledgement

We want to thank Dr. Orlans, Dr. Rose, Dr. Aitken and Dr. Parry for their kind supply of anti-chicken immunoglobulin-A sera, and Miss Renate Steiner for her competent and reliable technical assistance. This study was supported by grants from the Austrian Research Council (project 1997) and the Fund of the Austrian Cancer Society.

References

1. Bienenstock, J., Perey, D.Y.E., Gauldie, J. & Underdown, B.J. J. Immunol. 109: 403, 1972.
2. Lebacq-Verheyden, A. M., Vaerman, J.P. & Heremans, J.F. Immunology 22: 165, 1972.
3. Orlans, E. & Rose, M.E. Immunochemistry 9:833, 1972.
4. Aitken, I.D. & Parry, S.H. Abstr. 10th Int. Symp. Lab. Animals, Hruba Skala, CSSR, p. 21, 1973.
5. Watanabe, H. & Kobayashi, K. J. Immunol. 113:1405, 1974.
6. Kincade, P.W. & Cooper, M.D. Science 179:398, 1973.
7. Albini, B., Wick, G., Rose, E. & Orlans, E. Int. Arch. Allergy 47: 23, 1974.
8. Lebacq-Verheyden, A. M., Vaerman, J.P. & Heremans, J.F. Immunology 27: 683, 1974.
9. Albini, B. & Wick, G. Adv. Exp. Med. Biol. 29: 203, 1973.
10. Albini, B. & Wick, G. Int. Arch. Allergy 44: 804, 1973.
11. Moller, G. J. Exp. Med. 114: 415, 1961.
12. Albini, B. & Wick, G. J. Immunol. 112: 444, 1974.
13. Tufveson, G. & Alm, G.V. Int. Arch. Allergy 48: 537, 1975.
14. Martin, L.N. & Leslie, G.A. J. Immunol. 113: 120, 1974.

CONTRIBUTION OF THE BURSA OF FABRICIUS TO THE MATURATION OF THE B CELL SYSTEM IN CHICKENS

P. Nieuwenhuis

Department of Histology, University of Groningen

Oostersingel 69/1, Groningen, The Netherlands

In a previous paper (1) it was shown that in 6 week old chickens surgical bursectomy and X-irradiation (BX/600 rads) did not prevent *de novo* formation of germinal centres, in contrast to the well known effects of bursectomy and irradiation immediately post hatching. On the other hand a marked though transitory deficiency in the lymphocyte population surrounding Schweigger-Seidel sheaths (sheath lymphoid system, SLS) was noticed. This seemed to indicate that beyond a certain age the B cell system in chickens had matured to a stage where bursal influence (humoral?, cellular?) is less essential and the system had become self-perpetuating, suggesting a non-bursal site taking over (see also: 2, 3).

Experiments to be reported here were aimed at analysing this postulated maturation process in the early post-hatching period.

EFFECT OF BURSECTOMY AND X-IRRADIATION AT VARIOUS INTERVALS POST HATCHING ON THE DEVELOPMENT OF THE B CELL SYSTEM.

Experimental design: Female white leghorn (Shaver-Starcross strain no. 288) chickens were obtained at 1 day of age and surgically bursectomised on days 4, 7, 10 or 14 post hatching. Three days after surgery bursectomised and sham bursectomised controls were subjected to 600 rads whole body X-irradiation. Five weeks after the irradiation these two groups (BX/600 rads and SBX/600 rads resp.) as well as a normal control group were injected i.v. with 0.5 ml 10% SRBC in PBS. Seven days later animals were bled for anti-SRBC antibody titration and killed for microscopical investigation of the spleen, cecal tonsils and bursa of Fabricius (or bursal remnants: none could be found). Germinal centres were counted in two well separated mid-spleen sections per animal and numbers were

25

TABLE I

Surgery	BX day 4	BX day 7	BX day 10	BX day 14	SBX day 4	SBX day 14	-
X irr.(600 rads)	+	+	+	+	+	+	-
No. of animals	4	4	5	4	4	6	3
No. of Germinal Centres/sq. unit	2	0	129	111	95	126	151
Sheath lymphoid system	-	-	++	+++	+++	+++	+++
Titers (7th day) anti SRBC	1	0	10.2	10	9.5	11	11.3

calculated per standard area of spleen roughly equivalent to two spleen sections.

Results: As can be seen from table I early (day 4 or day 7) BX/600 rads animals did not respond to SRBC with detectable antibody formation nor germinal centre formation, in sharp contrast to the 10- and 14-day BX/600 rads groups. In the latter, germinal centre formation and anti-SRBC titers did not differ significantly from SBX/600 rads animals and were only slightly lower than in normal controls.

It is worth noticing that in the absence of the bursa (10- and 14-day BX/600 rads groups) the sheath lymphoid system (SLS) with high numbers of germinal centres present reaches normal scores, again suggesting these latter structures as an alternative source (next to the bursa) for the SLS.

EFFECT OF EARLY BURSECTOMY AND X-IRRADIATION ON THE DEVE-
LOPMENT OF THE ANTIGEN TRAPPING CAPACITY.

Experimental design: (i) ^{125}I-human fibrinogen (Fib*, 10μCi/ 20 gr. of body weight) was injected i.v. into 7-, 14- or 21-day old normal chickens. Three days later spleens were taken for histology and processed for autoradiography. (ii) Four day BX/600 rads and SBX/600 rads animals as well as normal controls of the same age were injected i.v. with Fib* (see above) three weeks after the irradia- tion. From each group half of the animals had been preimmunised one week earlier with 1 mg human fibrinogen i.v.. Twenty-four hours and 3 days after Fib* animals were killed and spleens were processed for autoradiography.

Results: (i) Autoradiographs from 7th day Fib* spleens (day 10) showed that by this time antigen trapping is still virtually nil. Occasional accumulations of grains were found in the white pulp (PALS) at the branching point of an arteriole. In 14th day Fib* spleens (day 17) antigen trapping was qualitatively normal as compared to controls (see (ii)). Twenty-first day Fib* spleens (day 24) showed essentially the same picture. It was concluded that between days 7 and 14 post hatching antigen trapping capacity from virtually nil reaches at least qualitatively full maturity by day 14. (ii) In normal animals (28 days old) early signs of antigen trapping by 24 hours were found in the white pulp near the branching point of the central arteriole. Two days later grains were found over the SLS just outside the Schweigger-Seidel sheaths proper as well as over and associated with newly formed germinal centres. In unprimed SBX/600 rads animals the same picture was obtained in con-trast to the preimmunised group were germinal centre formation and antigen trapping were slightly enhanced. In both BX/600 rads groups no germinal centres were found and no signs of antigen trapping could be detected.

RECONSTITUTION OF ANTIGEN TRAPPING CAPACITY BY PASSIVE ANTIBODY IN BURSECTOMISED/IRRADIATED CHICKENS?

Experimental design: Four day BX/600 rads and SBX/600 rads chickens were injected i.v. with Fib* at 4 weeks of age as described above. In each group some animals were reconstituted i.v. with either: (i) 2 ml of hyperimmune chicken anti human fibrinogen (ChaHuF) or (ii) 2 ml of normal chicken serum (NS) 24 hours before Fib* (see fig. 1) or (iii) 2 ml of early (7th day) ChaHuF 24 hours after Fib* from donor animals of the same age. Three days after Fib* blood (B) was collected in heparinised syringes and spleen (S) and pectoral muscle (M) were taken also. Radioactivity per mg sample was counted and plotted as percentage of the activity found in 1μl of blood from non reconstituted BX/600 rads animals. Spleens were processed for autoradiography (AR).

Results: In the BX/600 rads groups again no indications for antigen trapping were obtained (spleen/blood ratio's in all groups approx..36); spleen activity was probably due to contaminating blood in the sample. In all SBX/600 rads groups spleen/blood ratio's were always more than twice as high indicating antigen trapping in the spleen irrespective of the ChaHuF administered (ratio's approx. equal). These data were confirmed in the autoradiographs (see fig. 1), where antigen trapping was only readily observed in the non re-consituted SBX/600 rads group. In none of the BX/600 rads groups germinal centres were found.

RE-EVALUATION OF THE EFFECT OF BURSECTOMY AND IRRADIATION ON THE DEVELOPMENT OF THE B CELL SYSTEM.

Experimental design: The same experiment as described in the first paragraph was repeated, however, with sligtly different inter-vals (including 6 wks), early (6th day) and late (6 weeks) sham bursectomies and using a new X-ray machine.

Results: Mortality in this series was much higher than before (approx. 90-50% compared with 50-20% previously). As can be seen

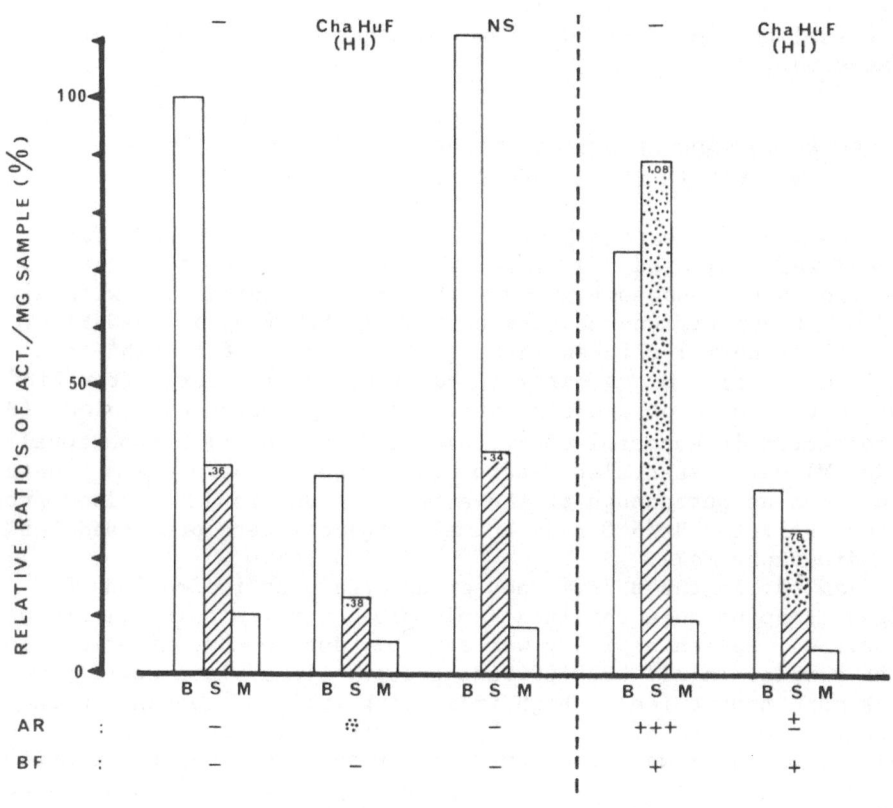

FIGURE 1

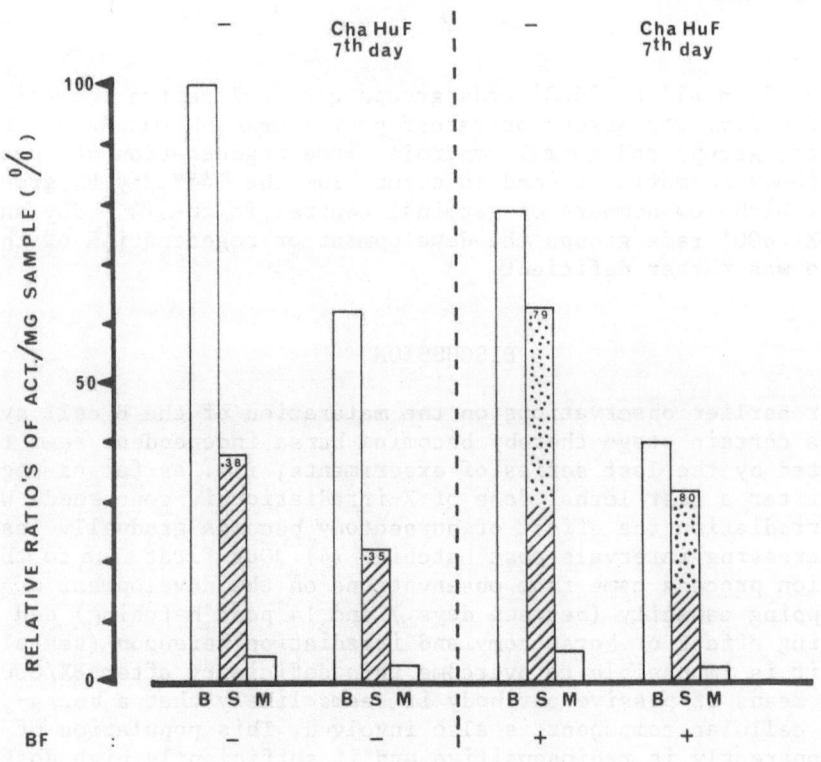

Figure 2

TABLE II

Surgery	BX day 6	BX day 10	BX day 14	BX 6 wks	SBX day 6	SBX 6 wks	–
X irr. ('600' rads)	+	+	+	+	+	+	–
No. of animals	11	4	6	5	4	4	6
No. of G.C./sq.u.	0	2	14	9	115	74	139
S.L.S.	–	–	+	±	+++	+++	+++
Titers (7th day) anti-SRBC	2.5	3.5	7	11.2	16	15.5	16

from fig. 2 in all BX/'600' rads groups germinal centre formation
after SRBC i.v. was absent or rather poor compared with both SBX/
'600' rads groups and normal controls. Some regeneration of specific antibody formation seemed to occur from the 14th day BX group
onwards. With low numbers of germinal centres in the 14th day and
6 wks BX/'600' rads groups the development or regeneration of the
SLS also was rather deficient.

DISCUSSION

Our earlier observations on the maturation of the B cell system
beyond a certain stage thereby becoming bursa independent seem to
be refuted by the last series of experiments, i.e. as far as regeneration after a near lethal dose of X-irradiation is concerned. Without X-irradiation the effect of bursectomy becomes gradually less
with increasing intervals post hatching (4). Our first clue to this
maturation process came from observations on the development of antigen trapping capacity (between days 7 and 14 post hatching) and the
abolishing effect of bursectomy and irradiation hereupon (see also:
5). As it is impossible to overcome this deficiency after BX/600
rads by means of passive antibody it seems likely that a bursa-
derived cellular component is also involved. This population of
cells apparently is radiosensitive and if sufficiently high doses
of X-irradiation are given can be wiped out completely even at 6
weeks of age.

These considerations have led to the following working hypothesis, implying that bursal influence is mediated by the production
of a population of lymphoid cells instrumental as antigen binding
cells (ABC's), antibody synthesizing cells (ex-AFCP's) or both in
the process of antigen trapping (in non gut associated lymphoid
tissues?), thereby providing a necessary condition for germinal
centre formation. This is assuming that antigen handling in the bursa
(see 6) is different from antigen handling in other lymphoid tissues.

Once germinal centre formation has started a new source of
ABC's (AFCP's?) has become available and bursal influence is less

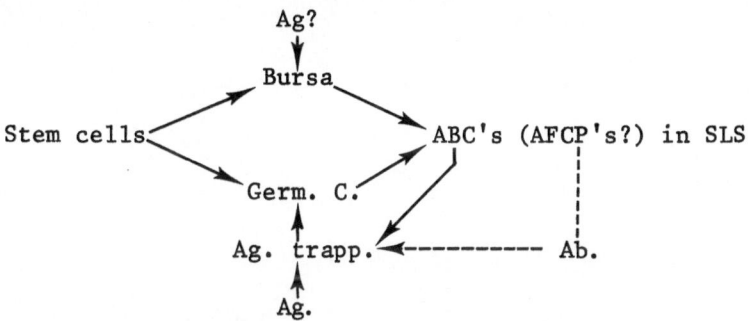

essential. Both bursa-derived and germinal centre derived ABC's (AFCP's?) would morphologically be represented by the lymphocyte population surrounding Schweigger-Seidel sheaths (SLS) (see also 1, 7).

Only if all ABC's and their alternative source somehow are completely eliminated, B cell system development cq. regeneration has to start anew, being reduced again to bursa-dependency.

ACKNOWLEDGEMENTS

It is a pleasure to acknowledge the competent technical assistance of the late Miss Willy Polman and Misses Jeanny Prins and Lineke Bos. The investigations were supported by the Foundation for Medical Research (FUNGO) which is subsidized by the Netherlands association for the Advancement of Pure Research (Z.W.O.).

REFERENCES

1. Nieuwenhuis, P., Adv. in Exp. Med. and Biol., 29, 95 (1973)
2. Lerner, K.G., Glick, B. and McDuffie, F.C., J. Immunol., 107, 493 (1971)
3. Bryant, B.J., Adler, H.E., Cordy, D.R., Eur. J. Immunol., 3, 9 (1973)
4. Greatzer, M.A., Cote, W.P. and Wolfe, H.R., J. Immunology, 91, 576 (1963)
5. White, R.G., Henderson, D.C., Eslami, M.B. and Nielsen, K.H., Immunology, 28, 1 (1975)
6. Schaffner, T., Mueller, J., Hess, M.W., Cottier, H., Sordat, B. and Ropke, C., Cellular Immunol., 13, 304 (1974)
7. De Kruyff, R.H., Durkin, H.G., Gilmour, D.G. and Thorbecke, G.J., Cellular Immunol., 16, 301 (1975).

BURSA OF FABRICIUS : UPTAKE OF RADIOACTIVE PARTICLES AND RADIOTOXIC "SEALING" OF BURSAL FOLLICLES *

T. Schaffner, J. Herring[1], H. Gerber and H. Cottier

Institute of Pathology, University of Bern, Switzerland, and [1]Biology Department, Battelle Pacific Northwest Laboratories, Richland, Wash., USA

Earlier studies have demonstrated that the avian bursa functions as a site of intense and selective uptake of particles through the tuft epithelium which overlies the follicles (1, 2). The bursa undergoes rhythmic compression in synchrony with respiration and shows slow, peristalsis-like movements which, in addition to a suction reflex elicited by contact of fluids or solids with the anal orifice, provides for a constant exchange of cloacal and bursal contents. These findings and indirect evidence in favor of bacterial mechanisms located in the tuft epithelial covering the bursal follicles (2) led to the postulate that the bursa may be primarily an immunologic contact organ where lymphoid cells become sensitized against intestinal antigens (3). The above observations have been confirmed and extended by other authors (4).

The present report deals with the uptake of radioactive, α-emitting particles by the bursa. The experiments were aimed at interfering with immunological functions of the chicken by radiotoxic damage to all follicles exposed to such particulates.

EXPERIMENTAL

Colloidal particles of ^{239}Pu(IV) with a molecular weight ranging from 10^5 to 10^7 and a diameter of approximately 100 Å were pre-

* This work was supported by the US Energy Research and Development Agency and the Swiss National Foundation for Scientific Research.

pared according to <u>Ockenden</u> and <u>Welch</u> (5) and 10 µCi were administered by gavage feeding to 10 newly hatched White Leghorn chickens.
In other animals, 1.5, 3, 10 or 100 µCi of the colloidal radionuclide were administered via the cloacal route. The ^{239}Pu(IV) particles used in our study are practically insoluble and radiolysis
is negligible. The isotope ^{239}Pu emits close to 100% of its decay
energy in the form of ∿5.14 MeV alpha particles with a tissue range
of approximately 50 µm.

Animals were killed by ether overdose at various time intervals
following administration of the radionuclide, and the bursa, the
liver, the gut and the carcass were examined with regard to weight,
radioactivity, histological changes and autoradiographically detectable localization of the radioactive particles.

Colloidal carbon in the form of India ink was given via the
cloacal route as described previously (2) to test the radiotoxic effect of ^{239}Pu(IV) located in the bursa on the uptake of particles
administered at later time intervals.

RESULTS AND DISCUSSION

The distribution of ^{239}Pu in different organs 7 days after

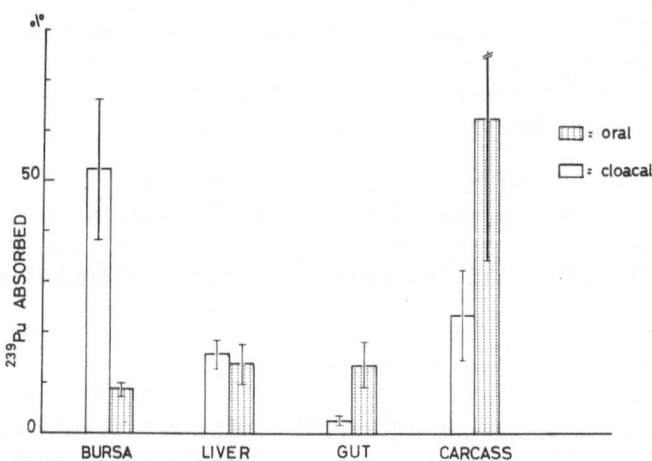

Fig. 1. Distribution of ^{239}Pu in different organs of chickens, 7
days after cloacal or peroral administration of 3 µCi of colloidal
^{239}Pu(IV) on the day of hatching.

cloacal or peroral administration of the radionuclide is shown in
Fig. 1. It is evident from these data that the cloacal route is by
far more efficient in achieving maximum relative concentration of
the radioactive particles in the bursa than the peroral application.
But even after peroral administration, the bursa contained more
than 10 times the amount of ^{239}Pu than the liver, and more than 50
times that in the gut if the content in ^{239}Pu was expressed on a
per unit weight basis.

   Histologic autoradiographs revealed that within 24 hours after
cloacal administration radioactive particles had penetrated the
tuft epithelium and occupied the entire medullary portion of the
bursal follicles at first in an intercellular localization, then
concentrated in macrophages. There were signs of considerable tuft
epithelial damage. This is not surprising since these structures
serve as restricted sites of entry and passage for practically all
the alpha emitting particles reaching the bursal medulla. Cell
death due to radiotoxicity was also important among the medullary
lymphoblasts and lymphocytes in the cortical areas adjacent to the
medulla. Although difficult to assess, it may be assumed that medullary macrophages were also damaged by the alpha rays.

   In the following period, up to at least 3 weeks after administration of ^{239}Pu, the particles showed an increasing tendency to

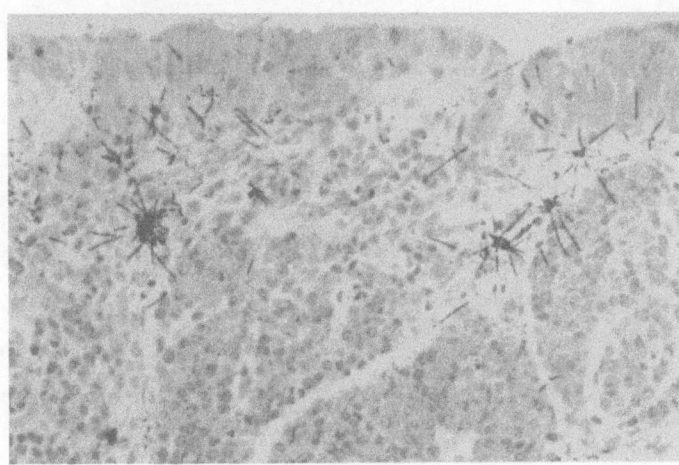

Fig. 2. Surface of bursal follicles, 7 days after peroral administration of 10 µCi of colloidal ^{239}Pu(IV). Some "hot spots" have already formed in extrafollicular localizations, also between the epithelium and the follicles (Autoradiograph, 12 weeks exposure time,
enlargement 350 x).

form aggregates. They were gradually translocated from the interior of the medulla to extrafollicular sites, where "hot spots" were found between the follicles and the overlying epithelium and lateral to the former (Fig. 2).

With time, due to radiation damage and consecutive repair processes, most bursal follicles were separated from the covering epithelium by a thin layer of connective tissue with a tendency for scarring. Concomitant with this change, the bursal follicles became smaller and smaller, the reduction in size being due to a substantial loss of lymphoid cells in both the medulla and the cortex (Fig. 3). Of importance, atrophied follicles, separated from the epithelium by a layer of fibrous tissue, contained medullary lymphoid cells with a significantly smaller median diameter than the untreated controls of the same age (Fig. 3), while no such difference in cellular size could be found in cortical lymphocytes. Some follicles disappeared completely.

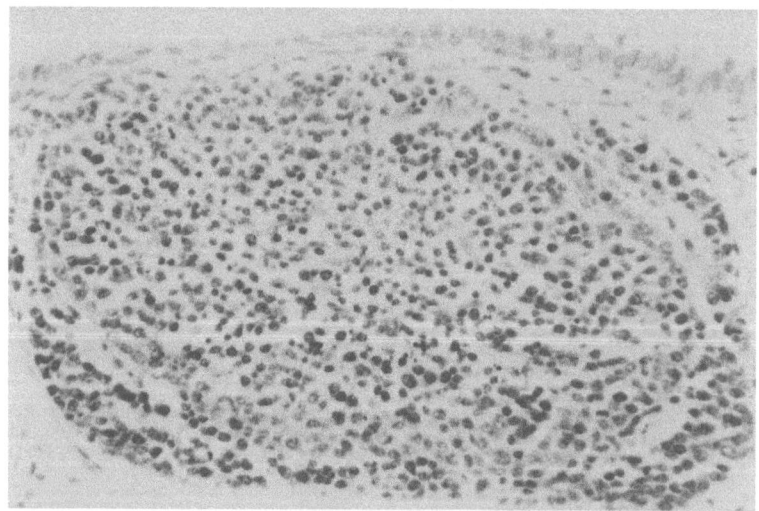

Fig. 3. Bursal follicle, 4 weeks after application of 100 μCi of colloidal ^{239}Pu(IV) via the cloacal route. Note the absence of typical tuft epithelium, the thin layer of connective tissue between the epithelium and the follicle, the relatively smaller size of medullary lymphoid cells and the thin cortex (enlargement 240 x).

As a consequence of these radiation-induced changes, the bursal weight underwent a dose-dependent reduction (Table I).

Table I. Estimated organ doses and radiation induced weight changes after transcloacal administration of two different doses of ^{239}Pu(IV) colloid.

µCi ^{239}Pu per animal	Organ	Estimated accumulated organ dose	Organ weight (% of controls)
3	Bursa	1.5×10^3 rads in 9 days	66 (p <0.05)
100	Bursa	7.8×10^3 rads in 21 days	30 (p <0.01)
100	Liver	8.3×10^3 rads in 21 days	100

Changes in body weight were not observed following cloacal application of 3 or 100 µCi of ^{239}Pu(IV).

When 0.1 ml of India ink was given via the cloaca to animals which, at hatching 4 weeks earlier, had received 100 µCi of colloidal ^{239}Pu(IV) via the same route, uptake of carbon particles by the atrophic bursa was barely noticeable. This was in marked contrast

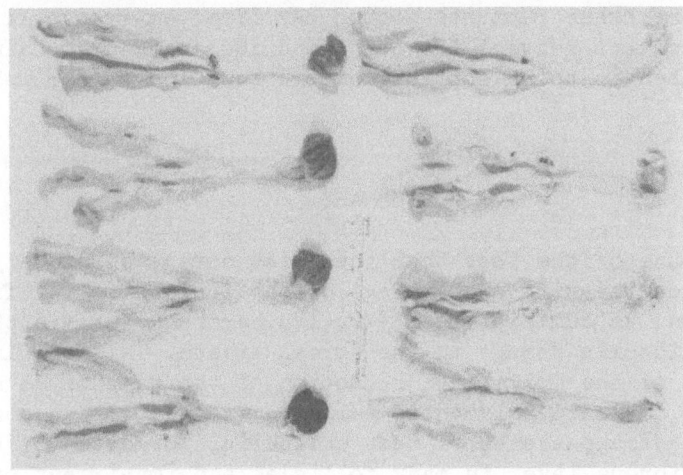

Fig. 4. Lower portions of the gastrointestinal tract of 4-week-old chickens, 1 day after administration of o.1 ml of India ink via the cloacal route. Specimens in the right half of the figure originate from animals that had received 100 µCi of colloidal ^{239}Pu(IV) on the day of hatching. Note the virtual absence of particle uptake by the bursae which were damaged by the radioactive material (1:3).

to untreated controls of the same age (Fig. 4). This "sealing effects" of the radioactive particulates taken up by the bursa was
most probably due to a) the virtual disappearance of tuft-type epithelia covering the bursal follicles and their replacement by flat
epithelial cells, and b) the interposition of a layer of connective
tissue between the epithelium and the follicular medulla, as described above. Chickens with bursae damaged and "sealed" by the radiotoxic effects of ^{239}Pu showed significantly lower serum concentrations of IgG than untreated controls.

Alterations in bursal structure and function similar to those
elicited by radioactive particles were recently observed in a different model. After ligation of the bursal duct on the day of hatching, leaving intact both innervation and blood supply of the bursa,
retarded development of the cortical zone, and depletion of the follicular medulla were noticed.

These observations and the long known fact that in birds transcloacal administration of antigens results in effective immunization in a number of model systems, leads one to postulate that the
bursa serves as a peripheral immunologic contact organ. If a generation of B cells by the bursa in the complete absence of antigens
is possible, cannot at present be answered, since the amniotic fluid
with which the bursa communicates from day 10 to 11 of embryogenesis
on, contains both maternal and environmental antigens. Furthermore,
the urodeal membrane ruptures around day 17 of embryonic life which
allows for contact between the bursa and the antigen-containing egg
yolk which then is being emptied through the cloaca (for review,
see 3).

SUMMARY

Making use of the fact that the avian bursa is uniquely equiped
for uptake, degradation and storage of particulate matter from the
cloacal lumen, we administered ^{239}Pu(IV) perorally or via the cloaca
to cause radiotoxic damage to the bursal tissue. This resulted in
a involution of the follicles, reduction of the lymphocyte mass,
predominance of smaller lymphoid cells in the medulla as compared
to controls, disappearance of tuft epithelia, formation of a sub-
epithelial fibrous layer in many follicles and impairment or an almost complete loss of the capacity of the bursa to take up particulate matter. Concomitant with these changes was a reduction in
the concentration of serum IgG. These findings are discussed in relation to the immunologic contact role of the bursa.

REFERENCES

1. Schaffner, Th., Sordat, B., Mueller, J., Miller, G.G., Hess, M.W. and Cottier, H. Abstract, Joint Meeting of European Societies for Immunology, Strasbourg, September 4-7, 1973, p. 68.

2. Schaffner, Th.,Mueller, J., Hess, M.W., Cottier, H., Sordat, B. and Ropke, C. Cellular Immunology, 13, 304 (1974).

3. Schaffner, Th., Hess, M.W. and Cottier, H. Ser. Haemat., VII, 4 (1974).

4. Sorvari, T., Sorvari, R., Ruotsalainen, P., Toivanen, A. and Toivanen, P. Nature, 253, 217 (1975).

5. Ockenden, D.W. and Welch, G.A. J. chem. Soc. 3358 (1956).

THE NEED FOR TRANSCRIPTION AND TRANSLATION FOR DIFFERENTIATION OF BONE MARROW CELLS BY THYMIC FACTORS IN MAN

G.S. INCEFY AND R.A. GOOD

Memorial Sloan-Kettering Cancer Center

New York, New York 10021

The exact mechanism by which the thymus influences differentiation of bone marrow precursor cells into thymocytes after their migration into its environment is not fully understood. Studies in vitro with normal human marrow cells (1,2) and peripheral blood lymphocytes (PBL) (3) have demonstrated that one or more small populations of cells are inducible to express T cell markers after incubation in the presence of human or calf thymic factors. The molecular nature of the steps induced by these factors prior to the appearance of specific markers on the cell membrane are unknown. In an attempt to elucidate the mode of action of thymic factors on precursor human marrow cells in vitro, we have studied the effect produced by partially purified human thymic factors (HTF) on RNA and protein synthesis in different marrow cell populations, isolated by discontinuous density gradient centrifugation (2). In addition, we have studied the effect of specific inhibitors of RNA and protein synthesis on these events during incubation of the different marrow cell populations with HTF.

The procedure followed for fractionation of human marrow cells is shown in Fig. 1. Marrow cells can be fractionated on BSA or Ficoll gradients (2) into 5 fractions. Precursor cells, defined as cells which can be induced to bear new T lymphocyte characteristics were found in layer III in a density range of 1.055-1.066 in normal adults. Inductions were carried out during a short incubation with HTF, fractions 3 or 5 (F3 or F5), purified according to the procedure of A. Goldstein (4). Since usually very few cells were present in layers I and II, appearance of lymphocyte markers on these cells could not always be determined after incubation with HTF. But it was possible to establish the existence of another

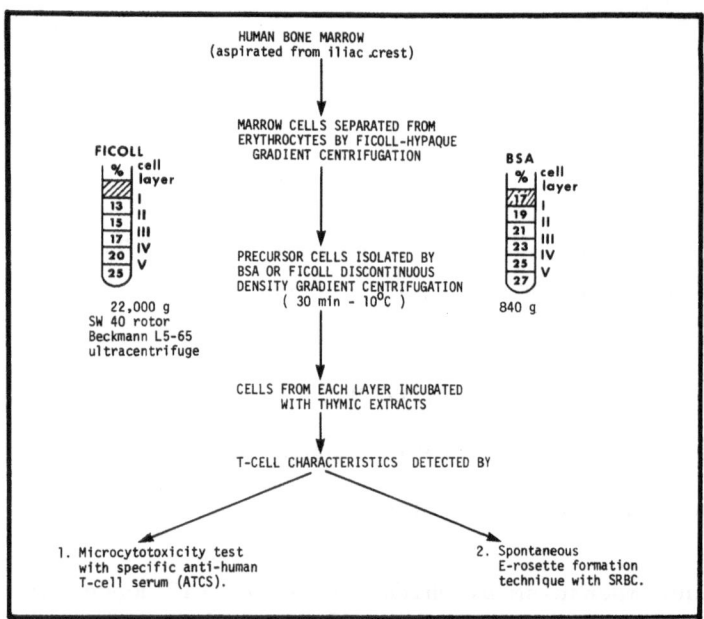

Fig. 1.   Procedure for the fractionation and characterization of
precursor marrow cells inducible in vitro by HTF to bear T lymphocyte characteristics.

precursor cell population in layer I, in a density range of 1.046-
1.055. Marrow cells from 18 healthy volunteers (21-50 years old)
have been studied. Precursor cells have been found in layer III
in 17/18 and in layer I in 12/18 of these individuals. The percentage of cells differentiated by HTF in layer I was smaller than
that in layer III.

     The appearance of T cell characteristics after incubation
with HTF was determined by two techniques: a microcytotoxicity
test using a specific anti-human T cell serum (ATCS) as indicator
(1,5) and spontaneous E-rosette formation with sheep red blood
cells (SRBC) (2). Results obtained with cells of layer III, isolated on a BSA gradient, are shown in Fig. 2. A marked increase
in cells bearing HTLA+ phenotypes (human T lymphocyte antigens)
were detected after a 2 hr incubation with either calf or HTF (F3).
A small increase of some significance was also apparent using the
E-rosette technique, difference from control value being at a P
level less than 0.01, as assessed by the Student t-test. When incubation was prolonged to 14 hr, a more pronounced increase could
be demonstrated by the E-rosette technique in the presence of HTF
(2).

     To determine the mode of action of HTF on marrow precursor
cells in vitro, the effect of specific inhibitors of RNA synthesis

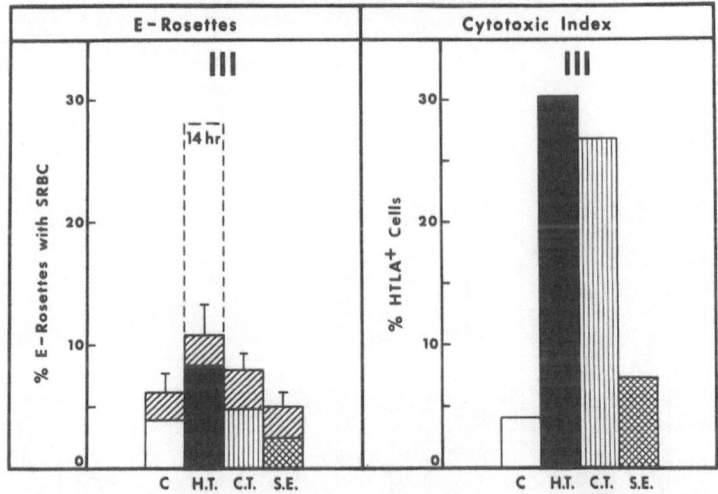

PRODUCTION OF T-CELL MARKERS ON NORMAL HUMAN
MARROW CELLS BY THYMIC EXTRACTS

Fig. 2. Differentiation of normal human marrow cells into cells
bearing T lymphocyte characteristics demonstrated after a 2 hr
incubation with human (H.T.) or calf (C.T.) thymic extracts (F3)
and human spleen (S.E.) (F3).

(actinomycin D, α-amanitin) and protein synthesis (puromycin) was
determined and compared to respective controls treated with inhibitors (2). Cells were treated with inhibitors as indicated on
Figs. 3 and 4 prior to addition of HTF (F3). Controls and inhi-
bitor-treated cells were then incubated for 2 hr in a 5% CO_2-95%
air humidified incubator. At the end of the incubation period
cells were washed twice with RPMI-1640 medium (RPMI) prior to formation of E-rosettes with SRBC or testing with ATCS and rabbit complement in a microcytotoxicity test. Viability was greater than
85% in all samples, as assessed by trypan blue exclusion. Both
actinomycin D and α-amanitin completely abolished the differentiation produced in cells of layer III by HTF. Actinomycin D seems
to increase somewhat the number of SRBC receptors in controls
treated with inhibitor, an effect demonstrated in other similar
experiments. However, this increase is small and is not significant. It could be due to derepression of some control mechanism
involved with synthesis of SRBC receptors. The inhibition of RNA
synthesis produced by α-amanitin is different from that
produced by actinomycin D. The latter inhibits transcription of
DNA into RNA by binding to the double-stranded DNA whereas α-amanitin inhibits RNA chain elongation by its effect on the DNA-depend-
ent RNA polymerase II (2). Puromycin, a protein synthesis inhibitor (2), inhibited markedly the synthesis of SRBC receptors and of

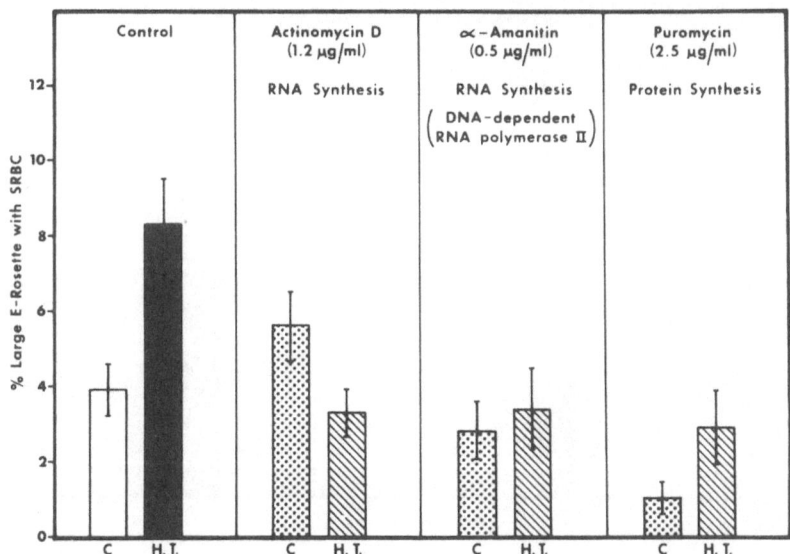

Fig. 3. Effect of inhibitors of RNA and protein synthesis on induction of receptors for SRBC in cells of layer III during a 2 hr
incubation with HTF (F3). The standard deviation is indicated by
the vertical line on top of each column. Open and black columns,
control (C) and HTF treated cells (H.T.) respectively; dotted and
striped columns, cells treated with inhibitors 5 min prior to addition of either RPMI (C) or HTF to (H.T.) respectively.

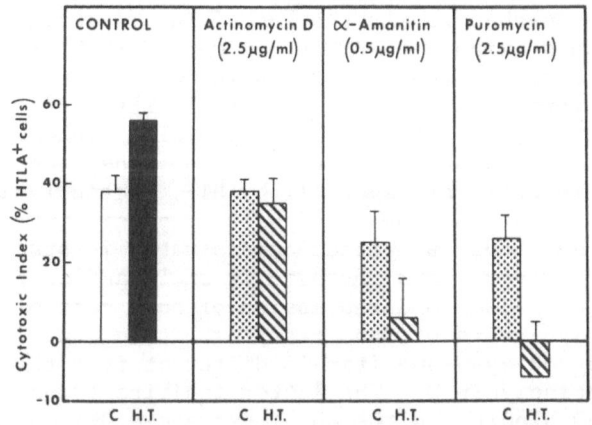

Fig. 4. Effect of inhibitors of RNA and protein synthesis on induction of HTLA[+] phenotypes in cells of layer III during a 2 hr
incubation with HTF (F3). See Fig. 3 for details.

HTLA[+] phenotypes at the low dose of 2.5 µg/ml both in controls and H.T.-treated cells. It did not, however, completely prevent induction by HTF as demonstrated in Fig. 3. This could indicate that the inhibitor concentration was too small to completely arrest translation of all mRNA required for synthesis of SRBC receptors after induction by HTF during 2 hr incubation. It might also suggest that other steps are involved prior to translation, such as RNA synthesis, for differentiation to occur, and that at the low and not cytotoxic doses of inhibitors used, RNA and protein synthesis were not completely abolished. These findings of inhibition of appearance of T cell markers are in contrast with those observed with PBL (3). When PBL were fractionated on a BSA gradient and cells of layer III were treated with the same inhibitors in the presence or absence of HTF, appearance of these markers still occurred, even when protein synthesis was inhibited 50% by higher concentrations of puromycin (25 µg/ml), as described by ^{14}C-leucine incorporation. It was demonstrated that the increase in E-rosette formation in layer III was due to conversion of cells forming small rosettes (PBL having 1 to 3 SRBC adhering) into cells forming large rosettes (PBL with 4 or more SRBC). In addition, in layer I, a very small population of PBL, 0.08% of the total number of cells applied on the gradient, was sensitive to the effect of puromycin and differentiation in these cells appeared to be inhibited. Cells of layer I, however, differed from those of layer III, since in layer I most E-rosettes were derived from cells not forming rosettes originally.

The studies conducted with the various inhibitors of RNA and protein synthesis prompted us to determine what direct effects HTF may have on RNA and protein synthesis in vitro. This was investigated during a short and long incubation of all marrow cell fractions with a more purified HTF (F5). RNA synthesis was studied during the last 2 hr of a 4 hr incubation period with HTF. As shown in Fig. 5, RNA synthesis is enhanced by the presence of HTF in cells of layer III, IV and V and inhibited in cells of the combined layers I + II. Inhibition by HTF in cells of layers I + II was confirmed in another experiment under similar conditions. Enhancement of RNA synthesis by HTF was sensitive to α-amanitin. This inhibitor diminished the increase in E-rosette formation observed in cells of layer III in the same experiment (Fig. 6) as demonstrated in Fig. 2 in other studies. Therefore, transcription of some mRNA seems required for induction of SRBC receptors by HTF (F5) in marrow cells but not in PBL. Alpha-amanitin had no effect on cells of layers I + II, where a 3% increase in E-rosette formation over control value was obtained after incubation with HTF. The presence of this inhibitor had a small stimulatory effect on protein synthesis in control and HTF-treated cells of layer III. When protein synthesis was studied in each cell layer during a 5 hr incubation with the same HTF (F5), a pattern different from that obtained with RNA synthesis was observed (Fig. 7). The

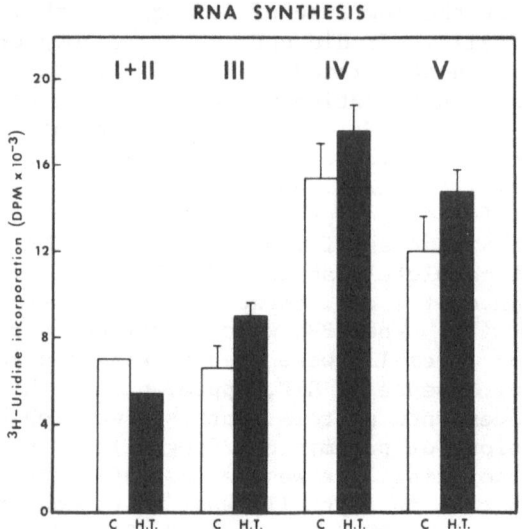

Fig. 5.   Effect of HTF (F5) on RNA synthesis in marrow cells of the various layers of a Ficoll gradient. Cells were incubated with HTF in microtest culture plates for 4 hr and labeled with ^{3}H-uridine for 2 hr prior to end of incubation. Cells were then collected on glass-fiber filters and counted in a Packard liquid scintillation spectrometer. Open and black columns represent control with RPMI (C) and HTF-treated cells (H.T.) respectively.

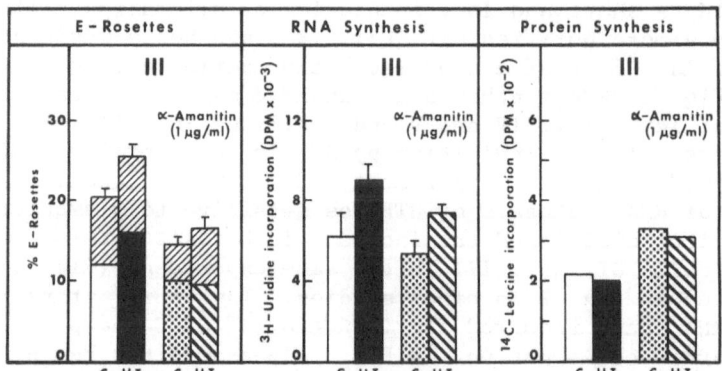

Fig. 6.   Effect of α-amanitin on E-rosette formation, RNA and protein synthesis in marrow cells of layer III of a Ficoll gradient during a 5 hr incubation with HTF (F5). Cells were labeled with ^{3}H-uridine or ^{14}C-leucine 2 hr prior to the end of incubation. Incorporation of label was determined as described in Fig. 5.

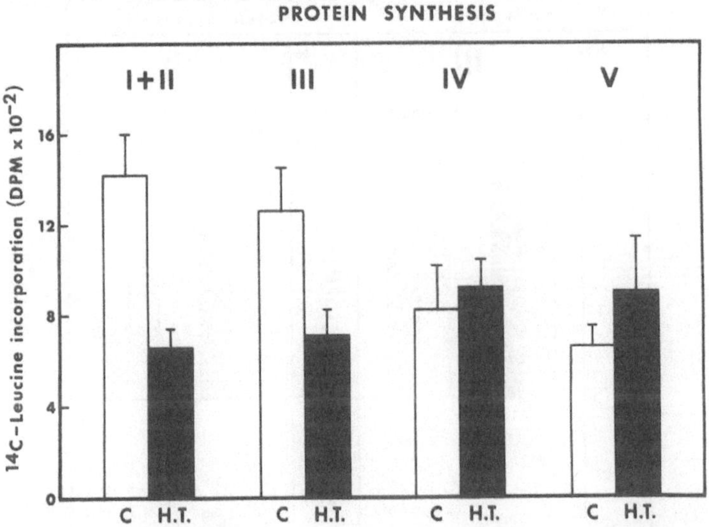

PROTEIN SYNTHESIS

Fig. 7. Effect of HTF (F5) on protein synthesis in marrow cells of layers I + II, III, IV and V of a Ficoll gradient. Cells were incubated 5 hr and labeled with ^{14}C-leucine (New England Nuclear) for 2 hr prior to end of incubation. Details on Fig. 5.

presence of HTF during incubation markedly inhibited protein synthesis in cells of layers I + II and layer III, but stimulated it somewhat in cells of layers IV + V.

The effect of higher concentrations of puromycin (20 µg/ml) on protein synthesis and E-rosette formation in marrow cells of layers III and V was then investigated. As shown in Fig. 8, the small increase in E-rosette formation produced by HTF is somewhat inhibited by the presence of puromycin in cells of layers III and V, but induction by HTF in cells of layer III was still present in puromycin-treated cells as shown previously in Fig. 3. Cells of layer V were also inhibited, but the percentage of E-rosette forming cells in that layer is small and possibly not significant. When protein synthesis was measured in both cell layers, it was found to be markedly inhibited by puromycin in controls and H.T.-treated cells, following the pattern observed in their respective controls not treated with inhibitors; inhibition of protein synthesis was still present in layer III but not in layer V.

To investigate further these effects, RNA, protein synthesis, and E-rosette formation were simultaneously studied in human marrow cells after 20 hr incubation with HTF (F5) (Fig. 9). A sharp increase in E-rosette formation was now present in cells of layer

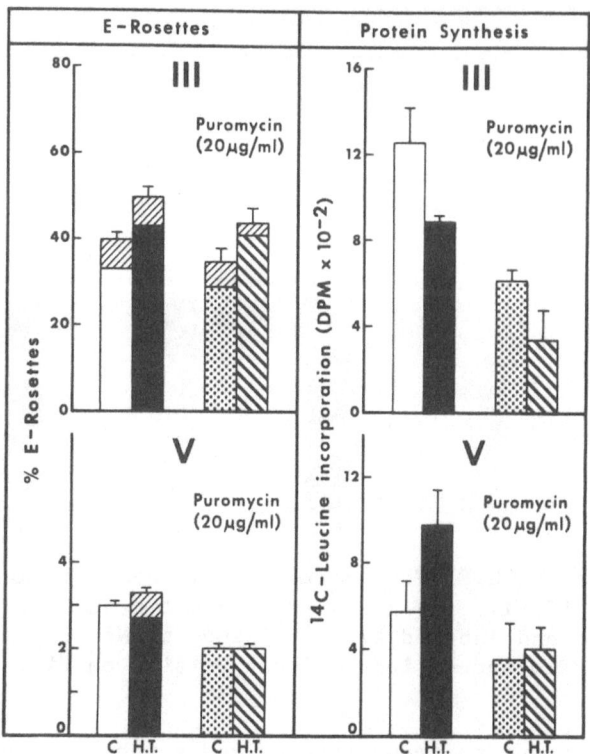

Fig. 8. Effect of puromycin on E-rosette formation and protein synthesis in marrow cells of a Ficoll gradient layers III and V during incubation with HTF (F5). Puromycin was added 5 min prior to addition of extract. Cells were incubated as described under Fig. 7. For other details see Fig. 5.

II, but not in layer III. RNA synthesis was stimulated in both layers II and III as shown, but it was found to be stimulated in all the layers except layer I (not shown). Thymic factors inhibited protein synthesis in cells of layer II and very markedly stimulated in cells of layer III and to a lesser degree in cells of layers IV and V, (not shown). At the times of incubation studied, it appears that protein synthesis is being turned off by HTF (F5), while E-rosette formation has been stimulated.

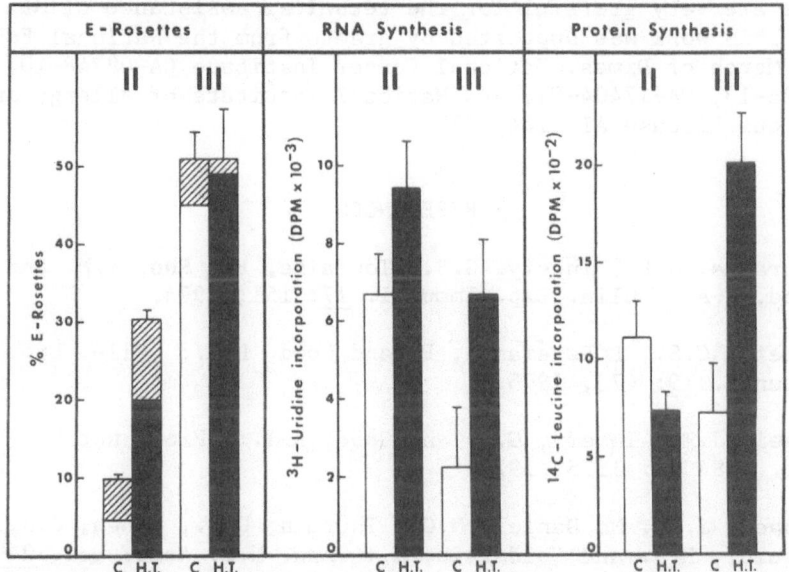

Fig. 9. Effect of HTF (F5) on E-rosette formation, RNA and protein synthesis after 20 hr incubation. Cells were treated as
described under Figs. 5 and 7.

In summary: 1. Two small populations of human marrow cells are
differentiated to cells bearing T-cell markers
by Thymosin F3 or F5.

2. Analysis with metabolic inhibitors indicates
that transcription and translation of RNA are
needed for induction of T cell markers (layer
III).

3. a) At 4 hours incubation RNA synthesis is enhanced in layers III, IV and V and inhibited in
layers I + II. b) At 20 hours incubation RNA
synthesis is markedly enhanced in all cell layers.

4. a) At 5 hours incubation protein synthesis is
suppressed in layers I + II and III, but not in
IV and V. b) At 20 hours incubation protein synthesis is markedly increased only in layer III.

Further studies are required to understand in more detail the mode
of action of thymic factors on precursor cells.

    We are very grateful for the technical assistance of Mr. R.L.
Chua. This work was supported by grants from the National Founda-
tion - March of Dimes, National Cancer Institute CA-08748-10,
CA-05826-13, CA-17404-01, and National Institute of Allergy and
Infectious Disease AI-11843-02.

REFERENCES

1. Touraine, J.L., Incefy, G.S., Touraine, F., Rho, Y.M. and
    Good, R.A.: Clin. Exp. Immunol. 17: 151, 1974.

2. Incefy, G.S., L'Espérance, P. and Good, R.A.: Clin. Exp.
    Immunol. 19: 475, 1975.

3. Vogel, J.E., Incefy, G.S. and Good, R.A.: Proc. Nat. Acad.
    Sci., USA 72: 1175, 1975.

4. Hooper, J.A., Mc Daniel, M.C., Thurman, G.B., Cohen, G.H.,
    Schulof, R.S. and Goldstein, A.: Ann. N.Y. Acad. Sci. 249:
    125, 1975.

5. Boumsell, L., Incefy, G.S., Bernard, A., Schwartz, S.,
    Smithwick, E. and Good, R.A.: J. Pediatrics, 1975 (in press).

IMMUNOLOGICAL POTENTIAL OF YOLK SAC CELLS

F. Hofman and A. Globerson

Department of Cell Biology, The Weizmann Institute of Science
Rehovot, Israel

Yolk sac cells have been shown to be the source of hemopoietic cells in the embryo (1) and to provide lymphoid precursor cells to the thymus (2), bursa of Fabricius (3) and embryonic liver (4). Accordingly, study of the ontogeny of the immune response should begin with analysis of the yolk sac cells. The questions raised in this respect are whether at this early stage of development the cells already have the potential to produce immune responses, and whether they can express such a potential. Answering this may advance the understanding of the generation of diversity.

The early work of Tyan (5) has demonstrated that yolk sac cells, when transferred to irradiated recipients, can cause mortality of secondary hosts, indicating that cells of yolk sac origin can elicit a GVH response. However, these studies did not answer the question whether a priori the yolk sac cells are capable of reacting. We employed for that purpose an in vitro GVH system (6) in which the cells could be assayed directly and found that 9-day embryonic yolk sac cells could elicit a splenomegaly reaction (7). Since the GVH response is attributed to T cell activity (8), we now attempted to test whether yolk sac cells are also capable of expressing other T cell activities.

Supported by a grant from the U. S. -Israel Binational Science Foundation and by the Minerva Foundation. The excellent technical assistance of Mrs. Claire Altman and Mr. Shalom Gahali is gratefully acknowledged.

51

MATERIALS AND METHODS

Mice. The mouse strains used in this study were Balb/c, C57Bl and F1(Balb/c x C57Bl). Yolk sac cells were obtained from embryos on day $9-9^{1}/2$ of gestation, unless otherwise stated. The date of plugging was considered day zero of gestation.

GVH assay. The modified local lymph node assay was described in detail (9). In short, experimental cells, in a volume of $5\,\mu l$, were injected into the foot pads of newborn mice. After 5—6 days, the local popliteal lymph nodes were removed, dissolved in 2N NaOH, and their protein content was measured by the optical density at 280 $m\mu$.

Mixed lymphocyte cultures and response to mitogens. Mixed lymphocyte reaction (MLR) and mitogen stimulation were performed in the microtiter plates. The culture media consisted of 5% FCS in RPMI and incubation in 10% CO_2/air. PHA (Welcome) and Con A (Miles-Yeda) were used in a range of concentrations in this culture system. The cytolytic assay was performed using ^{51}Cr-labelled mouse fibroblasts as the targets. The experimentally sensitized cells were incubated together with the target cells for 24 h. The supernatant was subsequently collected and measured for ^{51}Cr content.

RESULTS

Analysis of GVH response by yolk sac cells. We first attempted to test whether the GVH response expressed by yolk sac cells in vitro (7) can also manifest itself in other GVH assay systems. We, therefore, employed the local GVH assay, measuring enlargement of the popliteal lymph node in newborn host mice. An analysis of lymph node indices was initially made by injecting syngeneic spleen and lymph node cells at several concentrations into the foot pads of mice on the day of birth. Subsequently, the protein content of the lymph node from the injected side was evaluated and compared to that of the uninjected one. Under such conditions, relative enlargement never exceeded an index of 2 (Fig. 1). Therefore, a result was considered positive when the index was 2 or greater.

Balb/c yolk sac cells were then injected, at a dose of 10^5 cells into the right side foot pads of newborn F1(Balb/c x C57Bl) mice, while the left side was left untreated. As shown in Fig. 1, the yolk sac cells elicited lymph node enlargement in 4 out of 17 hosts. This result was constantly

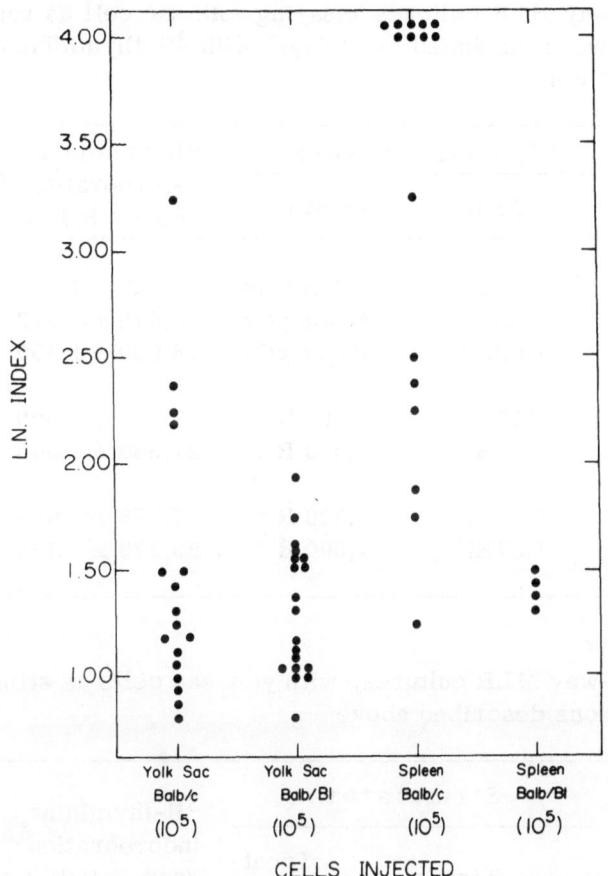

Fig. 1. Modified local lymph node graft versus host assay. Syngeneic or semiallogeneic cells were injected into the foot pad of newborn F1(Balb/Bl) mice. Each dot represents the lymph node (LN) index of a single host.

observed in repeated experiments. F1 yolk sac cells, when injected into the F1 newborn (Fig. 1), gave no such increase in size in all 19 cases, indicating that lymph node enlargement is not simply proliferation of the embryonic cells, nor is it due to maternal Balb/c contamination. F1(Balb/Bl) yolk sac cells injected into the foot pads of Balb/c newborns produced lymph node enlargement in 3 out of 12 hosts, indicating that the response was due to stimulation of the host tissue by the semi-allogeneic yolk sac cells, and not by maternal Balb/c cells.

TABLE 1. One-way MLR cultures assaying yolk sac cell as responders. Cell cultures were incubated for 3 days, with ^{3}H-thymidine present during the last 8 h

Responder cells	Stimulator spleen		^{3}H-thymidine incorporation (cpm ± S. E.)	Stimulation index
	Strain	Treatment		
Balb/c yolk sac	C57Bl	Mitomycin	12,936 ± 4,915	1.01
Balb/c yolk sac	Balb/c	Mitomycin	12,679 ± 573	0.94
C57Bl spleen	Balb/c	Mitomycin	18,699 ± 1,450	2.05
Balb/c yolk sac	C57Bl	1,500 R	3,650 ± 309	0.88
Balb/c LN	C57Bl	1,500 R	21,980 ± 1,560	1.46
Balb/c yolk sac	C57Bl	1,500 R	7,278 ± 604	1.15
Balb/c LN	C57Bl	1,500 R	23,279 ± 665	1.73

TABLE 2. One-way MLR cultures, with yolk sac cells as stimulators. Culture conditions described above

Responder LN	Stimulator		^{3}H-thymidine incorporation (cpm ± S. E.)	Stimulation index
	Tissue	Treatment		
C57Bl	F1* yolk sac	–	16,771 ± 2,016	1.13
F1	F1 yolk sac	–	18,148 ± 1,271	1.15
C57Bl	F1 spleen	–	5,906 ± 782	2.67
F1	F1 spleen	–	4,830 ± 908	1.50
C57Bl	Balb/c yolk sac	Mito.	12,712 ± 1,129	1.05
C57Bl	Balb/c LN	Mito.	14,923 ± 1,410	2.03
Balb/c	Balb/c LN	Mito.	9,484 ± 469	1.00
C57Bl	Balb/c yolk sac	Mito.	20,677 ± 1,363	1.30
C57Bl	Balb/c LN	Mito.	31,036 ± 2,112	2.88

*F1 = (Balb x C57Bl)F1.

MLC response. In the next series of experiments, yolk sac cells were examined for their ability to stimulate or be stimulated in the MLR, an in vitro correlate of the GVH response. Adult lymph node cells were incubated with F1 yolk sac cells, or mitomycin-treated allogeneic yolk sac cells, at a ratio of 1:1 for 2, 3, or 5 days. Stimulated cultures, as measured by ^{3}H-thymidine uptake, were pulsed for 8 or 12 h. It was found (Table 2) that yolk sac cells, semi-allogeneic or treated with 25 μg of mitomycin, did not cause stimulation in an MLR. Yolk sac cells were then tested for responding capacity in cultures of allogeneic mitomycin-treated or 1,500 Rad cobalt-treated spleen cells, at a ratio of 1:1. In one series, yolk sac cells with mitomycin-treated syngeneic spleen cells were used as control. As demonstrated in Table 1, yolk sac cells did not respond in the MLR. Yolk sac cells compared with allogeneic lymph node cells also showed no response. The cytolytic capacity of yolk sac cells possibly stimulated in an MLR was tested. Three-day cultures of Balb/c yolk sac cells and irradiated C57Bl spleen cells were exposed to ^{51}Cr labelled C57Bl target fibroblast cells for 24 h. The MLR cultures with yolk sac cells did not cause a significant amount of ^{51}Cr release, whereas the controls using adult cells did.

Response to mitogens. Finally, we measured the response of yolk sac cells to mitogens. Yolk sac cells at concentrations of 1.5—5.0 x 10^5 were cultured with PHA at doses ranging from 0.5 to 1.5 μg/ml. After 2 or or 3 days, the cultures were pulsed with ^{3}H-thymidine. The results indicate (Table 3) that yolk sac cells were not sensitive to PHA stimulation. In a second series of experiments we applied Con A to yolk sac cells of day 9 and day 10 of gestation, at concentrations of the drug ranging from 1.0 to 2.5 μg/ml. After three days, yolk sac cell cultures showed no significant incorporation of ^{3}H-thymidine above background, as compared with spleen cells (Table 3).

DISCUSSION

Yolk sac cells have been analyzed for properties attributed to T cell activities. In the in vitro GVH (7) and in vivo local GVH, yolk sac cells have been shown to cause a reaction. It thus seems that yolk sac cells have the capacity to recognize foreign cell surface antigens and cause the proliferation of the allogeneic cells. This capacity of yolk sac cells appears independently of the influence of the embryonic thymus, since the thymus develops only after day 13 of gestation. Nor is it affected by

TABLE 3. Mitogen stimulation. Cell cultures were incubated with PHA
or Con A for 3 days, with ^{3}H-thymidine present during the last 8 h

Cell source	Mitogen (µg/ml)	Cell concentration	^{3}H-thymidine incorporation (cpm ± S. E.)	Stimulation index
Incubation with PHA				
Yolk sac	2.5	10^5	8,976 ± 1,092	0.95
Yolk sac	1.3		8,451 ± 432	0.90
Yolk sac	0.5		8,123 ± 679	0.86
Spleen	2.5		8,718 ± 382	2.68
Spleen	1.3		10,001 ± 695	3,07
Spleen	0.5		7,780 ± 592	2.39
Incubation with Con A				
Yolk sac (day 9)	2.5	5×10^5	28,109 ± 641	0.97
Yolk sac (day 9)	1.3		20,631 ± 844	0.71
Yolk sac (day 10)	2.5		42,486 ± 2,625	1.13
Yolk sac (day 10)	1.3		39,250 ± 2,239	1.04
Spleen	2.5		51,796 ± 2,893	2.20
Spleen	1.3		51,849 ± 1,547	2.24
Yolk sac (day 9)	1.0		48,850 ± 4,721	1.08
Spleen	1.0		179,063 ± 3,613	3.42

maternal thymus, since thymectomized mothers have fostered embryos
with yolk sac tissue responding in the in vitro GVH (10). Evidently, the
full array of T cell functions has not been realized in the embryonic population. In the MLR, yolk sac cells could serve as neither stimulators nor
responders. In addition, PHA and Con A, T cell mitogens, could not activate yolk sac cells. Perhaps acquisition of the other immunological functions may require the migration and maturation of these cells in the
embryonic environment. It should be noted that the GVH assay involves

application of the cells onto spleen explants (6) or in vivo (the present study). In contrast to the cell cultures (MLR and response to mitogens), this procedure may enable a rapid, critical step of maturation of the yolk sac cells during the assay. Yet, regardless of this possibility, the present study indicates that yolk sac cells, still within the extra-embryonic membrane, have the potential to perform certain immunological functions, related to recognition of foreign H-2 antigens. An analysis of the range of recognition of stem cells as compared to that of adult is necessary for understanding of generation of diversity.

SUMMARY

Mouse yolk sac cells on day 9 of gestation were found to elicit a GVH response, measured by enlargement of the local popliteal lymph nodes. The response cannot be attributed to contaminating maternal cells, since F1(Balb/c x C57Bl) yolk sac cells did not cause a reaction in F1(Balb/c x C57Bl) hosts. On the other hand, yolk sac cells did not elicit a detectable MLC reaction, nor did they respond to PHA or Con A. Hence, mouse yolk sac cells have the potential to express a certain limited array of immunological reactivities, before the development of embryonic thymus and liver.

REFERENCES

1. Kirschbaum, K. and H. Downey, Anat. Rec. 68, 227 (1937)
2. Moore, M. A. S. and J. J. T. Owen, J. Exp. Med. 126, 715 (1967)
3. Moore, M. A. S. and J. J. T. Owen, Nature 215, 1081 (1967)
4. Moore, M. A. S. and D. Metcalf, Brit. J. Hematol. 18, 279 (1970)
5. Tyan, M. L., J. Immunol. 100, 535 (1968)
6. Auerbach, R. and A. Globerson, Exp. Cell Res. 42, 31 (1966)
7. Hofman, F. and A. Globerson, Eur. J. Immunol. 3, 179 (1973)
8. Cantor, H. and R. Assofsky, J. Exp. Med. 135, 764 (1972)
9. Arrenbrecht, S., submitted.
10. Hofman, F., unpublished observations.

ONTOGENY OF T LYMPHOCYTES STUDIED IN ATHYMIC AND FOETAL MICE

G.E. Roelants, K.S. Mayor, L.-B. Hägg and F. Loor

Basel Institute for Immunology

Grenzacherstr. 487, CH-4058 Basel, Switzerland

Earlier studies on T lineage lymphocytes in congenitally athymic nude mice (1,2) have been extended to surgically T deprived mice and early stages of embryogenesis. They permit the further characterisation of a new type of lymphocyte and its implication in T cell ontogeny.

CHARACTERISTICS OF T LINEAGE LYMPHOCYTES IN ATHYMIC MICE

T lineage lymphocytes are present in all lymphoid organs of athymic mice (spleen, lymph nodes, bone marrow, Peyer's patches, peripheral blood) but are usually more abundant in the spleen where they may represent 20% of all lymphocytes (2). They are negative for membrane Ig detected by immunofluorescence but have a low density of the θ (Thy 1) antigen which is detected by indirect immunofluorescence using either AKR anti-θC3H reagents or a rabbit antibody raised against mouse brain associated θ antigen made specific by absorption in vivo (1). The density of θ is lower than on the surface of usual thymocytes or peripheral T cells for it can not be detected by cytotoxicity or immunofluorescence using a directly conjugated TRITC-AKR IgG-α-θC3H reagent (1). It should be stressed that while in most experiments we used the rabbit reagent which allows the simultaneous detection of θ and /or Ig on the same cell sample one does not have to rely on this reagent only since θ is equally well detected on athymic mouse lymphocytes by the mouse reagent used in sandwich or even by the directly conjugated TRITC-AKR IgG-α-θC3H provided it is redistributed in patches by a second layer of unconjugated anti-mouse Ig reagent. In TL positive strains,

TL is also detected on those cells by anti- TL reagent prepared in
congenic mice (3) (TL negative strain of mice served as control) (4).
However, T lineage lymphocytes of the bone marrow are devoid of TL
(4). Other surface markers e.g. Ly have not yet been tested.

Other characteristics of these cells which differentiate them
from usual peripheral T cells of normal mice are their low electrophoretic mobility (2), their lack of recirculation through the
thoracic duct (2) and their very short life span of one to two days
(4).

PRODUCTION AND REGULATION

The cells described in section 1 are usually produced in the
bone marrow but may also be made by the spleen when the bone marrow
is destroyed by injection of ^{89}Sr (4). They represent 75-95% of the
lymphocytes present in embryo thymuses at 13 days of gestation,
typical θ positive cells appearing only between day 14 and 15 of
gestation. They also represent 1-2% of 13 days foetal liver cells
(4).

The production of these cells is under homeostatic control of
the thymus for they appear in the periphery in a matter of a few
days after thymic deprivation and their production in large numbers
stops after thymus grafting to either congenitally or surgically T
deprived mice (4). This control is mediated by humoral factor for
the grafted thymus may be inserted in a millipore chamber (4).
Spleen in a millipore chamber is not effective.

COMMITTMENT OF MULTIPOTENTIAL STEM CELLS TO THE T LINEAGE:
A THYMUS INDEPENDENT PROCESS

The many thymocytes characteristics (surface markers, turnover,
electrophoretic mobility) of T lineage lymphocytes in athymic mice,
their regulation by the thymus and the presence of similar cells
in the thymus early in embryogenesis strongly suggest a precursor
role for these cells. Most of our studies were done on surgically
T deprived mice or on nude mice born from nu/nu males and nu/+
heterozygous mothers and the possible influence of thymic factors
coming from the mother or from normal littermate during embryonic
life could not be assessed. However, recently in collaboration
with Dr. P. Dukor, we had the opportunity to study nude mice obtained
from a colony of homozygous nu/nu males and females. We found that
cells with the characteristics described above were present in those
animals as well (Table 1).

Table 1
θ^+ lymphocytes in nu/nu mice born from nu/nu parents

Mouse (Ref. No. and organ)	θ^+strong (2)	Types of cells detected (1)				
		θ^+ (3)	$Ig^-\theta^+$ (4)	$Ig^+\theta^+$ (4)	$Ig^+\theta^-$ (4)	$Ig^-\theta^-$ (4)
1 Spleen	–	1.7–10.1	8.4–12.6	1.7	67.5	18.2
2	–	1.2–9.2	5.4–8.1	1.5	67.5	22.9
3	–	1.3–8.9	8.0–8.8	1.2	60.0	30.0
4	0.6–1.4	–	6.4–8.0	2.8	68.8	20.4
5	0.4–1.3	–	6.3–9.1	1.0	65.0	24.9
6–10	0.4–0.9	0.7–2.8	~12.0	~3.0	~43.0	~34.0
1–3 Lymph Nodes	–	0.6–5.7	8.7–9.1	0.4	84.9	5.6
4–5 " "	0.3–1.5	–	3.9–4.9	0.3	81.9	12.9

(1) For complete experimental procedure see Ref. 1. When a range of percentage is given, the first number relates to the bright fluorescent cells only and the second number relates to all specifically fluorescent cells, the very faint ones included; (2): as detected by TRITC-AKR IgG-α-θC3H (rings); (3): as (2), but after a second layer of unlabelled SIgG-α-MIg to cluster the fluorescent α-θ into spots; (4) as detected by RIgG-α-MθBr (NRIg as control) followed by TRITC-SIgG-α-RIg and FITC-SIgG-α-MIg.

From these results and those of the litterature on T precursor in athymic mice (e.g. 5-9) the following picture of T cell ontogeny starts to emerge.

BONE MARROW   BLOOD   THYMUS

$Ig^-\theta^-TL^- \longrightarrow Ig^-\theta^{+weak}TL^- \rightarrow Ig^-\theta^{+weak}TL^+ \longrightarrow Ig^-\theta^{+strong}TL^+$

HOMEOSTATIC CONTROL

OTHER LINEAGES   SUBSETS

STEM CELL   PRE-THYMOCYTES   THYMOCYTES

Its most striking feature is that the crucial step of differentiation by which a multipotential stem cell becomes committed to the T pathway (pre-thymocyte) not only takes place outside the thymus but is even independent of any thymus factor, the thymus playing an essential role only in the further maturation of those cells.

REFERENCES

1. Loor, F., and G.E. Roelants, 1974. High frequency of T lineage lymphocytes in nude mouse spleen. Nature 251:229.

2. Roelants, G.E., F. Loor, H. von Boehmer, J. Sprent, L.-B. Hägg, K.S. Mayor and A. Rydén. 1975. Five types of lymphocytes (Ig$^-$ θ^-, Ig$^-$ θ^{+weak}, Ig$^-$ $\theta^{+strong}$, Ig$^+$ θ^- and Ig$^+$ θ^+) characterized by double immunofluorescence and electrophoretic mobility. Organ distribution in normal and nude mice. Eur. J. Immunol. 5:127.

3. Loor, F., N. Block and J.R. Little. 1975. Dynamics of the TL antigens on thymus and leukemia cells. Cell. Immunol. 17:351.

4. Roelants, G.E., K.S. Mayor, L.-B. Hägg and F. Loor. 1975. Immature T lineage lymphocytes in athymic mice. Presence of TL, lifespan and homeostatic regulation. Submitted for publication.

5. Bach, J.F., M. Dardenne, A.L. Goldstein, A. Guha and A. White. 1971. Appearance of T-cell markers in bone marrow rosette-forming cells after incubation with thymosin, a thymic hormone. Proc. Nat. Acad. Sci. (USA) 68:2734.

5. Scheid, M.P., M.K. Hoffmann, K. Komuro, O. Hämmerling, J. Abbott, E.A. Boyse, G.H. Cohen, J.A. Hooper, R.S. Schulof and A.L. Goldstein. 1973. Differentiation of T cells induced by preparations from thymus and by non-thymic agents. The determined state of the precursor cell. J. Exp. Med. 138:1027.

7. Loor, F., and B. Kindred. 1973. Differentiation of T cell precursors in nude mice demonstrated by immunofluorescence of membrane markers. J. Exp. Med. 138:1044.

8. Pritchard, H., and H.S. Micklem. 1973. Haemopoietic stem cells and progenitors of functional T-lymphocytes in the bone marrow of nude mice. Clin. Exp. Immunol. 14:597.

9. Kindred, B., and F. Loor. 1974. Activity of host-derived T cells which differentiate in nude mice grafed with co-isogenic or allogeneic thymuses. J. Exp. Med. 139:1215.

ONTOGENY OF T CELL FUNCTION IN THE FETAL LAMB

Arthur M. Silverstein and Shraga Segal

The Wilmer Institute, Johns Hopkins University School

of Medicine, Baltimore, Md., and Department of Cell

Biology, Weizmann Institute, Rehovot, Israel

The maturation of the ability of mammalian fetuses to mount active immunologic responses following antigen stimulus appears to follow a well-defined and precisely timed sequence. Competence to respond to some antigens arises very early in gestation, while other antigens are unable to stimulate active immune responses until later in gestation or even during the neonatal period. Thus, for each species or inbred strain, the earliest appearance of antibody formation to a given antigen, or of such other phenomena as allograft rejection, appears to represent a very discrete differentiative event. It would also seem clear that this type of stepwise immunologic maturation is based upon a series of individual developmental events, rather than the abrupt appearance of a single general immunologic control mechanism. The apparently general nature of this sequential maturation of immunologic competence is supported by data in such disparate species as the fetal lamb (1, 2), the opossum (3), and the mouse (4).

It has always been tempting to believe that the critical event responsible for the achievement of immunologic competence to a given antigen was the first appearance of specific immunoglobulin receptors for that antigen upon the surface of appropriate immunocytes. (The possibility that this stepwise maturation provides a direct temporal record of the first appearance of structural immunoglobulin genes by some sort of somatic mutation or recombination mechanism must be rejected, for reasons given elsewhere [2] .) Since most of the antigens in the developmental hierarchy of the fetal lamb (Table I) are widely recognized as thymus-dependent, the final event leading to the development of competence to form antibody against a given antigen could involve the first appearance of a T cell receptor, a B cell receptor, or both. In this report we will review the data on the ontogeny of T cell function in the fetal lamb.

MATURATION OF SPECIFIC HELPER T CELLS

In order to test whether the first appearance of antigen-specific functional T cells is the critical factor in the timing of immunologic competence to that antigen, an in vivo assessment of helper T cell function in anti-hapten responses was employed (5). This involves the administration of a non-immunogenic priming

TABLE I

Stepwise maturation of immunologic competence in the lamb. *

Antigen	Gestation age
	(days)
Bacteriophage ϕX 174	<40
Ferritin	56
Q-fever vaccine	<65
Skin allografts	75
Snail hemocyanin	80
Simian virus 40	90
Bacteriophage T4	105
Dinitro phenyl hapten (DNP)	<110
Arsanilate hapten	<110
Ovalbumin	120
Bluetongue virus	122
LCM virus	140
- - - - - - - BIRTH - - - - - - - -	150
Diphtheria toxoid	postpartum
Salmonella typhosa "O"	postpartum
BCG	postpartum

*Reproduced from reference 2.

dose (1 mg in saline given i. v.) of a hapten such as DNP on one carrier. One week later, an injection of 50 μg of unrelated protein antigen in complete Freund's adjuvant injected intramuscularly is given, in order to stimulate T cell reactivity against the second antigen. Some weeks later, the normally non-immunogenic dose of the hapten coupled to the second carrier antigen is administered (again 1 mg in saline i. v.). If functional helper T cells are stimulated to the second carrier protein by the adjuvant injection, they will collaborate with the hapten-specific B cells stimulated by the initial priming injection on the unrelated carrier to produce a strong booster anti-hapten antibody response following the final immunization (6, 7).

In the context of the developmental sequence observed in the fetal lamb (Table I), all of the immunizations were given between 80 and 105 days gestation, using DNP as the hapten, hemocyanin (to which the fetus shows competence at about 80 days gestation) as the first carrier antigen, and ovalbumin (to which the fetus does not develop competence until 120 days gestation) as the second carrier antigen.

The results of this study are illustrated in Table II. It will be seen that all of the animals receiving the full course of three injections (priming with DNP-ferritin, supplement of ovalbumin in adjuvant, and challenge with DNP-ovalbumin) formed a very strong booster anti-DNP response, as measured by DNP-T4 phage

TABLE II

Test for ovalbumin-specific helper T cells. Fetuses were primed with DNP-KLH and boosted with DNP-oval, with or without an intermediate oval-adjuvant supplement. [*]

Fetal lamb	Oval supplement	Anti-DNP titer
1	Yes	10, 000
2	Yes	>10, 000
3	Yes	3, 500
4	No	<10
5	No	<10
6	No	<10

[*]Adapted from reference 5.

neutralization assay (8) one week after the final immunization.
In contrast, controls receiving the priming and booster
injections, but deprived of the ovalbumin-in-adjuvant supplement
aimed at stimulating ovalbumin-specific helper T cells, were
unable to form a detectable anti-DNP antibody response.

It is clear from these results that the fetal lamb is able to
generate functional ovalbumin-specific helper T cells prior to
the earliest time (120 days gestation) at which it first shows
immunologic competence to form anti-ovalbumin antibody. Since
these helper T cells are antigen-specific, it must be assumed
a) that they act through the intercession of antigen-specific
receptors on the cell membrane; b) that these receptor molecules
are the products of V-region structural genes; and, finally,
c) that at least in the case of this one antigen, ovalbumin, the
ability to manifest full immunologic competence does not await
the first appearance of functional antigen-specific receptors
upon T cells.

The time of appearance in ontogeny of functional B cells with
antigen-specific receptors is somewhat less clear. A number of
investigators (9-12) have reported the very early appearance of
antigen-binding B cells in a variety of species, including the
presence of large numbers of ovalbumin-binding cells in the fetal
lamb long before 120 days gestation (12). In many of these studies,
the large proportion of cells found to bind any given antigen raises
a serious question about the specificity of the test employed.
However, if we grant the existence of some ovalbumin-binding
B cells in the fetal lamb prior to 120 days gestation, then the
sudden ability of the fetus to form anti-ovalbumin antibodies at
that later age might be due to: a) the earlier absence of some
ancillary participating cell type or other paraimmunologic process;
b) the earlier presence of some inhibitory mechanism such as a
specific suppressor T cell; or, what currently appears most
likely to us, c) a final differentiative stage in B cell development
which first permits the receptor-antigen complex to be translated
into an appropriate signal to stimulate full B cell function. Thus,
the demonstration by passive means of specific receptors upon the
surface of an immunocyte may be a necessary but probably not a
sufficient criterion of the ability of that cell to fulfill its
programmed functions.

THE CONTROL OF T CELL MATURATION

One other aspect of the ontogeny of T cell function deserves brief mention here. This concerns the demonstration in a large number of species of the critical role of the thymus in the development of the full T cell function (13). It has been found in the fetal lamb, however, that extirpation of the thymus, even early in gestation, has little effect on the subsequent immunologic maturation of the animal (14, 15). These animals, though henceforth somewhat lymphopenic, proceed with the normal stepwise maturation of the immunologic competencies as outlined in Table I, including the demonstration of such T cell functions as allograft rejection and the formation of antibodies against T-dependent antigens. Indeed, even an animal thymectomized very early in gestation and then massively treated with antilymphocyte serum to further deplete it of lymphoid cells is found to reconstitute full immunologic function during the neonatal period (16). This phenomenon is especially paradoxical in that, although the animals as they grow up present with what appears to be a set of lymphoid tissues that look morphologically purely B-dependent, yet they still are able to subserve all of the expected T cell functions, including a full set of antigen-specific helper T cells (17).

The ability of the fetal lamb to continue to develop all of its T-dependent functions following thymectomy, and the ability of the neonate to reconstitute its T-dependent functions in the absence of a thymus, raise interesting questions about the possible existence of alternative mechanisms to control the early maturation of T cell lines, their acquisition of antigen-specific receptors, and their attainment of full functional competence. Recent observations that children with the DiGeorge type of thymic alymphoplasia may slowly reconstitute their T cell functions after some years seem to point in the same direction (18).

ACKNOWLEDGMENTS

These studies were supported in part by U. S. Public Health Service Research Grant HD-07935 from the National Institute of Child Health and Human Development, an unrestricted gift from Alcon Laboratories, Inc. , and an Independent Order of Odd Fellows Research Professorship.

REFERENCES

1. A. M. Silverstein, J. W. Uhr, K. L. Kraner, and R. J. Lukes, J. Exp. Med. 117:799, 1963.

2. A. M. Silverstein, in: P. Liacopoulos and J. Panijel, Eds., Phylogenic and Ontogenic Study of the Immune Response and its Contribution to the Immunological Theory, p. 221. Paris, INSERM, 1973.

3. D. T. Rowlands, Jr., D. Blakeslee, and E. Angala, J. Immunol. 112:2148, 1974.

4. W. K. Sherwin and D. T. Rowlands, Jr., J. Immunol. 113:1353, 1974.

5. A. M. Silverstein and S. Segal, J. Exp. Med. (in press).

6. K. Rajewsky, V. Schirrmacher, S. Nase, and N. K. Jerne, J. Exp. Med. 129:1131, 1969.

7. D. H. Katz, W. E. Paul, E. A. Goidl, and B. Benacerraf, J. Exp. Med. 132:261, 1970.

8. O. Mäkelä, Immunology 10:81, 1966.

9. A. R. Hayward and J. F. Soothill, in: Ontogeny of Acquired Immunity, Ciba Foundation Symposium, New York, Elsevier, 1972.

10. J. M. Dwyer and I. R. Mackay, Immunology 23:870, 1972.

11. J. M. Decker, J. Clarke, L. M. Bradley, A. Miller, and E. E. Sercarz, J. Immunol. 113:1823, 1974.

12. J. M. Decker and E. E. Sercarz, Nature 252:416, 1974.

13. J. F. A. P. Miller and G. F. Mitchell, Transplantation Rev. 1:3, 1969.

14. A. M. Silverstein and R. A. Prendergast, in: J. Šterzl and I. Řiha, Eds., Developmental Aspects of Antibody Formation and Structure, p. 69. Prague, Czech Academy of Sciences, 1970.

15. G. J. Cole and B. Morris, Aust. J. Exp. Biol. Med. Sci. 49:33, 1971.

16. A. M. Silverstein and R. A. Prendergast, in: B. D. Jankovic and K. Isakovic, Eds., Microenvironmental Aspects of Immunity, p. 383, New York, Plenum Press, 1973.

17. A. M. Silverstein and S. Segal, unpublished observations.

18. F. S. Rosen, Ped. Clin. N. America 21:533, 1974.

INVOLVEMENT OF CELLS WITH 'B' PROPERTIES IN DEVELOPMENT OF T HELPERS

A. Globerson[1], S.M. Kirov[2] and C.R. Parish

Department of Microbiology, JCSMR, ANU Canberra

Australia

INTRODUCTION

The question as to whether T and B cell populations develop independently of each other, or whether they represent different stages of differentiation within the same cell lineage is so far unresolved. During ontogeny, T and B cells differentiate in different compartments (1). However, this distinction is not entirely clear cut. Mouse embryonic liver, which is supposedly a territory of B cell development (2,3) may give rise to cells with T properties upon treatment with thymic factors, as expressed in reactivity in a GvH response (4) or expression of membrane markers (5). The question is thus raised as to whether the embryonic liver contains cells which are uncommitted, and the pathways of development can be imposed by effects of micro-environmental or humoral factors, or whether cells with T properties develop from cells which already express B characteristics.

In the present study we therefore attempted to distinguish between these two possibilities.

[1]Recipient of EMBO long-term fellowship (1974). Permanent address: Department of Cell Biology, the Weizmann Institute of Science, Rehovot, Israel.

[2]Present address: Department of Medicine, Hobart Hospital, Tasmania, Australia.

MATERIALS AND METHODS

Animals. CBA/H and (CBA/H x C57B1/6)F_1 mice from breeding
colonies in the John Curtin School were used throughout these experiments. The adult mice employed were 7-8 weeks old. Embryos
were obtained from mice plugged daily, the day of plug being considered as day 0 of gestation.

Irradiation and cell transfers. Total body irradiation at a
dose of 750 R was applied from a ^{60}Co source at the CSIRO laboratory
in Canberra. Liver cell suspensions were prepared and washed as
previously described (6). Embryonic liver and adult bone marrow
cells (from 3-4 week old donors) were injected i.v. at a dose of
20-25 x 10^6 cells/mouse within 4 hours from irradiation. Flagellin
monomer (MON) was injected i.v. at a dose of 1.0 μg/mouse. Mice
treated with cells received the antigen admixed with the cell
suspension.

Culture procedure and assay of antibodies. Cell cultures were
employed as previously described (7). 'B' cells for cultures consisted of normal adult spleen cells treated with anti-θ and complement. Cultures were stimulated with DNP-MON and the response was
measured 3 days later. Assay for PFC involved SRBC coupled with DNP
by Fab (8). The slide technique was employed according to Cunningham
and Szenberg (9).

Treatment of cells with anti H-2 antibodies. Balb/c anti C57B1/6
ascitic fluid was kindly provided by Dr. R.M. Zinkernagel. The procedure of treatment to the cells was according to Miller & Sprent (10).

Rosetting technique. For separation of Ig bearing (Ig^+) from
non Ig bearing (Ig^-) cells we employed the rosetting technique as
recently described (11). The Ig^+ fraction was recovered by osmotic
shock to the erythrocytes (11) and washed twice before further use.

RESULTS AND DISCUSSION

We first attempted to find out whether embryonic liver cells
can give rise to development of T helper cells in the thymus of irradiated recipients. To encourage passage of the cells through the
thymus, we splenectomized the mice 1-7 days before irradiation
(Globerson, unpublished). Hence, splenectomized and irradiated
adult CBA/H mice were divided into 3 groups: receiving either 17-
day embryonic liver cells, or adult bone marrow (BM) as a positive
control since it is known to develop T cells upon passage through
thymus (12), or no cells. All the three groups were given MON to
produce a carrier effect, enhancing a subsequent in vitro response
to DNP-MON. Mice were sacrificed 10-11 days afterwards, their

Table 1. In vitro response to DNP-MON by cultures of anti θ treated spleen cells with thymus cells of mice receiving different treatments and immunized with MON.

Cells cultured		Anti DNP PFC/culture[a]
Spleen	Thymus Treatment to donor	
Anti θ treated	Spx[b], liver	975 ± 152
"	Spx, BM	1160 ± 84
"	Spx	487 ± 47
-	Spx, liver	< 20
Anti θ treated	-	450 ± 42
Untreated	-	2305 ± 162

[a] Mean values from results of 4 cultures, ± S.E.

[b] Spx = splenectomized, irradiated mice.

thymuses were removed and suspended in culture medium. They were then admixed with anti-θ treated ('B') spleen cells, and stimulated with DNP-MON. Four cultures were set up in every experimental and control group unless otherwise stated. The anti-DNP response was measured 3 days later, by assaying the number of PFC produced on DNP-SRBC.

As shown in Table 1, thymus cells of mice treated with liver, when cultured with 'B' cells, produced a response to DNP similar to that of BM-repopulated mice, although lower than that of normal spleen cells. In the absence of 'B' cells there was no response by thymuses of the liver-repopulated mice. Hence the treatment with embryonic livers gave rise in the thymus to helper cells which cooperated with 'B' cells in the response to DNP-MON.

We considered two alternative mechanisms to explain these observations: (a) the embryonic liver cells developed into helper cells in the thymic environment; (b) the donor cells enhanced recovery of the host thymus elements. These two possibilities are by no means mutually exclusive. To test whether donor cells participated directly in this activity, or whether the helper function is entirely related to the host, we employed immunogenetic markers to distinguish between donor and host components. Hence, the next experiment was performed in parallel in two types of combinations: (1) CBA/H liver cells were transferred to (CBA/H x C57Bl/6)F_1 recipients. (2) F_1(CBA/H x C57Bl/6) livers were injected to CBA/H mice. In both cases, thymus cells, harvested 10 days after irradiation, were treated with anti-C57Bl/6 antibodies and complement. Control samples were incubated with complement only. The treated as well as untreated cells were cultured with B cells and DNP-MON, and the response to DNP was assayed subsequently, as in the previous experiment. As shown in Table 2, elimination of donor cells interfered with the response to DNP whereas elimination of recipients' cells had no significant effect. The background level of the response (B cells only) was in general high in this experiment, yet the difference between the various groups was obvious. The experiment was repeated and the same type of results were obtained.

It was thus concluded that cells of embryonic liver origin can function as helpers in the response to the hapten-carrier conjugate.

We then designed to find out whether cells developing into 'helpers' in the thymus derive from precursors which manifest properties of 'B' populations. We therefore fractionated 17 day embryonic liver cells to separate Ig^+ cells from Ig^- cells. The separate fractions were transferred to splenectomized irradiated recipients, which were simultaneously treated with MON. Thymuses were tested 10-11 days later, as in the previous experiments. It was found that thymus cells of mice receiving the Ig^- fractions had no overt effect on the response to DNP, the results being similar to those of 'B' cells without any added thymus cells.

Table 2. Analysis of host and donor contribution to the helper function by thymus cells of irradiated recipients.

| | Cells cultured | | Anti DNP PFC/ |
| | | Thymus | |
Spleen	Treatment to donor	Treatment to cells	culture [a]
Anti θ treated	Fl [b] liver→ spx CBA	anti C57Bl+C' [c]	1325 + 112
"	"	C'	2185 + 115
Anti θ treated	CBA liver→ Spx Fl	anti C57Bl+C'	1555 + 79
"	"	C'.	1585 + 75
Anti θ treated	-	-	1125 + 175
Untreated	-	-	2333 + 165

[a] Mean values from results of 4 cultures, + S.E.

[b] Fl = (CBA/H x C57Bl/6)F1.

[c] C' = Guinea pig serum complement.

Table 3. In vitro response to DNP-MON by cultures of anti θ treated spleen cells with thymus cells of mice receiving fractionated embryonic liver or adult bone marrow cells.

Cells cultured		Anti DNP PFC/culture [a]
Spleen	Thymus Treatment to donor	
Anti θ treated	Spx, Ig$^+$ liver cells	1030 + 40
"	Spx, Ig$^-$ liver cells	530 [b]
"	Spx, Ig$^+$ BM cells	1100 + 42
"	Spx, Ig$^-$ BM cells	515 + 50
Anti θ treated	-	675 + 25
Untreated	-	1905 + 35

[a] Mean of results from 4 cultures + S.E.

[b] Mean of results from 2 cultures.

To test whether this observation represents a phenomenon unique to embryonic cells, or whether development of helper cells in the adult can also follow a similar pattern, we repeated this study with adult bone marrow cells. Table 3 shows the results of an experiment performed in parallel with bone marrow and embryonic liver cells. It appeared as if Ig$^+$ cells from bone marrow give rise to cells enhancing the in vitro response to DNP-MON, similar to the finding with the liver cells. In the subsequent experiments we employed, therefore, bone marrow cells to further analyze this observation.

Since it has been indicated that cells with 'B' properties may play a role in helper function in a response to hapten-carrier conjugates (13-14), we tested whether the thymus cells enhancing the response to DNP-MON have B or T properties. We approached this question by two types of assays. In the first, thymuses of BM treated recipients were incubated with anti θ serum before culture, to test whether the residual cells can manifest a response. In parallel, another portion of the same thymus cells was fractionated, and the Ig$^-$ cells were cultured to test whether they have any activity. As shown in Table 4, treatment with anti θ antibodies reduced the activity to the levels of control cultures containing 'B' cells only, or supplemented with thymocytes of splenectomized irradiated mice which did not receive any cells. On the other hand, it was found that Ig$^-$ cells were active, leading to an enhanced response to DNP-MON. It should be noted that the results in Table 4 represent two separate experiments. Although the background level of response of B cultures in expt. I were high, they are significantly different from those of

Table 4. Characterization of the cells performing helper function
in thymuses of repopulated recipients.

Cells cultured			Anti DNP PFC/culture [a]	
Spleen	Thymus			
	Treatment to donor	Treatment to cells	Experiment I	Experiment II
Anti θ treated	Spx, BM	–	NT [b]	765 + 108
"	"	Anti θ + C'	1305 + 141	NT
"	"	C'	2125 + 43	NT
"	"	Ig⁻ fraction	1705 + 28	810 [c]
Anti θ treated	Spx	–	1285 + 78	580 [c]
"	–	–	1125 + 176	480 + 101
Intact	–	–	2333 + 165	1585 + 111

[a] Mean of results from 4 cultures + S.E.

[b] NT = not tested

[c] Mean of results from 2 cultures

the control containing normal adult spleen cells. Thus, the helper
activity seems to depend on cells with T properties. To determine
whether the fraction of Ig$^+$ in the inoculated cells gives rise to Ig$^-$
helper cells, we transferred Ig$^+$ cells from normal BM into recipient
mice. Thymus cells were harvested as before, and divided into two
groups; one was cultured as an intact population, the other was
fractionated and Ig$^-$ cells were cultured. In a preliminary experiment it was found that in both cases the response was enhanced,
measuring 860 PFC/cltr in the former group and 800 in the latter,
which is a significant response as compared to 480 in the cultures
of 'B' cells only. It is thus suggested that Ig$^+$ cells may contribute
to the development of T helper cells. Although these observations
by no means demonstrate linkage between all T and B populations,
they may shed some light on the controversy concerning the existence
of Ig on T cells.

SUMMARY

Cells bearing Ig on the membrane, fractionated from either 17
day embryonic livers or from normal adult bone marrow, when transferred to splenectomized-irradiated mice, lead to development of
helper cells in the thymus of the recipients. The helper function
was expressed when the recipients were stimulated with flagellin-
MON and the thymus cells were cultured together with anti θ treated

spleen cells and stimulated with DNP-MON. The response to DNP was not enhanced when the irradiated mice were inoculated with non Ig bearing cells. Helper activity was related to cells which were eliminated with anti θ antibodies and did not have detectable Ig. Hence, cells with 'B' properties may be involved in development of T helpers.

Acknowledgment: The valuable technical assistance of Miss Janice Mundy is greatly appreciated.

REFERENCES

1. Greaves, M.F., J.J.T. Owen and M.C. Raff (1973) eds.: T and B lymphocytes, origins, properties and roles in immune responses. America Elsvier Pub. N.Y.
2. Nossal, G.J.V. and Pike, B.L. (1973) Immunol. 25, 33
3. Owen, J.J.T., M.D. Cooper and M.C. Raff (1974) Nature 249, 363
4. Globerson, A., T. Umiel and D. Friedman (1975) Ann. N.Y. Acad Sci. 249, 248
5. Komuro, K. and E.A. Boyse (1973) J. Exptl. Med. 138, 479
6. Umiel, T. and A. Globerson (1974) Differentiation 2, 169
7. Kirov, S.M. (1974) Europ. J. Immunol. 4, 739
8. Straussbach, P., A. Sulica and D. Givol (1970) Nature 227, 68
9. Cunningham, A.J. and A. Szenberg (1968) Immunol. 14, 599
10. Miller, J.F.A.P. and J. Sprent (1971) J. Exptl. Med. 134, 66
11. Parish, C.R., S.M. Kirov, N. Bowern and R.V. Blanden (1974) Europ. J. Immunol. 4, 808
12. Micklem, H.S. and Loutit, J.F. (1966) eds. Tissue grating and radiation. Academic Press.
13. del Guercio, P. and E. Leuchars (1972) J. Immunol. 109, 951
14. Kunin, S., G.M. Shearer, A. Globerson and M. Feldman (1973) Cell. Immunol. 8, 455

STUDIES ON THE DEVELOPMENT OF IMMUNITY: GENERAL CONSIDERATIONS

Robert Auerbach   in collaboration with C. Landahl,
A. Chakravarty and S. Wu
University of Wisconsin, Madison, Wisconsin 53706

Developmental aspects of immunity are so broad in scope that it is difficult to provide any meaningful synthesis or summation of the many studies in this area. The development of the immune system includes virtually all the key processes of differentiation including cell migration, inductive tissue interactions, maturational and divisional events from lymphoblasts to large, medium and small lymphocytes, development of surface receptors including immunoglobulins, determinants related to antigen recognition such as Ia gene products, development of tissue specific antigens such as θ, TL, or Ly-1 and2, development of capacity to produce and release various mediators of cellular immunity such as blastogenesis factor, angiogenesis factor or MIF, change in capacity to respond to stimulation by DNA synthesis, maturation and division, development of capacity to secrete immunoglobulins, to recognize complement components and to respond to antigen-induced signals.

In our own laboratory we have continued to examine functional maturation of the various cell types associated with immune reactions. Chakravarty (1) has demonstrated that embryonic thymus cells taken as early as the 16th day of embryonic development become helper cells following 24 hours of incubation in vitro in the presence of concanavlin-A. Con-A incubation is associated with a shift in surface antigen expression, with thymus cells showing an increase in expression of H-2 antigens with a corresponding reduction in expression of θ. Interestingly, maturation of thymus cells as measured by their capacity to evoke a graft-versus-host reaction in vitro is not accelerated by con-A treatment, thymus cells becoming mature for this function only around the time of birth.

Shaokee Wu has tried to compare the ontogeny of spleen cells in terms of their ability to stimulate or respond in mixed leukocyte culture (MLC) and in cell-mediated lytic capacity (CML). He has found (2) that while the spleen is immunocompetent at birth as measured by MLC, and can stimulate allogeneic cells at this time, it is not yet capable of CML activity; this arises only at day 7. Most provocative is his finding that even when CML of specific target cells is observed, the usual cross-reactive killing of third party cells is still absent; cross-reactive lysis was first found to occur at around day 21.

A less emphasized but potentially most important cell in immune reactions is the macrophage or adherent cell (A cell) known to be needed for immune reactions to take place in vitro. Carol Landahl (3) has been able to show that under rigorous test conditions the A-cell requirement is specific for spleen cells, in that it is not replaced by macrophages or adherent cells from most other organs including peritoneal exudate cells. Functional splenic A cells, as measured by response to sheep red blood cells (SRBC) in combination with adult spleen non-adherent cells, can first be found in the spleen 4 days after birth. This finding correlates well with the in vivo response of the mouse, since mice at younger ages do not normally respond to SRBC.

In contrast to the postnatal maturation of functional A cells measured by cooperation in the response to SRBC, splenic A cells from newborn mice can already support nonadherent cells in MLC. This is not too surprising since the A-cell requirement for MLC appears to be primarily a nutritional one, unlike its role in the humoral response where it has been variously considered as an acceptor of thymus-originating immunoglobulins, for antigen-processing, antigen-focussing or complement fixation. When Landahl tried to determine whether there are particular functions of A cells not present at birth but present one week later she found that the ability to bind complement, IgG and thymus-originating products secreted in vitro all appeared similar for neonatal and 7-day adherent cells. Thus the reason for the shift in competence occurring in A-cells during the first week of life remains obscure.

In discussing the ontogeny of immunity we have been remiss, however, in not emphasizing more the development of non-immunity or tolerance; indeed when we measure the rise of immunocompetence in various test systems we must be aware of the possibility - indeed the likelihood -- that immunosuppression may well be the rule during development, and that it is the selective escape from suppression that to large part we have been documenting in our studies. To open a discussion here of the whole range of immunosuppressive agents operative during development, including hormones, antibodies, immune complexes and suppressor cells, is simply not

Table 1

Effect of tolerization of mother on immune response of their young: Interval between tolerization and conception 2-5 weeks

Treatment	# of litters	# of assays	PFC/10^6 spleen cells SRBC	HRBC	Ratio SRBC/HRBC
SHS	14	29	67.8*	717.7	0.09
HHS	7	19	523.8	36.1**	14.51
Saline	6	16	697.1	353.3	1.97

* 9.7% of normal response to SRBC

**10.2% of normal response to HRBC

Table 2

Effect of tolerization of mother or foster mother on immune response of their young

Treatment of mother	nurse	# of litters	# of assays	PFC/10^6 spleen cells SRBC	HRBC	Ratio SRBC/HRBC
SHS	saline	4	5	853.4	427.5	2.0
HHS	saline	3	6	884.9*	264.5	3.3*
saline	SHS	3	4	33.2*	297.6	0.1
saline	HHS	4	5	596.2	26.0	22.9

*   one assay was unusually high for SRBC response

**   4% of normal response to SRBC

*** 8% of normal response to HRBC

possible ; a single example of work I have been carrying out this
past year, however, may serve to illustrate the potential importance of suppression to our understanding of the ontogeny of immune
function.

We had previously shown that unresponsiveness to SRBC or HRBC
can be induced by injection of a soluble component released from
erythrocytes by hypotonic lysis. Such unresponsiveness was found to
be long-lasting, specific, and not correlated with production of
significant amounts of detectable antibody. When female mice made
previously tolerant to SRBC or HRBC were mated to normal males,
their offspring were found to be tolerant as well, when tested at
28-45 days of age. (Table I)   Using an experimental protocol designed
to examine the role of nursing in transmission of tolerance we were
able to show that the tolerogenic influence was transmitted through
the milk (4) (Table II).   .

Since the gradual breaking of tolerance in the mother is
associated with a spontaneous synthesis of specific hemagglutinating
antibody the possibility that the induction of tolerance in the
young was antibody-mediated is a distinct possibility. Indeed in
experiments I have carried out recently it was possible to show
that immunization of female mice prior to their becoming pregnant
may lead to immunosuppression of their young, provided that a
high titer of antibody is still present during the nursing period.
The titer required for immunosuppression of young was, however,
several logs higher than that observed during the spontaneous break-
down of tolerance. Thus at the moment it appears more likely that
the tolerogenic influence transmitted by tolerized mice is an
antigen-antibody complex, or includes antibody not detected by the
methods used in our experiments.

In summary, many studies have emphasized the early maturation
of immunocompetence, some tracing back to the embryonic yolk sac.
Each functional capacity appears to have its own pattern of ontogeny,
as seen with respect to T-cells, B-cells and A-cells, with reference
to CML, MLC or GvH, and with delineation of the appearance of surface
markers and protein synthetic machinery. As an added complication
I have suggested that an additional factor for consideration is the
influence of the mother on the spectrum of immune responsiveness of
her young.

1 Chakravarty, A. PhD Dissertation, University of Wisconsin 1975
2 Wu, Shaokee MS Dissertation, University of Wisconsin 1975
3 Landahl, C. PhD Dissertation, University of Wisconsin 1974
4 Auerbach, R. and Clark, S. submitted for publication 1975

Research studies reported in this paper were supported by grants
from the National Institutes of Health and the National Science
Foundation

Surface Properties and
Activation of Lymphoid Cells

SURFACE PROPERTIES OF LYMPHOID CELLS - INTRODUCTION

Michael Schlesinger

Department of Experimental Medicine & Cancer Research

The Hebrew University-Hadassah Medical School
Jerusalem, Israel

The cell surface of lymphocytes plays a vital role in all of the functions of these cells. The recognition of antigens, the triggering of lymphocytes, their migration pattern, all reflect specialized activities of the lymphocyte surface. Indeed, the topic of "surface properties of lymphoid cells" is so broad and all-embracing that all of modern immunology can be comfortably discussed under this heading. This is amply illustrated by the wide scope of the papers to be presented in this session.

Many of the properties of the cell surface have a direct bearing on the functions of lymphocytes. A large number of cell surface structures are now known to function as distinct receptors (cf. 1). These include such moieties as cell surface immunoglobulins, Fc receptors, and C'_3 receptors. The electric charge of the cell surface of lymphocytes may affect the efficiency of the binding to these receptors. The mobility of cell surface receptors and the fluidity of the cell membrane may also determine the activity of lymphocytes. Additional cell surface markers, which have received intensive attention are cell-surface antigens (2). While such structures are useful for the identification of lymphocyte subpopulations their functional role is not clear as yet (3).

It cannot be overemphasized that great care has to be taken with each and any of the methods used for the identification of surface structures, both as far as methodological problems and interpretation of the results are concerned. There are many pertinant examples. Detection of antigens depends on the sensitivity of the analytical methods employed. TL-antigens were thought to be confined to the thymus of normal mice. But now it seems that sensitive

methods detect low concentrations of the TL-antigens in peripheral
lymphoid organs (4). Indeed TL-antigens may possibly.be characteristic for thymic stem cells (5). Recent studies with the scanning
electron microscope have indicated that T- and B-cells have distinct
cell surfaces (6). The differences in the appearance of the membrane
of lymphocyte subpopulations becomes obscured, however, when the
membrane is altered by changes in the temperature or by activation
of the cells.

Cell surface markers are useful for the detection of lymphocyte
subpopulation. In the thymus of mice the major population is rich
in the θ- and TL-antigens, but poor in H-2 antigenicity, while the
minor population has the reverse attributes. It has recently become clear that peripheral T-lymphocytes, engaged in cytotoxic reactions against allogeneic target cells are θ-positive, have a high
concentration of the Ly.2 and Ly.3 alloantigens, but are deficient
in their Ly.1 antigenicity (7). In contrast, T-cells capable of
killing syngeneic tumor cells may have a high Ly.1 antigenicity (8).

An open problem is that of the differentiation-pathways of
lymphocytes. Are the various subsets of T-cells, which we can
identify, merely sequential stages in the differentiation of a single
cell lineage, or do they constitute distinct subpopulations arising
by divergent differentiation? Is the differentiation of T-cells
complete within the thymus, or do immature cells leave the thymus
("immature post-thymic cells") to mature in the periphery? Similar
questions can be asked concerning the differentiation pathways of
subsets of B-lymphocytes. Roelants et al (5) have now shown that
pre-thymic cells may possess low quantities of the θ-antigen. It
is possible, therefore, that the θ-antigen may not necessarily be
restricted to thymus-derived cells, but rather may be a marker for
"thymus-dependent" lymphocytes.

An additional problem, to be borne in mind during studies of the
lymphocyte cell-surface, is the dynamic nature of the cell surface.
It should be remembered that cell membrane constituents turn over,
and that membrane fragments may be shed. Various reagents may affect
differentially either the synthesis of cell-membrane structures or
the transport and integration of new cell membrane constituents into
the pre-existing cell membrane. Finally, it should be taken into
account that following activation, cells may acquire "new" properties.
Activated T-cells, may for instance acquire Fc-receptors (9).

An intriguing question is that of the functional meaning of
surface constituents. The role of immunoglobulin molecules on the
surface of B-cells as antigen-receptors is well established. It is
not clear, however, how H-2 antigens are involved in the binding of
antigens by T-cells (10). What is the relationship of HLA antigens
and β_2-microglobulin to the T-cell receptor in man? How are Ia-

antigens related to the Fc-receptor? What is the functional meaning of the association of H-2 antigenicity and C'_3 receptors on the surface of microphages (3)?

Finally, we come to the problem of the relationship between cell-surface receptors and the triggering of cells. We still do not understand which interactions with cell-surface receptors lead to activation, and which, in turn, lead to suppression. Is more than one stimulus necessary for triggering? Can different degrees of stimulation of the same cell lead either to activation or to suppression?

These are some of the current questions relating to the surface properties of lymphoid cells and lymphocyte activation. We shall hear some of the answers in the present session. Answers to some of the questions may, however, have to wait for Germinal Center Conferences in the future.

REFERENCES

1. Schlesinger, M., Ser. Haemat. 7: 427, 1974.

2. Schlesinger, M., Progr. Allergy 16: 213, 1972.

3. Schlesinger, M., Israel, E., Chaouat, M., and Gery, I., Ann. N.Y. Acad. Sci. 249: 505, 1975.

4. Basch, R.S., Transpl. Proc. 7: 325, 1975.

5. Roelants, G.E., Mayor, K.S., Hagg, L.B., and Loor, F., Proc. 5th International Conference on Lymphatic Tissue and Germinal Centers in Immune Reactions (In Press).

6. Polliack, A., Lampen, N., Clarkson, B.D., de Harven, E., Bentwich, Z., and Kunkel, H.G., J. Exp. Med. 138: 607, 1973.

7. Shiku, H., Kisielow, P., Bean, M.A., Takahashi,T., Boyse, E.A., Oettgen, H.F., and Old, L.J., J. Exp. Med. 141: 227, 1975.

8. Shiku, H., Kisielow, P. Bean, M.A., Takahashi, T., Oettgen, H.F., and Old, L.J., American Association for Cancer Research - Abstracts 16: 67, 1975.

9. Yoshida, T.O., and Andersson, B., Scand. J. Immunol. 1: 401, 1972.

10. Hämmerling, G.J., and McDevitt, H.O., J. Immunol. 112: 1734, 1974.

IS A SPECIALIZED STIMULATOR CELL REQUIRED FOR THE INDUCTION OF
ALLOGRAFT IMMUNITY?

K.J. Lafferty, A. Bootes, G. Dart, G. Radovich, and

D.W. Talmage

John Curtin School of Medical Research, Canberra,

Australia, and Webb-Waring Lung Institute, Denver,

Colorado, U.S.A.

INTRODUCTION

The survival of thyroid transplants in allogeneic mice has
been strikingly prolonged by first culturing the grafts for several
weeks in vitro (1). Two alternative mechanisms have been proposed
for the prolonged survival:

(1) A modification of tissue antigens occurs during the in
vitro culture resulting in a loss of tissue antigenicity.

(2) Some of the leucocytes trapped in the graft are essential
for the activation of recipient T-lymphocytes, and are
gradually lost during the in vitro culture.

In relation to this second proposition, we have proposed that
the activation of specific T-lymphocytes is the function of a living
cell with special properties (2-4) and have reported evidence that
in mice the macrophage is the most efficient if not the only cell
with this stimulating activity (5). Others have reported similar
evidence for guinea pig and human macrophages (6,7).

We reasoned that if the loss of tissue macrophages was
responsible for the prolonged survival of cultured organ grafts,
then the injection into the recipient of macrophages syngeneic to
the graft should activate specific transplant immunity and cause
graft rejection. On the other hand, if the loss of tissue antigens

was responsible for the prolonged survival, the injection of macrophages would have little effect. We also used an alternative method
of reducing the number of blood leucocytes in the graft: x-radiation
of the donor two days before removal of the organs. This treatment
also prolonged allograft survival. With both the cultured and the
irradiated grafts we found that the I.V. injection of living peritoneal exudate cells (PEC, 50-80% macrophages), if syngeneic to the
graft stimulated its rejection. However the injection of the host
with antigen in the form of inactivated peritoneal cells, either
alone or emulsified with complete Freund's adjuvant, did not cause
the rejection of modified thyroid allografts.

MATERIALS AND METHODS

Thyroid organ culture and transplantation was carried out as
previously described (1). Graft function was assayed by 125I-
uptake (1) and kidneys having a count 4-fold or more higher than the
control kidney were scored as bearing a functional transplant.

RESULTS

The data in Table 1 shows the effect of culture time on the
20 day survival of Balb/c thyroid in Balb/c, CBA and C57Bl recipient
mice. All uncultured allografts were totally rejected by 20 days;
in fact C57Bl recipients reject Balb/c thyroid in about 10 to 11
days and CBA recipients reject such allografts in about 12 to 13
days. In contrast the majority of the cultured allografts were still
functioning 20 days after allotransplantation. The time of culture
has an effect on graft survival. Although the majority of the 12
day cultured thyroids were functional 20 days after transplantation,
histological examination showed most of these transplants were infiltrated with mononuclear cells. As the culture time is increased up
to 26 days, little or no infiltration is seen in the surviving
allografts. Thyroids held in culture for 33 days or more show

TABLE 1

Survival of Cultured Balb/c Thyroid 20 Days after Transplantation
into Syngeneic (Balb/c) and Allogeneic (CBA, C57Bl) Recipients

Time in Organ culture (days)	RECIPIENT		
	Balb/c	C57Bl	CBA
0	3/3	0/13	0/6
12	6/6	4/5	7/7
19	6/6	10/13	7/7
26	5/7	5/5	5/6

varying degrees of degeneration and very variable results were
obtained when this tissue was transplanted.

Although the cultured thyroid is weakly immunogenic, this tissue
retains tissue antigen and can be rejected when the recipient's
immune system is activated by peritoneal cells syngeneic to the
tissue transplant. Table 2 shows the experimental support for this
statement. Uncultured Balb/c thyroid was completely rejected 15 days
after transplantation into CBA recipients, while all 26 day cultured
allografts survived for this period. The intravenous injection of
CBA recipients with 10^5 CBA PEC at the time of transplantation had
no effect on the survival of Balb/c thyroid. However the injection
of Balb/c PEC into such recipients resulted in the rejection of all
transplants. Histologic examination showed little or no cellular
infiltration and normal structure in the two surviving groups while
complete destruction of normal structure was observed in the rejected
group.

If macrophages or other passenger leucocytes carried in the
transplant are responsible for the stimulation of allograft immunity,
treatments of the donor that might affect these cells should also
have an effect on allograft survival. Table 3 shows representative
data obtained when uncultured thyroids were transplanted directly
in Balb/c mice. In the first group, no treatment was given to the
allograft donor. A/J thyroids were uniformly rejected in 10 days
but most CAF_1 thyroids retained function for 10 days and were
rejected by 20 days.

The second group of experiments were performed with thyroid
grafts taken from CAF_1 mice injected intravenously (I.V.) with 0.3
ml of a 1:5 dilution of a stock colloidal carbon suspension (Pelikan,
C11/143a, 10% c) immediately before sacrifice. These transplants
were slightly grey from the carbon, which greatly facilitates

TABLE 2

Immunogenicity and Antigenicity of 26 Day Cultured Balb/c
Thyroid Transplanted into CBA Recipients

Thyroid Transplant	Cells Injected into Recipient	Graft Survival[2]
Uncultured	None	0/6
Cultured	None	7/7
Cultured	10^5 CBA PEC[1]	8/8
Cultured	10^5 Balb/c PEC	0/5

1. PEC, Peritoneal exudate cells
2. ^{125}I injected 15 days after transplantation

TABLE 3

Survival of Thyroid Allografts and Semiallografts in Balb/c
Mice - Effect of Donor Treatment

Donor	Treatment of Donor	Day of 125_I	Graft Survival
A/J	None	10	0/5
CAF$_1$	None	20	3/10
CAF$_1$	Carbon	20	4/4
CA/J	γ and C^1	10	5/5
CAF$_1$	γ and C	20	4/5

1. 750 r ^{60}Co γ-irradiation and colloidal carbon injection
   (see text).

their location after several weeks under the kidney capsule. The
carbon also appeared to enhance survival since four out of four
CAF$_1$ grafts retain function for 20 days, although histologic examination revealed moderate infiltration.

The third group of experiments were performed with thyroid
transplants taken from donors given 750 r ^{60}Co γ-radiation (whole
body) two days before removal of the thyroid and an I.V. injection
of carbon immediately before sacrifice. This treatment of the donor
grately enhanced survival of the allogeneic A/J grafts. All survived
10 days compared to no survival in the first group of untreated A/J
allografts. The effect of donor treatment on the CAF$_1$ transplants
was less striking because these grafts occasionally (3/10) survived
20 days in Balb/c recipients without such treatment.

On the basis of the above results, a more extensive set of
experiments was performed to demonstrate the importance of living
leucocytes of donor strain to the induction of transplant immunity.
Donor CAF$_1$ mice were uniformly treated with 520 r ^{60}Co two days
before grafting and injected with carbon immediately before sacrifice
125_I was injected on day 13, and kidneys counted on day 14. As
shown in Table 4 thirty-six CAF$_1$ grafts placed on Balb/c mice without injection of PEC all showed function at 14 days with a mean ratio
of radioactivities in grafted and control kidneys of 96 $\pm$ a S.E. of
12. Twenty-nine similar grafts placed in Balb/c recipients injected
with 1,000 CAF$_1$ PEC showed significant function in only 5 grafts
with a mean ratio of 2.7 $\pm$ 0.1. The highest ratio in the CAF$_1$ PEC
recipients was 16. Only 2 of the 36 uninjected recipients showed a
lower ratio; of these one was 8 and the other 14. Five CAF$_1$ grafts
in Balb/c recipients injected with 1,000 Balb/c PEC showed an
average ratio of 144 $\pm$ 9 which was not significantly different from
the uninjected group from the same experiment. The injection of

TABLE 4

14-Day Survival in Balb/c Mice of CAF_1 Thyroid from
Donors Pretreated with γ-Rays and Carbon

Cells Injected	Mean Ratio[1]	Fraction with Ratio > 4	> 16
None	96 $\pm$ 12	36/36	34/36
10^3 CAF_1 PEC	2.7 $\pm$ 0.7	5/29	0/29
10^3 Balb/c PEC	144 $\pm$ 9	5/5	5/5
10^3 C57Bl PEC	47 $\pm$ 15	5/5	4/5
Killed[2] CAF_1 PEC	81 $\pm$ 12	16/16	16/16

1. Ratio of counts in grafted kidney to control kidney
2. See text

1,000 C57Bl PEC into similar recipients resulted in a mean ratio of
47 $\pm$ 5 which was a significant reduction in graft function compared
to uninjected or Balb/c injected controls, but much more function
than seen in the group injected with donor CAF_1 PEC.

The injection of killed donor type PEC into Balb/c recipients
of CAF_1 thyroid grafts had no significant effect. The mean ratio
in this group was 81 $\pm$ 12. The cells injected were as follows:
10^4 cells heated to 56° C for one hour (3 recipients), 10^4 cells
treated with 1% formalin for one hour (3), 10^4 cells sonicated for
three 10-second intervals in a Branson Sonifier (3), 10^6 sonicated
cells (4) and 10^6 cells sonicated in complete Freund's adjuvant (3).

DISCUSSION

The data presented in this paper extend our previous studies
of the effect of organ culture on thyroid allograft survival (1).
Lengthening the organ culture period to approximately four weeks
results in a situation where cultured allografts are indistinguishable
from isografts 20 days after transplantation. The failure of the
cultured tissue to stimulate its own rejection is not due to an
inaccessibility to circulating lymphoid cells or an incapacity of the
latter to recognize the cultured tissue as foreign. Once the
recipient's immune system has been activated by peritoneal cells
syngeneic to the cultured allograft, this tissue is promptly rejected.

These findings are consistent with the concept that a living
stimulator cell is required for T-cell activation (2-4). It would
appear that during organ culture this stimulator cell either dies
or is inactivated. Irradiation of the thyroid donor, two days prior
to the removal of the thyroid for transplantation, also prolongs the

survival of this tissue in allogeneic and semiallogeneic recipients. This finding provides further support for the concept that passenger leucocytes carried in the transplant play an important role in the activation of the allograft response.

The requirement of a stimulator cell for T-cell activation provides an explanation for the specificity of T-cell phenomena where the activity of primed T-cell is assayed (8-9). If the T-cell must interact with antigen on the surface of a stimulator cell before it can be induced, it is possible that the T-cell receptor "sees" both the antigen and part of the surrounding cell surface components. Thus, these primed T-cells will now interact most efficiently with complexes of the type to which they were initially primed. Cells primed in a syngeneic system will be specific for antigen in combination with a syngeneic or semiallogeneic cell. No such restriction will be observed when allogeneic stimulator cells provide the inductive stimulus as is the case when cytotoxic cells are generated in mixed leucocyte culture. It may be for this reason that living allogeneic stimulator cells are much more efficient in the induction of allograft immunity than antigen presented on dead cells, either alone or emulsified in complete Freund's adjuvant. Antigen presented on allogeneic stimulator cells would activate T-cells specific for the allogeneic cells. Antigen derived from cells unable to stimulate themselves, would have to be presented to host T-cells via the host's own stimulator cells, and thus the T-cell response induced by such antigen may be specific for this material in combination with a cell of host genotype. Such T-cells may be relatively inefficient in their interaction with the same antigen presented on the surface of allogeneic target cells. This effect would be similar to the allogeneic restriction observed in the T-cell mediated killing the virus infected cells (8).

REFERENCES

(1)   Lafferty, K.J., Cooley, M.A., Woolnough, J., and Walker, K.Z., Science, 188, 259 (1975).

(2)   Lafferty, K.J., Walker, K.Z., Scollary, R.G. and Killby, J.A.A., Transplant. Rev. 12: 198 (1972).

(3)   Talmage, D.W., Radovich, J., LeFever, J. and Hemmingsen, H., Ann. N.Y. Acad. Sci. 207: 29 (1973).

(4)   Lafferty, K.J. and Cunningham, A.J., Aust. J. Exp. Biol. Med. Sci. 53: 27 (1975).

(5)   Talmage, D.W. and Hemmingsen, J., J. Allergy and Clin. Immunol. (in Press, 1975).

(6)   Greineder, D.K. and Rosenthal, A.S., J. Immunol. 114: 1541
      (1975).

(7)   Rode, H.R. and Gordon, J., Cell Immunology 13: 87 (1974).

(8)   Doherty, P.C. and Zinkernagel, R.M., Transplant. Rev. 19: 89
      (1974).

(9)   Katz, D.H. and Benacerraf, B., Transplant. Rev. 22: 175 (1975).

This work was supported by U.S. Public Health Service Grants
AI-03047 and CA 13419, National Science Foundation Grant GB-43219,
and a Fellowship from the International Union Against Cancer.

CELL SELECTION IN THE THYMUS OF MICE TREATED WITH ESCHERICHIA COLI LIPOPOLYSACCHARIDE (LPS) [+]

S. Uccini[1], L. Ruco[1], G. Soravito[1], L. Adorini[2], G. Doria[2] and C.D. Baroni[1]
[1]Inst. of Pathological Anatomy II, University of Rome
[2]CNEN-Euratom Immunogenetics Group, Lab. Radiopathology, C.S.N., Casaccia (Rome)

There is evidence that T-lymphocytes are not directly involved in the anti-LPS humoral immune response (1, 2, 3). However it has been shown that LPS has some biological effects on T-cell functions both in vitro (4, 5), and in vivo (6-10). The demonstration that LPS influences some T-cell functions requires further investigation.

In the present paper we report the results of an vivo study in which we have examined the anti-LPS antibody response and the effects of LPS on thymus cell killer and helper functions in mice.

6-12 week old (C57BL/10xDBA/2)F$_1$ mice (BDF$_1$) and inbred DBA/2 mice were used in three types of experiments (Experiment A, B and C).

A: Relationship between thymus weight and antibody response to LPS

45 day old male BDF$_1$ mice were injected i.p. with different doses of LPS (Lipopolysaccharide from Escherichia Coli 055:B5 method Westphal; Difco Detroit Mich.) in 0.1 ml of PBS. The effects of immunization on thymus weight and on the number of PFC anti-LPS in the spleen are illustrated in Fig.1. It is clear that there is a progressive dose-dependent thymus weight decrease

[+]Supported in part by a research contract from CNR (Rome, Italy) and by a CNEN-Euratom Association Contract, Publication n° 1208 of the Euratom Biology Division.

concomitant to an increase in the number of PFC, reaching plateau value at the dose of 20 μg. Analysis of all individual data revealed a statistically significant negative correlation (P=0.01)
between thymus weight and PFC anti-LPS.

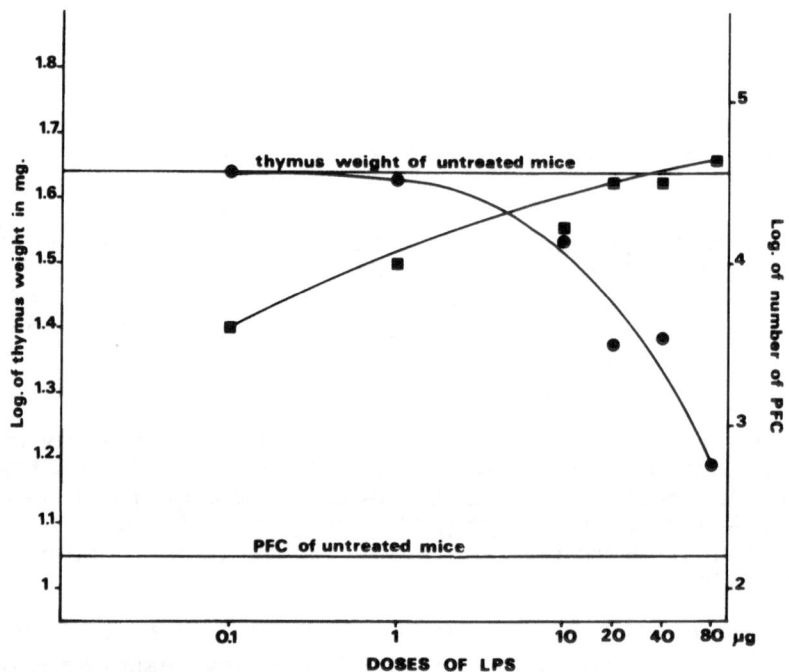

Fig. 1: Thymus weights (●—●) and number of PFC (■—■) four days
after immunization with different doses of LPS. Each
point represents the mean of at least 10 observations.

B: LPS enhances GVH activity of thymus cells

Thymus cells were prepared from 45 day old DBA/2 male mice given a single i.p. injection of 20 μg of LPS in 0.1 ml of PBS
and sacrificed 4 days later. Three groups (40 mice in each group)
of 90 day old BDF_1 male mice were given a total-body X ray dose
of 500 R (11). 1-2 hours after irradiation the animals were injected i.v. with 1 ml of Eagle's Medium or with 20×10^6 LPS-treated
DBA/2 thymus cells in 1 ml of Eagle's Medium, or with 20×10^6
DBA/2 untreated thymus cells in 1 ml of Eagle's Medium. The results of this experiment (Fig. 2) show the cumulative mortality caused by the GVH activity of thymus cells from LPS-treated or untreated donors.

It is clear that treatment <u>in vivo</u> with LPS significantly (P < 0.01) hastens and increases the GVH activity of thymus cells. No mortality was observed in irradiated F_1 mice which received no cells, and in DBA/2 irradiated controls injected either with un- treated or with LPS treated singeneic thymus cells.

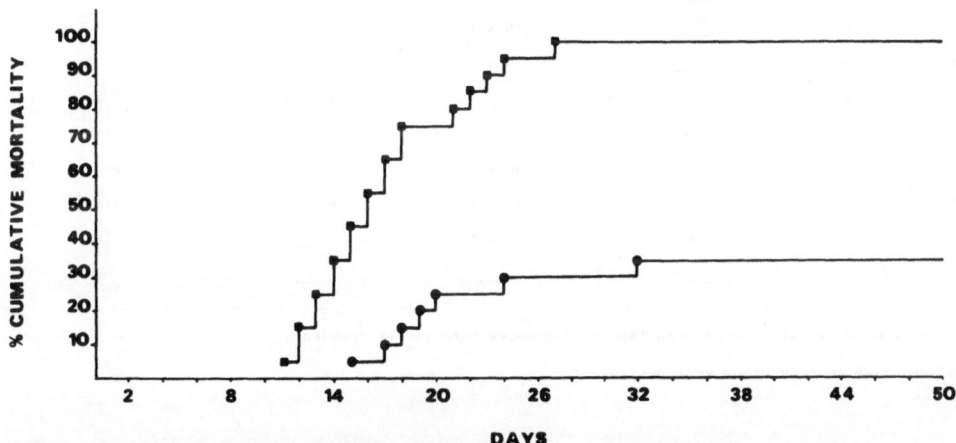

Fig. 2: Cumulative mortality observed in sublethally irradiated BDF$_1$ mice grafted with 20×10^6 DBA/2 thymus cells ob- tained from untreated (●—●) or LPS treated (■—■) donors.

C: LPS enhances helper activity of thymus cells

Lethally irradiated (900 R) BDF$_1$ mice were injected with sin- geneic cells as follows: a) thymus cells from LPS-treated donors and bone marrow cells from normal donors; b) normal thymus and bone marrow cells; c) thymus cells from LPS-treated donors; d) normal thymus cells; e) normal bone marrow cells; f) no cells. All recipients were immunized i.p. with 5×10^8 SRBC at time of cell transfer and boostered 3 days later. Treated donors were given i.p. 20 μg of LPS 4 days before sacrifice. Table 1 shows that thymus cells from LPS-pretreated mice are more efficient than normal thymocytes in cooperating with normal bone marrow cells in the response against SRBC.

TABLE 1

Helper Cell Activity of Thymus Cells from Untreated or 20 ug LPS Treated Donors in the Response to Sheep Red Blood Cells in BDF_1 Mice [*]

Group	N° mice/ group	Treatment of thymus donors	N° of thymus cells grafted	N° of marrow cells grafted	PFC/recipient spleen [**]
A	6	___	20×10^6	40×10^6	350
B	6	___	40×10^6	40×10^6	445
C	6	___	80×10^6	40×10^6	1235
D	6	___	80×10^6	___	2
E	6	___	___	40×10^6	42
F	6	LPS	20×10^6	40×10^6	445
G	6	LPS	40×10^6	40×10^6	1000
H	6	LPS	80×10^6	40×10^6	2245
I	6	LPS	80×10^6	___	22
L	6	___	___	___	0

[*] All mice were lethally irradiated (900 R) 1-2 hours before cell transfer.

[**] Spleen cells in each group were pooled.

CONCLUSIONS

The present data indicate that injection of LPS induces a decrease in thymus weight with selection of thymocytes more efficient in killer and helper activities. It has been reported (12) that two T-cell types may cooperate in the GVH reaction: the effector T_1 and the amplifier T_2. The maturation from T_1 to T_2 occurs mainly in the periphery, whereas immature cortex thymocytes differentiate to T_1 within the thymus (13). Our results, showing an LPS-dependent enhancement of thymocyte killing activity, suggest that LPS selects thymocytes mostly of the T_1 type.

LPS- treated thymocytes are more efficient in the reconstitution of the anti-SRBC response. These data can be explained considering that LPS, like cortisone (14), enriches the thymus with more immunocompetent helper cells.

Alternatively it may be suggested that LPS selects in the thymus cell populations characterized by high proliferative activity.

Unpublished observations showing that LPS-treatment in vivo increases the in vitro response of thymocytes to Con-A are consistent with this interpretation.

REFERENCES

(1) Müller G., Michael G., Cell Immunol., 2: 309, 1971

(2) Manning J. K., Reed N. D., Jutilia J. W., J. Immunol., 108: 1470, 1972

(3) Veit B. C., Michael J. G., J. Immunol., 109: 547, 1972

(4) Armerding D., Katz D. H., J. Exp. Med., 139: 24, 1974

(5) Kagnoff M. F., Billings P., Cohn M., J. Exp. Med., 139: 407, 1974

(6) Spitznagel J. K., Allison A. C., J. Immunol., 104: 119, 1970

(7) Allison A. C., Davies A. J. S., Nature, 233: 330, 1971

(8) Lagrange P. H., Mackaness G. B., Miller T. E., Pardon P. J. Immunol., 114: 442, 1975

(9) Lagrange P. H., Mackaness G. B., J. Immunol., 114: 447, 1975

(10) Skidmore B. J., Chiller J. M., Morrison D. C., Weigle W. O., J. Immunol., 114: 770, 1975

(11) Doria G., Agarossi G., Transplantation, 6: 218, 1968

(12) Cantor H., Asofsky R., J. Exp. Med., 135: 764, 1972

(13) Raff M. C., Cantor H., in: Progress in Immunology-Ed. by B. Amos- Academic Press, N.Y. London, 1971, pp. 83-93

(14) Cohen J. J., Claman H. N., J. Exp. Med., 133: 1026, 1971

Unpublished observations show that PS treatment in organ
cultures or in vitro completely abrogates the capacity to respond
and do not stimulate viruses.

(1) Sprent, J., Mi......

(2) ....

(3) ......

(4) ...... Ny, ...

(5) ...... Kappler, J.W., A ......

(6) Marrack, P. ......

(7) Zinkernagel, R.M., Callahan, G.M., Klein, J. and Dennert, G.,
J. Immunol. 130, 1427-1979.

(8) Bevan, M.J., Hodgkinson, P.A., J. Immunol. 119, 447,
1978.

(9) Sprent, J., Clarke, C.A., Alkmann, L.M., Marie, V.,
....

(10) Klein, J., Aspesilein, ...

(11) Bevan, M.J., ...

(12) ...... J. Exp. Med. 1055-1029, 1981.

CLONAL EXPANSION AND THYMUS DEPENDENCE.

MICROCULTURE EXPERIMENTS WITH TNP-LIPOPOLYSACCHARIDE

José Quintáns and Ivan Lefkovits

Basel Institute for Immunology

Grenzacherstrasse 487, CH-4058 Basel, Switzerland

INTRODUCTION

Lipopolysaccharide (LPS) is a potent polyclonal activator of B cells (1). We have shown that LPS can activate nude spleen cells in vitro to antibody production under conditions where a potential participation of T cells was practically excluded (2). Studying clonal events in vitro (2), we demonstrated that B cells specific for sheep red cells (SRC) were activated by LPS to undergo few cell divisions early in the culture period without sustained clonal expansion. However, if SRC were added to the cultures as well, further clonal expansion was observed. Hence, it seems that antigen is necessary for maintaining clonal proliferation. The specific B cell involved in giving rise to large clones clearly reacted to an antigen-mediated signal in addition to that provided by LPS.

In this paper we use TNP-LPS to investigate the relationship between clonal expansion and thymus dependence.

MATERIALS AND METHODS

Mice

Nude mice of both sexes partially backcrossed to C57BL/6 and Balb/C backgrounds were obtained from Dr. C.W. Friis, Gl. Bomholtgaard, Ltd., Ry, Denmark.

Culture Conditions

Conventional 1 ml cultures were set up according to Mishell-Dutton (3). Microculture experiments (4) followed the technique of Quintáns and Lefkovits (5).

Preparation of TNP-LPS

100 mg of LPS (lipopolysaccharide from E. Coli 055:135, Difco Laboratories, Detroit, Mi., USA) were disolved in 10 ml of a 10% solution of K_2CO_3. To this, 100 mg of trinitrobenzene sulfonic acid (Sigma, St. Louis, Mo., USA) were added and the mixture kept at room temperature under stirring for 4 hours. The conjugate was then extensively dialyzed against phosphate buffer saline.

Assay

For PFC tests the cultured cells were incorporated into a mixture of agarose, indicator red cells, and complement and spread on a microscope slide (2). As indicator cells SRC and lightly conjugated TNP-SRC (6) were used. The anti-TNP PFC were inhibitable by 10^{-4}M TNP-caproic acid.

RESULTS

TNP-LPS was first tested over a large dose range in the Mishell-Dutton system using nude spleen cells. The results are shown in Fig. 1. It can be seen that optimal immunogenic doses are found around 10^{-2} µg/ml whereas 1 g/ml or higher suppress the response. This suppression does not occur when unconjugated LPS is used. Such higher amounts of TNP-LPS at the same time cause an increase of the background response to SRC and H^3 Thy uptake as part of a nonspecific polyclonal activation (results not shown). We decided to use 0.05µg/ml TNP-LPS as this dose is immunogenic while the same amount of unconjugated LPS is generally ineffective - it does not induce anti-TNP PFC.

The time kinetics of the anti-TNP response induced by 0.05 µg/ml of TNP-LPS is illustrated in Fig. 2a. The response is noticeable by day 2, peaks at day 3 and declines thereafter. This pattern of a fast induction of the response (days 2-3) and early decline has been consistently found in all experiments carried out with different preparations of TNP-LPS. Although it has been reported (7) that the response to TNP-LPS can be increased by the addition of an allogeneic factor, Fig. 2b shows that when such effect occurs, it can be accounted for by an increase of background response.

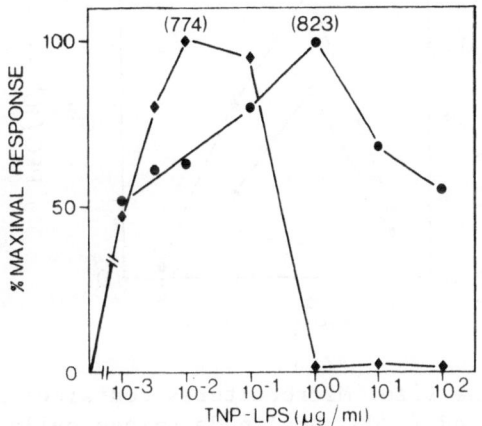

Fig. 1. Dose response curve of TNP-LPS in conventional Mishell-Dutton
cultures. Cultures contained 10^7 nude spleen cells per dish. 2 or 3
dishes were assayed for each experimental point on TNP-SRC and SRC.
Maximal numbers of PFC obtained are shown in parenthesis. ● day 2,
◆ day 3.

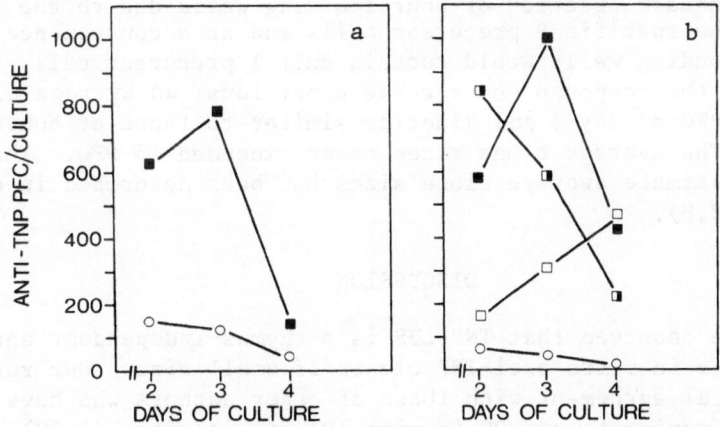

Fig. 2. Kinetics of anti-TNP response. 10^7 nude spleen cells cultured alone ○, or in the presence of 0.05 µg/ml TNP-LPS ■, allogeneic
factor □ or allogeneic factor + 0.05 µg/ml TNP-LPS ▣ .

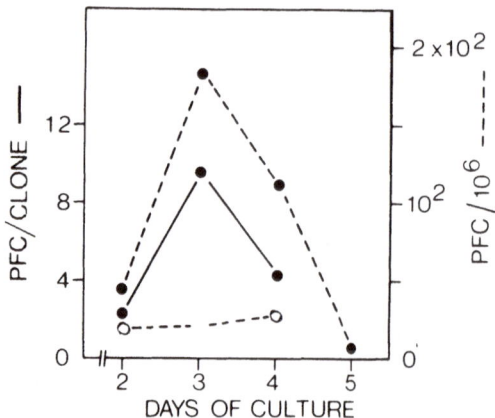

Fig. 3. Average clone size. Microcultures contained 2 x 10^4 active and 8 x 10^4 irradiated (1200 rads) nude spleen cells per well. ○ no addition, ● addition of 0.05 µg/ml of TNP-LPS.

The clonal expansion induced by this thymus-independent antigen was analysed in microcultures containing 2 x 10^4 active nude spleen cells per well. This input of active B cells was chosen because it gives an adequate fraction of nonresponding wells due to the limitation of the specific B precursor cells and as a consequence most of the responding wells would contain only 1 precursor cell. Fig. 3 illustrates the response under these conditions: an average clone size of 10 PFC on day 3 and kinetics similar to those of conventional cultures. The average clone sizes never exceeded 15 PFC. The procedure to estimate average clone sizes has been described in detail elsewhere (2,8).

DISCUSSION

We have observed that TNP-LPS is a thymus-independent antigen which induces in vitro anti-TNP clones of small size. Our results are in general agreement with those of other authors who have used this hapten conjugate of LPS in vivo (9) and in vitro (7,10). The dose of TNP-LPS used in our studies (0.05 µg/ml) had to be carefully chosen because mitogenic and immunogenic ranges of our preparations were partially overlapping.

Our initial interest was related to test whether TNP-LPS would provide only a nonspecific LPS-type of signal to the TNP specific B cells (in which case we would predict a small clone size) or whether it could furnish an antigen-mediated signal capable of sustaining clonal expansion further. The correlation between clone sizes and proliferative and/or maturational events has been dealt with elsewhere (8).

The average clone size and the kinetics of the response induced by 0.05 µg/ml of TNP-LPS are strongly reminiscent of those obtained with polyclonal activation by LPS: small clones with a peak on day 3. TNP-LPS at immunogenic doses behaves functionally as unconjugated LPS at mitogenic doses except that the response is now limited to the anti-TNP specific precursor cells. It appears then that TNP serves to put in contact LPS with the B cells, as suggested by others (11), but the contact of TNP-LPS with TNP-specific B cells does not bring forth any activating signal other than that provided by the LPS. This could be due to either a property of the subpopulation of B cells involved in this thymus-independent response or to a peculiarity of the antigen itself. It is conceivable, for instance, that the binding of LPS to its site is much stronger than that of TNP to the Ig receptor and this prevents the occurrence of any signal at this level. It is possible, on the other hand, that Ig receptors are not involved in triggering (12). In any case when studying activation of B cells by hapten-conjugates of LPS one is dealing with activation by LPS of LPS-reactive cells where such a kind of nonspecific signal leads to deficient clonal expansion, as shown here and previously (2).

Another interesting problem is that of the existence of a general relationship between clone sizes and thymus dependence. We have shown elsewhere that anti-SRC clones are amenable and dependent on quantity and quality of T cell help (8). We have furthermore seen that the thymus independent in vitro response to heat killed vaccine of pneumococci R36A (Pn) specific for phosphorylcholine (PC) consists of small clones (13), whereas the response to PC-KLH, which is also specific for PC but thymus-dependent (Quintáns and Cosenza, unpublished) gives rise to large clones. The observations reported here for TNP-LPS as well as the results with Pn indicate that thymus independence brings about small clones while T cell help favors clonal expansion. Nevertheless, the small clones observed with TNP-LPS and Pn might be attributable to other characteristics than thymus independence: direct mitogenicity in the case of TNP-LPS leading to exhaustive maturation of B cells and inefficiency of Pn to fully expand the clone.

ACKNOWLEDGEMENTS

Miss Susan Davies and Miss Alexandra Reid provided good technical help.

REFERENCES

1. Möller, G., ed.: Transpl. Rev. 11: 1, 1972.
2. Quintáns, J. and Lefkovits, I.: J. Immunol. 113: 1373, 1974.
3. Mishell, R.I. and Dutton, R.W.: J. exp. Med. 126:423, 1967.
4. Lefkovits, I.: Eur. J. Immunol. 2:365, 1972.
5. Quintáns, J. and Lefkovits, I.: Eur. J. Immunol. 3:392, 1973.
6. Rittenberg, M.B. and Pratt, K.L.: Proc. Soc. Exp. Biol. 132:575, 1969.
7. Hunter, Ph. and Kettman, J.R.: Proc. Nat. Acad. Sci. 71:512, 1974.
8. Quintáns, J. and Lefkovits, I.: Eur. J. Immunol. 4:617, 1974.
9. Fidler, J.M.: Cell. Immunol. 16:223, 1975.
10. Jacobs, D.M. and Morrison, D.C.: J. Immunol. 114:360, 1975.
11. Coutinho, A., Gronowicz, E., Bullock, W. and Möller, G.: J. exp. Med. 139:74, 1974.
12. Coutinho, A. and Möller, G.: Adv. Immunol. 1975, in press.
13. Cosenza, H., Quintáns, J. and Lefkovits, I.: Eur. J. Immunol. 5:343, 1975.

CELLULAR EVENTS INVOLVED IN THE TRUE PRIMARY IMMUNE RESPONSE OF

SPLENOCYTES IN VITRO

H. Friedman, I. Kamo and J. Kateley

Department of Microbiology and Immunology

Albert Einstein Medical Center, Philadelphia, Pa. USA

The immunization of lymphoid cells can be readily achieved in vitro with common antigens such as syngeneic erythrocytes, serum proteins or chemical haptens. More antibody forming cells (AFCs) usually are induced when lymphoid cells are derived from antigen primed donor animals. A "true" primary immune response by splenocytes from unprimed animals is difficult to induce. In general, pre-existing immunocytes to most antigens are present even before specific immunization. Furthermore, even in the absence of specific antigen, AFC usually appear in vitro to most antigens, including erythrocytes and bacterial antigens, suggesting that there is a cross-reacting antigen in the culture medium or environment (1-5).

Vibrio cholerae (VC) somatic antigens stimulate a true primary immune response in vivo; immunocytes to these bacteria appear only after specific immunization (6-8). For example, examination of the spleen and lymph nodes of mice of various strains prior to immunization with the cholera antigen has failed to reveal the presence of a single vibriolytic antibody secreting cell to the microorganism even by means of a highly sensitive plaque assay in agar gel with living vibrios as the target. In contrast, after immunization with VC large numbers of specific vibriolytic plaque forming cells appear in the spleen and lymph nodes of immunized animals. Peak numbers of 10^5 or more splenic AFC appear 12 to 14 days after immunization with as little as 1.0 ug VC. There is a distinct lag of at least 2 days before the appearance of the first AFC, followed by a rapid stepwise increase in number during the following four to six days (8). This distinctive kinetics of accumulation of AFC to vibrios in mice given a single immunization with VC is relatively

similar to what is considered a "true primary" immune response to
sheep red blood cells in germfree, cholostrum-free piglets given
SRBC as antigen for the first time (9,10).

After primary immunization of mice with cholera vaccine only
19S IgM PFCs are detected during the first two to three weeks. However, unlike the response to the somatic antigens of other gram negative organisms low efficiency IgG PFCs rapidly develop to the somatic antigen of the vibrios. The numbers of such IgG PFCs are relatively low and they occur late in the primary response (15-30 days).
Following booster immunization of mice primed 8 to 10 weeks earlier
with vibrio antigens a rapid appearance of 19S and 7S IgM PFCs occurs, with peak responses on days 7 to 8 (11,12). IgG PFCs
predominate during the secondary response. In the present study
the responses of splenocytes from normal non-immunized mice to
cholera somatic antigens were assessed in a completely in vitro
system in order to characterize some of the cellular events occurring during a "true" primary immune response as compared to a
secondary response.

METHODS AND MATERIALS

Inbred Balb/c mice obtained from Flow Laboratories, Dublin,
Va. were used for these studies. They were 6 to 8 weeks of age
and weighed approximately 18 gm. Antigen consisted of heat killed
vaccine derived from overnight cultures of V. cholerae, strain
Ogawa (6-8). Mice were immunized by i.p. injection of 50 to 100 ug
of the organisms. Vibriolytic PFCs were determined by a plaque
assay in agar gel utilizing living vibrios (approximately 10^8 organisms) incorporated into the soft agar gel containing dispersed
spleen cells from immunized mice (6-8). The agar-cell mixture
was poured onto the surface of a previously prepared petri plate
containing a base layer of nutrient agar and incubated for one hour
at 37^oC, followed by treatment with 3-5 ml sterile guinea pig complement. The plates were then incubated for an additional 3 to
6 hours until a "lawn" of microcolonies of vibrios appeared
except in those areas of "no growth" indicating the presence of
vibriolytic PFCs. These were considered due to 19S IgM secreting
immunocytes. For the indirect facilitation technique plates were
treated with diluted anti-mouse Ig serum as an additional step (11,
12). Those additional plaques which appeared in the antiserum
treated plates were considered due to low efficiency IgG PFCs
(12). Anti-Ig serum with specificity to IgG_{1a}, IgG_{2a} and IgA
were also used to enumerate specific classes of 7S PFCs (11).

For in vitro culture 5 x 10^6 splenocytes were incubated on a
dialysis membrane in 1 ml Minimal Essential Medium (MEM) fortified
with 10% fetal calf serum in the inner chamber of a Marbrook culture vessel (13,14). Eleven ml of medium were placed in the outer

chamber. For immunization 0.1 ml of graded amounts of cholera vaccine was added per chamber and the number of PFCs determined at various time intervals thereafter. In control experiments sheep RBC was used as the immunogen; i.e. 4×10^8 RBCs were injected i.p. into animals for in vivo immunization and 2×10^6 erythrocytes added to cultures for in vitro immunization. Specificity of the plaques to vibrios was determined by addition of phenol extracted vibrio LPS to the agar plate at the time of plaque assay (6-8).

EXPERIMENTAL RESULTS

Vibriolytic PFCs were conspicuously absent in spleen cell cultures from normal mice incubated in Marbrook vessels for up to 12 days unless vibrio antigen was specifically added. When 10^6 heat killed vibrios were added at the time of culture initiation vibriolytic PFCs appeared 3 to 4 days later, with peak numbers on days 7 to 8. There was a rapid decrease in number thereafter (Table 1).

Table 1. The effect of antigen dose on the in vitro immune response of spleen cells from normal, non-immunized mice.

Antigen dose[a]	Vibriolytic PFC response on day[b]				
	+2	+4	+6	+8	+10
10^4	–	0	0	0	0
10^5	–	1	4	21	8
10^6	0	2	46	135	63
10^7	0	0	12	47	16
10^8	0	0	2	18	12

[a]Indicated number of heat killed vibrios added in 0.1 ml volumes to 5×10^6 spleen cells from normal Balb/c mice at time of culture initiation.

[b]Average number of vibriolytic PFC/10^6 spleen cells for 5-6 cultures on day indicated after culture initiation.

These kinetics of the in vitro PFC response to vibrios were different from that occurring in vivo. However, it is important to note that viability of the cultures decreased rapidly after days 5 to 6 so that by day 10 there were fewer than 10-15% of the original numbers of viable cells per culture.

Addition of an unrelated antigen to the cultures, such as
sheep red cells or an E. coli vaccine, failed to stimulate a
single vibriolytic PFC. In contrast, large numbers of anti-SRBC
PFCs appeared in cultures of normal splenocytes immunized in vitro
with RBC. Peak numbers appeared on days 4 and 5 (Fig. 1).

Furthermore, relatively large numbers of hemolytic PFCs appeared in control cultures without antigen or after immunization
with cholera vaccine or E. coli. Although the numbers were lower
than those appearing in cultures immunized with SRBC, they were
still much higher than the original background and contrasted to
the total absence of "background" PFCs to the vibrios. The concentration of vibrios added to stimulate splenocytes directly influenced the magnitude of the vibriolytic PFC response. Maximum
numbers occurred with 10^6 vibrios per culture vessel. A ten-fold
increase or decrease in antigen concentration resulted in markedly
fewer PFCs.

Since IgG PFCs readily appeared in vivo late in the primary
and during the secondary response it was of interest to determine
whether such PFCs also develop in vitro. For this purpose spleen
cells were obtained from mice immunized with vibrios 8 to 10 weeks
earlier and placed in culture with or without added bacteria.
There were generally only 1 to 2 IgM PFCs and no detectable IgG
PFCs per million splenocytes at the time of culture initiation.
A rapid rise in both classes of PFCs occurred after in vitro immunization of the primed splenocytes (Table 2). Within 2 days
approximately two dozen IgM PFCs developed per million cultured
splenocytes. This number increased rapidly thereafter, reaching
peak levels by days 7 to 8 after secondary immunization in vitro.
Furthermore, the number of IgG PFCs increased even more rapidly
and reached larger peak numbers, which also occurred on day 7
after secondary immunization in vitro. Furthermore, the availability of mono-specific antisera permitted the detection of IgG
producing cells of different classes (Table 2). The main class
of low efficiency PFCs was due to IgG_1 immunoglobulins, although
large numbers of IgG_{2a} and Ig_{2b} secreting PFCs also developed.
The peak numbers always occurred on day 7. Very low numbers of
IgA PFCs developed, with the peak numbers also occurring on day 7.

Unlike the situation with unprimed spleen cells, low but significant numbers of vibriolytic IgM PFCs developed in cultures containing splenocytes from primed animals without the addition of
vibrios (Table 2, Figure 1). The number of such "background"
PFCs was relatively low as compared to the number of induced PFCs.
Nevertheless an increase in the number of IgM PFCs occurred over
a 7-10 day period in vitro reached levels like that occurring during
the primary immune response in vitro with splenocytes from normal
animals incubated with vibrio antigen. Also, as can be seen in

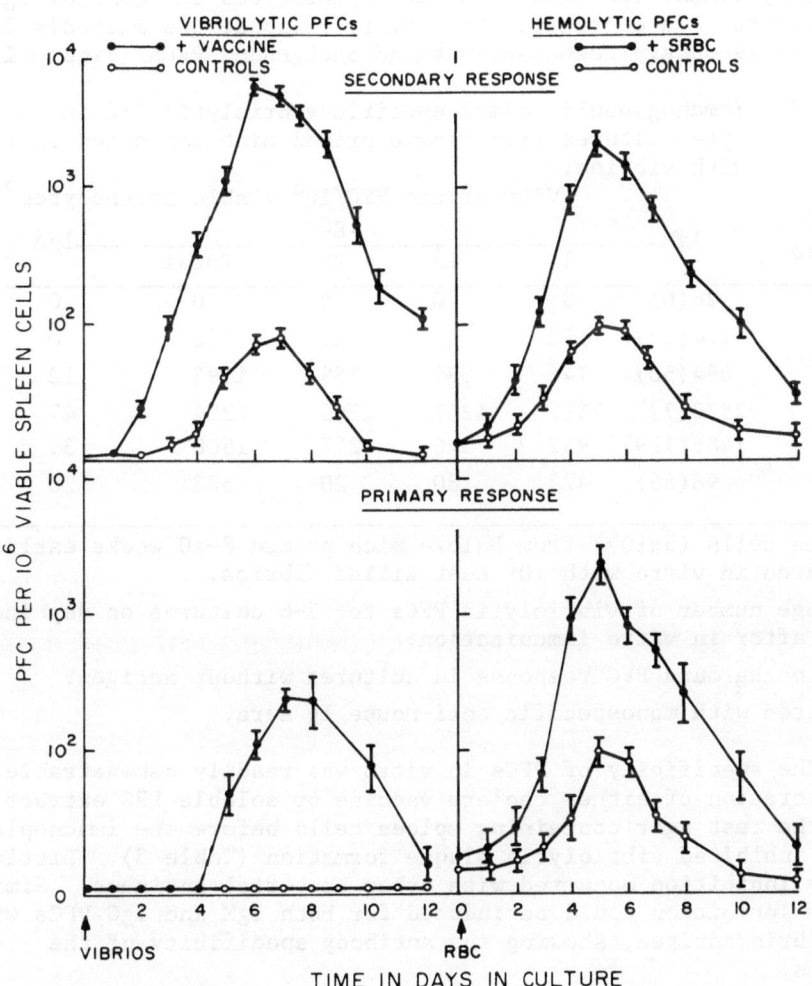

Figure 1. Cytokinetics of the primary and secondary in vitro immune response to vibrios or sheep RBC by spleen cells from normal
or antigen primed Balb/c mice. Each point represents the average
PFC response for 10^6 viable splenocytes on day indicated after in
vitro immunization. Primed mice immunized i.p. 6-8 weeks earlier
with either vibrios (10 ug) or SRBC (4×10^8 erythrocytes). Cultures consisted of 5×10^6 spleen cells immunized in vitro with
either 10^6 heat killed vibrios or 2×10^6 SRBCs.

Figure 1, the kinetics of the secondary immune response to vibrios
in vitro was quite similar to the kinetics of both the primary and
secondary immune response to sheep erythrocytes in terms of IgM
immunocytes. In contrast, the primary response was markedly lower
than the secondary response, with no background PFCs (Figure 1).

Table 2. Immunoglobulin class specific vibriolytic PFC in splenocyte cultures from vibrio primed mice immunized in vitro
with vibrios.

Day of culture	IgM	Vibriolytic PFC/10^6 viable splenocytes[b]				
		IgG[d]				IgA
		1	2a	2b	Total	
2	28(6)[c]	0	0	0	0	0
4	174(37)	192	55	25	272	0
6	684(56)	746	384	189	1593	12
7	2570(77)	1812	1257	1165	4234	47
8	1485(119)	932	346	222	1500	35
10	98(86)	423	80	20	523	20

[a]Spleen cells (5×10^6) from Balb/c mice primed 8–10 weeks earlier
cultured in vitro with 10^6 heat killed vibrios.

[b]Average number of vibriolytic PFCs for 3–6 cultures on day indicated after in vitro immunization.

[c]( )= background PFC response in cultures without antigen.

[d]Detected with monospecific anti-mouse Ig sera.

The specificity of PFCs in vitro was readily demonstrable.
Incorporation of either cholera vaccine or soluble LPS extract
into the test agar containing spleen cells before the immunoplaque
assay inhibited vibriolytic plaque formation (Table 3). Little
if any inhibition occurred with other bacterial antigens. Similar
plaque inhibition could be induced for both IgM and IgG PFCs with
the vibrio antigen, showing the antibody specificity of the
plaques.

DISCUSSION

The results of these studies show a marked difference in the
immune response in vitro of splenocytes exposed for the first time
to vibrio antigens as compared to the response of splenocytes from
mice primed in vivo with this bacterial antigen. Background vibriolytic PFCs were consistently absent in the spleen of normal non-
immunized mice, both in vivo and in vitro. No PFCs with specificity to the bacteria appeared in spleen cultures of unimmunized mice
for a period of up to 12 days. In contrast, marked increases in
the number of PFCs to erythrocyte antigens, as well as other bacterial antigens, occurred when non-immunized spleen cells from nor-

mal mice were cultured in medium alone. This is thought to be due
to cross-reacting antigens in the culture medium or to "non-
specific" stimulation of immunocompetent cells by mitogens present
in the medium. Splenocytes from vibrio primed mice when cultured
in medium without specific vibrio antigen, also developed increased
numbers of vibriolytic IgM PFCs. This increase seemed comparable
to the increase in the number of "background" immunocytes to SRBCs
(1-3). Thus the finding suggests that development of PFCs in medium alone without an antigen such as sheep red cells may be due to
the inapparent "priming" of lymphoid cells to either RBC antigen
per se or cross reacting antigens in the environment of mice long
before the animals are used for antibody studies.

Table 3.   Inhibition of vibriolytic PFCs stimulated in vitro with
            vibrio antigen.

Inhibitor in agar[a]		Vibriolytic PFC per 10^6 splenocytes[b]	Percent inhibition
None		86	–
cholera vaccine	1.0 ug	52	39
	10.0 ug	10	91
cholera LPS	1.0 ug	44	49
	10.0 ug	6	93
E. coli LPS	1.0 ug	81	5
	10.0 ug	77	10

[a]Indicated bacterial antigen added to immune splenocytes 30 minutes
  before plaque assay.

[b]Average number of PFC for 10^6 splenocytes pooled from Marbrook culture vessels 7 days after in vitro immunization with vibrios and
  tested in vibriolytic assay, with or without indicated inhibitor.

Although a primary IgM PFC response to vibrio antigens could
be induced readily in vitro, the kinetics of the response was significantly different from the primary response induced in vivo in
intact mice given the same dose of vibrio antigen (6-8). The
first PFCs appeared in vitro only after a lag of 3 to 4 days,
rather than the 2 day lag in vivo. Furthermore, peak numbers occurred on day 7-8 in vitro, whereas in vivo the peak response was
on days 12 to 14. This difference, however, could be due to the
possible inadequacy of the in vitro culture system. The Marbrook
chamber system permits longer survival of cells in vitro as compared to cultures of lymphocytes in a roller tube or petri plates.
Nevertheless, by days 7 to 10 after culture initiation only 15 to
20% of the cells are viable. By day 12 to 15 very few cells are
viable. Thus the peak response in vitro of seven days may be more
apparent than real since the ability of the cells to continue to
secrete antibody in vitro would be obviously compromised as cell
viability decreased.

Antibody forming cells of both IgM and IgG classes were
readily detected in cultures of vibrio primed splenocytes following
immunization in vitro with cholera antigen. However, differences
were also apparent between in vitro vs in vivo secondary responses.
For example, the peak secondary IgM response occurred on days 6
to 7 in vitro, 1 to 2 days after the peak IgM response in vivo.
In addition, the largest numbers of secondary IgG PFCs occurred
on the same day as the peak IgM response, while maximal IgG
responses occurring in vivo preceded the maximal IgM response.
Similar to responses in intact animals (11), immunocytes secreting
IgG_1 antibody were the most predominant subclass of 7S IgG antibody producing cells during the in vitro response.

Stimulation of antibody forming cells in vitro to a highly
immunogenic bacterial antigen in the absence of pre-existing
antibody forming cells provides a valuable model system to examine in detail the cellular events occurring in vitro after immunization of immunocytes from normal animals. The availability
of such a system will permit the examination of the role and interaction of T and B lymphocytes, as well as macrophages during
immunization under a variety of conditions without the complication of the presence of background antibody activity which increase in number non-specifically during experimental manipulation.

SUMMARY

An antibody response showing characteristics of a "true" primary response was readily induced in vitro with splenocytes from
normal non-immunized animals cultured with strongly immunogenic
Vibrio cholerae somatic antigens. Prior studies have shown that
the response to vibrios in intact animals appeared to be a true
primary response since no pre-existing antibody forming cells
were present in non-immunized animals and the antigen induced response, following a lag of two days, resulted thereafter in a rapid
stepwise increase in the number of specific PFCs, reaching a peak
at 12 to 14 days. Using the Marbrook culture system for antibody
formation a readily detected immunocyte response to vibrios was
induced with splenocytes from normal non-immunized animals. No
background antibody forming cells developed to the organisms
without addition of vibrios in vitro. After in vitro immunization with 10^6 bacteria significant numbers of IgM PFCs appeared
with a peak response on days 7 to 8. Splenocyte cultures from
mice primed earlier with vibrios developed a marked secondary
response, with appearance of both IgM and IgG PFCs. Large numbers of both classes of PFCs developed, with peak responses on
days 6 to 7, similar to the "primary" response to sheep erythrocytes. However, significant numbers of PFCs to vibrios developed
in cultures of vibrio-primed cultures even in the absence of vibrios during the 12 day culture period. The availability of a completely in vitro model system to induce a true primary immune

response without the complication of pre-existing background antibody forming cells will be of value for further studies concerning
various cellular pathways and interactions during the immune response to small amounts of strongly immunogenic bacterial antigens.

ACKNOWLEDGEMENT

The capable technical assistance of Mr. Navin Patel and Mr.
Chandu Patel during various phases of this study is acknowledged.
Supported by research grants from the U.S. National Science Foundation and the National Institute of Allergy and Infectious Diseases.

REFERENCES

1. Jerne, N.K., Nordin, A.A. and Henry, C. in Cell-bound Antibod-
    ies, ed. B. Amos and H. Koprowski, p. 109, Wistar Press, Phila.
    1963.
2. Ingraham, J.S., C.S. Acad. Sci., 256:5005, 1963.
3. Mishell, R.I. and Dutton, R.W., Science 153:1004, 1966.
4. Urzo, P. and Gengozian, N., J. Immunol. 111:712, 1973.
5. Jerne, N.K., Henry, C., Nordin, A.A., Fufi, H., Koros, M.C.A.
    and Lefkovits, F., Transpl. Rev. 18:130, 1974.
6. McAlack, R.F., Cerny, J., Allen, J.L. and Friedman, H. Science
    168:141, 1970.
7. McAlack, R.F., Cerny, J. and Friedman, H. J. Immunol. 107:
    1752, 1971.
8. Cerny, J., McAlack, R.F., Sazid, M.A., Fonton, J. and
    Friedman, H. J. Immunol. 106:1371, 1971.
9. Sterzl, J. and Silverstein, A.M. Adv. Immunol. 5:337, 1967.
10. Kim, Y.B. and Watson, D.W., Fed. Proc. 27:493, 1968.
11. Kateley, J.R., Patel, C. and Friedman, H. J. Immunol. 113:
    1811, 1974.
12. Friedman, H. Immunol. in press, 1975.
13. Marbrook, J. Lancet 2:1279, 1967.
14. Kateley, J.R., Kamo, I., Kaplan, G. and Friedman, H. J. Nat'l.
    Canc. Inst. 53:1371, 1974.

NONSPECIFIC ESTERASE ACTIVITY IN T CELLS

J. Mueller, H.U. Keller, G. Brun del Re, H. Buerki and
M.W. Hess
Department of Pathology, University of Bern
CH-3010 Bern, Switzerland

Histo- or cytochemical demonstration of non-specific acid
esterase activity in lymphocytes can be used to differentiate between two cell populations in mouse lymphoid tissue and in lymph
or peripheral blood. Using a standardized histochemical technique
with fixed incubation time, esterase activity was present in the

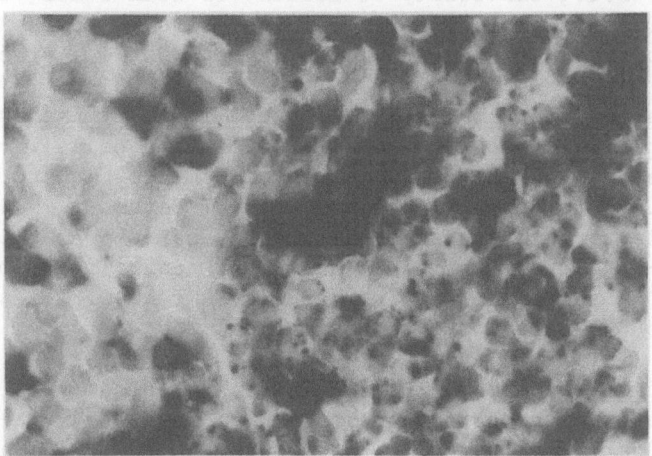

Fig. 1.   Demonstration of acid α-naphthyl acetate esterase activity in a section of a mouse (ICR strain) mesenteric lymph node.
Note dot-like reaction product in lymphocytes located in the diffuse cortical (paracortical) zone (right), indicating esterase
activity; esterase-positive cells are virtually absent in the
lymphoid follicle (left) (x 600).

vast majority of lymphocytes of so-called thymus-dependent areas, in particular the diffuse cortical (paracortical) zone of lymph nodes, and of the thoracic duct while most lymphocytes in primary follicles lacked esterase activity (Fig. 1). Based on this observation it was suggested that non-specific acid esterase activity may be used as a criterion for differentiation of peripheral T and B lymphocytes in tissue sections and smears of mouse lymph nodes (1).

In this report we describe results of an extension of these earlier studies: in a series of in vitro experiments, esterase activity in lymphocytes was correlated with allo- and xenoantigens of mouse T cells as well as with B cells carrying surface immuno-globulin. Individual lymphocytes of mouse lymph nodes or peripheral blood were scored for the presence or absence of T cell surface antigens and surface Ig, respectively. Following incubation of fixed smear preparations with α-naphthyl acetate, positive or negative reaction for esterase activity was recorded for these identical cells.

MATERIALS AND METHODS

Animals. Colony-bred Charles-River albino mice (ICR strain; Tierzuchtinstitut, University of Zürich) of both sexes, aged 1/2 to 1 month, were used. The animals received standard pellet food and water ad libitum. Mice were killed by an overdose of ether.

Preparation of cell suspensions from mouse lymph nodes and peripheral blood. Suspensions of living, single cells were made by teasing mesenteric lymph nodes in medium RPMI 1640 containing L-glutamin (Microbiological Associates, Inc., Bethesda, Md.). Mono-nuclear cells were separated from citrated peripheral blood using an Isopaque-Ficoll mixture. The cells were centrifuged for 10 minutes at 650 g and suspended in ice-cold RPMI 1640. All suspensions were kept at 4°C throughout the experiments.

Immunofluorescence. Thy-1(θ C3H) was revealed by successive incubation of a lymphocyte suspension with mouse anti-theta serum (batch 17, Searle Laboratories, High Wycombe, England) and FITC-labeled swine anti-mouse-Ig (SEVAC, Prague) as described earlier (2). Indirect immunofluorescence was used to detect Ig-bearing lymphocytes: successive incubation was carried out with rabbit anti-mouse Ig (Behring, Marburg) and FITC-labeled goat anti-rabbit Ig (SEVAC, Prague).

Direct immunofluorescence was employed in a double staining

assay in which mesenteric lymph node lymphocytes were incubated
with TRITC-labeled rabbit anti-MTLA* (3) and a mixture of FITC-
labeled goat anti-mouse IgG$_1$, -IgG$_{2A}$ and IgG$_{2B}$ (Meloy Laboratories,
Springfield, Va.).

Evaluation of cells in suspension or in smear preparations was
carried out by incident uv-light microscopy (Leitz OPAK).

Demonstration of non-specific, acid esterase activity. Since
irregular, and in particular, slow drying of the preparations interferes with the cytochemical demonstration of esterase activity, cytocentrifuge smears were prepared under standardized conditions
and used throughout the present study. Samples of 0.2 ml of a suspension containing 1.5 x 10^6 cells/ml were spun on a slide by centrifugation at 500 rpm for 5 seconds (Shandon-Elliot Cytocentrifuge
SCA-0020; Shandon Scientific Company, London). Immediately after
the centrifuge had stopped, smears were fixed in 0.1 M phosphate-
buffered 2.5% glutaraldehyde (pH 7.4) for 10 minutes at 4°C. The
preparations were then rinsed 10 times in distilled water. Following scoring the cells by immunofluorescence and recording their
exact position, staining for esterase activity was carried out with
the incubation mixtures described previously (1). With this protocol, incubation for 1 hour at 37°C was sufficient to obtain the
characteristic red-brown reaction product indicating presence of
non-specific acid esterase. Cells previously scored by immunofluorescence for presence of surface antigens or Ig were then re-
located, and the presence or absence of esterase activity was evaluated by light microscopy.

RESULTS AND DISCUSSION

Preliminary experiments showed that the relative proportion
of lymphocytes carrying the surface antigens Thy-1 (θ C3H) and MTLA
or surface Ig was identical on glutaraldehyde-fixed smear preparations to that found in suspensions of non-fixed cells. Similarly,
the number of lymphocytes exhibiting esterase activity was not altered by preincubation of the cells with fluorochrome-labeled antisera, provided that the protocol for preparation of smears was
strictly adhered to.

Results of individual cell scorings are presented in Table I.

---

* TRITC-labeled anti-MTLA was a gift from Dr. C. Bron, Institut de
Biochimie, University of Lausanne.

Table I: Individual cell scoring of mouse lymph node and peripheral blood lymphocytes.

Surface characteristics	Percentage of lymphocytes with esterase activity	
	Peripheral blood	Lymph node
θ+	80%	95%
Ig+	4%	n.d.
IgG+	n.d.	6%

Over 90% of both lymph node and blood lymphocytes with esterase activity carry the Thy-1(θ) surface antigen, while only 5.5% of lymph node lymphocytes and 2% of lymphocytes in peripheral blood are positive for surface Ig and esterase activity.

The results obtained in the experiment in which lymphocytes from mesenteric lymph nodes were double stained with TRITC-anti-MTLA and FITC-anti-IgG and subsequently tested for esterase activity are presented in Fig. 2. Most esterase-positive cells were found to be MTLA-positive. MTLA-positivity was recorded in 10% of esterase-negative lymphocytes. Not a single cell carrying surface IgG was either MTLA- or esterase-positive. A total of 20% of all lymphocytes carried neither MTLA nor surface IgG; in none of these could esterase activity be detected. Since in this study only surface IgG was included for technical reasons, a fraction of this esterase-negative population of lymphocytes may carry other surface

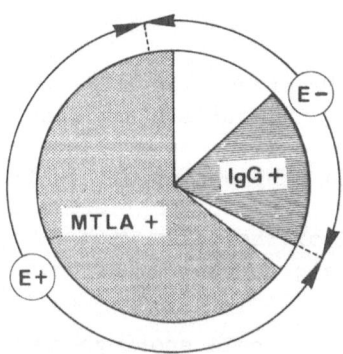

Fig. 2. Relative distribution of MTLA+, IgG+ and esterase-positive lymphocytes in mouse (ICR strain) mesenteric lymph node. Values are based on individual cell scoring (see Materials and Methods).

immunoglobulins. The esterase activity of so-called "null" cells (4), the relative proportion of which could not be determined, can not be assessed at present.

θ-positive cells with no esterase activity were present among both lymph node and peripheral blood lymphocytes, though the low numbers evaluated preclude definite judgment as to whether or not they represent a major proportion of esterase-negative lymphocytes. Lymphoid cells in the outer thymic cortex are virtually all esterase-negative (1). Esterase activity, therefore, appears to be acquired by thymic lymphocytes shortly before or after leaving the thymus or in the periphery. This interpretation is supported by the observation that most of the E- θ+ cells in mouse peripheral blood exhibited either full or 3/4 ring fluorescence with anti-θ serum. In the lymph nodes a more close correlation between esterase activity and the presence of θ-antigen is found as compared to the peripheral blood. This may indicate that esterase activity is to a particular degree associated with long-lived populations of T lymphocytes.

A small proportion of lymphocytes was found to be esterase-positive and negative for either θ or MTLA. This population may contain peripheralized T cells which had gradually lost their complement of thymic surface antigens to an extent that it is not detectable by the methods used (2) and/or may represent $Ig-\theta^{+weak}$ lymphocytes (5).

It remains to be examined whether or not the very small fraction of E+Ig+ lymphocytes are identical with activated T cells carrying Fc-receptors (4).

SUMMARY

Acid α-naphthyl acetate esterase activity characterizes the majority of peripheral T cells in mice. In addition to the simplicity of the cyto- or histochemical demonstration of esterase activity and the fact that this method may be applied to tissue sections and smears, the present study indicates that combination with lymphocyte surface markers may offer an important approach to the examination of differentiation pathways of peripheral T cells.

REFERENCES

1. J. Mueller, G. Brun del Re, H. Buerki, H.U. Keller, M.W. Hess and H. Cottier; Europ. J. Immunol. 5, 270, 1975.

2. A.D. Chanana, J. Schaedeli, M.W. Hess and H. Cottier; Cellular Immunology 13, 216, 1974.

3. C. Bron and D. Sauser; J. Immunol. 110, 384, 1973.

4. G. Brown and M.F. Greaves; Europ. J. Immunol. 4, 302, 1974.

5. G.E. Roelants, F. Loor, H. von Boehmer, J. Sprent, L.-B. Hägg, K.S. Mayor and A. Rydén; Europ. J. Immunol. 5, 127, 1975.

THYMOCYTE SUBPOPULATIONS AS STIMULATORS IN THE MIXED LYMPHOCYTE REACTION

D.B. Lausé, S.D. Waksal, H.W. Waksal, R.L. St. Pierre

The Ohio State University, Department of Anatomy
333 West Tenth Avenue
Columbus, Ohio 43210   USA

INTRODUCTION

Recent studies involving the mixed lymphocyte reaction (MLR) have suggested that genes which map in the I region, and are expressed predominately on B-lymphocytes, are responsible for stimulation of allogeneic responding cells (1). It has been shown, however, that both T- and B-lymphocytes stimulate in the MLR, albeit T-lymphocytes are less stimulatory than B-lymphocytes (2).

The present study defines a subpopulation of cortisone-resistant thymocytes and thymocytes separated on discontinuous gradients of bovine serum albumin (BSA) which act as stimulating and responding cells in an allogeneic MLR.

MATERIALS AND METHODS

Animals used throughout this study were 4-6 week old C57B1/6 and Balb/c mice. All cell combinations were cultivated in Eagle's minimum essential medium supplemented with 15% fetal calf serum. All cultures were performed in triplicate in Falcon Microtest tissue culture plates and incubated for 72 hours at 37°C and 10% CO_2. Mixed cell reactions contained 5×10^5 responding cells and 5×10^5 Mitomycin-C treated syngeneic and allogeneic stimulating cells.

Incorporation of ^{3}H-thymidine was assayed for the proliferative response in MLR. One microcurie per 0.1 ml of ^{3}H-thymidine (6 Ci/mmole) was added for the final 10 hours of culture. Cultured cells were harvested on glass wool filter paper with a multiple

automatic sample harvester and ^{3}H-thymidine incorporation expressed
as counts per minute for both allogeneic and syngeneic cultures.

Unseparated thymocytes and thymocytes separated on discontinuous gradients of BSA according to the method of Raidt et al (3)
were used as stimulating and responding cells against syngeneic
and allogeneic spleen cells. Animals received an injection of 2.5
mg of hydrocortisone 48 hours before the harvesting of thymocytes.

RESULTS

As seen in Table 1, 4-6 week old untreated and unseparated
C57Bl/6 thymocytes did not respond significantly to Mitomycin-C
treated Balb/c spleen cells over syngeneic controls. In fact, the
thymocytes collected from the A-B layers of BSA gradients responded
4.4 times greater than Balb/c A-B layer thymocytes against Balb/c
spleen cells. A dramatic increase in response of A-B layer cells
is seen when compared to unseparated thymocytes in which A-B layer
thymocytes responded significantly greater. C layer thymocytes responded significantly to allogeneic cells, however, this response
was approximately 3 times less than the response of A-B layer thymocytes. Thymocytes collected from the D layer of the gradient did
not significantly respond to allogeneic cells.

TABLE I

THYMOCYTE SUBPOPULATIONS AS RESPONDING CELLS IN MLR

Responder Cell Population	cpm[a]			ratio	$\dfrac{\text{allogeneic}[b]}{\text{syngeneic}}$
Untreated thymocytes	141	±	11		1.5
Syngeneic Control	93	±	16		
A-B layer thymocytes	8,232	±	888		4.4
Syngeneic Control	1,881	±	330		
C layer thymocytes	294	±	14		2.3
Syngeneic Control	127	±	25		
D layer thymocytes	165	±	20		1.5
Syngeneic Control	108	±	18		

[a] counts per minute of incorporation of ^{3}H-thymidine in cultures of
4×10^5 responding spleen lymphocytes and 4×10^5 allogeneic and syngeneic stimulating thymocytes.

[b] stimulation ratios were computed by dividing the allogeneic spleen
cell response by the syngeneic control.

Table 2 shows that untreated and unseparated thymocytes did not stimulate allogeneic spleen cells above syngeneic controls. The response of Balb/c spleen cells to A-B layer thymocytes is significantly greater than Balb/c spleen cells responding to A-B layer Balb/c thymocytes stimulated only 1.6 times greater. Thymocytes collected from the C and D layers of the gradient did not affect a significant response to allogeneic cells.

TABLE 2

THYMOCYTE SUBPOPULATIONS AS STIMULATOR CELLS IN MLR

Target Cell Population	cpm[a]	Ratio allogeneic[b]
		syngeneic
Untreated thymocytes	1,952 ± 177	1.02
Syngeneic Control	1,911 ± 344	
A-B layer thymocytes	3,075 ± 125	2.10
Syngeneic Control	1,479 ± 141	
C layer thymocytes	1,685 ± 142	1.14
Syngeneic Control	1,480 ± 294	
D layer thymocytes	1,147 ± 178	0.67
Syngeneic Control	1,697 ± 313	

[a]counts per minute of incorporation of ^{3}H-thymidine in cultures of 4×10^5 responding spleen lymphocytes and 4×10^5 allogeneic and syngeneic stimulating thymocytes.

[b]stimulation ratios were computed by dividing the allogeneic spleen cell response by the syngeneic control.

As seen in Table 3, untreated thymocytes demonstrated no significant stimulation of allogeneic spleen cells. However, cortisone-resistant thymocytes effected 2.7 times more stimulation than syngeneic controls and were 1.5 times more effective than untreated thymocytes. In comparing the target cell activity of A-B layer cells and cortisone-resistant cells, both populations exhibit approximately the same stimulatory ratios over syngeneic controls.

TABLE 3

UNTREATED AND CORTISONE-RESISTANT THYMOCYTES
STIMULATOR CELLS IN MLR

Target Cell Population	cpm[a]			Ratio	allogeneic[b]
					syngeneic
Untreated thymocytes	11,920	±	767		1.8
Syngeneic Control	6,663	±	943		
Cortisone-Resistant thymocytes	14,575	±	1,178		2.7
Syngeneic Control	5,449	±	32		

[a]counts per minute of incorporation of ^{3}H-thymidine in cultures of 4×10^5 stimulating cortisone-resistant and untreated allogeneic and syngeneic thymocytes.

[b]stimulation ratios were computed by dividing the allogeneic spleen cell response by the syngeneic control.

DISCUSSION

The present study shows that unseparated and untreated thymocytes respond poorly to allogeneic spleen cells whereas A-B layer thymocytes demonstrate the strongest response. These findings are consistent with the studies of Konda et al (4) suggesting that this minor subpopulation of thymocytes exist as an immunocompetent population prior to peripheralization.

A major problem in recent studies on MLR has been the identification of the lymphocyte class possessing surface antigens which stimulate allogeneic cells. The present results using cortisone-resistant and albumin gradient separated thymocytes indicate that, within the thymus, stimulatory activity is associated with the minor subpopulation of thymocytes which are cortisone-resistant, are of low density and responsive to alloantigens and phytomitogens (5).

Products of the Ir region (Ia antigens) have been suggested as the stimulating antigens in the MLR (1). Recent studies have shown that a minor population of Fc positive thymocytes exist (6). These cells appear to be within the A-B layer and cortisone-resistant population discussed above. Anti-Ia sera inhibit the binding of aggregated immunoglobulin to the Fc receptor on B-lymphocytes (7). If Ia is also intimately associated with the Fc receptor on

T-lymphocytes, the Fc positive thymocyte subpopulation may be responsible for thymocyte stimulation in the MLR.

REFERENCES

1. Lozner, E.C., D.H. Sachs, G.M. Shearer and W.D. Terry.
        Science 183:757, 1974.
2. Lonai, P. and H.O. McDevitt. J. Exp. Med., 140:1317, 1974.
3. Raidt, D.J., R.I. Mishell and R.W. Dutton. J. Exp. Med.,
        128:681, 1968.
4. Konda, S., E. Stockert and R.T. Smith. Cell. Immunol.,
        7:275, 1973.
5. Lause, D.B.   Anat. Rec., 181:406, 1975.
6. Stout, R., Waksal, S.D., Sato, V. and L.A. Herzenberg.
        Proc. 10th Leukocyte Culture Conference, IN PRESS
7. Dickler, H. and D.H. Sachs. J. Exp. Med., 140:779, 1974.

CLONAL PROLIFERATION OF HUMAN STIMULATED LYMPHOCYTES ON AGAR CULTURE

Rozenszajn, L.A., Shoham, D. and Kalechman, I.

Hematological Laboratories, Meir Hospital, and

Dept. of Life Sciences, Bar-Ilan University, Israel

INTRODUCTION

In order to investigate the process of proliferation, differentiation and maturation of hemopoietic cells, colony development of human bone marrow or peripheral blood cells has been studied. This was accomplished by the addition of stimulating factors or feeder layers which permit growth of colonies, such as macrophages-monocytes, granulocytes and eosinophils to soft agar culture media (1-4). Clonal responses of lymphocytes in vitro have been described in a suspension culture medium where the lymphocytes were activated by mitogens (5-7). These clonal responses provide the rationale for the use of mitogens to stimulate a responsive human lymphocyte population to induce clonal proliferation of lymphocytes in a two layer soft agar system. The convenience of the soft agar method is the advantage of locating colonies, thus making possible the study of the conditions for formation of clones made up of cells originating from one precursor cell.

MATERIALS AND METHODS

Suspension culture: Three different kinds of cell suspensions were used: 1) Human venous blood lymphocytes separated on glass columns, 2) nucleated human bone marrow cells were used when their stained smears were diagnosed as normal and the number of lymphocytes was evaluated by differential counting of 10^3 nucleated cells, 3)normal spleen cells obtained from patients after traumatic rupture of the spleen.

Nucleated cells, 10^6/ml, were cultured in a suspension culture medium (8) using 0.1 ml bactophytohemagglutinin M (PHA) in duplicate tubes. One of them was used after 15-18 hours of incubation to culture the cells in soft agar, and the other one for estimation of lymphocyte transformation after 72 hours of culture.

Soft agar culture: The PHA sensitized lymphocytes were seeded in amounts of 10^6 cells per one 15x60 mm Petri dish according to the two soft agar layer technique (9,10). Additionally the lower agar layer contained PHA in a concentration of 0.0625 ml per 5 ml medium. The dishes were incubated at 37^0C in a water-saturated atmosphere with 5-7.5% CO_2. As controls, cultures were set up with unsensitized cells or in the absence of PHA in the Petri dish.

Assays for culture conditions of colony development: The assays were based on determination of the optimal time of preceding sensitization of lymphocytes with PHA, the varying concentration of PHA in the soft agar layer, the appropriate number of PHA-sensitized lymphocytes seeded, and a comparison between the action of fetal calf serum (FCS) and autologous plasma in the soft agar on colony development.

Examination of cultures: In order to follow the development of clones, isolated blast-like cells from the cultures were selected and observed under an inverted microscope every three to four hours for a period of 40 hours, beginning with the third day after seed-ing. The development of colonies and their morphology was observed during 3-7 days of culturing. Small and large lymphocyte colonies from culture medium were sampled by means of a capillary tube in order to evaluate the morphological properties of the cells, and their membrane markers. The rate of transformation of lymphocytes in the suspension culture after 72 h. was determined by counting 200 cells in smears stained with May-Grünwald Giemsa staining (MGG).

Cell surface markers: Suspended lymphocytes from the colonies were washed three times in phosphate buffered saline and used for spon-taneous E-rosette formation with sheep red blood cells (SRBC) (T-cells) (11), for rosette formation with mouse red blood cells $C_{57}Bl$ strain (MRBC) (B-cells) (12), and for lymphocyte bearing membrane associated immunoglobulin determination (B-cells) (13).

As control for rosette formation, PHA-stimulated and trans-formed lymphocytes, leukocytes from patients suffering from chronic lymphatic leukemia (CLL), as well as granulocytes and macrophages obtained from colonies of human bone marrow, cultured in soft agar, were used.

RESULTS

Human lymphocytes from peripheral blood, bone marrow, and spleen which were stimulated with PHA prior to being seeded in soft agar, developed into clones containing at least 50 cells each, 3 to 5 days after seeding. By means of repeated observations it was possible to follow the development of a colony starting from one single cell until it reached 50 to 60 cells. Two types of colonies developed: large colonies which appeared after 3 to 4 days on the bottom of the upper agar layer and comprised, after 5 to 6 days, 200 to 500 or more cells; and small colonies which were seen in a higher plane in the upper agar layer after 6 to 7 days of culture resulting in production of 50 to 150 cells. After ten days, the colonies degenerated and the cells were lysed. No other types of colonies, such as monocytes-macrophages or granulocytes, were found during the development of lymphocyte colonies or after their degeneration. The number of colonies per 10^6 cells seeded ranged, for peripheral blood, between 250 and 500, and for spleen from 60 to 150 colonies. From 60 to 100 colonies were obtained from 10^6 nucleated bone marrow cells. It should be noted that morphologic study disclosed the presence of 7 to 13 per cent of lymphocytes among the bone marrow cells.

Colonies of lymphocytes developed only in continuous presence of PHA, both in the preliminary suspension medium and in the soft agar layer. No colonies developed in control cultures. The optimal PHA-sensitization time was found to be no less than 12 hours. Incubation periods in liquid medium with PHA, exceeding 12 hours, did not lead to any further significant increase in the number of developing colonies. Optimal concentrations of PHA were 0.0125 ml per ml medium for PHA present in the lower layer. Higher concentrations of PHA depressed colony formation, and no colonies developed when PHA concentration reached 0.3 ml per ml of medium (Fig. 1). It should be noted that FCS enhanced the number of colonies (Fig. 2). A linear relation between the number of cells seeded and the number of resulting colonies was observed. Thus, one out of 2×10^3 or 3×10^3 lymphocytes in peripheral blood has the potential to develop as colony.

The MGG stained cells of the colonies which appeared after 3 to 4 days and 6 to 7 days of culture showed that all cells were large pyroninophilic and blast-like, some of them in mitosis. The mitotic index determined in the colonies was 4 to 5 per cent; in the suspension culture it was 0.1 per cent.

Under phase microscopy the cells had a characteristic morphology manifested by prominent nucleoli and cytoplasmic vacuoles, thus resembling transformed normal human lymphocytes stimulated by PHA in liquid culture media (Fig. 3). The E-rosette-forming ability of the colonies' cells was manifested by 50 to 75 per cent

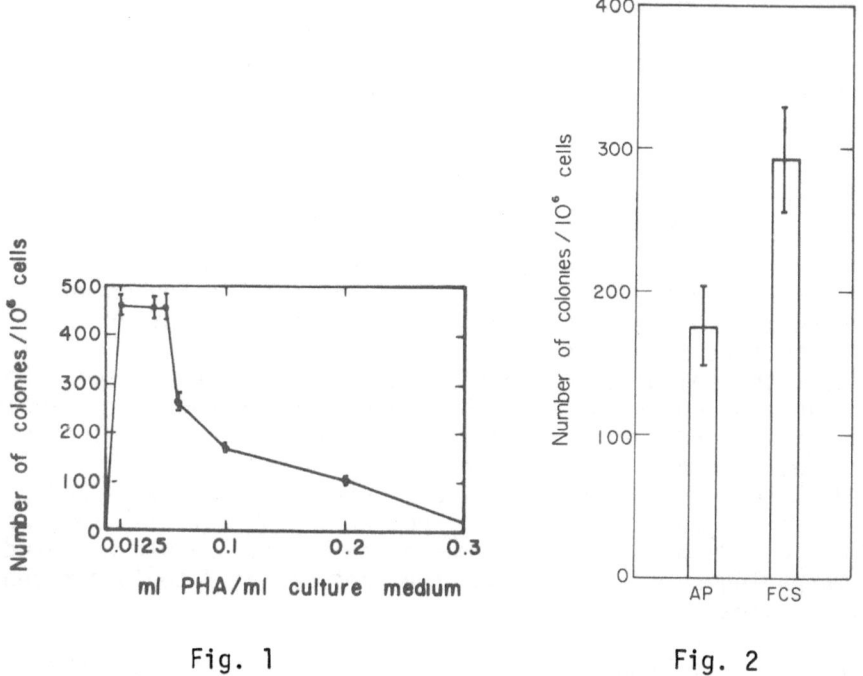

Fig. 1   Fig. 2

Figs. 1 and 2. Lymphocytic colony formation. Fig. 1 (left), comparison of autologous plasma (AP) with fetal calf serum (FCS).
Fig. 2 (right), effect of varying concentrations of PHA.

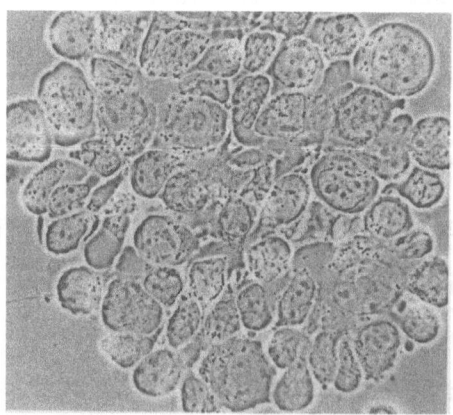

Fig. 3. Appearance in phase contrast microscope of cells derived
from small colony after 5 days of culture.

SRBC rosettes and by 0 to 2 per cent MRBC rosettes. Similar results were obtained from lymphocytes cultured in liquid medium.
The lymphocytes from CLL showed 80 to 90 per cent of MRBC rosettes
and 1 to 4 per cent SRBC rosettes. No rosette-forming ability was
found by using monocytes-macrophages and eosinophils from soft
agar cultures.

No significant immunofluorescence of lymphocytes was detected.

DISCUSSION

The ability of human lymphocytes to grow and develop as colonies in soft agar is demonstrated in the present study. In our
results the colony-forming lymphocytes represent lower values than
those reported by others (5,6). These differences may be explained
by variations in techniques, and by our definition of a colony as
requiring the presence of 50 cells or more. The advantage of the
soft agar system over liquid medium is the ability of locating
colonies made up of cells originating from one blast-like cell.
The mitotic index, under these conditions, exceeds that in liquid
medium by a factor of 50. The difference in the appearance of the
two types of colonies is due to the depth of growth, with small
colonies developing on the surface of the upper agar layer. It is
likely that the earlier developing larger colonies act as feeder
layer stimulating the development of the small colonies. The relationship between the number of colonies and the number of
lymphocytes seeded shows that only a limited proportion of transformed lymphocytes has the potential to divide and grow as colony.

Essential conditions for colony formation are preceding sensitization of lymphocytes with PHA and continuous presence of PHA in
the soft agar culture. Presence of PHA in the agar is required for
completion and resumption of the mitotic cycle, even when lymphocytes had been stimulated with PHA for 72 hours prior to seeding
in agar culture.

A comparison between the number of colonies developing from
cultured bone marrow cells with those from peripheral blood shows
that in proportion to the number of lymphocytes seeded, a larger
number of colonies developed from bone marrow cells. A possible
explanation may be that non-lymphocytic nucleated bone marrow
cells act as feeder layer, thus stimulating clone development.

On the other hand, the lower number of colonies developing
from seeding spleen cells as compared with peripheral blood, may
reflect the higher proportion of B-cells in the spleen (14).
This assumption is supported by our observation that about 20 per
cent of human spleen cells form SRBC rosettes, by contrast with
about 75 per cent of lymphocytes from peripheral blood.

The nature of the colonies cells was determined by studying their rosette forming ability, and by tests for surface immunoglobulin. As judged by the SRBC rosette-forming ability, their morphologic identification by phase contrast microscopy, as well as the MGG staining, the colonies were composed of typical transformed cells similar to those obtained by culturing peripheral blood lymphocytes in presence of PHA in liquid culture media (15). It may be concluded from our results that the colonies are composed of T lymphocytes.

REFERENCES

1. Paran, M., Sachs, L., Barak, Y. and Resnitzky, P.: Proc. Nat. Acad. Sci. 67: 1542, 1970.

2. Chervernick, P.A. and Boggs, D.R.: Blood 37: 131, 1971.

3. Iscove, N., Senn, J.S., Till, J.E. and McCulloch, E.A.: Blood 37: 1, 1971.

4. Shoham, D., Ben David, E. and Rozenszajn, L.A.: Blood 44: 221, 1974.

5. Marshall, W.H., Valentine, F.T. and Lawrence, H.S.: J. Exp. Med. 130: 327, 1969.

6. Chi, K.W. and Bloom, A.O.: Nature 227: 171, 1970.

7. Coulson, A.S., Turk, A., Glade, P.R. and Chessin, L.N.: Lancet I: 89, 1968.

8. Moorhead, P.A., Nowell, P.C., Mellman, W.Y., Battips, D.M. and Hungerford, D.A.: Exp. Cell. Res. 20: 613, 1970.

9. Pluznik, D.H. and Sachs, L.: J. Cell. Comp. Physiol. 66: 319, 1965.

10. Bradley, T.R. and Metcalf, D.: Aust. J. Exp. Biol. Med. Sci. 44: 287, 1966.

11. Wybran, J., Carr, M.C. and Fudenberg, H.H.: J. Clin. Invest. 51: 2537, 1972.

12. Stathopoulos, G. and Elliott, E.: Lancet I: 600, 1974.

13. Aisenberg, A.C. and Bloch, K.J.: New Engl. J. Med. 287: 272, 1972.

14. Rabellino, E., Colon, S., Grey, H.M. and Unanue, E.R.: J. Exp. Med. 133: 156, 1971.

15. Tanaka, Y., Epstein, L.B., Brecher, G. and Stohlman, F.: Blood 22: 614, 1963.

SPONTANEOUS AND INDUCED CHANGES IN THYMUS PATTERN

N. Haran-Ghera, R. Chazan and M. Ben-Yaakov

Department of Chemical Immunology

The Weizmann Institute of Science, Rehovot, Israel

Two major thymocyte subpopulations have been identified within the thymus of different mice strains irrespective of age. The major subpopulation (about 85%) which resides mainly in the cortex is immunoincompetent, cortisone and radiation sensitive, rich in theta (θ) antigen but bears little or no H-2 antigen. The minor subpopulation is immunocompetent, cortisone and radiation resistant, rich in H-2 but low in theta (1-4). In recent studies (5) we have shown that the majority of radiation and radiation leukemia virus induced lymphatic leukemias, consisted of T lymphocytes bearing high levels of surface H-2 alloantigens. Similar findings were obtained recently with spontaneous AKR T lymphatic leukemias. Since the target organ for overt lymphatic leukemia expression is the thymus, the possibility that the different leukemogenic agents could change the pattern of the normal thymus subpopulations and thereby provide the lymphoid population susceptible to neoplastic transformation and/or proliferation was further studied. Tests were performed to find out whether administration of the radiation leukemia virus (injected intraperitoneally or directly into the thymus of C57BL/6 mice) or fractionated whole body irradiation, both agents inducing a high incidence of lymphatic T leukemia in the C57BL strain of mice, could change the thymus pattern transiently for several weeks after leukemogenic treatment. The presence of θ antigen and high levels of H-2 alloantigen on thymocytes within 40-50 days following the leukemogenic treatment was determined using a cytotoxic test (trypan blue dye exclusion test). Anti θ C3H serum (prepared by 6 weekly injections of 10^8 C3H thymus cells into AKR mice) and H-2 alloantiserum - shown to be cytotoxic only to thymocytes having high levels of H-2 antigen (obtained following 6 weekly injections 10^8 C57BL/6 spleen cells into C3H mice), were used in this analysis.

The results are summarized in Fig. 1. Two virus preparations, having different leukemogenic potency (p. 136 being more potent),
were injected intraperitoneally (0.5 ml i.p.) or directly into
both thymus lobes (0.01 ml into each lobe) and the mean percentage
of high H-2 bearing thymocytes was evaluated within 50 days following virus injection. This treatment did indeed change, for several
weeks, the pattern of the normal thymus population, namely, an
abundance of high H-2 thymus derived lymphocytes were present in
the thymus, in spite of the fact that the thymus had already regenerated and almost regained its initial normal weight (Fig. 1 upper
right angle).

    Similar results were obtained when 6-8 week old female C57BL/6
mice were exposed to fractionated irradiation (four weekly doses of
170 R whole body exposure). The mean percentage of high H-2 thymocytes ranged between 50-80% for about 25 days after the last radiation exposure. An interesting observation was obtained when isologous bone marrow cells were injected intravenously within several
hours after the last radiation treatment (a procedure reducing

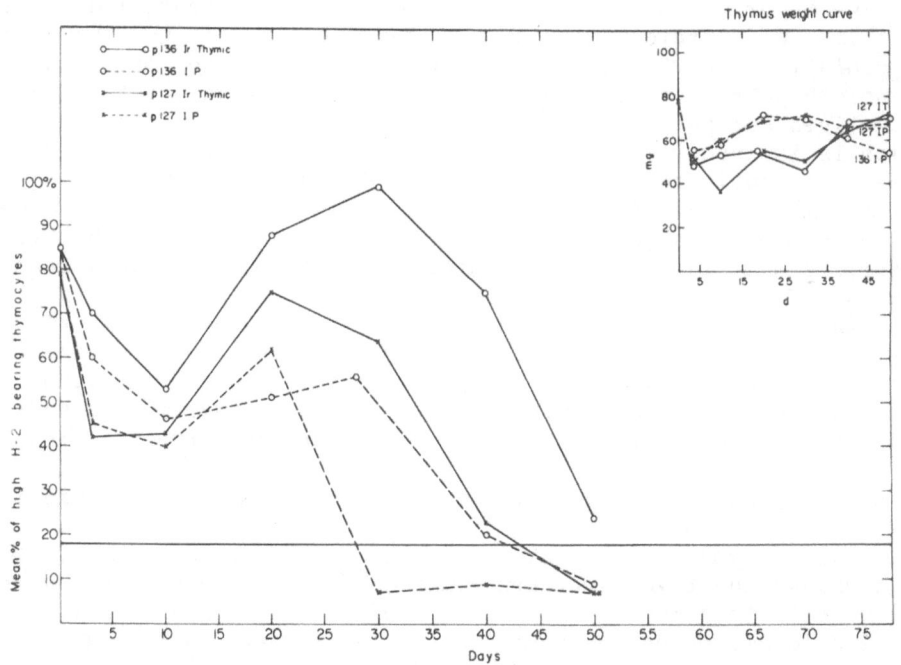

Fig. 1. Mean incidence of high H-2^b alloantigen bearing thymocytes
in C57BL/6 female mice following intraperitoneal (I.P.) or intrathymic (Ir.Thymic) injection of radiation leukemia virus (two
different virus preparations tested). Thymus weight curve (mg)
following virus inoculation is charted in the upper right angle.

TABLE 1. Graft versus host reaction induced by thymus cells from normal and radiation leukemia virus inoculated C57BL/6 mice

No. of cells injected i.p.	Thymus-normal		Thymus-virus inoculated (p.136)		P value
	Number tested	Spleen index	Number tested	Spleen index	
1×10^7	8	1.10 ± 0.07	8	1.03 ± 0.06	P<0.5
2×10^7	5	1.28 ± 0.07	6	1.54 ± 0.11	P<0.1
3×10^7	7	1.21 ± 0.09	7	1.39 ± 0.05	P<0.1
4×10^7	6	1.44 ± 0.14	6	1.67 ± 0.11	P<0.2
5×10^7	6	1.71 ± 0.13	7	2.22 ± 0.13	P<0.05
10^7 normal spleen cells	5	2.28 ± 0.08			

markedly radiation induced leukemia incidence). This treatment reduced drastically the radiation induced elevated high H-2 population pattern; within 7 days following radiation the high H-2 thymocyte population was below the observed normal levels and this decreased level was mainteined at least for 40 days. The lack of the high H-2 thymus subpopulation following radiation and bone marrow treatment could, perhaps, be considered as a factor in preventing leukemic cell proliferation since it might be assumed that a certain level of this population is a prerequisit for overt leukemia development.

Thymocytes bearing low levels of θ antigen and high levels of H-2 are considered to be the immunocompetent cells able to cause a GVH response (6). We therefore tested whether the virus related increase within the thymus of the H-2 population could be correlated with an increased capacity of these thymocytes to induce a GVH response. Thymus cells (10^7-5 x 10^7) taken from virus inoculated C57BL/6 mice (20 days after virus injection) or from normal controls (2 month old), as well as 10^7 normal spleen cells (from 2 month old normal donors) were injected into 10 day old (Balb/c x C57BL/6)F_1 mice and their spleen index was estimated 10 days later. An increase in the ability of thymocytes from virus injected mice as compared to normal thymocytes to evoke a GVH response was indicated (Table 1).

The incidence of spontaneous T lymphoid leukemia in AKR mice exceeds 90% at an average latent period of 12 months. Infectious virus was demonstrated in many tissues of the embryo or the non-leukemic adult AKR mouse, though the thymus, in spite of its being the target organ for overt leukemia development, was shown to have a reduced virus titer when compared to other organs (7,8). Since the administration of a leukemogenic virus was shown previously to

change the thymus population pattern, it seemed of interest to test
the age related thymus population of AKR mice which have an intrinsic leukemogenic virus source responsible for the development of
spontaneous leukemia. The mean percent of high H-2 and θ bearing
thymocytes was evaluated in non leukemic AKR thymuses taken from 1
day old to 15 month old mice. A similar parallel study was carried
out testing C57BL/6 thymuses of similar ages. The results are
summarized in Fig. 2. In normal C57BL/6 mice we found a consistent
low level of 8-22% thymocytes bearing high levels of H-2 throughout
life. In AKR mice a significant spontaneous increase in the high
H-2 thymus subpopulation was observed from 5 month onwards, reaching a 50% incidence in 8 month old non leukemic thymuses and 70%
in one year old non leukemic mice. These age related spontaneous
changes in the pattern of nonleukemic AKR thymuses could contribute
to the ultimate gross proliferation of the disease in the thymus
(providing the susceptible population for leukemic cell proliferation). The long latent period needed for spontaneous leukemia
development in the AKR strain of mice could be affected by the
timing of the spontaneous changes in the thymus pattern.

The general thymus growth pattern involves maximal development
early in life followed by marked involution at the age of several
months. In SJL/J mice a secondary increase in thymus weight is
observed from 7 months onwards. It seemed therefore of interest to

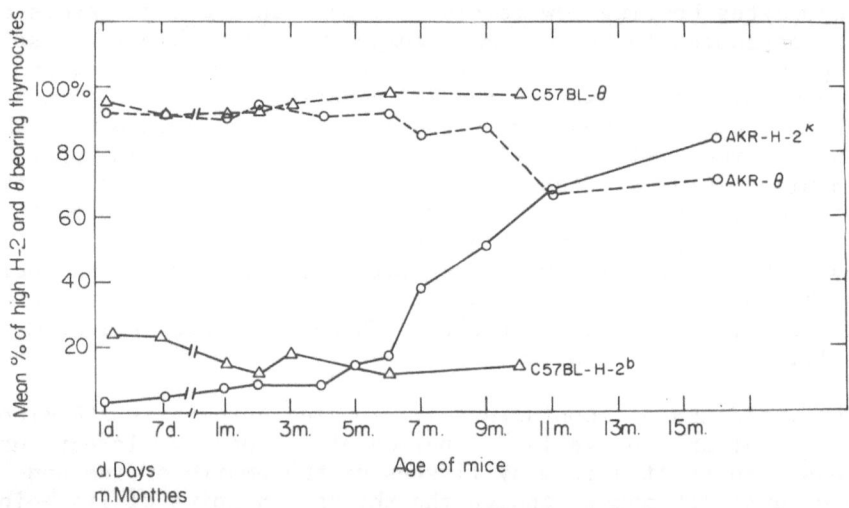

Fig. 2. A comparative age related mean incidence of high H-2 and θ
bearing thymocytes in AKR and C57BL/6 mice.

analyse the thymus population pattern in SJL/J mice in relation to
age increase using membranal antigenic markers. The presence of θ
antigen and high levels of H-2 alloantigen on thymocytes was determined using the cytotoxic test. The incidence of immunoglobulin-
bearing cells was evaluated using the direct immunofluorescent
technique (9). The results obtained are summarized in Fig. 3.
From the age of 4 months onwards a decrease in the percentage of θ
bearing cells and a progressive age related increase in the percentage of thymocytes carrying high levels of the H-2 alloantigen
could be detected in the thymus of SJL/J mice. Increasing incidence of immunoglobulin bearing cells could also be detected in SJL/J
thymuses from the age of 5 months, reaching a 50% incidence of IgG
and 22% IgM bearing cells in the thymus of 15 month old SJL/J mice.
The functional abilities of these B cells present in older SJL/J
thymuses (possessing functions of a peripheral lymphoid organ) have
been described recently (10). The age dependent thymus pattern of
a year old mouse (its thymus analysis indicating mean values of

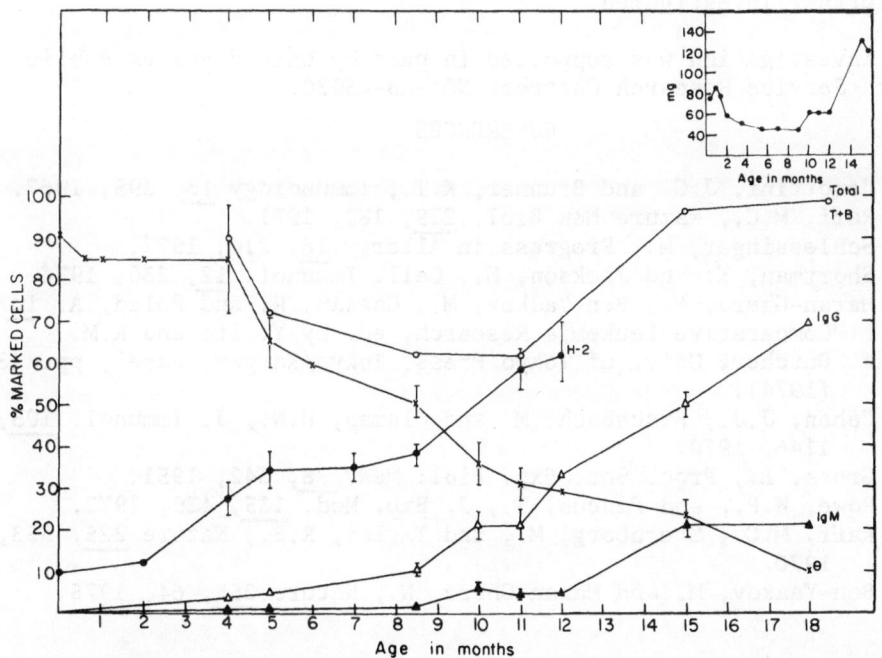

Fig. 3. Changes in weight and cellular composition of SJL/J thymuses with increasing age. Percentage of θ bearing cells and high H-2^S
bearing cells was determined using AKR/J anti θ C3H/eb serum or
C3H/eb anti SJL/J H-2^S serum respectively. The percentage of IgG
and IgM bearing cells was determined by direct immunofluorescence
testing with goat anti mouse IgG or IgM sera. Thymus weight curve
at right angle.

about 30% θ bearing thymocytes, 50% high H-2 bearing thymocytes and 20% immunoglobulin bearing cells) could be reproduced in a newborn isologous thymus grafted under the kidney capsule of 12 month old intact SJL/J mice but not in 12 month old thymectomized mice. Weekly analysis of the subpopulations in these thymus grafts in old intact hosts indicated a progressive drop in the θ bearing thymocytes and an increase in the high H-2 and immunoglobulin bearing cells reaching the level of 40% θ, 40% high H-2 and 15% immunoglobulin bearing lymphoid cells in four week old thymus grafts (the second lobe of each newborn thymus was grafted under the kidney capsule of a two month old intact or thymectomized SJL/J mice and their population pattern was always normal, namely, 90% θ bearing thymocytes and 20% high H-2 bearing thymocytes and no immunoglobulin bearing lymphoid cells). The four week old intrarenal thymus grafts in 12 month old thymectomized mice had the normal thymus population pattern of young mice (86% θ bearing thymocytes and 20% high H-2 bearing thymocytes). These results might suggest the presence of a "thymus regulating factor" in the aging SJL/J thymus which is now further investigated.

This investigation was supported in part by United States Public Health Service Research Contract NO1-CB-43930.

REFERENCES

1. Cerottini, J.C. and Brunner, K.T., Immunology 13, 395, 1967.
2. Raff, M.C., Nature New Biol. 229, 182, 1971.
3. Schlessinger, M., Progress in Allergy 16, 214, 1972.
4. Shortman, K. and Jackson, H., Cell. Immunol. 12, 230, 1974.
5. Haran-Ghera, N., Ben-Yaakov, M., Chazan, R. and Peled, A. in "Comparative Leukemia Research, ed. by Y. Ito and R.M. Dutcher, Univ. of Tokyo Press, Tokyo/Karger, Basel, pp. 133 (1974).
6. Cohen, J.J., Fischbach, M. and Claman, H.N., J. Immunol. 105, 1146, 1970.
7. Gross, L., Proc. Soc. Exp. Biol. Med. 78, 342, 1951.
8. Rowe, W.P., and Pincus, T., J. Exp. Med. 135, 429, 1972.
9. Raff, M.C., Sternberg, M., and Taylor, R.B., Nature 225, 553, 1970.
10. Ben-Yaakov, M. and Haran-Ghera, N., Nature 255, 64, 1975.

THYMOCYTE MATURATION IN AKR LEUKEMIA

Waksal, S.D.*, S. Smolinsky, I.R. Cohen, R.L. St. Pierre, M. Feldman
Weizmann Institute of Science and the Ohio State University. Rehovot, Israel and Columbus, Ohio USA

INTRODUCTION

The central role played by the thymus during leukemogenesis in the AKR mouse is well established (1, 2). The AKR mouse develops lymphocytic lymphoma and leukemia with an incidence of 90% (2). Although this strain is infected with gross virus prior to birth, manifestations of the disease are not apparent until six months of age (3). Therefore, there appears to be a latent period before the onset of thymoma in these animals. The intrathymic events during this latent period are of prime importance since neonatal thymectomy reduces the incidence of leukemia (4).

Differentiation of thymocytes within the thymus leads to the development of immunocompetent, thymus-derived lymphocytes (T-lymphocytes) [5, 6]. The majority of thymocytes contain large amounts of Thy-1 and smaller amounts of H-2 antigens on their surfaces. A smaller population of thymocytes possess small amounts of Thy-1 and larger amounts of H-2 on their surfaces. The former population is considered less mature and predominates in the cortical regions of the thymus while the latter population is more mature and is found largely in medullary regions. Normal thymocytes respond well in vitro to the mitogen concanavalin A and respond poorly to phytohemagglutinin.

The present study examines Thy-1 and H-2 surface antigens as well as mitogen responsiveness of thymocytes in aging AKR mice compared with the low leukemic strain of mouse C3H/hej.

MATERIALS AND METHODS

Animals

Female AKR/J and C3H/hej mice were obtained from Jackson Laboratory in Bar Harbor, Maine and were maintained on Purina Laboratory Chow and water ad libitum.

Antisera

Anti-mouse brain serum was made according to the method of Golub with slight modification. Details of this procedure are described elsewhere (7). Anti-H-2K serum was prepared by injecting C3H.SW mice with lymphocytes from C3H mice.

Mitogens

Concanavalin A (Con A) from Pharmacia Fine Chemicals, Uppsala, Sweden, phytohemagglutinin P (PHA) Difco Laboratories, Detroit, Michigan, lipopolysaccharide, E coli (LPS) were used as phytomitogens.

Cultures

All cultures were performed in triplicate in Microtest II culture plates (Falcon Plastics). Each well contained 8×10^5 thymocytes obtained from each of the different groups of AKR/J and C3H/hej mice suspended in 100 lambda of Dulbecco's modified Eagle's medium (GIBCO, Grand Island, N.Y.) supplemented with 5% fetal calf serum (GIBCO).

Incorporation of ^{3}H-thymidine was assayed for proliferative response in MLR. One microcurie per 0.1 ml of ^{3}H-thymidine (6 Ci/mmole) was added for the final 10 hours of culture. Cultured cells were harvested on glass wool filter paper with a multiple automatic sample harvester and ^{3}H-thymidine incorporation expressed as counts per minute.

Cytotoxicity Test

The test of cytotoxicity of the antisera was a modification of the technique of Gorer and O'Gorman (8). Single cell suspen-

sions of thymocytes were prepared. The concentration was adjusted
to $5x10^6$ viable cells/ml, as determined by trypan blue exclusion.
Five hundredths ml quantities of antisera, of thymocytes
($5x10^6$/ml), and of guinea pig complement (diluted 1:4) were placed
in tubes and incubated for 45 minutes at 37°C in 5% CO_2. Viability
was determined by trypan blue exclusion. Titers were recorded as
the reciprocal of the dilutions of anti-mouse brain serum (anti-
MB) and anti-H-2K serum causing 50% cell death.

RESULTS

Mitogen Responsiveness

Thymocyte populations (Table 1) derived from C3H/hej mice aged
6-8 weeks, 16-24 weeks and greater than 24 weeks uniformly exhibited
a very high response to Con A and a significantly lower response to
PHA as expressed in the low PHA/Con A ratio. No significant response was elicited in any of these groups by LPS, a B-lymphocyte
mitogen. A similar response to these mitogens was observed in AKR
mice aged 6-8 weeks. Thymocytes from AKR mice 16-24 weeks of age
showed a significant decrease in Con A responsiveness as well as
a significant and dramatic increase in PHA responsiveness, while
LPS responsiveness remained low. Thymocytes from animals aged 16-
24 weeks exhibited a further decrease in Con A responsiveness and
further increase in PHA responsiveness. Thymocytes from this latter
age group showed a negligible response to LPS.

Analysis of Thy-1 and H-2

Thymocyte populations from C3H mice showed no decrease in
concentration of Thy-1 (brain-associated) until after 18 weeks of
age and then only showed a slight decrease (Table 2). Thymocytes
from AKR mice at 6-8 weeks of age contain a large amount of Thy-1
on their surface. At the 16-24 week stage, AKR thymocytes begin
to show a reduction in Thy-1. This reduction continues into the
thymoma (24 week) stage in which the majority of cells demonstrate
low concentrations of Thy-1. Concentrations of H-2 are low in the
early stages of examination of C3H thymocytes, and there is only a
slight increase with age. AKR thymocytes bear low concentrations
of H-2 antigens at 6-8 weeks of age. At 16 weeks of age, thymocytes from AKR mice demonstrate a significant increase in H-2.
This increase continues steadily into the thymoma stage (Table 2).

TABLE 1

MITOGEN RESPONSES OF THYMOCYTE POPULATIONS FROM AKR AND C3H MICE
UPTAKE OF H^3-THYMIDINE IN CPM[a]

Thymocyte Source	Control	PHA	Con A	LPS	PHA/Con A ratio[b]
AKR 6–8 weeks of age	57±16	990±87	6973±2214	396±94	0.12
AKR 16–24 weeks of age	89±37	5297±185	4562±241	598±256	1.16
AKR 24+ leuke-mic	377±43	6921±385	2422±185	323±41	2.85
C3H 6–8 weeks of age	89±27	957±154	6663±502	367±88	0.14
C3H 16–24 weeks of age	145±36	703±96	6001±307	509±103	0.11
C3H 24+	167±45	1027±102	5760±239	617±95	0.18

[a]counts per minute of incorporation of ^{3}H-thymidine in cultures of 8×10^5 responding thymocytes.

[b]ratios were computed by dividing responses in cpm of PHA by cpm of Con A.

TABLE 2

CYTOTOXIC TITERS OF ANTI-H-2K AND ANTI-MOUSE
BRAIN SERA AGAINST AKR AND C3H THYMOCYTE POPULATIONS

	CYTOTOXIC TITERS[a]						
	AKR Age in Weeks				C3H Age in Weeks		
	6–12	16	20	24+ (leukemic)	6–12	6–24	24+
Anti-H-2K	32	128	256	512	32	32	64
Anti-MB	256	128	64	32	512	512	256

[a]Titers were recorded as the reciprocal of the dilution of anti-mouse brain serum (anti-MB) and anti-H-2K serum causing 50% cell death.

DISCUSSION

The present study shows AKR thymocytes undergo changes in the concentration of surface antigens and in mitogen reactivity during their aging process. These changes include a decrease in the concentration of Thy-1 antigen and an increase in the concentration of H-2 antigens. Additionally, these changes in Thy-1 and H-2 antigens have also been shown using a fluorescence activated cell sorter (Waksal, S.D. et al., in preparation). Thymocytes from 16-24 week old AKR mice also show a dramatic shift in the PHA/Con A ratio. These changes correlate well with the observed cortical-medullary inversion in the thymus of pre-leukemic AKR mice (9).

Earlier studies on AKR leukemic have shown that the neoplastic cells are of T-lymphocyte origin and mimic many characteristics of normal T-lymphocytes (10). The thymus is responsible for the differentiation and maturation of precursor cells to peripheral T-lymphocytes (5). During this differentiation process Thy-1 antigen concentration decreases in order from the large subcapsular cells, small cortical, and mid-sized medullary cells. H-2 antigen concentration increases in this order (6). It has been postulated that the thymus epithelium and/or its product is responsible for these intrathymic events (11). The changes in the pre-leukemic AKR thymus indicate an increase in the normal process of thymocyte differentiation. These changes may be due to an accelerated maturational process induced by the AKR thymus epithelium.

It has been shown that the AKR thymus is more effective in stimulating lymphopoiesis and inducing T-lymphocyte differentiation than the thymus of low leukemic strains (12, Waksal, S.D. et al., in preparation). The reticuloepithelial cells of the AKR thymus grow more rapidly than those from low leukemic strains, with the most rapid growth observed in epithelium from thymomas. (Waksal, S.D., unpublished observations).

Thus the T-lymphocyte lymphoma in this system may involve a basic defect in the thymus reticuloepithelium and/or its product which may allow the triggering of the viral oncogene present in the precursor cells.

ACKNOWLEDGEMENTS

The authors wish to express their appreciation to E. A. Latham-Griffin for excellent technical assistance and Barbara Jordan for typing the manuscript.

REFERENCES

1. Miller, J.F.A.P. Nature 191:248, 1961.
2. Metcalf, D. The Thymus, Recent Results in Cancer Research,
        Vol. 5, Springer-Verlag, Inc., New York, 1966.
3. Gross, L.   Proc. Soc. Exp. Biol. Med., 78:342, 1951.
4. Miller, J.F.A.P. Br. J. Cancer 14:93, 1960.
5. Raff, M.C. and Wortis, H.H. Immunology 18:931, 1970.
6. Weissman, I.L., Small, M., Fathman, C.G. and Herzenberg, L.A.
        Fed. Proc., 34:143, 1975
7. Waksal, S.D., R.L. St. Pierre, J.R. Hostetler, and R.M. Folk.
        Cell. Immunol., 12:66, 1974.
8. Gorer, P.A. and O'Gorman, P. Transplant. Bull., 3:142, 1956.
9. Metcalf, D. J. Nat. Cancer Inst., 37:425, 1966.
10. Barker, A.D. and Waksal, S.D. Cell. Immunol., 12:140, 1974.
11. Waksal, S.D., Cohen, I.R., Waksal, H.W., St. Pierre, R.L. and
        Feldman, M. Ann. N.Y. Acad. Sci., 249:492, 1975.
12. Auerbach, R. IN: Epithelial Mesechymal Interactions. (R.
        Fleischmajer and R.G. Billingham, eds.), p. 200, 1968.

*Dr. Waksal's present address:
    Immunology Branch
    National Cancer Institute
    National Institutes of Health
    Bethesda, Maryland 20014

LYMPHOCYTES AND HEMOPOIETIC BONE MARROW CELLS - ANTIGENIC RELATIONSHIPS BETWEEN THESE CELLS AND LYMPHATIC TISSUE REPOPULATION FROM STEM CELLS

W.Müller-Ruchholtz, H.-U.Wottge, H.K.Müller-Hermelink

Immunol.Unit, Inst.of Hygiene and Dept. of Pathology

Med.School of the Univ.,D-23 Kiel, Fed. Rep. Germany

Attempts to separate bone marrow (BM) lymphocytes from hemopoietic BM cells are of increasing interest but opposed by many difficulties. A complete separation would allow for better understanding of the relationship between these cells, including the early events of lymphocyte formation. The most important practical aspects can be expected in BM transplantation since complete elimination of lymphocytes could prevent GVHR. Our separation attempts were based on the observation that different types of cells within the same organism can exhibit different patterns of surface antigenic determinants. Thus the following questions were asked:(1)To what extent do lymphocyte cell surface antigens,i.e.physiologically accessible antigens, share determinants with the surfaces of the different hemopoietic cells and consequently, how can cell type-specific antilymphocyte sera be prepared? (2)To what extent and how fast does repopulation of lymphatic organs occur in lethally irradiated rats after restitution with lymphocyte-free as compared to untreated BM in syngeneic or strongly allogeneic donor/recipient combinations?

MATERIALS AND METHODS

Specimens of rabbit antisera against rat thymic lymphocytes were used unabsorbed (ALS-O) or after absorption with equal vol. of rat erythrocytes (ALS-E), $5 \cdot 10^8$/ml cultivated peritoneal exudate cells (ALS-EP), and $2 \cdot 10^8$/ml liver cells from 20-day old fetuses (ALS-EPLf). Unless indicated a serum pool was used and each absorption done 3 times. 10^8 rat BM cells/ml were incubated in undil. antiserum; for in vivo experiments undil. fresh rat serum was added as the source of complement;incubation time was 30 min.at 37°C. For antibody-labeling of incubated BM cells, sheep-anti-rabbit IgG was conjugated with peroxidase and evaluat-

ed electron microscopically. Restoration of lethally irradiated
(1275 rads from a ^{60}Co source)LEW rats was achieved with 2·10^8 syngeneic or 6·10^8 strongly and fully allogeneic CAP BM cells,half
of them being injected i.v.after 2 and 18 hrs. resp. Lymphatic
chimerism was tested with a lymphocytotoxic LEW-anti-CAP-serum
in trypan-blue dye exclusion tests.

RESULTS

The first question asked above was answered by in vitro experiments. The serological absorption data are shown in Fig.1,
indicating the same for 19 different antisera:(1) Each absorption was done exhaustively, as indicated by the maintenance of
a titer plateau upon repetition. (2) Erythrocytes and peritoneal cells eliminated different antibodies, as indicated by the titer drop upon changing the absorbens. This demonstrates the presence of 3 different antibody specifities in ALS-O, one of which
is reactive with the descendants of the erythropoietic cell line,
the other being reactive with myelopoiesis derived cells (peritoneal cells, i.e. macrophages and granulocytes).

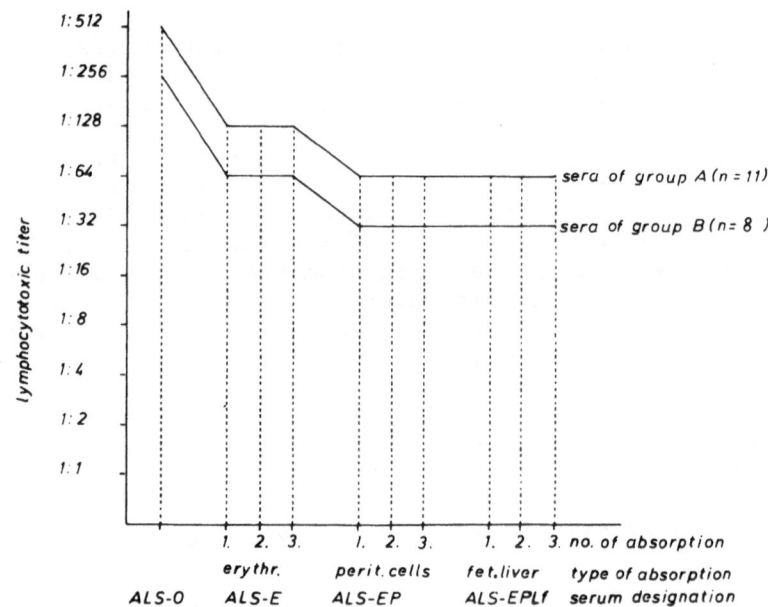

Fig.1: Lymphocytotoxicity of differently absorbed ALS.

The relevance of these absorptions for BM cells could be
shown morphologically after addition of peroxidase-conjugated
anti-rabbit IgG to ALS-incubated BM (Fig.2 and Tab.1). The following was found:(1) After incubation in ALS-O the surfaces of
all cells are labeled by a continuous layer of peroxidase reaction products. (2) ALS-E leaves unlabeled erythrocytes and late
normoblasts. (3) ALS-EP leaves additionally unlabeled mature my-

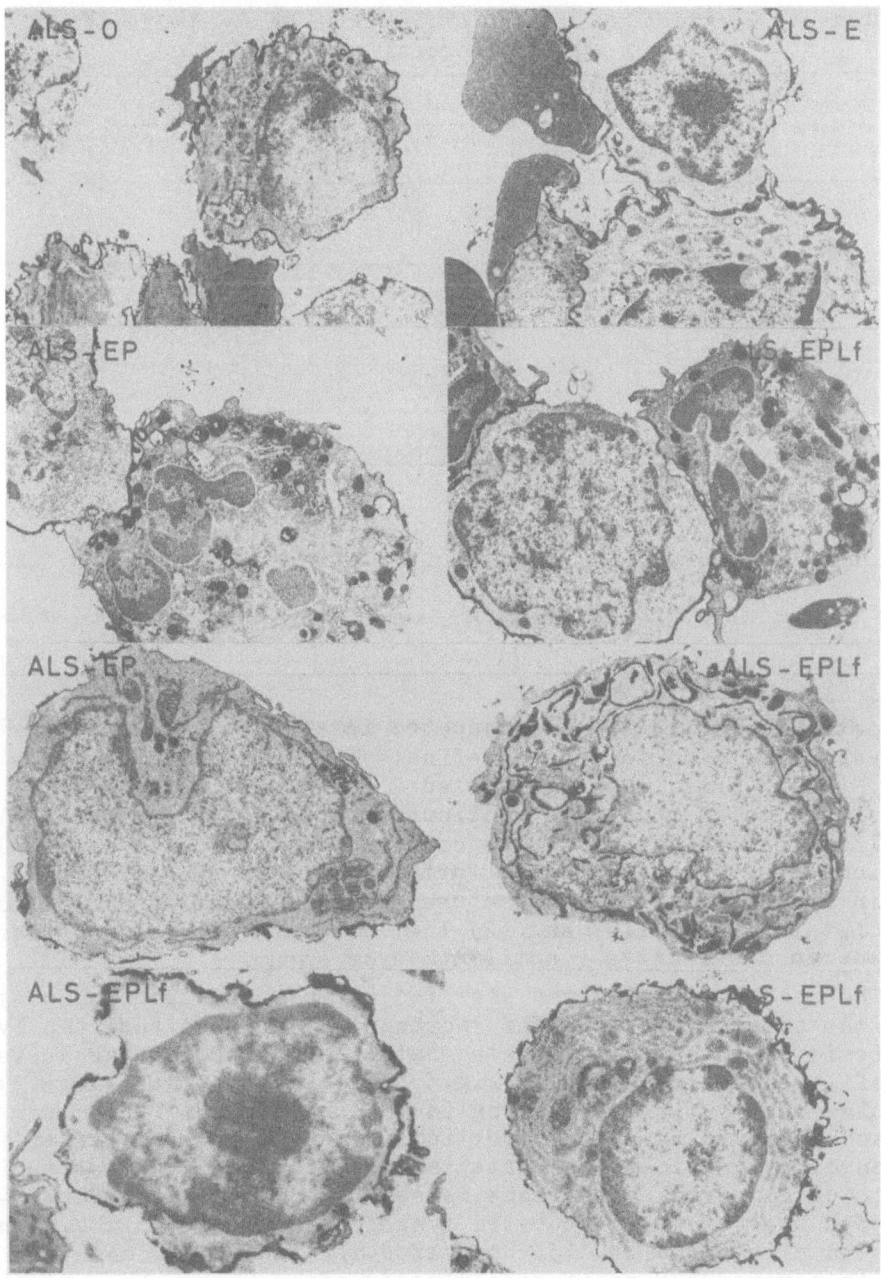

Fig.2: Peroxidase labeling of the surfaces of different hemopoietic cells, BM lymphocytes (second right and lower left) and
plasma cells (lower right) after incubation in differently absorbed ALS.

Table 1:   Peroxidase-Labeling of Rat Bone Marrow Cells after
           Incubation with Differently Absorbed ALS

Rabbit-Anti-Rat Lymphocyte-Serum (ALS)	Lymphoid Cells			Myelopoietic Cells		Erythropoietic Cells		Megakaryo-cytes
	Lympho-cytes	Blasts	Plasma-cells	early	late	early	late	
ALS unabsorbed	+	+	+	+	+	+	+	+
ALS - E	+	+	+	+	+	+	Ø	(+)
ALS - EP	+	+	+	(+)	Ø	(+)	0	Ø
ALS - EPL	+	+	+	Ø	0	Ø	0	0
Controls RtNS , RbNS - EP	0	0	0	0	0	0	0	0

elopoietic cells. (4)ALS-EP incubated immature erythropoietic
and myelopoietic cells show a definite but only patchy surface
label. (5)ALS-EPLf leaves unlabeled all hemopoietic cells but
still leads to an unchanged continuous labeling of lymphocytes
and plasma cells. These results confirm the serological data. In
addition, they show (1) that a further antibody specificity exists in ALS, reactive with immature hemopoietic cells and absorbed by fetal liver cells, and (2) that combined absorption definitely leads to a selectively antilymphocyte serum.

The second question was answered by in vivo experiments studying the capacity of ALS-EPLf incubated BM to restitute the lymphopoiesis of lethally irradiated rats. The morphological appearance of lymph nodes, shown in Fig.3, revealed the following:(1)
A regular restitution, beginning in the B-dependent follicular
zone and followed by the paracortical zone, takes place after injection of syngeneic or incubated allogeneic BM. (2) The time interval, until normal appearance is seen, varies considerably:3-5
wks. with untreated or incubated syngeneic BM, but 6-8 wks.with
incubated allogeneic BM. (3) Untreated allogeneic BM, however,
leads to severe GVHR manifested already after 2 wks. by a gross
enlargement of the lymph nodes with infiltration of the paracortical zone by activated macrophages and immunoblasts, and still
expressed by lymphocyte deprivation after 6-8 wks. in the small
group of survivors. Correspondingly, the thymus showed lymphatic

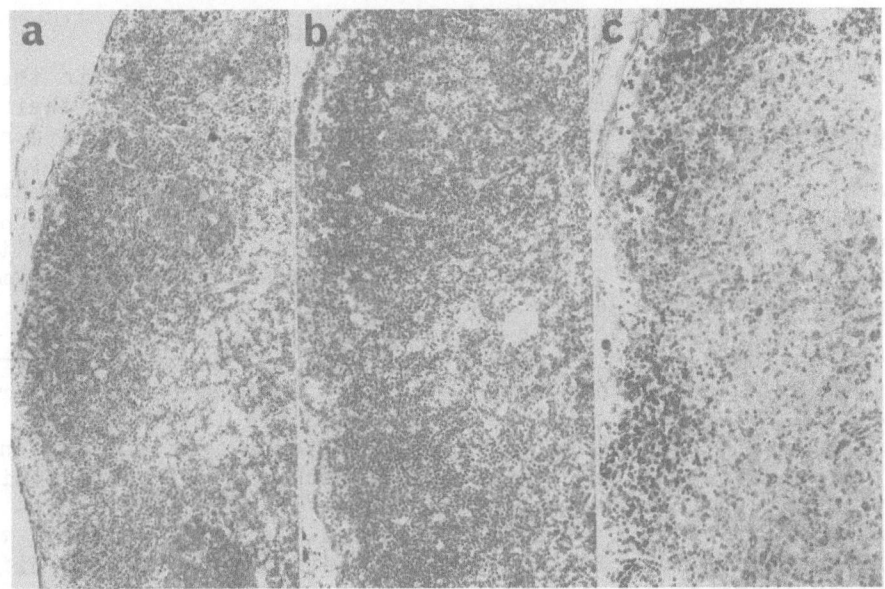

Fig.3: Appearance of lymph nodes 42 days after lethal irradia-
       tion and grafting of syngeneic (a), incubated allogeneic
       (b), or untreated allogeneic (c) BM. (140 x)

restitution in the former groups but infiltration leading to a-
trophy in the group of untreated allogeneic BM recipients.

      Lymphatic chimerism in the LEW recipients of incubated allo-
geneic (CAP) BM was proven by alloantisera, as shown in Tab.2.
The percentage of CAP cells, detectable by cytotoxicity tests
in lymph nodes and spleen, increased remarkably with time after
restitution. Since the CAP control values average only 80%, the
chimerism data are to be considered as lower limit figures.

Tab.2: Cytotoxic effects of LEW-anti-CAP-serum.

			time after restitution (weeks)		
			2	4	52
% killed cells	restituted animals	lymph-node	11 — 13	19 — 22	47 — 55
		spleen	5 — 10	11 — 14	53 — 57
	bone marrow donors	lymph-node	78 — 82	79 — 84	78 — 83
		spleen	72 — 78	74 — 80	75 — 77

DISCUSSION AND CONCLUSIONS

The general rule that different types of cells within the
same organism can be distinguished by the differences in their
surface antigenic determinant patterns has attracted our attention in earlier extensive studies on cell type specificity of
xenogeneic antilymphocyte and antimacrophage sera. The presented
data demonstrate its applicability for the distinction between
lymphocytes and the different hemopoietic cells: In addition to
other antibodies, ALS contains antibodies against at least 3 lymphocyte membrane antigens which are shared by mature erythropoietic or myelopoietic or by immature hemopoietic cells; at
least one of these antigens is absent from the mentioned mature
cells. This suggests that lymphocytes are antigenically more related to hemopoietic cells the less mature the latter are and
is in line with the contention that (a) lymphocytes are descendants of hemopoietic stem cells and (b) each line of hemopoietic
differentiation includes a loss or hiding of some and the appearance of other cell surface structures. As to be expected the
described absorptions did not lead to distinctions between different sublines of lymphocytes: ALS-EPLf was still cytotoxic
for all lymph node lymphocytes at 1:32 dil.

This observation indicates the usefulness of ALS-EPLf for
the study of lymphatic tissue repopulation following restitution
of lethally irradiated animals with lymphocyte-free BM. The most
direct evidence for repopulation from grafted cells is derived
from the chimerism tests using allotransplantation antigens as
markers. The remarkable potential of lymphocyte-free BM to restore lymphatic tissue may best be seen by comparing the recipients of syngeneic untreated and incubated BM: the latter
showed only marginal delay of restoration. The 3-4 wks. delay
of recovery of lymphatic tissues after injection of incubated
allogeneic as compared to syngeneic BM, in spite of 3 times more
cells, may be due to some as yet unexplained inhibitory effect
of the allogeneic environment, which appears to be relatively
limited in view of the strongly and fully (not semi-) allogeneic strain combination used.

GVHR was found only after grafting of untreated allogeneic
BM. This may indicate that those attempts to allograft BM, which
have been reported in literature as being complicated by early
or late GVHR, did not succeed in a complete elimination of lymphocytes and/or their determined precursors. Our data do not
support the contention that newly derived lymphatic descendants
of stem cells initiate GVHR in an allogeneic environment: The
long standing (> 1 year) lymphatic chimeras with normal morphological appearance of lymphatic tissues accepted skin grafts
of BM donors lifelong but rejected third party grafts at nearly
normal speed.

DEMONSTRATION OF TWO DISTINCT MACROPHAGE SPECIFIC ANTIGENIC DETERMINANTS IN RATS

O. Förster and G. Nitulescu

Inst. for General and Exptl. Pathology

Univ. of Vienna, A 1090 Vienna, Austria

Several authors have demonstrated differences in the reactivity of antimacrophage sera with various types of macrophages (1, 2, 3, 4). Interest has been primarily focussed on alveolar and peritoneal macrophages. Some of the authors, however, have claimed to detect basic antigenic differences between free and fixed macrophages (1, 2).

Our studies were intended to investigate, whether such differences in the antigenic structure of various macrophage populations are qualitative or merely quantitative. This question can be answered by the performance of exhaustive cross absorptions, a study which has not been done by previous investigators.

Materials and methods:
Antisera against rat alveolar (ARAMS) and peritoneal (ARPMS) macrophages were raised in rabbits by repeated intradermal inoculation with adherent cells from lavage fluid of rat lungs or peritoneal cavity, respectively. The rats were male, 250 grams, of an outbred strain (SIV 50, S. Ivanovas, Kisslegg/Allgäu, West Germany). They were stimulated intraperitoneally with 10 ml 10 % proteose—peptone 4 days before sacrifice. After killing the animals with ether the peritoneal cavity was rinsed with 40 ml heparinized Hanks—BSS containing 1 % fetal bovine serum (FBS). The alveolar cells were harvested by rinsing the lungs through the trachea with the same fluid containing 0,25 % EDTA. After centrifugation for 5 minutes at 120 x g and two washes in Hanks—BSS + 1 % FBS the cells were resuspended in TC—medium 199 + 10 % FBS to a concentration of 10^7 cells per 10 ml of medium and plated into TC—Petri dishes and cultured at 37°C in a 95 % air – 5 % CO_2 athmo—

sphere. After 3 hours non adherent cells were removed and culture continued for 20 hours. Then the cells were rinsed again and brought into suspension in PBS with rubber policemen, washed twice in PBS and incorporated in complete Freund's adjuvant (Difco). 3 rabbits were immunized 5 times in weekly intervals with a total of $17,1 \times 10^7$ rat peritoneal macrophages (RPM), 3 rabbits in the same course with $18,1 \times 10^7$ rat alveolar macrophages (RAM). Before the third and each of the following boosters 40 ml blood was drawn, the sera heat-inactivated (56°C – 30 minutes) and stored frozen until use. Before testing their reactivity with various cells in indirect membrane immunofluorescence (IMF) (5) the sera were absorbed with glutaraldehyde treated (6) rat plasma (4×40 mg/ml), with rat erythrocytes (RBC) ($4 \times 1:5$ v/v) and nonadherent, mechanically isolated kidney cells ($4 \times 1:10$ v/v). Where indicated, cell preparations were incubated with nylon wool (Leuko–Pak, Fenwal Labs) to remove adherent cells. For each absorption with RAM and RPM 10^8 washed, unfractionated, packed cells of alveolar or peritoneal lavage fluid per ml antiserum was used.

To demonstrate binding of antibodies in IMF tests (or indirect immunofluorescence on cryostat sections) a FITC-conjugated goat-anti-rabbit gammaglobulin-serum (Behringwerke, Marburg/Lahn, West Germany, Ch. Nr. F 458) with a F/P ratio of 3,0 and an antibody content of 16 precipitation units was used in a final concentration of 1:64.

Results:

Immunization of rabbits with adherent cells from rat alveolar or peritoneal lavage fluids elicited antibodies reacting with a variety of cells and with plasma proteins. After absorption of the antisera with nonadherent rat kidney cells – to remove species specific antigens – with insolubilized plasma proteins, and with RBCs they were tested in IMF using five-fold dilutions on adherent and nonadherent cells of various tissues. The results are summarized in tables 1 and 2.

Titers were constant after the first bleeding. Sera from the first bleeding, although somewhat lower in titer, did not seem to be more specific for the immunizing cell type. All sera reacted not only with macrophages but also with lymphocytes of spleen, thymus, bone marrow and peripheral blood. Repeated absorptions with nonadherent spleen- and thymus cells removed this reactivity with lymphocytes, in some cases without a loss in titer against macrophages. A small fraction (about 5 %) of nonadherent bone marrow cells, however, still showed some straining with these lymphocyte-absorbed sera. This staining could be removed by absorption with nonadherent bone marrow cells.

Table 1:   IMF – titers of P–E–K absorbed* antimacrophage sera
on the cell type used for immunization.

	ARAMS			ARPMS	
rabbit Nr.	bleeding Nr.	titer (log 5)	rabbit Nr.	bleeding Nr.	titer (log 5)
122	1	8	181	1	6
	4	9		4	7
123	1	8	182	1	6
	4	9		4	7
124	1	8	183	1	6
	4	9		4	7

* absorbed with insolubilized rat plasma, erythrocytes and
nonadherent kidney cells.

Table 2:   IMF – titers of P–E–K absorbed* antimacrophage sera
(4th bleeding) on various cell types.

cell type	ARAMS Nr.			ARPMS Nr.		
	122/4	123/4	124/4	181/4	182/4	183/4
	titer (log5)			titer (log5)		
alveolar	9	9	9	5	5	5
peritoneal	6	6	6	7	7	7
liver**	5	5	6	5	5	5
spleen total	5	5	5	4	4	4
spleen nonadherent	4	4	4	4	4	4
thymus total	4	4	5	4	4	4
thymus nonadherent	4	4	4	4	3	4
bone marrow total	4	5	5	4	4	4
bone marrow nonadherent	4	4	4	4	3	4
PBL***	4	4	4	3	4	4
kidney total	4	4	4	4	3	3
kidney nonadherent	0****	0	0	0	0	0

* absorbed as in table 1,   ** indirect immunofluorescence on liver
cryostat sections. Only sinusoidal lining cells were stained
*** peripheral blood lymphocytes
****   0 = no reaction with 1:5 diluted antiserum

Sera absorbed with plasmaproteins, erythrocytes and nonadherent cells from kidney, spleen and thymus (P-E-K-L) still showed differences in titer between alveolar and peritoneal macrophages. ARAMS gave higher titers on RAM, ARPMS higher titers on RPM. If repeated cross-absorptions of these sera were performed with RAM or RPM, respectively, the titers were successively lowered on both cell types, approximately in parallel. A transient specificity for the cell type not used for absorptions could be obtained, further cross-absorptions, however, abolished all IMF-staining on both cell types. An example for one ARAMS and for one ARPMS is given in tables 3 and 4. The results with all the other sera - whether taken from early or from late bleedings - were basically identical.

Conclusions

Previous reports about differences in the reactivity of anti-macrophage sera with alveolar and peritoneal macrophages were confirmed by our results. Such differences could be explained in several ways. They could be caused by the occurrence of determinants specific for one cell type - in addition to those common to both cell types. On the other hand, they can be due to a different distribution of two or more macrophage specific determinants in the two cell populations - either present on different cells or on the same cell.

Our results of the cross absorptions seem to exclude the first possibility of RAM- and RPM-specific determinants. They also show the importance of exhaustive absorptions: after seven absorptions of ARPMS 183/4 with RAM the serum reacted only with RPM, not with RAM. On the other hand a specificity for RAM was obtained after seven absorptions of ARAMS 124/4 with RPM. At this point the occurrence of RAM- and RPM-specific determinants could have been postulated. Further cross-absorptions, however, removed also this reactivity.

Therefore, the existence of at least two different macrophage specific determinants with different distribution in various macrophage populations has to be assumed. It cannot be decided from our experiments, whether these determinants are common to all macrophages on which they are present in different density, or whether they are specific for one cell type, which contributes in different numbers to the various macrophage populations.

Furthermore, our results seem not to justify the division of macrophages into two antigenically distinct categories as has been proposed (1, 2). Macrophages from other organs behave quite differently in their reactivity with ARAMS and ARPMS, as judged from their IMF- and IIF-titers.

Table 3:   IMF-titers (log 5) on RAM and RPM of P-E-K-L absorbed*
           ARAMS 124/4 after repeated absorptions with RAM and RPM.

number of absorption with RAM	IMF-titers on		number of absorption with RPM	IMF-titers on	
	RAM	RPM		RAM	RPM
0	8	5	0	8	5
1	7	5	1	7	4
2	6	4	2	7	4
3	5	4	3	6	3
4	4	3	4	5	3
5	3	3	5	4	2
6	2	2	6	3	1
7	1	2	7	2	0
8	0**	1	8	1	0
9	0	0	9	0	0

* absorbed with insolubilized rat plasma, erythrocytes, nonadherent
kidney-, spleen- and thymus cells.

** 0 = no reaction with 1:5 diluted antiserum.

Table 4:   IMF-titers (log 5) on RAM and RPM of P-E-K-L absorbed*
           ARPMS 183/4 after repeated absorptions with RAM and RPM.

number of absorption with RAM	IMF-titers on		number of absorption with RPM	IMF-titers on	
	RAM	RPM		RAM	RPM
0	5	7	0	5	7
1	4	6	1	5	6
2	4	6	2	4	5
3	3	5	3	4	4
4	3	4	4	3	4
5	2	4	5	3	3
6	1	3	6	2	2
7	0**	2	7	2	1
8	0	1	8	1	0
9	0	0	9	0	0

* and ** = see table 3

Interestingly, kidneys contained adherent cells, which reacted with antimacrophage sera after absorption with nonadherent kidney cells. The nature of these cells has not been identified.

Nonadherent bone marrow cells retain some reactivity even after absorption of antimacrophage sera with other nonadherent cells, particularly lymphocytes. These cells may be promonocytes, which do not adhere to nylon fibers but possess already antigenic determinants of the mononuclear phagocyte system.

The reactivity of P–E–K–absorbed antimacrophage sera with lymphocytes may be due to antilymphocyte–antibodies elicited by a contamination of the immunizing cell population by some lymphocytes. Some authors, however, have postulated common antigenic determinants for rat lymphocytes and macrophages (7, 8). Additional experiments should answer this question.

Summary:

Exhaustive cross–absorptions of rabbit anti–rat alveolar macrophage sera with peritoneal macrophages and of anti–rat peritoneal macrophage sera with alveolar macrophages did not prove the existence of antigenic determinants specific for alveolar or peritoneal macrophages. Titer–differences of these sera on RAM and RPM seem to be caused by a different distribution of two or more macrophage specific determinants present in both cell populations.

Macrophages from other rat tissues show reactivity with these two sera different as well from alveolar as from peritoneal macrophages.

Acknowledgements:

This study has been supported by a grant from the Austrian Research Council, project Nr. 2595.

R e f e r e n c e s

1) Montfort, I. and Tamayo, R.P. (1971)
        Proc. Soc. Exp. Biol. Med. 138, 204–207
2) Martinez, R.D. and Montfort, I. (1973). Immunology 25, 197–204
3) Feldman, J.D., Tubergen, D.G., Pollock, E.M. and Unanue, E.R.
        (1972). Cell. Immunol. 5, 325–337
4) Dressler, D. and Skornik, W.A. (1974). J. Reticuloendothel.Soc.
        15, 55a
5) Möller, G. (1961). J. Exp. Med. 114, 415–432
6) Avrameas, S. and Ternynck, T. (1969). Immunochemistry 6, 53–66
7) MacLaurin, B.P. and Humm, J.A. (1970). Clin.exp.Immun.6, 125–136
8) Jasin, H.E., Lennard, D. and Ziff, M.(1971).Clin.exp.I.8,801–814

SURFACE PROPERTIES OF LYMPHOID CELLS - SUMMING UP

Michael Schlesinger

Department of Experimental Medicine & Cancer Research

The Hebrew University-Hadassah Medical School
Jerusalem, Israel

Great efforts have been made to deliniate the cell surface properties of distinct populations of lymphocytes in experimental animals and in man. To the many tools at our disposal for discrimination between T- and B-cells, a new technique has now been added. The demonstration of non-specific esterase activity in T-lymphocytes promises not only to serve as a useful marker, but may also shed light on the distinct biochemical activity of lymphocyte populations. It now remains to be seen in what T-specific reactions the esterase activity may be of importance.

There is a great heterogeneity among the lymphocytes in the thymus. The murine thymus contains a minor population of TL-negative cells, which possess a low θ- and Ly-antigenicity and are rich in H-2 antigenicity and a major population, rich in the TL, θ and Ly-antigens but poor in H-2. Closer analysis of the major population by fractionation on BSA-gradients reveals, however, a whole spectrum of cells, bearing different quantities of thymus-distinctive antigens (1).

We have heard today that the thymus of AKR mice with leukemic changes shows an increase of the minor thymic population, possessing a relatively low θ-antigenicity and high H-2 antigenicity. The thymus of leukemic animals showed an increased PHA responsiveness and greater reactivity in the mixed lymphocyte reaction. These changes, reminiscent of those occurring in the thymus of cortisone-treated mice, may be attributed to leukemogenic factors. Some of the age-related changes in the thymus may occur, however, in the absence of leukemic transformation.

Age-dependent changes are very striking in the thymus of man. The responsiveness to PHA and Con A of human thymus cells increases

markedly with advancing age (2). Another striking age-dependent
change is the proportion of thymus cells forming stable E-rosettes.
In man the majority of the thymus cells differ from the majority of
human peripheral T-lymphocytes in their capacity to form E-rosettes
with sheep red blood cells which do not disintegrate upon incubation
at 37°C. Examination of thymus cell suspensions of individuals
of various ages shows that with increasing age the proportion of
thymus cells forming "stable" rosettes decreases gradually (2).

Thymus subpopulations also differ in their capacity to stimulate in mixed lymphocyte reactions. Cells belonging to the minor
immunocompetent population in the thymus of either mice or man,
stimulate the blastogenic response of allogeneic lymphocytes, while
cells of the major thymus population fail to do so. The literature
has seen a heated debate in recent years concerning the question of
the expression of Ir-genes, and of MLC stimulating capacity of lymphocyte subpopulations. Various studies have attributed these properties
exclusively to either T- or B-cells, or to both populations. It
remains to be seen whether thymic cells express MLC determinants
associated with all parts of the H-2 complex, and whether they express the "M" antigen.

The thymus undergoes involution under various conditions, such
as stress, administration of corticosteroid hormone, cancer, or administration of LPS. The thymus cells eliminated preferentially in
involution belong to the major population of thymus cells, which
migrates selectively to the spleen, and may give rise to suppresser
T-cells (3). In contrast, thymic involution increases the proportion
of immunocompetent, lymph-node seeking lymphocytes. We heard today
that LPS administration which causes considerable involution of the
thymus results in a relative increase of the proportion of "helper
cells" in the thymus. It is beginning to appear as if the involution
of the thymus may serve a useful purpose. It can be speculated that
most of the cells which are eliminated during thymic involution are
the progenitors of suppressor T-cells. The selective depletion of
such potentially suppressive cells may be of advantage under conditions in which the organism is required to mount a vigorous immune
response.

Turning our attention to the peripheral lymphoid system - it
is becoming clear that there is an enormous heterogeneity among T-
lymphocyte subpopulations. Subpopulations differ quantitatively or
qualitatively in the expression of T-distinctive cell surface markers. The discovery that the θ- and Ly-antigens are distinctive for
mouse T-cells (4) enabled the demonstration that subpopulations
of T-cells differ in the concentration of these antigens. It has
recently been shown that T-cells capable of cytotoxic reactivity
against allogeneic targets, are θ + Ly.2 +, Ly.3 +, but have a low
Ly. 1 antigenicity (5). We have recently shown that subpopulations
of T-cells responding to various lectin concentrations differ in

their cell-surface antigenicity. T-cells in the lymph-nodes which
respond to low concentrations of PHA were found to be characterized
by their high θ-antigenicity but low Ly-1 antigenicity. In contrast
the T-cells responding to high concentrations of PHA have a high cell
surface concentration of both the θ- and Ly-1 antigenicity (6).
Spleen cells responding to various concentrations of PHA differ in
their H-2 antigenicity - the cells responding to low PHA concentrations have a high H-2 antigenicity, while those responding to high
PHA concentrations have a low H-2 antigenicity (7).

The heterogeneity of the cell surface proportion of T-lymphocytes seems to be correlated with a heterogeneity of their functional capacities. It remains, however, unclear if there is any causal
correlation between these two parameters. The question of the T-cell
receptor for the recognition of antigens, either upon initial exposure
or after repeated immunizations, is still open for debate.

Activated T-cells may become coated with an immunoglobulin
coat, be it through the appearance of cell-surface F_c receptors, or
by other mechanisms. In man, activated T-cells formed either in vitro
(8) or in vivo (9) were recently found to be characterized by their
capacity of forming stable E-rosettes, resistant to incubation at
37°C for 30 minutes. Rabbit anti-human immunoglobulin serum, which
did not inhibit the formation of regular E-rosettes (10), was found
to inhibit the formation of stable E-rosettes by activated T-cells.
The immunoglobulin coat of human T-cells activated in vitro could
be shown to be derived from the culture medium (8).

These studies, and those presented throughout the session,
indicate that subpopulations of lymphocytes differ in their cell-
surface properties, that heterogeneity of the cell-surface is correlated with differences in the responsiveness of these subpopulations to various mitogenic stimuli, and that following activation
of the cells the properties of the cell-surface are changed profoundly.

References

1. Schlesinger, M., Gottesfeld, S., and Korzash, Z.
       Cell. Immunol. 6:49, 1973.

2. Galili, U. and Schlesinger, M. J. Immunol. (In Press).

3. Gershon, R.K., Lance, E.M. and Konda, S.
       J. Immunol. 112: 546, 1974.

4. Schlesinger, M., and Yron, I. J. Immunol. 104: 798, 1970.

5. Shiku, H., Kisielow, P., Bean, M.A., Takahashi, T., Boyse, E.A.,
       Oettgen, H.F., and Old, L.J. J. Exp. Med. 141: 227, 1975.

6. Rabinowitz, R., Laskov, R., and Schlesinger, M. (In Preparation).

7. Schlesinger, M., Israel, E., Chaouat, M., and Gery, I.
       Ann. N.Y. Acad. Sci. 249: 505, 1975.

8. Galili, U. and Schlesinger, M. (Unpublished data).

9. Galili, U., Slavin, S., Eliakim, M., and Schlesinger, M.
      Clin. Immunol. Immunopathol. (In Press).

10. Galili, U. and Schlesinger, M. J. Immunol. <u>112</u>: 1628, 1974.

Homing of Cells and Inductive Effects
of Microenvironment and of Humoral Factors

MICROENVIRONMENT TO A LYMPHOID CELL IS NOTHING MORE THAN INTERACTION WITH ITS NEIGHBOURS

Maria de Sousa

Department of Bacteriology & Immunology, Glasgow

University & Western Infirmary, Glasgow G11 6NT (U.K.)

In 1966 the Rockefeller University Review published the Speech made by Rene Dubos after receiving the Arches of Science Award (1). The article has two illustrations; one, the conventional picture of Dubos being congratulated by the Chairman of the committee at the announcement luncheon, the other a delightful cartoon consisting of 3 simple line drawings of a worried, thinking man, sitting at a lonely desk, slowly metamorphosing into a turnip. The caption accompanying the drawing reads 'Deprivation of environmental Stimuli can turn man into a mental turnip!' In the article Dubos also makes the statement 'Human beings are as much the product of their environment as of their genetic endowment'. When one talks of environment to a human being we all have a fair idea of what is meant, but do we know what we mean when we talk of environment to a cell?

As the introduction to this session on 'The homing of cells and the inductive effects of microenvironment and of humoral factors' (the title got bigger as the organizers themselves thought about it) I shall propose that 'environment to a cell is nothing more than interaction with its neighbours', and hope that as the session unfolds the papers will either give or deny support to the proposition.

To illustrate it I shall start by saying that a turnip in the boot of a jeep in the Sahara is as likely to be stimulated to think as a turnip in the vegetable compartment of a Manhattan refrigerator, meaning that the capacity to stimulate resides as much in stimulation as in the ability to be stimulated. Thus, even in the simple process of acknowledging the existence of an environment,

interaction, between the one that acknowledges and that which is
acknowledged, is already implicit.

What form or forms does interaction take in the case of
lymphoid cells?

To a T precursor cell, genetically endowed with the ability to
differentiate and express a number of surface antigens (2), to find
itself in the environment of the thymus, today means, thanks to the
work of J.F. Bach's group (3) and others (4), not something vague
and obscure but interaction with neighbour cells in the thymus, most
probably cells of the epithelial reticular framework of the thymus
medulla. Moreover, in the case of T cell differentiation, we know
not only the cells involved in the process of interaction, but we
are making progress in the understanding of the molecular basis and
regulatory mechanism of the interaction (5-8). I hope that at the
end of the session we will know a lot more about thymus microenvironment after listening to the papers to be presented by Alm,
Kook and A. Goldstein.

Let us now follow the fate of a fully differentiated T cell.
Sooner or later this cell is going to find itself in specific environments within the spleen and lymph nodes, a phenomenon which I
have called ecotaxis (9). But what is that? What is the basis of
specific positioning? From my experiments with Curtis (10) I shall
say again that it is interaction with neighbours, moreover, I
think we can divide neighbours into obvious and underlying neighbours. An obvious neighbour to a T cell is another T cell or a B
cell at the boundary between the T and B territories. The underlying neighbours are those cells of the stroma of the peripheral
lymphoid organs about which we know so little and hope to learn more
from Drs.Müller-Hermelink and Rozing.

There are in the literature the expressions 'spleen seeking cells'
and 'lymph node seeking cells' (11). What do we mean by that? Are
there in the body direct separate routes to lymph nodes or spleen
which escaped the fine eye of William Harvey (12)? Or do we mean to
say that a lymph node seeking cell is a cell that interacted briefly
with other cells in the spleen, found them 'uninteresting', and
quickly reached the lymph nodes; by contrast, a spleen seeking cell
is a cell whose membrane characteristics will make it more prone to
interact with the resident spleen cell population?

The cell membrane has been implicated in one of the interactions
known to take place when a lymphocyte enters a lymph node, through
the post-capillary venule (13). I understand Dr. Van Ewijk will be
showing us the changes that occur during this process, as revealed
by the scanning electron microscope. Gesner and Ginsburgh (13)
proposed that the sugars on the surface of the lymphocyte are of

importance for the recognition of the endothelial cell in the post-
capillary venule.   And a number of experiments modifying the sugars
on lymphocytes by pretreatment with enzymes or plant lectins (14-19)
have shown a reduction of migration of cells into the lymph nodes,
with increase in the liver in the case of neuraminidase, or in the
spleen after treatment with trypsin or Con A.   These experiments
have been interpreted in the light of Gesner's proposal.   Dr. de
Freitas, in my laboratory has also examined this question following
the fate of Con A treated lymphocytes in splenectomised recipients
(19); not surprisingly, perhaps,under these circumstances, treated
cells enter the lymph nodes in the same quantities as untreated
ones (Table 1).

Thus, lack of entry into a lymph node is not the result of a
"cell decision" not to enter the lymph node, but more likely the
result of being "delayed", as it were, in the spleen.   Autoradiographs of spleens containing Con A treated cells indicate that they
are in the white pulp (Fig. 1) and not in the red pulp as one might
expect if phagocytosis of the cells were involved.

If environment to a cell is interaction with its neighbours
and interaction is more likely to occur within solid organs, how
will being delayed by an antigen or as the result of a minor membrane change be reflected in the 'fluid compartments' of the circulating system?   Scollay will be raising this question and
illustrating the importance of the study of distribution of functional classes of cells in different compartments; Balfour will be
talking to us about the role of the lymph itself in the development
of a contact sensitivity response, and Wallis will take us into the
unknown world of feedback mechanisms.

TABLE 1   Effect of splenectomy on lymph node entry of Con A
           treated lymphocytes*

Donor cells	Recipients	Spleen	Lymph nodes	Liver
untreated	intact	21 + 2	14 + 2	14 + 2
Con A treated	intact	35 + 3	7 + 1	16 + 1
untreated	Splx	-	18 + 2	27 + 1
Con A treated	Splx	-	18 + 3	27 + 2

* ^{51}Cr labelled, results expressed as % of injected radioactivity.

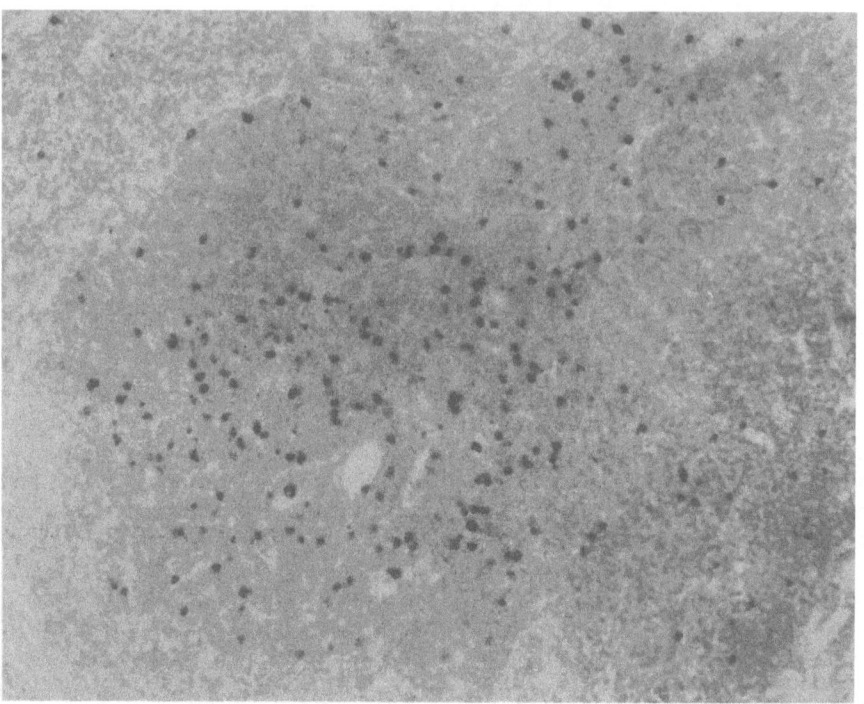

Fig. 1 .   Autoradiograph of spleen removed from recipient (mouse)
of ^{3}H-adenosine labelled syngeneic lymph node cells pretreated
in vitro with Con A.   Note that the majority of the labelled cells
is in the white pulp.   Stain: methyl-green pyronin.
Magnification: x 150

        Finally, if the primary basis of lymphoid tissue organization is
interaction between circulating and resident cells, and lymphocyte
traffic controlled by such an interaction, then we shall all look
forward to Weissman's paper on T/B cell interactions in lymphoid
tissues during the development of an immune response.

        His contribution will bring us back to the reality that this is
a Conference on Germinal Centres. Mine will end by bringing us back
to the reality that it is taking place in Israel. In what land better
than this should we be discussing the proposition that reaching a
destination may be the result of genetic determination, but to be
allowed to survive in it and allow others to survive round it is only
possible as the environmental result of a congenial interaction between
neighbours.

REFERENCES

1. Dubos, R., Rockefeller University Review 4:1, 1966.
2. Greaves, M.F., Owen J.J.T. and Raff, M.C. T and B lymphocytes,
    p. 39, Excerpta Medica, Amsterdam, 1974.
3. Dardenne, M., Papiernik, M., Bach, J.F. and Stutman, O.
    Immunology 27:299, 1974.
4. Pike, K.W. and Gelfand, E.W. Nature 251:421, 1974.
5. Goldstein, A.L. and White, A. Contemporary Topics in
    Immunobiology, 2:339. Eds. A.J.S. Davies and R.L.
    Carter, Plenum Press, New York, 1973.
6. Trainin, N. and Small, M. Contemporary Topics in
    Immunobiology, 2:321. Eds. A.J.S. Davies and R.L.
    Carter, Plenum Press, New York, 1973.
7. Goldstein, G., Scheid, M., Hammerling, U., Boyse, E.A.,
    Schlesinger, D.H. and Miall, H.D. Proc. Nat. Acad. Sci.
    72:11, 1975.
8. de Sousa, M. and Incefy, G.S. Biologic Activity of Thymic
    Hormones, p. 21. Ed. D. van Bekkum, Kooyker Scientific
    Publications, Rotterdam.
9. de Sousa, M. Clin. exp. Immunol. 9:371, 1971.
10. Curtis, A.S.G. and de Sousa, M. Cell. Immunol. (in press).
11. Zatz, M.M. and Lance, E.M. Cell. Immunol. 1:3, 1970.
12. Elkana, Y. and Goodfield, G.J.   ISIS, 59:63, 1968.
13. Gesner, B.M. and Ginsburgh, V. Proc. Nat. Acad. Sci.
    52, 750, 1964.
14. Woodruff, J.J. and Gesner, B.M. J. exp. Med. 129:551, 1969.
15. Woodruff, J.J. Cell. Immunol. 13:378, 1974.
16. Gillette, R.W., McKenzie, G.O. and Swanson, M.H. J. Immunol.
    111:1902, 1973.
17. Taub, R.N. Cell. Immunol. 12:263, 1974.
18. Schlesinger, M. and Israel, E. Cell. Immunol. 14:66, 1974.
19. de Freitas, A.A. and de Sousa, M. Eur. J. Immunol., in press.

SCANNING ELECTRON MICROSCOPY OF B- AND T-CELLS IN PERIPHERAL LYMPHOID ORGANS OF THE MOUSE

W. van Ewijk and N. H. C. Brons

Department of Cell Biology and Genetics, Erasmus University of Rotterdam, P. O. Box 1738, Rotterdam, The Netherlands

Scanning electron microscopy (SEM) was recently presented as an appropriate technique to distinguish between B and T lymphocytes (1, 2, 3). B cells generally showed many microvilli on the cell surface, whereas T cells had a smooth surface. These observations were based on SEM studies of lymphoid cells, isolated from peripheral blood by Ficoll-Hypaque density gradient centrifugation. The present report deals with the surface morphology of B and T cells in vivo. We studied the spleen and mesenteric lymph node of 4 groups of male mice: (a) adult thymectomized, lethally irradiated, bone marrow reconstituted (DBA/2 x C57BL/Rij)F1 mice, briefly indicated as TxBM mice, (b) nude mice (nu/nu, the outcome of fourth backcross matings to B10.LP/JPh mice, obtained from Centraal Proefdierenbedrijf TNO, Zeist, The Netherlands), (c) adult, lethally irradiated (DBA/2 x C57BL/Rij)F1 mice, reconstituted with syngeneic thymocytes, indicated as T mice and (d) adult, lethally irradiated (DBA/2 x C57BL/Rij)F1 mice reconstituted with syngeneic cortisone-resistant thymocytes, referred to as CRT mice. Fixation was performed by total body perfusion with a solution of 1.5 percent glutaraldehyde in 0.075 M sodium cacodylate buffer, a technique described in detail before (4). TxBM mice were fixed at 4 weeks after bone marrow reconstitution, T mice and CRT mice were fixed 6 days after reconstitution. Nude mice were fixed at 6 weeks of age. The spleen and mesenteric lymph node of the perfused mice were excised and slices of the fixed tissue were dehydrated in graded series of ethanol. The specimens were transferred to amylacetate and dried in a critical point drying apparatus. The dried specimens were mounted on specimen stages, covered with gold with a sputter coater and examined in a Cambridge, MK II A scanning electron

microscope. During examination, attention was focussed on areas where
B and T lymphocytes are known to localize and areas where recirculation
of lymphocytes is known to occur. In the spleen, B cells localize at the
periphery of the periarteriolar lymphatic sheath (PALS) and in follicles
(5); in lymph nodes B cells populate the outer cortex and cortico-medullary junction (6, 7, 8). T cells, on the other hand, home in the spleen in
the central PALS (4); in lymph nodes they populate the paracortical area
(9). Lymphocyte recirculation is known to occur in the marginal zone of
the spleen (10) and in postcapillary venules and medullary sinuses of
lymph nodes (11).

Examination of the peripheral PALS and follicles in the spleen of TxBM
mice revealed mainly lymphocytes with a smooth surface. In contrast,
lymphocytes present in the marginal zone exhibited numerous microvilli
(12). Similar observations were obtained in SEM studies of the spleen of
nude mice. B lymphocytes in the mesenteric lymph node of TxBM mice
and nude mice also showed both types of surface morphology: in the outer
cortex, they were smooth surface; in postcapillary venules and medullary
sinus, they exposed many microvilli. SEM studies of T mice and CRT
mice gave analogous results. In their specific microenvironment in the
spleen (PALS) and mesenteric lymph node (paracortical area) T cells
were smooth surfaced; recirculating T cells exposed microvilli. Lymphocytes in the medullary sinus of the mesenteric lymph node of TxBM mice,
nude mice (Fig. 1) and T mice were equal in size $(4.5\mu \pm 0.5\mu)$ and showed
microvilli up to 1μ in length. However, lymphocytes present in the medullary sinus of CRT mice (Fig. 2) were frequently found to be larger $(6\mu \pm
1\mu)$. Their microvilli were found to be approximately 0.4μ in length. In
postcapillary venules about one-third of the lymphoid cells attached to the
wall of the venule was smooth surfaced. These cells were always settled
in the ridges between adjacent high endothelial cells and were probably in
the process of passing the endothelial lining. It seems likely that the surface morphology of recirculating lymphocytes changes from villous to
smooth during this transition (12).

Fig. 1. Medullary sinus of the mesenteric lymph node of a nude mouse.
Lymphocytes (ly) are present between macrophages (m) and reticulum cells
(r). Lymphocytes show microvilli of about 1μ in length.

Fig. 2. Medullary sinus of the mesenteric lymph node of a CRT mouse.
Lymphocytes (ly) are in close contact with macrophages (m) and the endothelial lining (e) of the sinus. They exhibit microvilli of about 4μ in length.
Macrophages show a ruffling membrane, or a villous membrane. The
endothelial lining also shows a ruffling membrane at this site of the
medullary sinus.

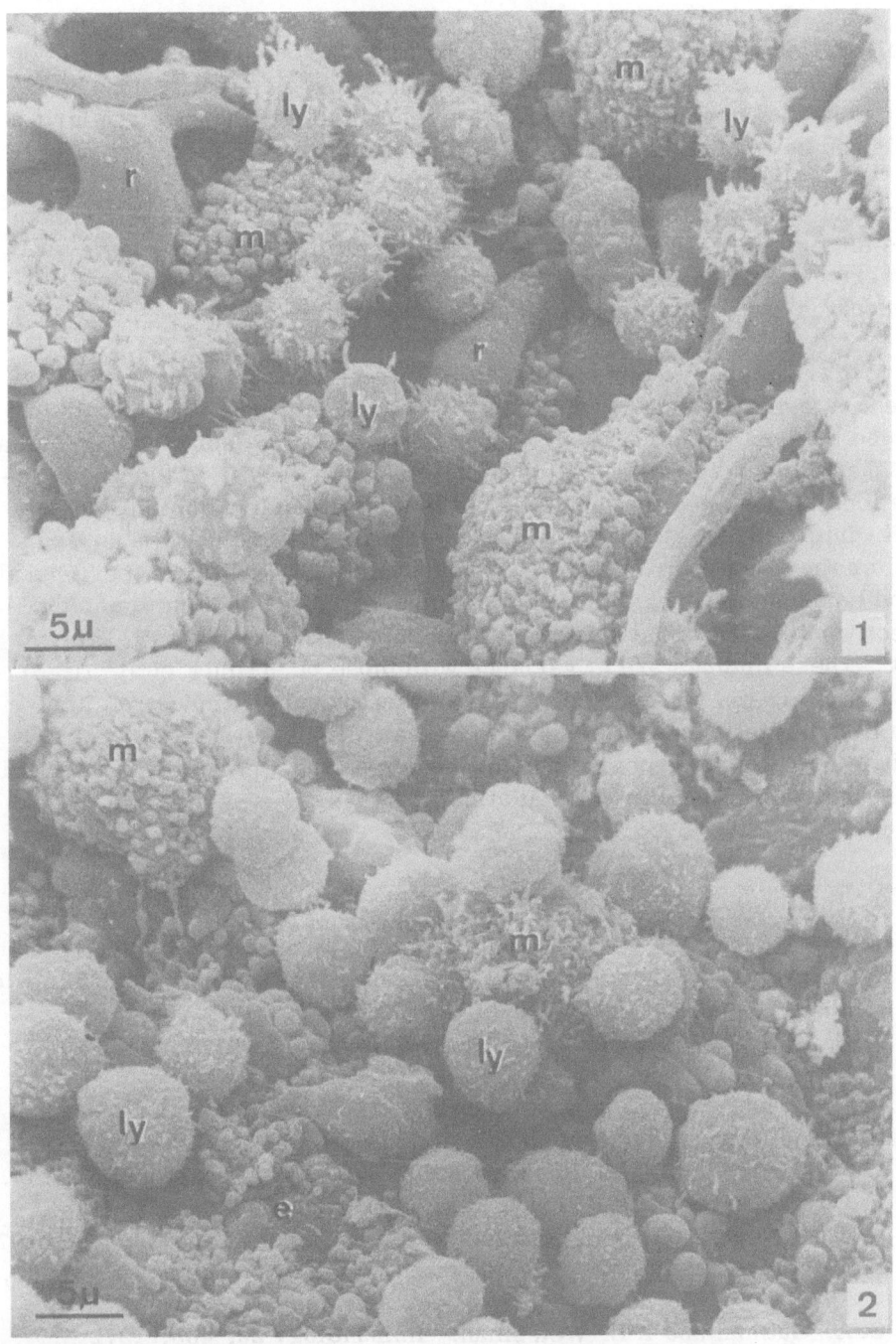

From the observations reported here it is obvious that a reliable identification of T and B cells in vivo by their surface morphology is not possible. However, circumstantial evidence suggests that lymphocytes of CRT mice, because of their cellular size and the length of their micro-villi, can be distinguished from other lymphocytes. SEM studies of cri-tical point-dried suspensions of thymocytes, cortisone-resistant thymo-cytes and suspensions of the mesenteric lymph node of TxBM mice and nude mice are now in progress in our laboratory. Up to now, however, we were not able to find significant differences in the morphology of thymocytes and cortisone-resistant thymocytes.

With reference to our observations on recirculating lymphocytes, recent data of Alexander and Wetzel (13) are of interest. These authors studied the surface morphology of mononuclear cells, isolated from human peripheral blood before and after Ficoll-Hypaque density gradient centri-fugation. They noted that about 90 percent of the cells exhibited micro-villi. Interestingly, the Ficoll-Hypaque separation method was not found to alter the villous surface of the lymphocytes. Passing of the peripheral blood lymphocytes over nylon wool columns, a method known to enrich selectively T cells (14), increased the number of villous cells to 95 per-cent. These findings are at variance with those of Polliack et al. (1, 3) and Lin et al. (2). In conclusion, the present results demonstrate that in vivo B and T cells exhibit smooth as well as villous surfaces. Their surface morphology appears to be dependent on their presence in specific microenvironments or in recirculating pathways.

REFERENCES

1. A. Polliack, N. Lampen, B. D. Clarkson, E. de Harven, Z. Bentwich, F. P. Siegal and H. G. Kunkel. J. Exp. Med. 138, 607, 1973

2. P. S. Lin, A. G. Cooper and H. H. Wortis. N. Engl. J. Med. 289, 548, 1973

3. A. Polliack, S. M. Fu, S. D. Douglas, Z. Bentwich, N. Lampen and E. de Harven. J. Exp. Med. 140, 146, 1974

4. W. van Ewijk, J. H. M. Verzijden, Th. H. van der Kwast and S. W. M. Luycx-Meyer. Cell Tissue Res. 149, 43, 1974

5. A. J. P. Veerman and W. van Ewijk. Cell Tissue Res. 156, 417, 1975

6. D. M. V. Parrot and M. A. B. de Sousa. Clin. exp. Immunol. 8, 663, 1971.

7. G. A. Gutman and I. L. Weissman. Immunology 23, 465, 1972

8.   J. Sprent. Cell. Immunol. 7, 10, 1973

9.   J. E. Veldman, Ph. D. Thesis, Dijkstra Niemeijer, Groningen, The Netherlands, 1970

10. W. L. Ford and P. Nieuwenhuis. Schweiz. med. Wschr. 104, 1348, 1974

11. J. L. Gowans and E. J. Knight. Proc. Roy. Soc. (London) Ser. B, 159, 257, 1964

12. W. van Ewijk, N. H. C. Brons and J. Rozing. Cell. Immunol., in press

13. E. L. Alexander and B. Wetzel. Science 188, 732, 1975

14. S. A. Eisen, H. J. Wedner and C. U. Parker. Immunol. Commun. 1, 571, 1972

HUMAN LYMPHATIC MICROECOLOGY - SPECIFICITY, CHARACTERIZATION AND ONTOGENY OF DIFFERENT RETICULUM CELLS IN THE B CELL AND T CELL REGIONS

H.K.MÜLLER-HERMELINK, U.HEUSERMANN, E.KAISERLING
and H.-J. STUTTE

Dept. of Pathology, Univ.of Kiel,Fed.Rep.Germany

The well-known phenomenon that the circulating B and T lymphocytes reach the lymphatic tissue by similar routes but dissociate thereafter according to their functional differentiation and localize at different sites, can hardly be understood if lymphocytes alone are considered as responsible. The evidence for specific microenvironments in the lymphatic tissue defining the structural component of a microecological relationship between migrating and resting cells, has been indirect and. up to now. a theoretical chalenge. The term "reticulum cell" is used as a common name for all structural cells in the lymphoreticular tissue, in spite of the fact that 1) different functional definitions, that have been proposed, may determine different cell types (e.g. fiber formation vs. phagocytosis) and 2) new cell types have been described in the lymphatic tissue of rodents and man, which neither phagocytose nore form fibers. These cells have been called dendritic reticulum cells (DRC)(1) and intergitating reticulum cells (IDC) (2). Our study deals with the morphological demonstration of different structural ("reticulum") cells in human lymphatic tissue, which as a microecological pattern, may give a formal explanation for the different localization of T and B lymphocytes.

MATERIAL AND METHODS

Material: 1.) human peripheral lymphatic tissue from spleen lymph node, tonsil and Peyer's patches without pathological changes. 2.) Thymus tissue of children removed during cardiac surgery. 3.) lymphatic tissue from thymus, spleen. lymph node, tonsil and Peyer's patches of 35 human fetuses of 8 - 30 weeks gestational age.

Methods: Described in detail elsewhere (4). In the first
step the distribution of B cell regions (BCR) was identified on
cryostat sections by the EAC-rosette technique (3). This was
correlated to enzymehistochemical findings on serial sections by
applying the demonstration of ATPase, 5'-nucleotidase(5'-n'ase),
nonspecific esterase, acid phosphatase and alkaline phosphatase.
In the second step this has been correlated to ultrastructure
by ultrahistochemical demonstration of ATPase, 5'-n'ase, and alkaline phosphatase.

RESULTS

Fig.1 shows the correlation of the EAC-binding region with
the demonstration of 5'-n'ase and ATPase activities on lymph
node sections. The 5'-n'ase reaction leads to a demonstration of
the BCR. A positive reaction is seen in the lymphocytes of the
corona and in a mesh-like distribution within the germinal center. Germinoblasts are negative as well as the lymphocytes and
other cells of the T cell region (TCR). ATPase activity is found
not only on lymphocytes of the primary follicle but also on cells
of the TCR. By applying a combined demonstration of ATPase and
nonspecific esterase or acid phosphatase activities it may be
shown that the cells in the TCR reacting positive for ATPase are
not the lymphocytes but reticulum cells with a weak nonspecific
esterase and acid phosphatase activity. ATPase is negative in
germinal centers.

The demonstration of alkaline phosphatase activity leads
to a positive reaction at the borderline of the TCR. Here, a linear reaction is found along the reticulin fibers. Strong acid
phosphatase and nonspecific esterase activities are found in macrophages of the BCR and TCR. These findings are confirmed in
all peripheral lymphatic tissues.

For the identification of the cell types responsible for
this characteristic enzyme pattern of BCR and TCR, the enzyme
activities are correlated to ultrastructural findings by ultrahistochemical demonstration of 5'-n'ase, ATPase and alkaline
phosphatase (Fig.2). 5'-n'ase activity of germinal centers is
confined to a linear reaction product on the surface of dendritic reticulum cells (DCR). ATPase activity of the TCR is found
on the surface of a characteristic cell type that VELDMAN (2)
in a study of lymphatic tissue of rabbits named interdigitating
reticulum cell (IDC). As shown here, IDC are confined to TCR in
all human lymphatic tissues. IDC are characterized by gross inter-
digitations of cell processes and by a typical tubulo-vesicular
system of the endoplasmic reticulum. The nucleus is often very
irregular with deep indentations. Alkaline phosphatase activity
is found on the cell surface of fibroblastic reticulum cells and
in reticulin fibers.

If a comparison of the enzyme patterns of reticulum cells

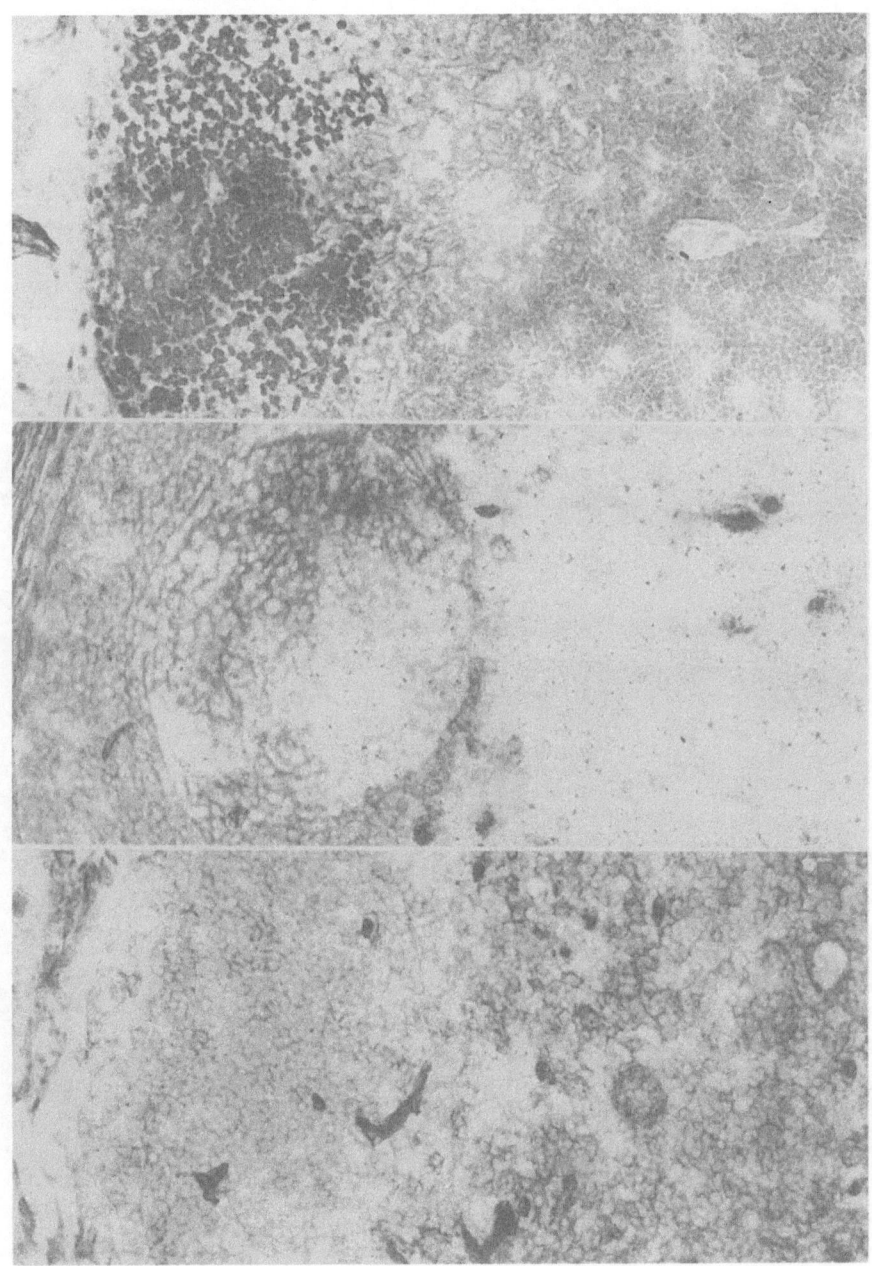

Fig.1: Correlation of EAC-rosette binding region (a) with the enzymehistochemical demonstration of 5'-n'ase (b) and ATPase on subserial cryostat sections of a human lymph node. For explanation see text 140 X.

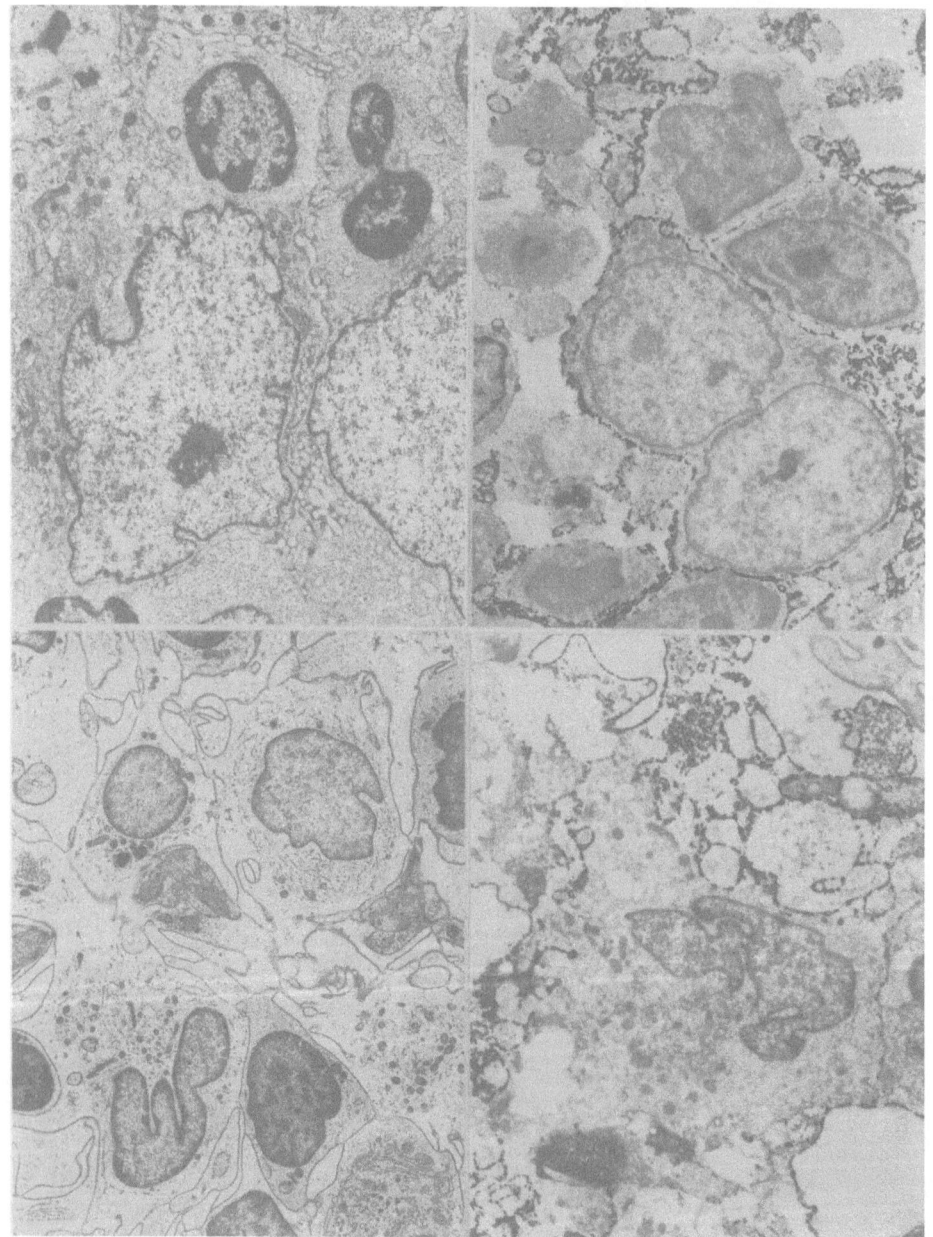

Fig.2: Ultrastructure of DRC and IDC. a) Normal electron microscopical appearance of DRC (5000 X) b) 5'-n'ase activity on the
cell surface of DRC (4000 X) c) IDC in the paracortical TCR of
lymph node (3000 X) d) ATPase activity on the cell surface of
IDC (5000 X).

is made, four rather than one cell type can be distinguished
(Tab.1). As a constant finding in all lymphatic tissues DRC are
specific for BCR and IDC for TCR. In addition, IDC are also found
at the corticomedullary boundary of the thymus, where no DCR are
found.

Tab.1: Enzyme histochemical patterns of different reticulum
cells in human lymphatic tissue.

reticulum cells	localization	nonspec. esterase	acid phosphat.	alkaline phosphat.	5'-n'ase	ATP ase
dendritic	B cell region	+	-	-	+	-
interdigitating	T cell region	((+))	(+)	-	-	+
fibroblastic	esp. border of T cell region	(+)	(+)	+	-	-/+
histiocytic	uncharacteristic	+++	+++	-	-	-/+

Tab.2: Ontogenetic appearance of different reticulum cells in
human lymphatic tissue.

gestational age	thymus	lymph node	spleen
8 - 9 weeks	first appearance of IDC in perivascular spaces		
12-14 weeks	demarcation of medulla . IDC ++	hemopoiesis, esp. myelopoiesis , first lymphatic cells	
16 weeks	"normal"	IDC ++ , typical T cell region	
20 weeks	"	"	first lymphocytes in periarteriolar region IDC +/-
26-30 weeks	"	in some : B cell region with DRC	B cell and T cell regions with IDC and DRC

In a further study the ontogenetic appearance of the different reticulum cells was studied in relation to the structural
maturation of the lymphatic tissue. The results are summarized
in Tab.2. IDC are found at the corticomedullary boundary of the
thymus almost as early as lymphocytes (at 8 week gestational
age). Lymphocytes appear in peripheral lymphatic tissue slightly earlier than these reticulum cells. They are found at this
place at a time when mainly hemopoietic, especially myelopoietic
cells are found. However, the appearance of typical TCR and BCR
is delayed until IDC and DRC are formed. Then hemopoiesis is no
longer found. TCR are formed earlier than BCR, the latter being
somewhat more variable in time of formation (16 vs. 25 - 30
weeks gestational age).

DISCUSSION AND CONCLUSION

BCR and TCR of human lymphatic tissue can easily be distinguished by different patterns of cell surface enzymes. Nonphago-
cytic reticulum cells of BCR and TCR can be differentiated from
each other as well as from fibroblasts and phagocytes by enzyme
histochemical methods. The time of ontogenetic appearance of
these cells fits rather well with the build-up of immunological
reactivity. TCR are formed very constantly between the 12. and
16. week of gestation, whereas the time of BCR appearance is delayed and more variable. It may be suggested that the formation
of typical BCR may be accelerated or delayed to some degree dependent of antigenic stimulation. These findings provide a direct approach to the investigation of alterations of the lymphatic microenvironment in human diseases. As a preliminary result
we found no IDC in the epithelial thymus remnant in thymic dys-
plasia, suggesting that these cells are involved in T cell formation and/or maturation. The applicability of these results on
problems of malignant lymphomas and other diseases is under
study.

LITERATURE

1) MILANESI, S.: Boll.Soc.ital.Biol.Sper. 41, 1223 (1965)
2) VELDMAN, J.E.: Histophysiology and electron microscopy of
                  the immune response. N.V.Boekdrukkeij Dijks-
                  tra Niemeyer, Groningen (1970)
3) DUKOR, P.; BIANCO, C.; NUSSENZWEIG, V.:
                  Proc.Nat.Acad. Sci USA 67, 991 (1970)
4) MÜLLER-HERMELINK, H.K.; HEUSERMANN, U.; STUTTE, H.-J.:
                  Cell.Tiss.Res. 154, 167 (1974)

'HYPERLYMPHOID' MICE

V.Wallis, E.Leuchars, D.Collavo and A.J.S.Davies

Chester Beatty Research Institute, Institute of Cancer
Research: Royal Cancer Hospital
Fulham Road, London SW3 6JB, England

We have previously shown that following the intravenous
introduction of lymphocytes into normal adult mice a state of T-
cell chimaerism results which is long lasting (1). The experiments
presented here investigate the fate of the injected cells during
the first day after injection and also the effect of multiple
injections of spleen or lymph node cells on the degree of T-cell
chimaerism. In addition to estimates of the numbers of T cells in
these chimaeras their antibody responses to sheep erythrocytes and
mitotic responses to oxazolone have been quantitated.

METHODS

Washed cell suspensions of spleens or lymph nodes from
CBA/H-T6T6 (T6T6) mice were injected intravenously into mice of the
syngeneic but chromosomally distinguishable CBA/H strain. In order
to display the chromosomes so that cells could be scored as being
of host or donor origin T cells were stimulated in vitro with
phytohaemagglutinin (PHA) (2). To quantitate the total number of
T cells in different organs cytotoxicity tests with anti-θ antiserum were performed by the trypan blue dye uptake method using a
two stage assay (3,4).

RESULTS

Fate of Injected Spleen Cells

CBA/H mice were injected with 10^8 washed T6T6 spleen cells.
At various times later the mice were killed and peripheral blood,

183

V. WALLIS, E. LEUCHARS, D. COLLAVO, AND A.J.S. DAVIES

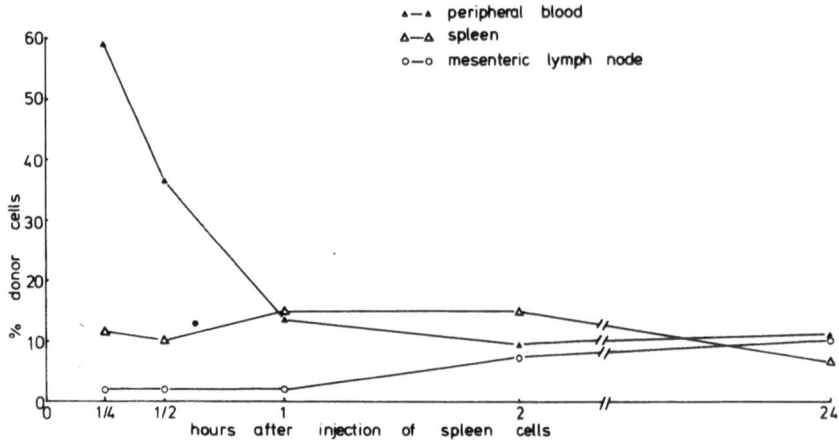

Fig.1   Mean percentage of donor cells in PHA-stimulated cultures
of blood, spleen and lymph node.

spleen and mesenteric lymph node were cultured with PHA. The
dividing cells at 3 days were scored as being of host or donor
origin. Figure 1 shows the percent of donor cells scored in the
cultures from each of the three tissues.

It can be seen that at 15 minutes a large proportion of the
dividing cells in the blood cultures are derived from the donor
inoculum. This proportion decreases rapidly over the next 45
minutes and slowly over the next hour to stabilise at about 10%.
The injected cells reach the spleen by 15 minutes after injection,
increase in proportion by 1hr but after 2hrs the proportion appears
to drop again. The cells take considerably longer to reach the
mesenteric lymph node – they constitute only 2% of the T cells up
to 1hr after injection but thereafter increase to levels of about
10%. Thus it seems that injected cells clear from the blood into
the spleen and to a lesser extent into the lymph nodes. The final
equilibrium perhaps involves some shift from spleen into lymph
nodes.

Multiple Injections of Spleen Cells

CBA/H mice were injected intravenously 9 times at weekly
intervals with 10^8 spleen cells from T6T6 mice. One week after
each injection blood was taken and cultured with PHA. The percent
of donor cells is plotted in Figure 2.

In general each injection of spleen cells resulted in an
increase in the level of chimaerism which reached nearly 40% after
9 injections. This level of chimaerism declined slowly and was

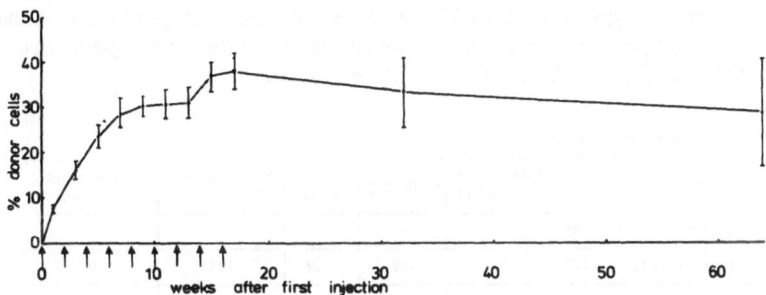

Fig.2 Mean percentage (± S.D.) of donor cells in PHA-stimulated
       cultures of blood. The arrows indicate the times of
       injection.

still nearly 30% 48 weeks after the last injection. This indicates
not only that you can produce a high level of T-cell chimaerism in
normal mice by the injection of normal spleen cells but also that
the chimaerism is very long lasting.

In another experiment some mice were injected 10 times with
10^8 lymph node cells and some 10 times with 10^8 spleen cells. They
were killed and blood, spleen and lymph node were cultured with PHA
to stimulate T cells, and spleen cells were also cultured with
E.coli polysaccharide to stimulate B cells. The degree of T-cell
chimaerism was the same in blood, spleen and lymph nodes, but
injection of lymph node cells resulted in higher levels of
chimaerism (66%) than injection of spleen cells (49%). The level
of B-cell chimaerism was higher in spleen-injected mice (40%) than
in lymph node-injected mice (13%). This probably reflects the
different proportions of T and B cells in the donor spleen and
lymph node inocula.

In the following 3 experiments CBA/H mice were injected 4
times with 10^8 T6T6 lymph node cells which resulted in about 50%
T-cell chimaerism. They were kept in the same boxes as uninjected
control mice of the same age. In the first experiment mice were
killed 15 and 45 days after the last injection, and in the other
experiments they were injected with sheep erythrocytes or painted
with oxazolone 13 days after the last injection.

                   Estimate of the Number of Lymphoid Cells

In Table 1 the organ weights and cell counts of lymphoid organs
from lymph-node injected mice are expressed as the percent of the
values obtained from the control mice.

It can be seen that, except for the axillary lymph nodes, the

Table 1 Organ weights and cell counts of mice injected 4 times with 10^8 lymph node cells, expressed as the mean percent of the values for uninjected control mice.

Injected as % control

	Weight	Nucleated cell count	Cells/mg	% θ +ve cells	Total number θ +ve cells	Total number θ -ve cells
Body weight	95	-	-	-	-	-
Axillary LN (4)	127	164	129	102	161	170
Mesenteric LN	104	115	110	107	122	100
Spleen	103	111	108	145	160	95
Thymus	91	101	111	-	-	-
Bone-marrow (1 femur)	-	104	-	-	-	-

% chimaerism = 47%

organ weights are similar to control values, but the number of cells in the lymph nodes and spleen are greater. The lymph nodes had a slightly higher percent of θ-+ve cells but the spleen was considerably higher. By totalling the number of cells from lymph nodes and spleen it is possible to obtain an estimate of the 'hyperlymphoidism' of these mice. There are 47% more T-lymphocytes in the lymph-node injected mice than normal, but the number of B cells is the same, although their distribution between lymph nodes and spleen seems to have been altered.

Table 2 Mean of $\log_{10}$ number of plaque forming cells ($\pm$ S.D.) in spleens of mice injected 5 days previously with sheep erythrocytes.

	Nucleated cells/spleen	IgM/10^6	IgG/10^6	IgM/Sp	IgG/Sp
Control	2.15±0.04	3.42±0.05	3.53±0.18	5.58±0.09	5.69±0.18
LN injected (50% chimaera)	2.30±0.08 < 0.01	3.37±0.10 NS	3.70±0.11 NS	5.67±0.12 NS	6.00±0.17 < 0.05
% control	140	88	148	122	206
Control	2.22±0.05	3.54±0.10	3.99±0.04	5.76±0.06	6.21±0.06
LN injected (51% chimaera)	2.35±0.05 < 0.01	3.52±0.14 NS	4.07±0.11 NS	5.87±0.17 NS	6.42±0.14 NS
% control	134	96	120	129	161

Response to Sheep Erythrocytes

The number of plaque-forming cells in the spleens of mice injected 5 days previously with 5×10^8 sheep erythrocytes intra-peritoneally was assayed by the Cunningham technique (5). The results of 2 experiments are shown in Table 2.

It can be seen that in both experiments the mean number of cells per spleen was significantly higher in the lymph-node injected mice. The number of IgM producing cells per million spleen cells was somewhat reduced in the lymph-node injected mice, but the number of IgG producing cells was higher. The total number of IgM producing cells per spleen was higher in the lymph-node injected mice while the total number of IgG producing cells was considerably higher.

Response to Oxazolone

Mice were painted with 3% oxazolone in absolute ethanol on the fore-paws and the front and the 4 draining lymph nodes were removed 3 days later (at this time all mitotic cells are T cells (6)). Cell suspensions were made, counted and then mixed in the ratio of 2:1 with a suspension of cells from the draining lymph nodes from oxazolone-painted F_1 mice (which have only 1 T6 marker chromosome) before making chromosome preparations. This was in order to make a comparison of the mitotic rates in the lymph nodes of hyper-lymphoid and normal control mice by measuring each against the same yardstick. The results are shown in Figure 3.

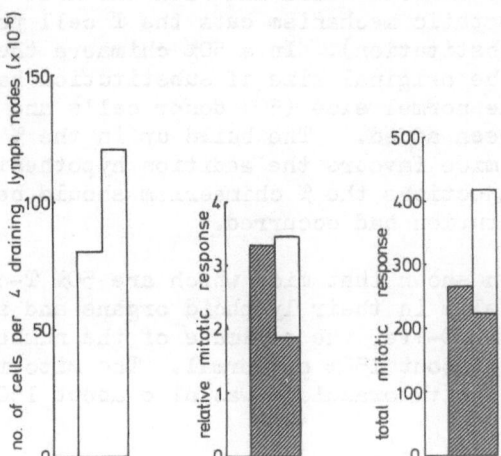

Fig.3 Number of cells and the mitotic rate in lymph nodes taken from control mice (1st column) and lymph-node injected mice (2nd column) painted 3 days previously with oxazolone. The shaded areas show the mitotic response of host cells.

It can be seen that there are considerably more cells in the draining lymph nodes of lymph-node injected mice. The relative mitotic rate (expressed as the ratio of the number of mitotic cells from experimental mice to the number of mitotic cells from the yardstick population), was the same in both groups, although it should be noted that the mitotic rate of host cells was decreased in the lymph-node injected mice. In the final part of the figure the total mitotic response has been estimated by multiplying the relative mitotic response by the total number of cells in the lymph nodes. It can be seen that the total number of host cell mitoses in the two groups is similar, but in the lymph-node injected group there are an equal number of donor T-cell mitoses. The overall response in the lymph-node injected is more than 50% greater than the control group.

DISCUSSION

The experiments reported here have shown that when lymphoid cells are injected intravenously into normal mice a permanent state of T-cell chimaerism results, in which the donor T cells appear to be incorporated into the recirculating pool so that similar proportions of donor cells are found in lymph nodes, spleen and blood. When multiple injections of lymphocytes are given a high level of T-cell chimaerism results. It seems to us that there are two hypotheses to account for the incorporation of donor T cells into a normal animal: 1) the donor T cells are added to the host T cell pool, resulting in an increased number of T cells in the animal (addition), and 2) the donor T cells mix with the host T cells and then an unknown homeostatic mechanism cuts the T cell pool down to its original size (substitution). In a 50% chimaera the T cell pool would still be the original size if substitution had occurred but would be twice the normal size (50% donor cells and 50% host cells) if cells had been added. The build up in the % chimaerism in multiply-injected mice favours the addition hypothesis. After the same number of injections the % chimaerism should be considerably higher if substitution had occurred.

While it has been shown that mice which are 50% T-cell chimaeras have more cells in their lymphoid organs and a greater proportion of these are θ-+ve, the estimate of the number of T cells in the animal is about 150% of normal. The mitotic response of the animals painted with oxazolone was also about 150% of normal.

The question remains, if the T-cell chimaerism results from addition of cells to the host T-cell pool why don't the 50% T-cell chimaeric mice have twice as many T cells as normal? It is possible that the rest of the T cells are sequestrated somewhere (histological examination of gut and Peyer's patches did not reveal them) or not all the θ−+ve cells are PHA responsive. If only about half of the θ−+ve cells were PHA responsive, and the donor cells were incorporated into the PHA responsive population exclusively this would explain the results obtained here.

ACKNOWLEDGEMENTS

    This work was supported by grants to the Chester Beatty Research Institute (Institute of Cancer Research: Royal Cancer Hospital) from the Medical Research Council and the Cancer Research Campaign.   The authors wish to thank Ken Gomer for technical assistance and Marjorie Butt for typing the manuscript.

REFERENCES

1) Doenhoff, M.J., Davies, A.J.S., Leuchars, E., Wallis, V.
    Nature, 227, 1352 (1970).
2) Doenhoff, M.J., Davies, A.J.S., Leuchars, E., Wallis, V.
    Proc.Roy.Soc.Lond.B., 176, 69 (1970).
3) Boyse, E.A., Old, L.J., Chouroulinkov, I. Meth.Med.Res., 10,
    39 (1964).
4) Schlesinger, M. J.Immunol., 94, 359 (1965).
5) Cunningham, A.J., Szenberg, A. Immunology, 14, 599 (1968).
6) Kerbel, R.S., Elliott, E.V., Wallis, V.J.   Cell.Immunol.,
    11, 146 (1974).

THE ROLE OF THE AFFERENT LYMPH IN THE INDUCTION OF CONTACT

SENSITIVITY

Bjørn Søeberg[*], Tatjana Sumerska[**], and Brigid M.Balfour[***]

[*]Department of Clinical Immunology, Rikshospitalet 7111, Copenhagen, Denmark, [**] (Wellcome Trust Fellow), Center for Infectious and Parasitic Diseases, Bul."Zaimov" 26, Sofia, Bulgaria, [***] National Institute for Medical Research, Mill Hill, London NW7 1AA, UK

Since it is known that destruction of the afferent lymph pathway can prevent the induction of contact sensitivity by skin painting the lymph must contain some essential element. In earlier experiments on pigs (McFarlin 1973) lymph was collected following skin painting with DNFB. Whole lymph was infused into an afferent lymphatic in a normal animal and shown to be capable of inducing contact sensitivity. In the experiments reported here pigs were painted with 50 microlitres of a 10% solution of DNFB in a mixture of equal parts of acetone and DMSO, a dose which was sufficient to sensitise the majority of animals.

Afferent Lymph Cells

In 6 out of 8 animals the skin became inflamed 2-5 hours after painting and the cell concentration in the lymph increased after

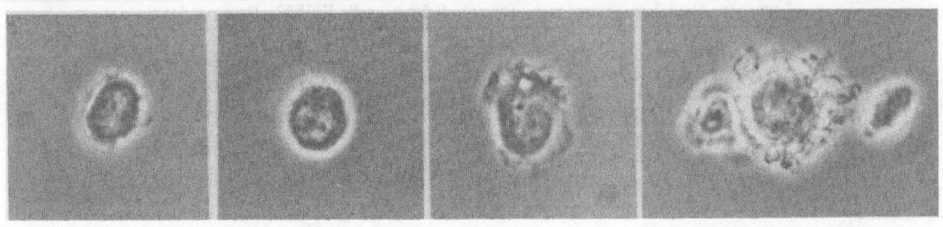

Lymphoid Cell   Lymphoid Cell   Macrophage   Aggregate containing Macrophage-like Cell

Figure 1. Afferent Lymph Cells following Skin Painting
with DNFB x 1000

9-11 hours, sometimes as much as 20 times above the normal level
50-100,000 cells/ml. The initial increase was almost entirely due
to polymorphonuclear leucocytes but later, 18-19 hours after painting, the cellular composition began to change, there were increased
numbers of lymphoid cells with small hair-like processes, macrophage-
like cells with long villi, a type of cell which is present in small
numbers in normal lymph and typical macrophages. Later still aggregates of cells were observed, containing one or more macrophage-
like cell with lymphoid cells attached to the surface villi. In
order to investigate the sensitising ability of the afferent lymph
cells, lymph was collected during the first 12 hours after painting, the cells were separated, washed and infused into an afferent
lymphatic in a normal animal. The first transfers were carried out
in outbred animals and the results are shown in Table I. 40% of
the animals developed contact sensitivity, but there was no obvious
correlation between the number of cells transferred and sensitisation. The second series of transfers were carried out between animals
who were compatible at the major locus (PLA matched). These animals
were obtained from the Animal Physiology Research Centre and the experiments were done in collaboration with Dr.Richard Binns and Dr.
David White. However the proportion of animals sensitised was the
same as in the outbred transfers.

The results suggested that the cells travelling to the node
during the first 12 hours after painting are capable of inducing
contact sensitivity and that histocompatibility at the major locus
is not an essential requirement.

The cells carried a small amount of DNP about 7-11 nanograms/10^6
cells and their sensitising ability may have been due to the presence
of antigen, if so they were very efficient carriers being able to
sensitise with as little as 90 nanograms DNP. The cells travelling
to the node during the second 12 hours after painting carried about
the same amount of DNP.

Table I. Induction of Contact Sensitivity by Transfer of Afferent
          Lymph Cells coming from Site of DNFB Painting

Cells collected during 1st 12 hours after painting

PLA Matched		Outbred	
No. of Cells Transferred	Response to Challenge	No. of Cells Transferred	Response to Challenge
11 x 10^6	−	10 x 10^6	−
19 x 10^6	+	10 x 10^6	+
28 x 10^6	+	17 x 10^6	−
37 x 10^6	−	23 x 10^6	−
42 x 10^6	−	44 x 10^6	+

Table II.   Induction of Contact Sensitivity by DNP Conjugated
                    Peripheral White Cells

Total DNP	DNP/10^6 Cells	Response to Challenge	
		Autologous	Heterologous
0.19 ug	0.004 ug	++	-
0.20 "	0.004 "	+	+
16.50 "	0.760 "	+	+
20.70 "	0.370 "	+	$\pm$
20.70 "	0.370 "		$\mp$
25.00 "	0.140 "	$\pm$	
25.00 "	0.600 "		+
25.00 "	1.000 "	++	

Cells other than Afferent Lymph Cells

Peripheral white cells were obtained from an animal 18 hours
after painting with DNFB. At this time the DNP content was about
4 nanograms/10^6 cells. The cells were divided into two portions,
one of which was X irradiated at a level of 3000R. Aliquots containing 5 x 10^7 unirradiated cells were infused into 2 outbred
and one PLA matched recipient and similar aliquots of irradiated
cells were infused into outbred recipients. It was found that irradiated as well as unirradiated cells were able to sensitise outbred recipients, but unirradiated cells failed to sensitise the PLA
matched recipient.

In order to determine whether the sensitising ability of cells
carrying a small amount of DNP could be attributed to their function
as antigen carriers, blood lymphocytes were conjugated in vitro with
DNP at a level of 4 nanograms/10^6 cells, that is at about the same

Table III.   Induction of Contact Sensitivity by DNP Conjugated
                     Heat Killed Peripheral White Cells

Total DNP	DNP/10^6 Cells	Response to Challenge	
		Autologous	Heterologous
0.2 ug	0.004 ug	$\pm$	+
0.2 "	0.004 "	-	-
19.0 "	0.170 "		-
25.0 "	0.150 "	-	+
30.0 "	0.230 "		+
30.0 "	0.230 "		+
33.0 "	0.170 "	+	

Table IV.   Induction of Contact Sensitivity by DNP Conjugated
                        Lymph Node Cells

Total DNP	DNP/10^6 Cells	Response to Challenge		
		Autologous	Heterologous	Heterologous X irradiated
5.0 ug	0.38 ug	–		
5.0 "	0.38 "	–		
25.0 "	0.33 "		++	
25.0 "	0.40 "	–	+	+
25.0 "	0.40 "	–		–
25.0 "	0.45 "		+	
25.0 "	0.50 "		++	
25.0 "	0.67 "			++

level as the afferent lymph cells. The viability of these lightly
conjugated cells was over 95% and they were able to make a partial
response to PHA.   It was found that these conjugated cells were able
to sensitise autologous and heterologous recipients, with as little
as 200 nanograms of DNP.   In other experiments blood lymphocytes
were conjugated at a higher level, between 100 and 1000 nanograms
DNP/10^6 cells.   These cells were much damaged, their viability immediately after conjugation was about 65% and they failed to respond
to PHA.   However they were still able to induce contact sensitivity
in autologous and heterologous recipients, though the amount of DNP
required was much greater, about 16-25 micrograms.   Heat killing
of lightly conjugated blood lymphocytes diminished their ability
to sensitise autologous recipients but had little effect on the
ability of highly conjugated cells to sensitise autologous and
heterologous recipients.

    In earlier experiments (McFarlin 1973) it was shown that auto-
logous lymph node cells conjugated at a low level of DNP were able
to sensitise. The experiments were repeated using highly conjugated
lymph node cells and it was found that the activity of the autologous cells was diminshed whereas heterologous cells were still able
to sensitise and their ability was not destroyed by X irradiation
with 3000R.   Thymocytes were obtained by partial thymectomy and conjugated in vitro at a level of 300-400 nanograms/10^6 cells. In
these experiments heterologous cells again proved to be more efficient sensitising agents than autologous cells.

    Peritoneal macrophages were conjugated at a level of 380 nan-
ograms/10^6 cells. These cells were able to sensitise heterologous
recipients but their efficiency was no greater than that of other
cell types.

Cell Membranes and Proteins

Lymph node cell and thymocyte plasma membranes (Allan and Crumpton 1970) and also red cell membranes were conjugated with DNP and infused into heterologous recipients. It was found that lymph node cell and red cell membranes were able to sensitise normal animals, whereas thymocyte membranes were almost inactive. However the minimum sensitising dose of DNP attached to membranes was 400 micrograms, very much greater than the minimum dose attached to cells, 0.2 micrograms. The conjugated membrane preparations were treated with glycylglycine in order to remove any unreacted DNFB which might have been retained inside the membrane vesicles, but this did not alter their sensitising ability.

DNP conjugated proteins were detected in the lymph in almost all animals. Earlier experiments had shown that the sensitising ability of the cell free fraction was mainly concentrated in the small molecular weight fraction (Balfour et al.1974). However in the experiments reported here it was found that the protein fraction was also able to sensitise, provided very large amounts were infused, containing 280 micrograms DNP. Treatment with glycylglycine again had no effect on the activity of the preparation.

In other experiments DNP conjugated pig serum was prepared at a level of 54 micrograms DNP/mg protein. This preparation was also able to sensitise and the minimum sensitising dose contained 133 micrograms DNP. Treatment with glycylglycine had no effect on its sensitising ability.

Since the small molecular weight fraction of the lymph contained up to 50% of the total radioactivity in lymph collected during the first 6-8 hours after skin painting with ^{3}H DNFB, the activity of DNFB itself and of the small molecular weight derivatives likely to be present in this fraction were investigated.

DNFB proved to be a potent sensitising agent when infused up an afferent lymphatic, as little as 500 nanograms would sensitise a normal animal, dinitrophenol would also sensitise but was about 200 times less efficient: DNP amino acids, including those capable of donating a DNP group, di-DNP cysteine and di-DNP tyrosine were either very inefficient or inactive.

A sensitive method for detecting DNFB was developed in collaboration with Dr.David Button and Dr.Ilina Bineva and preliminary results indicated that free DNFB was present in the lymph during the first 1-3 hours after skin painting in 40% of animals: all these animals developed strong inflammation 2-5 hours after painting. DNFB was not detected in lymph obtained from animals in whom the skin reaction was mild or delayed. Dinitrophenol was present in the

lymph in quite large quantities in about 60% of animals. Assuming
that the flow of lymph from the skin site to be about 3 mls/hour
it was calculated that 30% of animals would receive a sensitising
dose of DNFB during the first 3 hours after painting and these
animals plus a further 10-20% of animals would receive a sensitising
dose of dinitrophenol. In order to investigate this possibility the
painted skin site was excised 1-3 hours after painting and it was
found that 90% of the animals developed contact sensitivity. However
if the skin site was excised 12-18 hours after painting only 30-40%
of the animals were sensitised. When excision was delayed for 24
hours all animals were sensitised.

We conclude that the afferent lymph draining from skin
painted with DNFB contains a number of sensitising agents, DNFB,
dinitrophenol, DNP conjugated proteins and DNP conjugated cells.
The lymph reaching the draining node during the first few hours after
painting probably contains a sensitising dose of one or more of
these agents, since 90% of animals developed contact sensitivity
when the skin site was excised after 1-3 hours. However excision
at 12-18 hours reduced this proportion and it seems possible that
lymph secreted during the period 6-20 hours after painting also
contained inhibitory factors, but that the inhibition was normally
overcome by the arrival of activated cells during the period 18-24
hours after painting.

On the other hand significant numbers of immuno-competent
cells may have been concentrated in the skin during the period
6-18 hours after painting and their removal caused the animals to
become unresponsive. The experiments also indicated that conjugated cells of various types, afferent lymph cells, peripheral white
cells, lymph node cells and thymocytes were capable of inducing
contact sensitivity in autologous and heterologous recipients
(Baumgarten and Geczy 1970; Dennert and Harten 1975; Shearer et al.
1975). The ability to sensitise autologous versus heterologous
recipients was related to the degree of conjugation and to the
viability of the cell, for example highly conjugated heterologous
lymph node cells and thymocytes proved to be more efficient sensitising agents than highly conjugated autologous cells.

REFERENCES

1.   McFarlin, D.E. and Balfour, B.M., Immunology 25, 995 (1973).
2.   Allan, D. and Crumpton, M.J., Biochem.J. 120, 133 (1970).
3.   Balfour, B.M., McFarlin, D.E., Sumerska, T. and Parker, D.,
        Monogr.Allergy 8, 27 (1974).
4.   Baumgarten, A. and Geczy, A.F., Immunology Lond. 19, 205 (1970).
5.   Shearer, G.M., Rehn, T.G. and Garbarino, C.A., J.exp.Med. 141,
        1348 (1975).
6.   Dennert, G. and Hatlen, L.E., J.Immunol. 114, 1705 (1975).

STUDIES ON THE EFFECT OF ENVIRONMENT ON THE GVH

REACTIVITY OF RECIRCULATING LYMPHOCYTES

R.G. SCOLLAY and J.G. HALL

CHESTER BEATTY RESEARCH INSTITUTE

CLIFTON AVENUE, SUTTON, SURREY, ENGLAND

We have found qualitative and quantitative differences in the graft versus host (GVH) reactivity of lymphocytes from the blood, efferent lymph and peripheral lymph (afferent to the popliteal node) of sheep.

Blood cells were prepared from heparinised venous blood by spining through Ficoll-triosil, and about 80% of the cells had the appearance of small lymphocytes (see Table 1). Cells from afferent and efferent lymph were collected from chronically draining catheters placed in the appropriate lymphatic ducts (ref. 1). Peripheral (afferent) lymph contains cells which have passed from the blood into the tissues and then into the lymphatic system, but which have not been through a lymph node. About 80% of the cells are small lymphocytes, the remainder being mostly macrophages with a few immunoblasts and polymorphonuclear granulocytes. Normal efferent lymph consists almost entirely of small lymphocytes (Table 1) which have recirculated from blood to lymph via the post capillary venules of the lymph node.

Since there is no 'T' cell marker in the sheep, we have attempted to assess the T and B cell populations by using an anti immunoglobulin (Ig) stain, and assuming that most non Ig bearing small lymphocytes are T cells.

The washed cells were stained with a polyvalent rabbit
anti-sheep Ig, and counterstained with a sheep anti-
rabbit Ig conjugated to horseradish peroxidase (ref. 2).
Cells labelled with conjugate were shown by developing
the smears with benzidine in the usual manner.   The
results are shown in Table 1, and show that the three
cell populations contain about the same proportions of
T small lymphocytes.

Table 1
(bracketed Figures show range)

Compartment	Small lympho-cytes, % of total	Ig bearing cells, % of small cells	Presumed T cells, % of total
Blood mononuclear cell preparation	80% (70-90)	20-35%	60% (50-70)
Efferent lymph	95-99%	25-30%	70%
Afferent lymph	80% (65-90)	5-15%	70% (60-85)

Another point of interest is the recirculation
pattern of the two lymph cell populations.   Figure 1
shows the results of 4 experiments in which efferent
lymph cells were labelled with Na^{51}Cr and injected
intravenously back into the same animal.   The appearance of ^{51}Cr labelled cells in afferent and efferent
lymph was followed for 24 hours.   There is greater
variation in the afferent lymph samples because the
cell numbers in afferent lymph are very low and the
cell counts and isotope counts are proportionately
less accurate.   However, the general picture is the
same in the 4 experiments.   The curves for the
recirculation of cells into afferent and efferent lymph
are essentially the same, and reach the same plateau, so
although there is a tendency for labelled cells to appear
more rapidly in the afferent lymph, it is probably fair
to say that the recirculation patterns are not grossly
dissimilar.

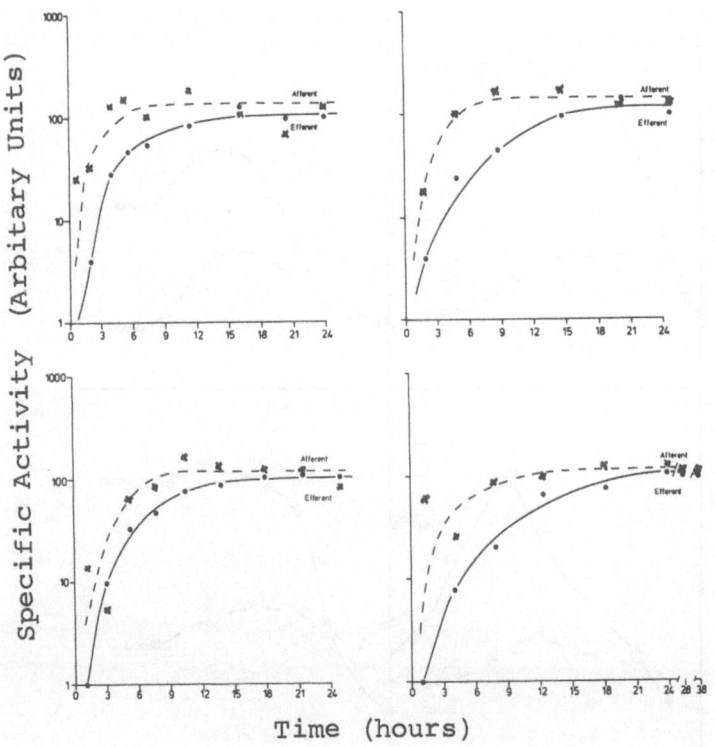

Figure 1. Recirculation of lymphocytes through afferent (x) and efferent (•) lymphatics: the appearance of lymphocyte associated label in afferent and efferent lymph following the intravenous injection of ^{51}Cr labelled autochthonous lymphocytes collected from efferent lymph. Four different sheep are shown. Afferent ducts were popliteal, efferent ducts prefemoral.

These then are our three populations of recirculating cells, each of which contains about 70% non Ig bearing lymphocytes. However, the behaviour of the three populations in the normal lymphocyte transfer (NLT) reaction is very different. The NLT reaction is a characteristic skin reaction which results when allogeneic lymphoid cells are injected intradermally into a normal (non-immune) recipient (ref. 3) and 4 typical examples can be seen in Figure 2, which compares the

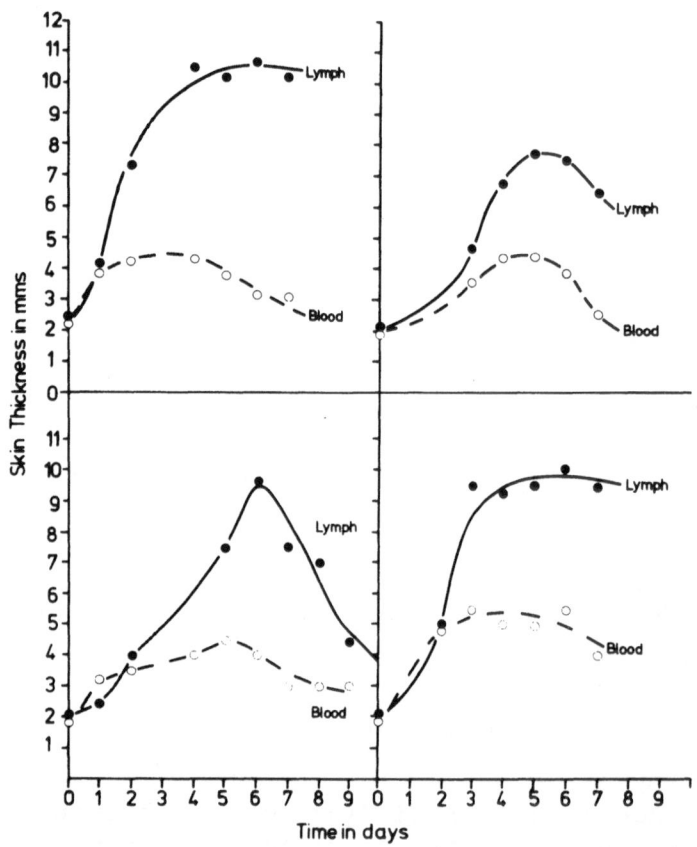

Figure 2. NLT with blood and efferent cells: a comparison of increases in skin thickness resulting from a primary intradermal innoculation of allogeneic cells (10^7 per site) from blood or efferent lymph of a single donor. The four boxes show four different pairs of sheep. Each point is the mean of triplicate lesions.

reaction induced by blood or efferent lymph cells from the same animal in a single recipient, in 4 donor/ recipient combinations. The reaction induced by blood cells is much less than that induced by efferent lymph cells (the reduction is equivalent to a 3-5 fold reduction in cell numbers) and the possibility of a Ficoll-triosil effect has been excluded.

Similarly a comparison between afferent and efferent lymph cells shows an afferent cell deficiency of a proportion equal to or greater than that shown by blood cells. Details of this afferent/efferent difference have been published elsewhere (ref. 4), and include histological evidence that the lesions are also qualitatively different.

The point should be made here that afferent lymph and blood cells are not non-reactive and do in fact cause lesions, as has been shown in the guinea pig (ref. 5). The differences are due to the relatively high reactivity of efferent lymph cells.

Mixed lymphocyte reaction (MLR's) using these cell populations have also been studied, and show that while blood and afferent lymph cells are better stimulators than efferent cells, in terms of MLR ratio (experimental CPM : control CPM), they are much worse as responders. However, these results require some qualification, since the very high backgrounds observed when blood and afferent lymph cells are used as responders may obscure quite brisk reactions. In addition, the presence of macrophages and monocytes in these preparations may non-specifically enhance reactions when they are used as stimulators.

These points are being further investigated, but they do indicate some of the problems associated with experiments of this sort.

We have shown then, that three different populations of recirculating lymphoid cells, taken from a single animal, at the same time, can, in at least one kind of immune reaction, behave in quite different ways, and that these differences cannot be explained on the basis of the T and B cell content of the cell populations, or on the macrophage content. Due care should therefore be taken before one assumes that results obtained with any one population reflect the immune capabilities of the entire animal.

The reasons for the great differences in the three populations described above are not yet clear, but it

should be borne in mind that they are continually inter-
mixing. Indeed the highly reactive lymph cells pour
into the blood from the thoracic duct at about 10^9 cells
per hour, sufficient to replace the entire lymphocyte
content of the blood in less than 10 hours. Any
mechanisms operating must do so fairly rapidly.
Experiments are in progress to try and resolve some
of these questions.

REFERENCES

1)   Smith, J. B., G. H. McIntosh and Bede Morris
          (1970). J. Anat., 107; 87
2)   Nakana, P. K. and A. Kawaoi (1974).
          J. Histochem. Cytochem., 22; 1084.
3)   Jones, M. A. S. and K. J. Lafferty (1969).
          Aust. J. exp. Biol. med. Sci. 47; 159.
4)   Scollay, R., and K. J. Lafferty (1975).
          Transplant. 19; 170.
5)   Brent, L. and P. Medawar (1968).
          Proc. Roy. Soc. B. 165; 281.

THE RECOVERY OF THE B CELL COMPARTMENT IN LETHALLY

IRRADIATED AND RECONSTITUTED MICE

J. Rozing and R. Benner

Dept. of Cell Biology and Genetics
Erasmus University
Rotterdam, The Netherlands

Reappearance of immunological responsiveness after lethal irradiation and reconstitution with hemopoietic stem cells is dependent on the recovery of two types of lymphoid cells: B and T cells. The B cell compartment seems to recover faster than the T cell compartment (1,2). Nossal and Pike compared the rate of recovery of anti-immunoglobulin binding cells in different lymphoid organs. They found a somewhat faster repopulation in the spleen than in lymph nodes and bone marrow (3,4). Everett and Tyler (5) provided evidence that in normal mice the marrow is the major site of lymphocyte production. These lymphocytes are probably immature stages of the B cell line (6).

In the present study the contribution of spleen and bone marrow to the recovery of the B cell compartment in irradiated and reconstituted mice was investigated by means of membrane fluorescence. Furthermore the rate of recovery of the B cell and T cell compartment in the spleen was studied.

MATERIALS AND METHODS

(C57BL/Rij x CBA/Rij)F1 female mice were used at 10-12 weeks of age. The animals were lethally irradiated (875 rad; 250 kV; 1 mm Cu filter added) and reconstituted with 1.5×10^6 fetal liver cells intraveneously. These liver cells were derived from embryos at 14 days gestation. These cells were chosen as a source of hemopoietic stem cells because by means of membrane fluorescence we never found B cells in these fetal livers at that time.

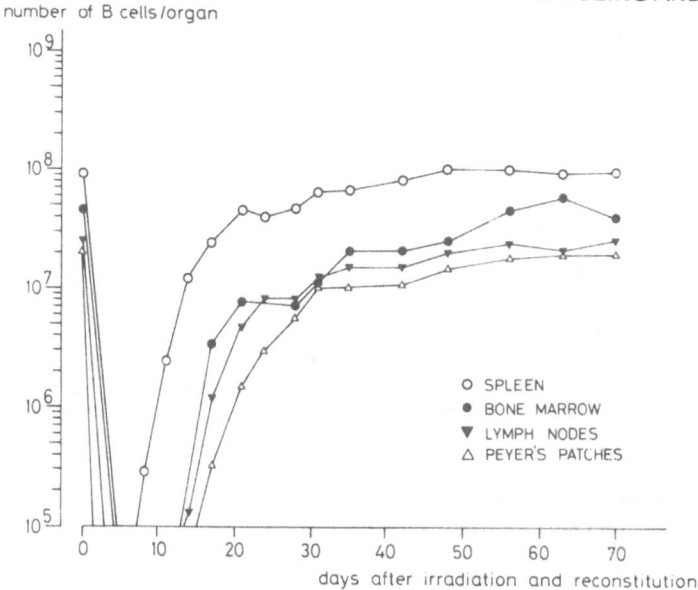

Fig. 1. Recovery of the number of B cells in various
         lymphoid organs after irradiation and reconsti-
         tution with fetal liver cells.

        B cells were assayed by means of a direct membrane
immunofluorescence procedure, described in detail by
Knapp et al. (7). A TRITC-goat anti mouse-immunoglobulin
conjugate (Nordic, Tilburg, The Netherlands) was used
for the demonstration of B cells.
        T cells were assayed by means of an indirect mem-
brane immunofluorescence technique. The cells were first
incubated with a rabbit anti mouse-thymocyte serum, kindly provided by Dr. J.M.N. Willers (University of Utrecht,
The Netherlands). Subsequently the cells were treated with
a TRITC-goat anti rabbit-immunoglobulin conjugate (Nordic,
Tilburg, The Netherlands). The slides were examined with
a Zeiss microscope equipped with a vertical illuminator
IV/F and an Osram HBO 50 mercury lamp.
        Splenectomy (Sx) and sham-splenectomy (ShSx) were
performed when mice were at 10-12 weeks of age. Approximately 2 months later these Sx- and ShSx-mice were used
for irradiation and reconstitution.
        To prevent cell production in the bone marrow, mice
were treated with a dose of 3 μCi [89]Sr (Amersham-Searle
Corp., Arlington Heights, Ill.)/gm bodyweight. These mice
were lethally irradiated and reconstituted immediately
before treatment with [89]Sr. Full details of the experimental approach will be published elsewhere.

RESULTS

After irradiation and reconstitution with fetal liver cells a sharp decline of the number of B cells was found in the spleen, bone marrow, lymph nodes (mesenteric, inguinal, axillary and brachial) and Peyer's patches (Fig. 1). At six days after reconstitution a recovery of the total cellularity was found in spleen and bone marrow (data not shown in figure). Another three days later an increased number of B cells could be demonstrated in the spleen. In the other lymphoid organs tested a rise of the number of B cells was found at 17 days after reconstitution. The number of B cells in all the organs tested proved to be completely or nearly completely restored at 60 days after irradiation and reconstitution. The development of the B cell compartment in the spleen was found to be much faster than the recovery of the T cell compartment (Fig. 2).

In splenectomized (Sx), irradiated and reconstituted mice also recovery of the B cell population was found in the bone marrow, lymph nodes, Peyer's patches and peripheral blood (Table I). Compared with control mice numbers of B cells in organs of Sx-mice were even higher at day 50.

In the bone marrow of mice treated with ^{89}Sr both the total number of nucleated cells and the number of B cells remained at an extremely low level (Table II). In spite of the absence of an increase of the number of nucleated cells

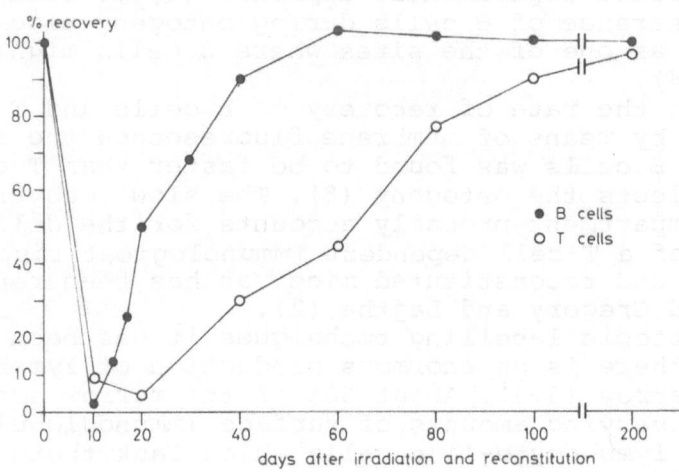

Fig. 2. Proportional recovery of B cells and T cells in the spleen after irradiation and reconstitution with fetal liver cells.

TABLE I

Number of B cells in various organs of splenectomized (Sx) and sham-splenectomized (ShSx) mice 50 days after irradiation and reconstitution.

Organ	Sx	ShSx
spleen	-	10.90 ± 1.15[a]
bone marrow	7.81 ± 0.90	2.97 ± 0.59
Peyer's patches	2.10 ± 0.17	1.37 ± 0.23
lymph nodes	2.82 ± 0.14	2.32 ± 0.36
blood	1.73 ± 0.18	0.86 ± 0.12

[a]Number of B cells per organ $(x10^{-7}) \pm 1$ S.E.M. (5 mice tested).

in the bone marrow a recovery of the B cell compartment in the spleen of the ^{89}Sr-mice was found. However, the number of B cells in the spleen of the ^{89}Sr-mice remained at a lower level than in the spleen of control mice.

DISCUSSION

After irradiation and reconstitution of mice with fetal liver cells B cells were found to reappear primarily in the spleen. In bone marrow, lymph nodes and Peyer's patches recovery of the B cell compartment started about 8 days later. Such a marked difference between spleen and other lymphoid organs was not found by Nossal and Pike, using a comparable experimental approach (3,4). Studies about the appearance of B cells during ontogeny also point to the spleen as one of the sites where B cells might be generated (3,4).

Comparing the rate of recovery of B cells and T cells in the spleen by means of membrane fluorescence the reappearance of B cells was found to be faster than T cells. This also reflects the ontogeny (8). The slow recovery of the T cell compartment probably accounts for the delayed reappearance of a T cell dependent immunological response in irradiated and reconstituted mice, as has been reported by Vos (1) and Gregory and Lajtha (2).

Using isotopic labelling techniques it has been demonstrated that there is an enormous production of lymphocytes in the bone marrow (5,9). About 50% of the marrow small lymphocytes show varying amounts of surface immunoglobulins (Ig) (6). The lymphocyte-like cells which lack theta-antigen, readily demonstrable Ig or complement receptors on their surface are suggested to be predominantly immature B lymphocytes (6). Osmond and Nossal recently studied the appearance of surface-Ig on short-lived bone marrow lym-

TABLE II

Number of nucleated cells and B cells in spleen and bone
marrow of ^{89}Sr-treated mice 25 days after irradiation and
reconstitution.

Organ	control mice		[89]Sr mice	
	nucl. cells	B cells	nucl. cells	B cells
spleen	19.4 ± 0.6^a	7.7 ± 0.4	16.3 ± 0.9	3.3 ± 0.1
marrow	43.5 ± 1.6	2.2 ± 0.1	2.8 ± 0.4	0.003 ± 0.001

[a]Number of cells per organ (x 10^{-7}) $\pm$ 1 S.E.M. (5 mice tested).

phocytes in mice (9). These authors provided evidence
that small lymphocytes in the marrow are initially Ig-
negative but rapidly express increasing amounts of surface-Ig during differentiation and proliferation. Basten
and coworkers using a radioactively labeled antigen "suicide" technique have shown that, in conditions in which
thymocytes and spleen B cells are inactivated, bone marrow
lymphocytes are unaffected (10). This could be interpreted
as suggesting that maturation to the antigen-binding stage
takes place predominantly after the cells have migrated
from the marrow. Everett and Tyler indeed provided evidence for a continuous transport of recently generated
small lymphocytes from the bone marrow to the spleen (4).
In our experiments the recovery of the B cell compartment
started some days after the first increase of nucleated
cells in bone marrow and spleen. This observation together
with the appearance of B cells in the spleen before they
could be demonstrated in the other lymphoid organs would
be consistent with the above line of evidence about B
cell differentiation. Since the B cell population in bone
marrow, lymph nodes, Peyer's patches and blood recovered
in control mice as well as in mice splenectomized before
irradiation and reconstitution, it can be concluded that
the spleen is not the only site where B cells mature.
    Supply of immature B cells by the bone marrow to the
other lymphoid organs can be excluded by using the bone-
seeking isotope [89]Sr (11). Phillips and Miller (11), using
[89]Sr-treated, irradiated and reconstituted mice, have shown
that such mice can evoke a PFC response in the spleen.
They suggest that B cell differentiation can occur without
lymphopoiesis in the bone marrow. Our data about the influence of ^{89}Sr treatment of the recipient mice upon the appearance of B cells in the spleen confirms this. In our
experiments total B cell count in the spleen by means of
membrane fluorescence allowed a quantitative study of the
influence of excluding the generation of cells in the bone

marrow. The number of B cells in ^{89}Sr-treated mice raised
up to only 50% of control mice at 25 days. For this phenomenon various explanations can be given:
(1) in normal mice there is probably a migration of immature B cells from the bone marrow into the spleen which is
absent in ^{89}Sr-treated mice.
(2) haemopoiesis in ^{89}Sr-treated mice only occurs in the
spleen. Therefore competition for stem cells might occur
between the various cell lines generated in this organ.
Although virgin B cells are reported to be non-recirculating cells (12), it can not be excluded that some B cells
are eliminated while circulating in the blood through the
marrow cavity. In conclusion it can be stated that ^{89}Sr-
treated mice are unable to compensate completely for the
absence of lymphocyte production in the bone marrow.

ACKNOWLEDGEMENTS

    The experiments with ^{89}Sr were performed in the Radio-
biological Institute (Rijswijk, The Netherlands) under su-
pervision of Prof. Dr. L.M. van Putten, to whom we are very
indebted for the facilities provided.
    This investigation was supported by the Interuniver-
sitary Institute of Radiationpathology and Radiation
Protection (Leiden, The Netherlands).

REFERENCES

1. O. Vos. In "Effects of radiation on cellular proliferation and differentiation". I.A.E.A., Vienna, p. 149,
   1968.
2. C.J. Gregory and L.G. Lajtha. Int. J. Radiat. Biol.,
   17, 117, 1970.
3. G.J.V. Nossal and B.L. Pike. Immunology, 25, 33, 1973.
4. G.J.V. Nossal and B.L. Pike. In "Microenvironmental aspects of immunity". p. 11, 1973.
5. N.B. Everett and R.W. Tyler. Int. Rev. Cytol. 22, 205,
   1967.
6. D.G. Osmond and G.J.V. Nossal. Cell. Immunol. 13,
   117, 1974.
7. W. Knapp, H.R.E. Schuit, R.L.H. Bolhuis and W. Hijmans.
   Clin. Exp. Immunol. 16, 541, 1974.
8. M.O. Chiscon and E.S. Golub. J. Immunol. 108, 1379, 1972
9. D.G. Osmond and G.J.V. Nossal, Cell. Immunol. 13,
   134, 1974.
10. A. Basten, J.F.A.P. Miller, N.L. Warner and J. Pye.
    Nature New Biol. 231, 104, 1971.
11. R.A. Phillips and R.G. Miller. Nature 251, 444, 1974.
12. J. Sprent and A. Basten. Cell Immunol. 7, 40, 1973.

REGULATION OF THYMIC LYMPHOPOIESIS IN VITRO

R. Juhlin, J.F. Sällström and G.V. Alm

Department of Histology

University of Uppsala, Uppsala, Sweden

The fundamental mechanisms involved in the regulation of thymic lymphopoiesis are largely unknown, including the properties of the lymphoid precursor cells and the factors that determine lymphoid cell proliferation and differentiation. We have therefore attempted to analyze possible regulatory mechanisms acting in thymic lympho- poiesis. Our experimental model has been the embryonic thymus in organ culture. In this system lymphoid cell development may be in- fluenced both by the thymic microenvironment, including locally produced thymic hormone(s), and by factors present in the serum supplement of the organ culture medium. We have thus demonstrated and characterized a factor in chicken (1,2) and mammalian sera (3) essential for chicken respectively mouse thymic lymphopoiesis in vitro. Other work suggested an internal control of lymphoid cell proliferation and development in the thymus (1,4).

The present communication concerns mainly the microenvironment- al aspects of lymphopoiesis in the chicken and mouse thymus in organ culture.

TIME DEPENDENT DEVELOPMENT OF THYMIC LYMPHOID CELLS IN VITRO

The time dependent development of lymphoid cells in organ cul- tures of the thymus of 10-day-old chick embryos and 14-day-old CBA mouse embryos was characterized. Details of the organ culture tech- nique as well as determination of lymphoid cell numbers per thymus, incorporation of ^{3}H-thymidine (^{3}H-TdR) during a 4 h pulse and cell sizes are given elsewhere (1,4,5). Chicken cultures contained 10% chicken serum and mouse cultures 10% fetal calf serum (FCS).

Supported by grants from the Swedish Cancer Society (511-B74-04XC) and Prenatalforskningsnämnden, Stockholm.

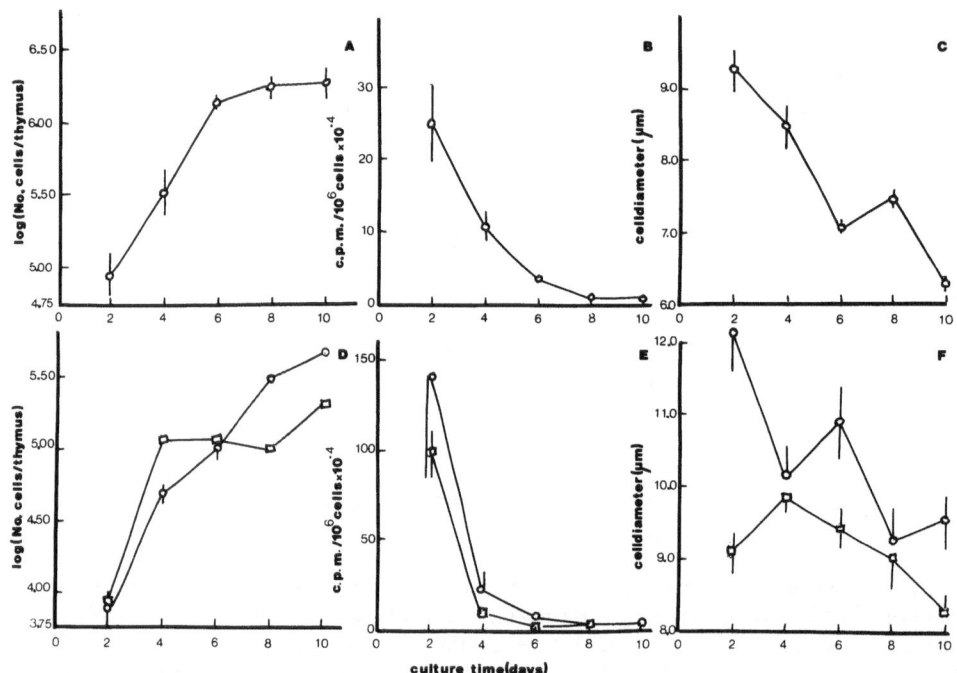

Figure 1. Growth characteristics of the embryonic chicken (A,B,C) and mouse (D,E,F) thymus in organ culture. (A,D), lymphoid cell number per thymus (B,E), ^{3}H-TdR incorporation per 10^6 cells. (C,F), mean cell diameters. The mouse thymus was cultured in high (o—o) and low (□—□) O_2 concentration.

Fig. 1 shows that in both the chicken thymus grown in 57% O_2 and the mouse thymus grown in 20% O_2 (5% CO_2, balance N_2) the number of cells increased initially rapidly with culture time and then reached a plateau value (Fig. 1 A,D). Thereafter (approx. on d. 14) the number of cells decreased (not shown). The incorporation of ^{3}H-TdR per 10^6 thymus cells, an estimate of the proportion of proliferating cells, decreased rapidly and reached a low basal value (Fig. 1 B,E). The mean sizes of the lymphoid cells also decreased with time, particularly in the chicken thymus (Fig. 1 C,F). Mouse thymus cultures maintained at high O_2 concentration (57%) showed initially lower lymphoid cell numbers than at 20% O_2, but continued to increase over approximately 14 days and then reached a plateau value. The ^{3}H-TdR incorporation was slightly higher and the lymphoid cells larger at high O_2 concentration. Furthermore we found that under such conditions lymphopoiesis was sustained for at least 8 weeks (Table 1).

Table 1. Long term culture of the thymus of the 14-day-old CBA mouse embryo at high O_2 concentration. Mean number of lymphoid cells (x 10^6) per thymus ± S.D. Six thymuses assayed each time.

Culture time (weeks)					
3	4	5	6	7	8
0.33±0.12	0.29±0.06	0.30±0.15	0.17±0.05	0.18±0.11	0.15±0.14

ATTEMPTS TO EXPERIMENTALLY INFLUENCE LYMPHOPOIESIS

The number of proliferating lymphoid precursor cells was reduced at the initiation of chick thymus organ cultures by a short (60 min) hot pulse with ^{3}H-TdR of high specific activity (4,5, for details). Pulsed thymuses initially showed reduced lymphoid cell numbers, but these increased and attained the plateau cell number of non-pulsed controls, although later than in these (Fig. 2 A).

A reduction of lymphoid cell number at the begin of the plateau phase (day 6) by hypoxia resulted in a recovery of the number of lymphoid cells back to the plateau level (Fig. 2 B). The recovery was associated with increased cell proliferation as measured by 16 h pulses with ^{125}Iodo-deoxyuridine (^{125}I-UdR) (Fig. 2 C). A 6 h ^{3}H-TdR hot pulse on culture day 6 during hypoxic treatment prevented the recovery of the cell depleted thymus (Fig. 2 B,C). Similar experiments started on culture days 8 or 10, did not result in such a recovery of the thymus (results not shown). Technical details are given elsewhere (5).

These results and those of the previous section are compatible with the hypothesis that lymphoid cell density (number of cells per unit volume thymus) limits lymphoid cell proliferation and promotes the differentiation of small nonproliferating lymphocytes. These cells, although capable of reacting to mitogens such as concanavalin A and phytohemagglutinin (6) may not be able to enter cell cycle again within the thymus. Any replacement of cell loss from the thymus originates from a pool of dividing lymphoid precursor cells. This pool may be depleted at lasting high cell densities, after which lymphopoiesis is irreversibly terminated. One of many conceivable factors which could regulate lymphopoiesis in vitro is the microenvironmental O_2 tension explaining the prolonged lymphopoietic activity in the mouse thymus cultured at high O_2 concentration. Such a mechanism could also operate in vivo.

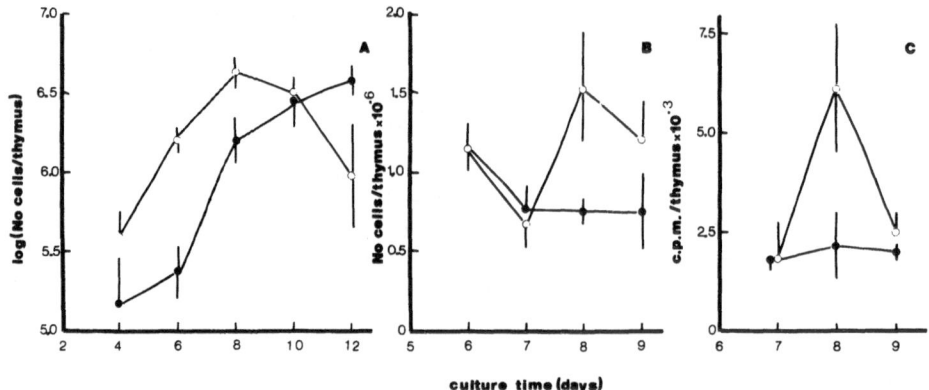

Figure 2. (A) Effect of a 60 min ^{3}H-TdR hot pulse on culture day 0
on cell numbers in organ cultured chicken thymus (●—●, pulse;
o—o, control). (B) Effect of hypoxia on d.6 on the cell numbers
in 6 h ^{3}H-TdR hot pulsed (●—●) and control (o—o) thymuses. (C)
Effect of hypoxia on the ^{125}I-UdR incorporation, otherwise as in
(B).

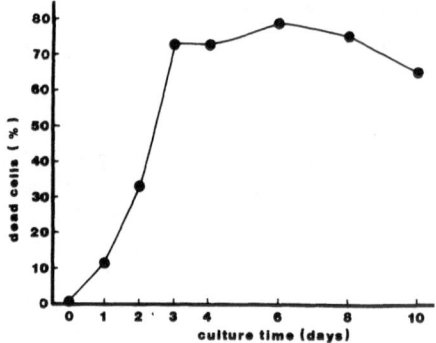

Figure 3. Development of θ-positive lymphoid cells in the embryonic
mouse thymus in organ culture (% cells killed by anti-θ antiserum).

ANTIGENIC AND FUNCTIONAL DEVELOPMENT OF MOUSE THYMIC LYMPHOID CELLS

    Work was initiated to define the antigenic and functional matu-
ration of lymphoid cells in the embryonic mouse thymus in organ culture. The well defined antigenic markers on murine T lymphocytes
makes this species particularly useful in studies of the differentiation of thymic cells.

    Previous work (7) showed that the thymus of the 14-day CBA
embryo contains no θ-positive cells and that such cells develop
during the following days. In the present investigation a conventional cytotoxic assay using AKR-anti-θCBA antiserum, rabbit com-

Table 2. In vitro Con A response of mouse thymic lymphoid cells derived from organ cultures or newborn and 1-month-old mice.

Cell source	^{3}H-thymidine uptake (cpm/culture)	
	No mitogen	Con A[1]
Org. cult. d.6, MS suppl.	347 ± 31	10313 ± 840 (2.5)
Org. cult. d.6, FCS suppl.	255 ± 41	578 ± 26 (2.5)
Org. cult. d.14, MS suppl.	158 ± 21	4947 ± 312 (5.0)
Org. cult. d.14, FCS suppl	61 ± 6	643 ± 21 (5.0)
Newborn mice	90 ± 9	14352 ± 3194 (0.625)
1-month-old mice	34 ± 4	6047 ± 673 (1.25)

[1] Figures in parentheses represent the optimal Con A conc. (μg/ ml).

plement and trypan blue stain was employed to determine the frequency of θ-positive cells during the organ culture of the thymus of the 14-day-old CBA mouse embryo. As shown in Fig. 3 the proportion of θ-positive cells increased rapidly during the first 3-4 days of culture and was thereafter relatively constant.

To exclude the presence of thymic hormone in the supplementary FCS of the organ cultures, 2.5% supplementary serum from normal or nude NMRI mice and from adult thymectomized CBA mice was tested. The thymus stimulating activity locating in the albumin fraction after separation of ammonium sulphate precipitated human serum on Sephadex G-150 was also tried as medium supplement (3). These supplements resulted in 85-93% θ-positive cells on culture day 7.

The rapid changes in the proportion of θ-positive lymphoid cells are seen simultaneously with the rapid increase of the number of lymphoid cells per thymus and the decrease of the proportion of proliferating cells. Thus rapid and marked changes in lymphopoietic activity and cellular composition of the mouse thymus occur in vitro. The relation between these as well as the action of thymic hormones in lymphopoiesis is further investigated.

The development of mitogen reactive lymphoid cells in the embryonic CBA mouse thymus in organ culture was also investigated. The thymuses of 14-day embryos were cultured with medium supplements of either 2.5% CBA mouse serum (MS) or 10% FCS and in 5% CO_2

and 95% air. At day 6 and 14 suspensions of lymphoid cells were
prepared from the organ cultures and maintained for 48 h in serum-
free semi-microscale cultures (8) with concanavalin A (Con A) in
different concentrations. Cell proliferation was measured with a
terminal 4 h pulse of ^{3}H-TdR. Control thymus cells were obtained
from newborn and 1-month-old mice.

Table 2 shows that the lymphoid cells from organ cultures
supplemented with mouse serum responded well to Con A. The responses were equivalent to those of the control thymic lymphoid cells,
although the maximum stimulation occurred at somewhat higher Con A
concentrations. However, cells obtained from FCS supplemented organ
cultures always showed much lower responses than cells from organ
cultures supplemented with mouse serum. The two types of supplementary sera gave equivalent lymphoid cell numbers per thymus, and
the viability of the cells did not differ. These results therefore
indicate that mitogen reactive lymphoid cells develop in the mouse
thymus in organ culture but that the supplementary serum appears
critical. The inferior results obtained with FCS may be associated
with its content of lymphocyte inhibitory fetuin (9).

These results suggest that the functional differentiation of
mouse thymic lymphoid cells in the lymphopoiesis can be further
studied in the organ cultures.

REFERENCES

1. Sällström, J.F. and Alm, G.V., Acta Path. Microbiol. Scand.,
   Sect. A 82: 287, 1974.

2. Sällström, J.F., Acta Path. Microbiol. Scand., Sect. A 82: 589,
   1974.

3. Sällström, J.F. and Alm, G.V., to be published.

4. Juhlin, R. and Alm, G.V., Cell Tissue Kinet., in press.

5. Juhlin, R. and Alm, G.V., Cell Tissue Kinet. 7: 327, 1974.

6. Sällström, J.F. and Alm, G.V., Int. Arch. Allergy 47: 388, 1974.

7. Owen, J.J.T. and Raff, M.C., J. Exp. Med. 132: 1216, 1970.

8. Tufveson, G. and Alm, G.V., Immunology, in press.

9. Yachnin, S., J. Exp. Med. 141: 242, 1975.

ISOLATION AND PARTIAL CHEMICAL CHARACTERIZATION OF THF, A THYMUS HORMONE INVOLVED IN IMMUNE MATURATION OF LYMPHOID CELLS

A.I.KOOK, Y. YAKIR and N. TRAININ

Department of Cell Biology

The Weizmann Institute of Science, Rehovot, Israel

Humoral factors of the thymus participate in the processes which lead to maturation and acquisition of immunocompetence of cells of the lymphoid system (1,2). We have demonstrated that THF, a thymic factor partially purified in our laboratory (3,4), induces immune maturation of thymus derived lymphoid cells via an obligatory rise in cellular levels of cAMP and in membranal adenyl cyclase activity (5,6). We have now isolated and partially characterized the chemical properties of THF with the aim to further understand the processes which lead to differentiation of thymus derived cells.

The bioassay routinely used to evaluate the activity of THF is the in vitro graft-versus-host (GVH) model adopted from Auerbach and Globerson (7). In this assay the relative enlargement of a newborn (C3H/eb x C57BL/6)F_1 spleen explant challenged by parental C57BL/6 spleen cells as compared with a paired explant exposed to spleen cells of syngeneic (C3H/eb x C57BL/6)F_1 origin in the same culture, reflects the response to allogeneic challenge by immuno-competent cells. The relative size of the cultures is determined 4 days after the addition of cells. The calculated area of each test spleen fragment divided by the corresponding area of its paired reference fragment, provides a numerical index of splenome-galy. Cultures are considered reactive when the index of splenome-galy obtained is 1.2 or more (7). We have previously shown that spleen cells from neonatally thymectomized (NTx) mice are totally incompetent to react in the above GVH assay which is an all or none test (3). Therefore, the biological activity of the THF preparations is expressed by its ability to induce competence in these cells to react in the in vitro GVH assay (3-6). In the following isolation procedure, cultures of parental spleen cells of NTx mice and of

syngeneic control spleen cells were simultaneously exposed to THF
preparations from calf thymus (THF activity was also found in
extracts prepared from syngeneic or allogeneic thymuses (4)). The
crude THF preparations as well as the various fractions obtained
during the isolation procedure were routinely sterilized before
assayed for activity by filtration through 0.45 μm millipore
filters. The standard preparation procedure used in our laboratory
involves homogenization of fresh calf thymus in x 2 volumes of
0.005 M sodium phosphate buffer pH 7.4 and centrifugation at 2500
g for 20 min. The supernatant is further centrifuged at 105,000 g
for 5 h and diluted to a standard protein concentration. This
active extract is then exhaustively dialyzed against a 20 times
larger volume of water for 60 h in the cold. The THF passes
through Union Carbide dialysis sacs No. 27/32 or 23/32 while the
portion retained in the dialysis sacs is devoid of activity,
suggesting that the molecular weight (M.W.) of the active agent is
roughly 6000 or less (3,4). Protein, RNA, DNA and reducing carbohydrates contents of the dialyzate which has been concentrated by
lyophylization were determined chemically. No DNA could be detected. However, a constant ratio of about 7 mg protein to 2 mg reducing carbohydrates and 1 mg RNA was obtained. This lyophylized
dialyzate was treated with both DNase and RNase and these enzymes
did not abolish the activity of the preparation. In contrast, the
preparation was inactivated by pronase. This partially purified
preparation of THF was stable when kept at -20°C for several months,
but lost activity after 48 h at room temperature. The lyophylized
preparation was then dissolved in 0.1 M ammonium bicarbonate pH 8.0
and fractionated by gel filtration on Sephadex G-10 column (Pharmacia) (Fig. 1).

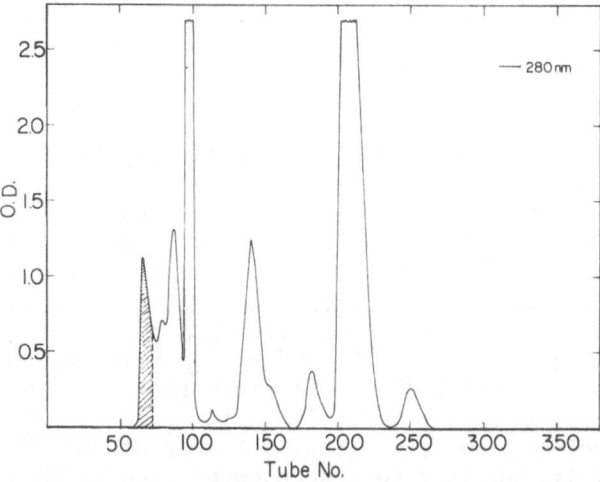

Fig. 1

Each of the protein peaks obtained was lyophylized, redissolved in ammonium bicarbonate and checked for activity. It was found that only substances which were eluted in the void volume of the column (shaded area) possess the ability to induce spleen cells from NTx mice to react in the in vitro GVH assay (Fig. 1, and Table 1).

TABLE 1

The Induction of In Vitro GVH Response in Spleen Cells of NTx C57BL/6 Mice by Active Fractions Obtained during various Steps of the Procedure for Isolation of THF

Fraction tested (20 μg protein/ ml)	Source of spleen cells	Incidence of reactive cultures			Culture response (%)
-	NTx	0/5	0/5	1/5	7
-	Intact	4/5	4/5	5/5	87
Dialyzate of thymus extract	NTx	3/5	3/5	3/5	60
Active peak of Sephadex G-10 column	NTx	5/5	4/5	4/5	87
Active peak of Sephadex G-25 column	NTx	5/5	5/5	4/5	93
Active peak of DEAE Sephadex A-25 column	NTx	4/5	4/5		80

The M.W. of THF thus appears to be greated than 700 since substances with M.W. above 700 are eluted in the void volume of G-10 Sephadex columns.

The material eluted with the void volume of the G-10 column was further fractionated by gel filtration on Sephadex G-25 fine column (Pharmacia) (Fig. 2). The column was eluted with 0.1 M ammonium bicarbonate pH 8.0. The resulting peaks were again lyophylized, redissolved and checked for their activity in the in vitro GVH assay system. Activity was consistently found in one peak only (shaded area, Fig. 2, and Table 1). The g-25 Sephadex column was calibrated with insulin (Sigma) (M.W. 5700), glucagon (Eli Lilly) (M.W. 3460) and bacitracin (Teva, Israel) (M.W. 1400). The elution volume of these substances was found to be inversely proportional to their molecular weights. The active material of the thymus extract (THF) was eluted immediately after glucagon. It hus appears that the M.W. of THF is about 3000.

The components of the active peak eluted from the G-25 Sephadex
column were further fractionated by anion exchange chromatography
on DEAE-Sephadex A-25 (Pharmacia) in 0.1 M ammonium bicarbonate
pH 8.0.   The column was developed with a linear concentration
gradient of NaCl (Fig. 3).   When the peaks obtained from the anion
exchange column were tested, it was found that the peak eluted in
0.15 M NaCl contained all the activity (shaded area, Fig. 3, and
Table 1).   This material was filtered through a G-10 Sephadex
column to remove salts and the activity was recovered in the void
volume of the column.   Starting with 400-500 gr wet weight of
calf thymus, 2-3 mg of active material can be obtained following
this step.   The material was concentrated by lyophylization and its
degree of purity was analyzed by isoelectric focusing (pH gradient
3.5 - 8.4) on polyacrylamide gels (8).   Eighty µg of protein were
applied to the gels.   The gels were subsequently stained either for
proteins with Coomassie brilliant blue (8) or for glycoproteins
with Alcian blue (9) (Fig. 4).   The pattern of the protein of the
crude active thymus extract is shown in gel A.   The active peak
obtained from the anion exchange chromatography column revealed the
presence of one band only which stained for protein (gel B) while
no glycopeptides were detected (gel C).

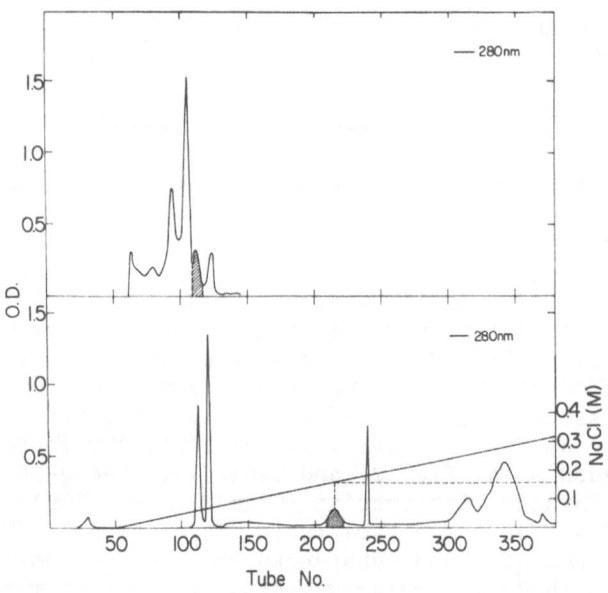

Figs. 2 and 3

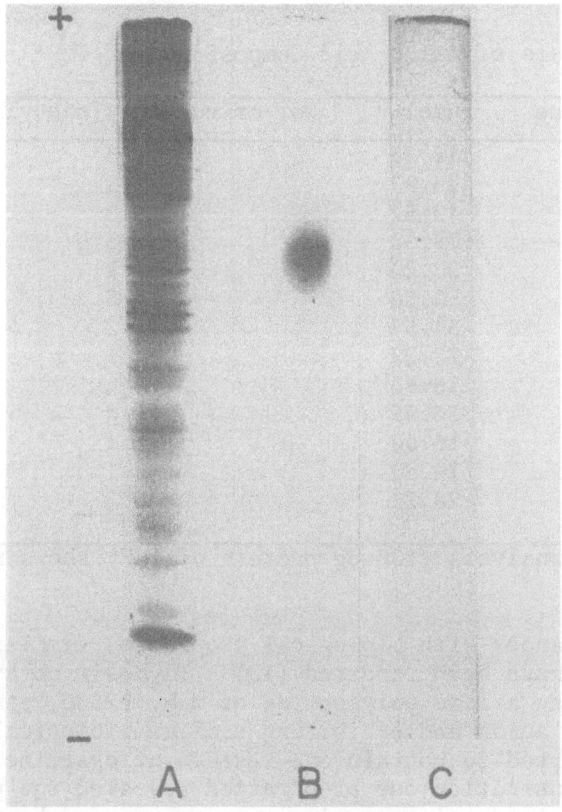

Fig. 4

The isoelectric point obtained for this polypeptide in three
different runs ranged between 5.66 - 5.90. In parallel, polyacrylamide gels which were not fixed and stained following the run, were
sliced and the contents allowed to diffuse into water in the cold.
Biological activity was recovered in the section corresponding to
the protein band. Thus it appears that the active peak eluted from
the anion exchange chromatography column contains THF which is an
acidic polypeptide having a M.W. of about 3000. The amino acid
composition of THF is shown in Table 2.

     No tryptophan is present in the amino acid composition of the
active polypeptide. 22, 48 and 72 hr hydrolysis were conducted to
evaluate the content of serine and threonine. Based on phenyl-
alanine as a unit, the M.W. is estimated at 2900. A high proportion of acidic amino acids can be observed.

TABLE 2

Analysis of Amino Acid Composition of THF*

Amino acid residue	nmol	No. of residue (phenylalanine=1)
Asp:	42.23	3
Thr:	23.94	2
Ser:	42.52	3
Glu:	78.52	5
Pro:	22.20	1
Gly:	50.80	3
Ala:	34.57	2
Half-Cyst:	22.27	1
Val:	18.83	1
Leu:	34.95	2
Phe:	16.00	1
Lys:	19.30	1
Arg:	28.32	2
		Sum: 27

*The amino acid analysis (100 µg protein of THF) shows no unusual
amino acids.

Other substances with biological properties similar to those
described by us have been reported (10). Thymosin obtained from
calf thymus, is an acidic polypeptide of M.W. 12500, containing the
same major amino acids and exhibiting similar biological activities.
Thymosin is reported to contain one residue of cysteine. Though in
the present communication our preparation revealed the presence of
this amino acid, in previous analysis cysteine was absent in the
active polypeptide (10).

In view of the differences in the number of amino acid residues and the M.W., it appears that THF possibly represent the active subunit of Thymosin.

REFERENCES
1. Trainin, N., Physiological Rev., 54, 272, 1974.
2. Trainin, N., Small, M., Zipori, D., Umiel, T., Kook, A.I. and
   Rotter, V. In: Thymic Hormones. (D.W. van Bekkum and A.M.Kruis-
   beck, eds.) 1975, in press.
3. Trainin, N., Small,M. and Globerson, A. J. Exp. Med. 130,765,1969
4. Trainin, N. and Small, M. J. Exp. Med. 132, 885, 1970.
5. Kook, A.I. and Trainin, N. J. Exp. Med. 139, 193, 1974.
6. Kook, A.I. and Trainin, N. J. Immunol., in press.
7. Auerbach, R. and Globerson, A. Exp. Cell. Res. 42, 31, 1966.
8. Eder, J. J. Immunol. Methods 2, 67, 1972.
9. Wardi, A.H. and Michos, G.A. Anal. Biochem. 49, 607, 1972.
10 "Biological activity of thymic hormones" D.W. van Bekkum and A.
   M.Kruisbeck, eds., Kooyker Scientific Publ., Rotterdam 1975,
   in press.

REGULATION OF IMMUNE BALANCE BY THYMOSIN: POTENTIAL ROLE IN THE DEVELOPMENT OF SUPPRESSOR T-CELLS

Allan L. Goldstein, Geraldine H. Cohen, Gary B. Thurman,
John A. Hooper and Jeffrey L. Rossio
Department of Human Biological Chemistry and Genetics,
Division of Biochemistry, University of Texas Medical
Branch, Galveston, Texas 77550

INTRODUCTION

Although the mechanism of action of thymosin has yet to be definitively established, it is clear that thymosin can activate immature lymphoid cells and induce their differentiation into immunologically competent T-lymphocytes in vitro and in vivo (1-5). It appears that one subpopulation of T-cells, the so-called "suppressor" or "regulator" T-cells, may be dependent upon thymosin for their differentiation and perhaps maintenance as a cell population (2,3). In this paper we review the results of animal and clinical experimentation which support the hypothesis that an imbalance in thymosin production and/or secretion may be part of the pathological mechanisms in certain autoimmune diseases. This deficiency is thought to lead to inadequate production of subpopulations of T-cells, such as the suppressor or regulator cells which appear to exert, in as yet an undefined manner, fine control over the immune system.

IMMUNE IMBALANCE AND THE DEVELOPMENT OF AUTOIMMUNE DISEASE

Several investigators have used the NZB mouse strain as a model for autoimmune disease (c.f. ref. 6). Talal et al. (15) demonstrated that neonatal thymectomy exacerbates and accelerates the course of autoimmune manifestations in NZB mice. Dauphinee et al. (2,3) reported that the development of suppressor T-cells in this strain, which spontaneously develops a syndrome similar to systemic lupus erythematosus (SLE) in humans, is dependent upon the endocrine thymus and that suppressor T-cell activity rapidly disappears prior to overt manifestation of autoimmune disease. These findings seem to imply that thymosin-dependent suppressor cells can exert fine control over other subpopulations of T and B-cells and may thus be involved in the

pathological mechanisms of immune disease in NZB mice. Other studies
by Gershwin et al. (7) and by Bach et al. (8) document aberrant T and
B-cell function, apparently related to thymosin deficiencies in NZB
mice. Many of these aberrant functions can be corrected by thymosin
administration. As indicated in Figure 1, decrease in thymosin production envisioned as a result of stress or of pathogen invasion, e.g.
viral infection, could ultimately lead to deficient numbers of suppressor cells responsible for regulation of other specialized T and
B-cell functions. For example, T-cells could become autoaggressive,
or, B-cell activity could be unleashed in the form of pathological B-
cell germinal centers as found in the thymus of many patients with
myasthenia gravis and SLE.

   Monier et al. (9) documented a qualitative abnormality
in thymic epithelial cells which is unique to Swiss/Gif (SWAN) mice
with antinuclear antibodies. They find that these thymus cells contain large crystalline granules which they hypothesize to be a non-
secreted form of thymosin. Studies by Mellors et al. (10) and by
Proffitt et al. (11) demonstrate the presence of viruses in NZB or in
other strains of mice, some of which can induce signs of autoimmune
disease, thymic abnormalities or neoplasia in normal animals. Although evidence for a viral etiology of aberrant T-cell function is
not yet conclusive, it is conceivable that a virus could provoke pathogenic processes resulting in autoimmune disease in genetically

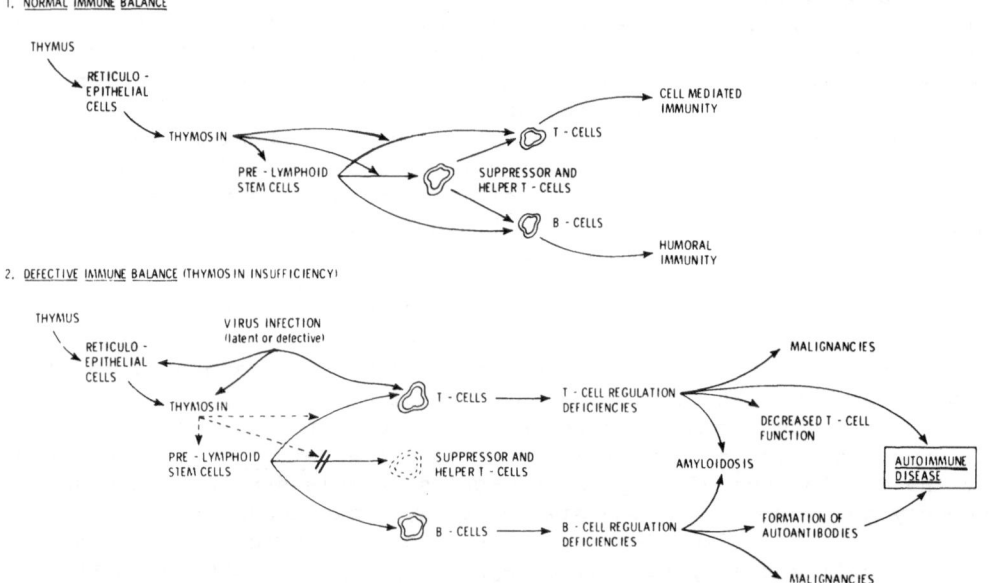

Figure 1. Decrease in thymosin levels and/or T-cells in autoimmune
disease.

susceptible hosts. We now know of a number of autoimmune diseases in humans which display familial patterns of incidence. These include Hashimoto's disease, SLE, Graves' disease and myasthenia gravis.

Beneficial effects of early thymectomy in patients with myasthenia gravis (12) and increased levels of thymosin-like factor in the blood of individuals with rheumatoid arthritis (13) point to the possibility that a hyperactive thymus gland may sustain certain autoimmune processes. Alternatively, it is possible that the apparent surplus of circulating thymosin may result from decreased hormone binding and consumption by immature target lymphoid cells which have lost their hormone receptors perhaps as a result of viral activation. With respect to the first possibility, over-production of thymosin could lead to the appearance of too many specialized T-cells of a given type, resulting in the reduced production of other needed specialized T-cell populations. Peltier, for example, reported (14) increased specialized T-cell function in patients with rheumatoid arthritis. Other studies showed that patients with rheumatoid arthritis respond favorably to thoracic duct drainage (15), thymic irradiation (16), and azathioprine immunosuppression (17). In another investigation, Waldmann et al. (18) showed that individuals with variable common immunodeficiency disease have excessive numbers of suppressor T-cells which apparently prevent the maturation of B-cells, and hence, these individuals have deficient levels of immunoglobulins. The above findings support the notion that suppressor or regulator cells play a key role in maintaining normal immune balance and homeostasis, and that loss of suppressor T-cell control along with virus-stimulated production of auto-aggressive cells, may result in gross T-cell deficiencies, autoimmune disease and possibly lymphoid tissue malignancy. Loss of fine T-cell control over B-cell populations could result in B-cell functional abnormalities including formation of auto-antibodies and possibly B-cell neoplasia.

There is some evidence that the target for thymosin in the peripheral blood is the so-called null cell, a cell having neither demonstrable T or B-cell type surface markers. In NZB mice shown in other studies to be deficient in serum thymosin-like activity, Stobo et al. (19) find an increase in the number of such null cells during the first few months of life. It is also interesting that patients with active SLE show an increase in null cells which are exquisitely responsive to thymosin in vitro (20).

THYMOSIN STUDIES IN HUMANS

In Vitro Studies

Our most recent studies show that the number of E-rosettes formed by purified peripheral blood lymphocytes obtained from patients with some primary and secondary immunodeficiency diseases can be increased _in vitro_ after short-term incubation with thymosin (21). This is seldom the case for lymphocytes from normal individuals. This observation led to the development of a new _in vitro_ test to identify patients with possible thymosin-related immunodeficiency diseases. The test is outlined in Figure 2. Thymosin fraction 5 increases the number of E-rosette forming cells (T-cells) from patients with a variety of serious clinical disorders including thymic hypoplasia, ataxia telangiectasia, Wiskott-Aldrich syndrome, SLE, cancer, chronic uremia, severe burns, as well as minor viral infections and allergy. Representative data from our studies are shown in Table 1. This assay, which we refer to as the Wara-Ammann rosette assay has been particularly useful in identifying immunodeficient patients who may be candidates for _in vivo_ thymosin therapy. As indicated in Figure 2, failure to increase the number of E-rosettes with thymosin _in vitro_ may indicate that the patient has adequate endogenous levels of thymosin or that we are dealing with a thymosin-independent disorder (e.g. stem cell deficiency).

Clinical Studies with Thymosin

On the basis of 10 years of well documented physiological studies with thymosin in a variety of animal models and completion of extensive toxicity studies using thymosin fraction 5 in mice and dogs, clinical trials have been initiated at a number of medical centers in the United States. To date, over 50 patients have received or are presently receiving thymosin under phase 1 protocols. These patients include children with DiGeorge syndrome, thymic hypoplasia, Wiskott-Aldrich, ataxia telangiectasia, and a variety of combined and common

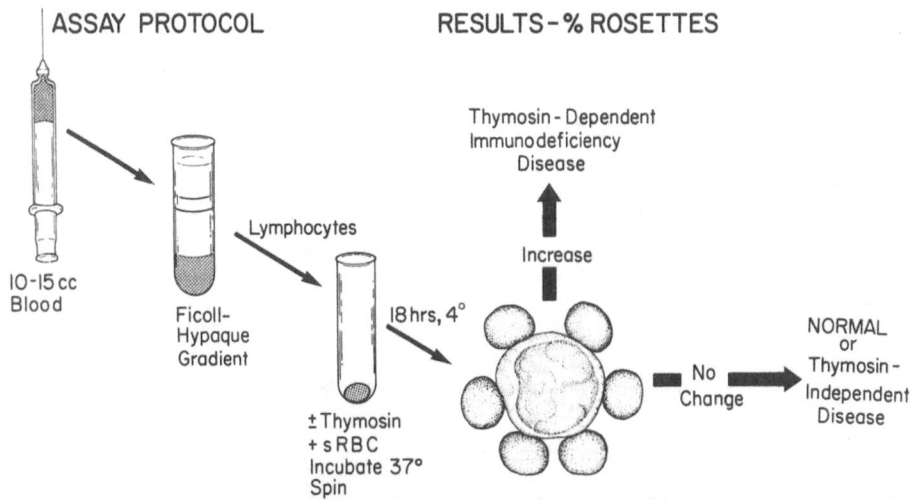

Figure 2.   Wara-Ammann E-rosette bioassay

TABLE 1.   Effect of thymosin (fraction 5) on human T-cell rosettes
of immunodeficient patients

Investigators, Disease and Number of Patients	Baseline	Thymosin Treatment	Significant Increase
Wara et al. (21)			
Normals (20)	50-65%	45-65%	-
Thymic hypoplasia	20%	45%	+
DiGeorge syndrome	25%	49%	+
Thymic hypoplasia and successful thymus transplant	32%	38%	-
Ataxia telangiectasia	27%	43%	+
Wiskott-Aldrich syndrome	28%	45%	+
Combined immunodeficiency	17%	20%	-
Sakai et al. (22)			
Normals (8)	34-71%	43-72%	-
Lung carcinoma (undifferentiated adenocarcinoma)	24%	42%	+
Hodgkin's disease, IV-B	34%	47%	+
Acute lymphocytic leukemia	35%	52%	+
Acute myelomonocytic leukemia	23%	54%	+
Disseminated melanoma	23%	37%	+
Stem cell leukemia (complete remission)	71%	74%	-
Endometrial carcinoma (no metastasis found)	62%	70%	-
Acute myelogenous leukemia	2%	17%	+
Scheinberg et al. (20)			
Normals (8)	58-67%	58-69%	-
Active systemic lupus erythematosis (6)	23-47%	35-72%	+
Inactive systemic lupus erythematosis (5)	52-70%	59-71%	-
Rheumatoid arthritis (5)	60-69%	58-67%	-
Harris et al. (23)			
Normals (8)	70-92%	65-85%	-
Chronic glomerulonephritis (2)	57-59%	76-78%	+
Nephrotic syndrome	71%	89%	+
Diabetic nephropathy	53%	63%	+
Chronic pyelonephritis	65%	76%	+

immunodeficiency diseases as well as immunologically anergic terminal cancer patients. Of the 50 patients treated with thymosin, 38 have been cancer patients with a variety of malignancies including Hodgkin's disease, chronic lymphocytic leukemia, lung carcinoma, leiomyosarcoma, melanoma, multiple myeloma and other lymphoid and nonlymphoid tumors. Patients in this study have received daily doses ranging from 1 to 400 mg/M^2 for 7 days or longer. To date there have been no indications of toxicity at any dose studied. The percentage of endogenous peripheral blood E-rosettes has increased in most thymosin-treated patients including those with primary as well as secondary immunodeficiency diseases (21,24-26). The capacity to respond to recall antigens during thymosin administration has increased in some patients and decreased in a few.

There has been marked clinical improvement during and following thymosin treatment in several patients with primary immunodeficiency diseases (21,24 and personal communications from A. Ammann, University of California Medical Center, C. August, University of Colorado Medical Center, T. Waldmann, National Cancer Institute, C. Griscelli, Necker Hospital and H. Hill, University of Utah Medical Center). Although there have been improvements in the clinical status in a few of the cancer patients receiving thymosin, we are unable to reach any definitive conclusions at this time (24-26).

Based upon the encouraging preliminary clinical results, large broad-based clinical trials with thymosin are presently underway in cooperation with a number of centers in the United States and Europe. The purpose of this study is to determine toxicity, effective dose, and to establish the efficacy of thymosin in enhancing T-cell immunity in patients with depressed or anergic immune systems.

SUMMARY

Studies in a variety of animal and human models indicate that thymosin plays a role in the differentiation of a number of T-cell subpopulations. The hypothesis presented is that a normal immune balance depends heavily upon the presence of thymosin-activated suppressor or regulator T-cells. A major thrust in our present research program is to determine whether or not the various disorders discussed here are causally related to abnormal thymosin production by the thymus gland. We are also assessing in animal models the potential value of thymosin in the treatment of specific autoimmune diseases. This information may yield new insights for the management of autoimmune type disorders such as SLE. Results from clinical trials to date suggest that thymosin will have a role in boosting the immune responses of patients with specific thymic malfunctions and may indeed exert an influence via the production of suppressor or regulator T-cells.

ACKNOWLEDGMENTS

These studies are supported in part by grants from the National Cancer Institute (CA 14108, CA 15419, CA 16964) and The John A. Hartford Fdn., Inc.

REFERENCES

1. Hooper, J.A., McDaniel, M.C., Thurman, G.B., Cohen, G.H., Schulof, R.S. and Goldstein, A.L. 1975. Ann. N.Y. Acad. Sci. 249:125.

2. Dauphinee, M.J., Talal,N., Goldstein, A.L. and White, A. 1974. Proc. Nat. Acad. Sci., 71:2637.

3. Dauphinee, M.J. and Talal, N. 1975. J. Immunol. 114:1713.

4. Goldstein, A.L., Guha, A., Howe, M.L. and White, A. 1971. J. Immunol. 106:773.

5. Bach, J.F., Dardenne, M., Goldstein, A.L., Guha, A. and White, A. 1971. Proc. Nat. Acad. Sci. 68:2734.

6. Talal, N. 1974. Progress in Clinical Immunology 2:101.

7. Gershwin, M.E., Ahmed, A., Steinberg, A.B., Thurman, G.B. and Goldstein, A.L. 1974. J. Immunol. 113:1068.

8. Bach, J.F., Dardenne, M. and Salomon, J.C. 1973. Clin. Exp. Immunol. 14:247.

9. Monier, J.C. and Robert, M. 1974. Ann. Immunol. (Inst. Pasteur) 125:405.

10. Mellors, R.C., Aoki, T. and Huebner, R.J. 1969. J. Exp. Med. 129:1045.

11. Proffitt, M. R., Hirsch, M.S. and Block, P.H. 1973. Science 182: 821.

12. Genkins, G., Papetestas, A.E., Horowitz, S.H. and Kornfeld, P. 1975. Ann. J. of Med. 58:517.

13. Bach, J.F., Dardenne, M. and Clot, J. 1974. International Symposium Immunol. Aspects of Rheumatic Diseases (In press).

14. Peltier, A. 1962. Rev. France et Clin. Biol. 7:770.

15. Paulus, H.E., Mackleader, H.I., Peter, J.B., Goldberg, L., Levy, J., Pearson, C.N. 1973. Arth. Rheum. 16:562.

16. Szanto, L., Fülöp, J., Feher, M. and Görgeny, I.F. 1973. Acta Med. Acad. Sci. (Hung) 30:11.

17. Urowitz, M.B., Gordon, P.A. Smythe, M.A., Pruzanski, W. and Ogryzlo, M.A. 1973. Arthr. Rheum. 16:411.

18. Waldmann, T., Broder, S., Durm, M., Blackmon, M., Blase, R.M. and Strober, W. 1974. Lancet II:609.

19. Stobo, J.D., Talal, N. and Paul, W.E. 1972. J. Immunol. 109:710.

20. Scheinberg, M.A., Cathcart, E.S. and Goldstein, A.L. 1975. Lancet I:424.

21. Wara, D.W., Goldstein, A.L., Doyle, N.E. and Ammann, A.J. 1975. New Eng. J. Med. 292:70.

22. Sakai, H., Costanzi, J.J., Loukas, D.F., Gagliano, R.G., Ritzmann, S.E. and Goldstein, A.L. Cancer (In press).

23. Harris, J., Sengar, P., Roshid, A., Hyslop, D., Green, L. and Goldstein, A.L. Transplantation (In press).

24. Goldstein, A.L., Sakai, H., Harris, N.S., Thurman, G.B., Goldman, A.S., Costanzi, J.J., Hersh, E. and Schafer, L. 1975. Fed. Proc. 34:529.

25. Costanzi, J.J., Gagliano, R., Loukas, D., Sakai, H., Thurman, G.B., Harris, N.S., and Goldstein, A.L. 1975. Proc. Amer. Assoc. Cancer Res. 16:135.

26. Schafer, L.A., Washington, M.L. and Goldstein, A.L. 1975. Proc. Amer. Assoc. Cancer Res. 16:233.

LYMPHOID TISSUE ARCHITECTURE. III. GERMINAL CENTERS, T CELLS, AND THYMUS-DEPENDENT VS THYMUS-INDEPENDENT ANTIGENS

I.L.WEISSMAN,G.A.GUTMAN,S.H.FRIEDBERG & L.JERABEK

Laboratory of Experimental Oncology, Dept. of
Pathology, Stanford Medical School, Calif. 94305

Supported by NIH grant AI-09072; ILW is a Faculty
Research Awardee of the American Cancer Society

Although the genesis and constituents of lymphoid
tissue germinal centers are not clearly defined, there is
evidence that they are induced by antigen, and may play
a role in T-B cell cooperation (1-3), generation of immunological memory (4), and differentiation of antibody-forming
cells (5-6). Since we had previously demonstrated T
antigen positive cells as constituents of germinal centers,
we wished to test their induction in "oligosynthetic"
lymph nodes with defined antigens. We chose three classes
of antigen – thymus dependent antigens, thymus-independent
antigens which induce antibodies limited to the IgM class,
and a newly-described thymus-independent antigen, DNP_{32}-
Ficoll, which induces both IgM and IgG antibodies.

Materials and Methods

In all experiments 4-6 week old BALB/c mice or Nu/Nu
mice were injected in a rear footpad with an immunogenic
dose of the following antigens: SRBC's, 1 x 10^7; human γ
globulin (HGG), 10 µg; bacterial lipopolysaccharide (LPS)
(DIFCO), 10 µg; polyvinylpyrrolidone (PVP) 2 µg; and
DNP_{32}-Ficoll, 10 µg (kindly provided as DNP-lysine-ficoll
prepared by the cyanuric chloride technique by Drs. W. Paul,
D. Mosier, and P. McMaster). Lymph nodes were removed
2-10 days after injection, and frozen sections were

prepared for immunofluorescence as previously described
(1,2). Anti-T antisera were prepared and absorbed as
described previously (1,2). This antiserum is specific
in immunofluorescence and cytotoxicity for the "T" subclass of lymphocytes (1,2); it prevents the in vitro
genesis of immune responses to SRBC's and this deficit can
be replaced by thymocytes or T cells (Chan, E., Gutman,G.,
and Weissman, I.L. - unpublished data); it is not cytotoxic
for antibody plaque-forming cells, various mouse myeloma
cells, or pluripotential spleen colony-forming cells.
It is not absorbed by brain, liver, bone marrow or "B"
spleens, and is absorbed equally well by thymocytes from
BALB/c (Thy 1.2) or AKR/J (Thy 1.1) mice. It reacts with
only one of the several components represented on thymocyte and T-lymphoma cell membranes (Bevan, M., Trowbridge,
I., and Weissman, I.L. - Nature, in press). In frozen
section immunofluorescence it stains thymic lymphoid cells
and cells in the T-dependent regions of peripheral lymphoid
tissues; it does not stain cells in skin, salivary gland,
kidney (7), muscle or liver (whereas cells in skin and
brain are Thy-1 positive). All of the immunofluorescence
or cytotoxic reactions with this reagent are fully
absorbed with murine thymocytes. Thus, this is a highly
specific reagent for the detection and localization of T
cells, and has, as yet, detected no known antigens on
non-T cells.

Frozen sections were either stained with α T, rabbit
α mouse Ig, or acridine orange (2) to define the location
and cellular composition of germinal centers. Lymph nodes
from mice immunized in parallel were stained with either
hematoxylin and eosin or methyl green pyronine. Hosts
were sacrificed 2,3,5,6, 8 and 10 days after antigen
injection and popliteal nodes draining the footpad injection sites were removed for processing. Immunized mice
were bled at sacrifice and antibody titres determined by
direct or indirect hemagglutination.

Results and Discussion

Early germinal centers are induced by thymus-dependent antigens in normal mice.

Germinal centers were only rarely found in control
hosts. Mice injected with SRBC and HGG developed germinal centers in association with almost every lymphoid
follicle; these were first apparent as foci of pyroninophilic blast cells at the margin between the primary
follicle and diffuse cortex by 2 or 3 days. By 4 days

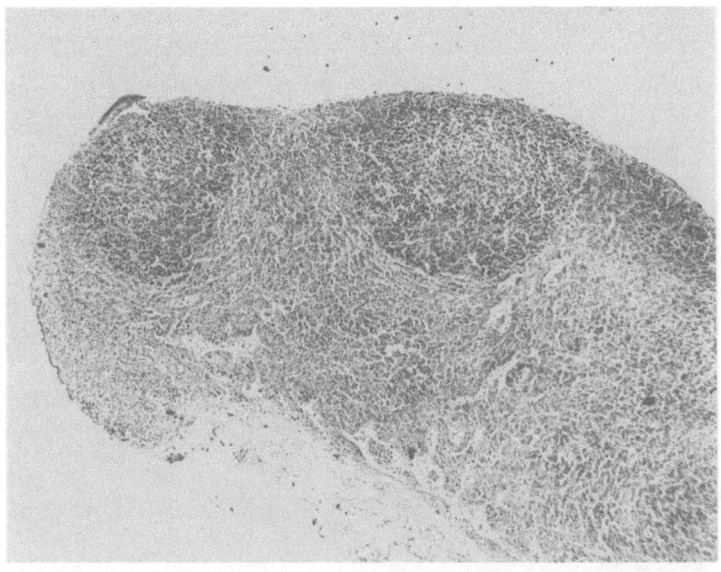

Fig. 1. Popliteal lymph node draining site of injection of 1×10^7 SRBC's 6 days before. Two large germinal centers are seen in the medullary pole of the two follicles. Methyl-green pyronine stain.

and thereafter, all germinal centers were prominent and occupied a central position in the medullary pole of these secondary follicles (Fig. 1).

Of the thymus-dependent antigens, LPS induced a massive lymphoid hyperplasia, with a diffuse pyronino-philic cell accumulation in follicles by the second day (Fig. 2), followed on days 4-5 by depletion of follicles. These changes are consistent with the role of this mole-cule as a polyclonal mitogen (8). At this time accumu-lations of plasma cells were observed in the medulla; this infiltration increased massively within the next few days and "plugging" of medullary lymphatics was observed (9). Small germinal centers were apparent after stimulation with this antigen by day 8 and were conspicu-ous in about a third of the follicles, although these never approached the size of those induced by the thymus-dependent antigens used in this study.

PVP induced germinal centers of about the same size and frequency as LPS. The response to DNP-ficoll was

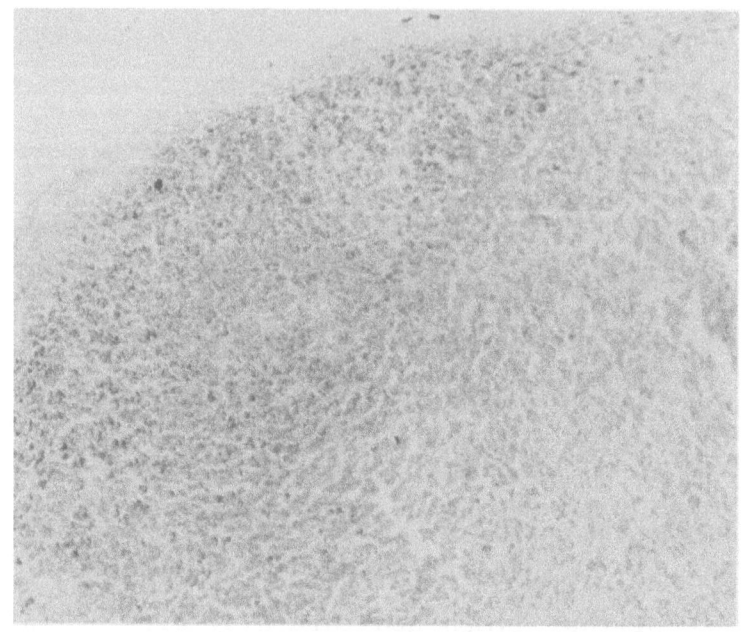

Fig. 2. Popliteal lymph node draining site of injection
of 10 μg LPS two days before. The dark staining cells
throughout the primary follicle are large pyroninophilic
cells. Only a few of these are found in the paracortex
(lower right). Methyl-green pyronine.

erratic; the first batch (March, 1974) regularly induced
early (4-6 day) germinal centers, but in animals injected
with a second batch (1975) germinal centers were observed
in low frequency and later (7-10 days) in most animals.

     Athymic (Nu/Nu) mice did not respond by germinal
center formation to stimulation with SRC'c, LPS, DNP-
ficoll or PVP. In the latter 3 cases, circulating
antibodies to these antigens were observed with titers
comparable to those observed in immunized normal animals.

All germinal centers have T antigen positive cells,
irrespective of the thymus dependence of the inducing
antigen

     Frozen sections of antigen-draining popliteal lymph
nodes were prepared at days 3,5,8 and 10 after antigen
injection. In all cases in which germinal centers were
induced, T antigen positive cells were present and

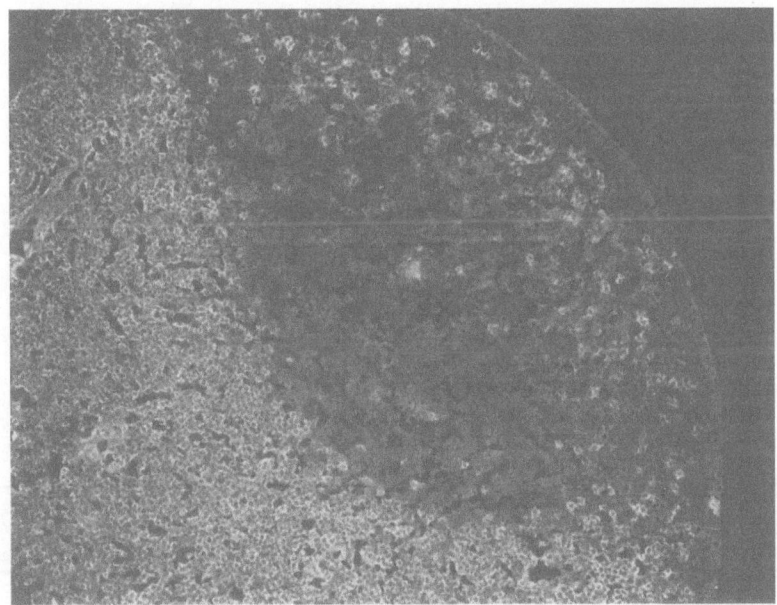

Fig. 3. (a) Popliteal lymph node with germinal center
in 2⁰ follicle on the top right, and paracortex in the
lower left. Anti-T stain. T positive cells in paracortex and cortical third of germinal center.

localized predominantly in the cortical pole of the
germinal center. (The medullary pole is, surprisingly,
both T-negative and Ig-negative.) Photographic evidence
of this is presented from mice 8 days after immunization
with SRBC's (Figure 3a,b,c).

The number of T cells (Table I) in secondary follicles induced by SRC's clearly exceeds their frequency
in primary follicles. On the other hand, the number and
specificity of T cells in secondary follicles induced by
thymus-dependent versus thymus-independent antigens has
yet to be explored.

While no germinal centers were induced by deliber-
ate antigenic stimulation of nude mice in this study, we
found after scanning lymphoid tissues from several Nu/Nu
animals, one germinal center in a mesenteric lymph node.
Although these mice are quantitatively depleted in T
cells, the single germinal center found contained T
antigen positive cells in a location and frequently

Table 1

T cell frequency in primary and secondary follicles

		% T cells
Primary follicle		4.7 ± 1.8
Secondary follicle (SRC induced)	Mantle	6.3 ± 1.0
Germinal center	Cortical pole	14.2 ± 4.4
	Medullary pole	2.8 ± 0.9

The results represent mean $\pm$ S.D. of counts done on photographed sections of five primary and secondary follicles. The secondary follicles were in draining lymph nodes of BALB/c mice injected in the footpad 8 days before with 1×10^7 SRBC.

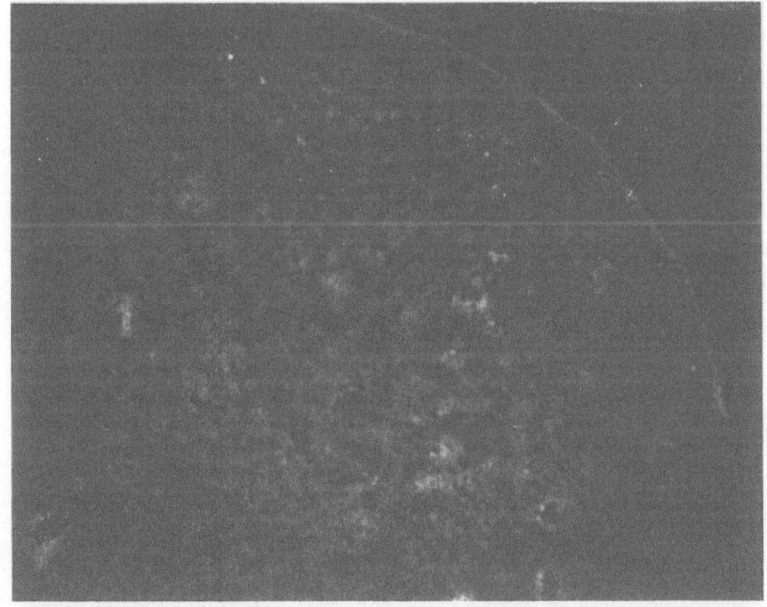

Fig. 3. (b) Same as (a), absorbed with thymocytes.

comparable to conventional thymus-containing littermates.
(The frequency, location, and derivation of Nu/Nu peripheral T cells is the subject of another communication
(Gutman, G.A., Sato, V., and Weissman, I.L., in preparation)). In all of the above cases, both germinal center
and diffuse cortex cellular fluorescence with α T serum
is completely removed by preabsorption of the serum with
BALB/c thymocytes (Fig. 3b). We thus tentatively
conclude that T antigen positive cells are obligate
constituents of germinal centers, whether induced by
thymus-dependent or thymus-independent antigens, or in
thymus-deprived hosts.

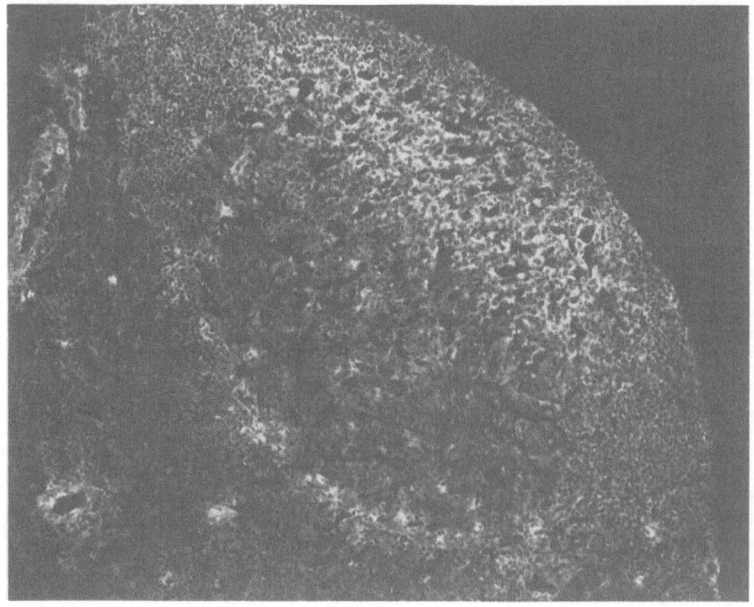

Fig.3.(c) Same as (a), stained with anti-Ig. The Ig
negative cells are in the paracortex and lower pole of
the germinal center. Ig positive small lymphocytes
are present in the mantle "capping" the germinal center
and extending on either side down to the paracortex.
The mantle is only a few cells thick under the capsule.
Very bright patterns of Ig positivity are found in the
cortical pole of the germinal center, in blast cells
and in a dendritic array. Scattered Ig positive blast
cells are present in the medullary pole of the germinal
center.

References

1. Gutman, G., and Weissman, I. Advances in Experimental Medicine and Biology, Morphological and Functional Aspects of Immunity 12: 595, 1971.

2. Gutman, G., and Weissman, I. Immunology 23: 465. 1972.

3. Weissman, I.L., Gutman, G.A., and Friedberg, S.H. Series Haematologica 7: 482, 1974.

4. Wakefield, J.D., and Thorbecke, G.J. J. Exp. Med. 128: 153, 1968.

5. White, R.G. In the Immunologically Competent Cell, Little, Brown and Co., Boston, 1963, p. 6.

6. Ellis, S.T., Gowans, J.L., and Howard, J.C. Cold Spr. Harb. Symp. Quant. Biol. 32: 395, 1967.

7. Greenspan, J.S., Gutman, G.A., Weissman, I.L., and Talal, N. Clin. Immunol. and Immunopath. 3: 16, 1974.

8. Coutinho, A., and Möller, G. Nature New Biol. 245: 12, 1973.

9. Kelly, R.H. Nature 227: 510, 1970.

References

1.

2.

3.

4.

5.

6.

7.

8.

9.

10.

SUMMARY AND AFTERTHOUGHTS ON SESSION 3: HOMING OF CELLS AND

INDUCTIVE EFFECTS OF MICROENVIRONMENT AND OF HUMORAL FACTORS

I.L. Weissman

Department of Pathology, Stanford University Medical

Center, Stanford, California 94305, U. S. A.

This session was characterized by considerations of structural
and fluid phase microenvironments in the antigen <u>independent</u> development and traffic patterns of T and B lymphocytes, as well as alterations in traffic and location of these cells following antigenic
stimulation. Maria de Sousa introduced the session by reviewing concepts of the specific recognition between circulating lymphocytes
and specialized endothelial cells (via post capillary venules in
lymph nodes and Peyer's patches; marginal sinuses in the spleen)
which allows entry of these lymphocytes (but not other blood borne
cells) into lymphoid tissue parenchyma. She demonstrated that the
failure to observe positive lymphoid tissue entry in some experimental
situations need not imply the lack of proper recognition between
lymphocytes and specialized endothelium; rather, augmented trapping
by nonlymphoid reticuloendothelial tissues may remove these cells
from the available pool. She also reviewed the evidence that
specific homing to T and B cell regions of lymphoid tissues occurs,
and this implies a second discriminative recognition process. Later
in the session, Weissman reviewed work by Gutman and Friedberg in his
lab that both T^+ and Ig^+ lymphocytes enter lymphoid tissues via
these specialized vessels in a random fashion. That is, T^+ cells
are as likely to enter the spleen in an Ig^+ cell region as a T^+ cell
region. Furthermore, Ig^+ cells enter a lymph node postcapillary
venule as frequently away from as toward the Ig^+ follicular pole.
Thus signals that determine Ig^+ cell homing to follicles, and T^+
cells to lymph node paracortex and splenic periarteriolar white pulp
occur sometime after lymphocyte contact with these specialized
endothelial cells.

van Ewijk then presented a scanning electron microscope
analysis of the morphology of lymphocytes <u>in situ</u> in "T" and "B"

mice.   Both T and B cells appear to have numerous surface microvilli
when in the blood circulation, and these microvilli can be shown to
be in contact with the luminal side of the aforementioned specialized
endothelial cells in traffic vessels of lymphoid tissues.   Surprisingly, no microvilli are found on lymphoid cells in T or B dependent
areas of lymphoid tissues;   cells in the medullary sinuses of lymph
nodes (presumably en route to the efferent lymphatics) possess these
microvilli.   van Ewijk proposed that lymphocyte microvilli are involved in the vessel recognition process, and that they are lost on
passage into the lymph node, only to be regained as these cells re-
enter the circulating pool.   He also reported that "T" mice prepared by injection of 5 x 10^7 cortisone resistant thymocytes
(rather than the whole thymocyte suspensions used in the first study)
contained an unusual population in lymph node medullary sinuses -
large cells with stubby microvilli, as contrasted with small cells
with long microvilli in the two above studies and in untreated mice.
This served as a caution to those who equate cortisone-resistant
thymocytes with peripheral T cells in experimental situations.
Demonstration that cortisone-resistant thymocytes may not contribute significantly to the thymus cell migration process was
presented in a later session by Weissman.   He presented data that
in situ labeling of thymus cells in a cortisone treated host results in appearance of less than 0.1% of normal levels of peripheral
thymus cell migrants.   Furthermore, over 95% of recently migrated
cells from an intact thymus are themselves sensitive to lytic
concentrations of corticosteroids.

     Returning to the theme of postvascular signals for specific T
and B cell homing, Müller-Hermelink presented data (in collaboration
with Heusermann, Kaiserling and Stutte) that structures exist which
may act as specific guiderails for these cells.   B cell regions are
rich in a class of dendritic reticulum cells which are histo-
chemically positive for alkaline phosphatase and 5'-nucleotidase
but lack detectable concentrations of ATPase or acid phosphatase.
On the other hand, T cell regions are distinguished by interdigitating reticulum cells which are ATPase and acid phosphatase
positive, and alkaline phosphatase and 5'-nucleotidase negative.
These interdigitating reticulum cells are also found at the cor-
tiɕomedullary junction in the thymus, an area rich in high walled
postcapillary venules.   It shall be interesting to see if T and B
lymphocytes possess specific substrates for these membrane enzymes,
and if specific removal of these substrates results in loss of
postvascular lymphoid tissue homing.

     Three papers on (antigen-independent?) T cell maturation were
presented.   Alm presented experiments (in collaboration with Juhlin
and Sällström) on the conditions necessary for the establishment and
maintenance of in vitro thymic organ cultures.   Species-specific
serum stimulating factors were demonstrated, which allow long term

(at least 8 weeks) thymic lymphocyte proliferation and differentiation.
During any period of "steady-state" culture a 6 hour exposure to
^{3}H-thymidine will abolish lymphopoiesis only if preceded by an
hypoxic stimulus. Thus it is possible that a reserve of G_O thymic
stem cells exists which are recruitable by environmental conditions.
Dr. Alm pointed out the potential value of this model for the systematic analysis of cellular and microenvironmental events which
contribute to normal and neoplastic T cell development. One of the
humoral factors (described by Trainin's group) which may substitute
for the thymus in T cell development is thymic humoral factor (THF).
This factor, upon addition to spleen cells from neonatally thymectomized mice, induces both a rapid rise in cellular cyclic AMP
levels and the induction and/or augmentation of the ability of these
cells to recognize and react against alloantigens. (In a later
session Small gave evidence that this conversion to alloreactivity
occurs in concert with a loss of anti-self reactivity.) Using the
assay of GvH reactivity, Yakir presented evidence (in collaboration
with Kook and Trainin) that the active principle in THF is a 3200
molecular weight acidic protein (27 amino acids) which lacks
detectable nucleic acids and carbohydrates. They now have a molecule
which should enable both further molecular analysis and identification
of the target cell(s) of its action.

     Using a somewhat less well defined higher molecular weight
thymic factor, thymosin, Goldstein (with Cohen, Thurman and Hooper)
presented evidence that circulating thymosin levels are often altered in a number of human conditions, including immunodeficiency,
malignancy, autoimmunity and aging. He proposed that these disease
states might reflect a primary imbalance in thymosin production,
resulting in excess or deficient numbers of helper or suppressor
T cells. Of course, the growing evidence that subpopulations of T
cells may augment and/or suppress both humoral and cell mediated
immune responses now allows a T cell hypothesis for any disease
involving abberations of the immune apparatus. It is the difficult
task of the proposers of these comprehensive hypotheses to demonstrate primary immunopathological lesions in each instance.

     Antigen independent (?) B cell maturation was studied in a well
controlled system by Rozing and Benner. They found that irradiated
mice injected with spleen colony hematopoietic cells showed a rapid
regeneration of Ig$^+$ cells. This regeneration occurred in several
hematopoeitic and lymphoid organs, but was always earlier and more
prominent in the spleen. Either splenic or other hematopoietic
sites are sufficient to allow this maturation, but neither bone marrow
nor gut associated lymphoid tissues are necessary. Thus B cell
development in mice is multifocal and occurs in organs of hematopoiesis.
In an earlier session, Cottier presented evidence that the avian bursa
of Fabricius was a site of considerable antigenic contact and lymphoid
cell reaction, and that radiotoxic "sealing" of the bursa could be

accomplished by a single administration of radioactive colloids to the cloacal lip. If the bursa is merely a site of contact between intestinal luminal antigens and the chicken lymphoid system, how good is the evidence that the bursa is the sole (or even significant) site of virgin B cell differentiation, especially if the site of virgin B cell maturation is accomplished in mice with a system possessed by birds, i.e., hematopoietic organs? As proposed elsewhere (Transplant. Reviews 24:159, 1975), these experiments require us to re-examine the possibility that homologous hematopoietic sites of virgin B cell maturation exist in birds, rather than the current hypothesis that B cell maturation is controlled by gut associated lymphoid tissues in birds and hematopoietic tissues in mammals.

A "bridge" paper between antigen-independent and antigen dependent movement of lymphoid cells was presented by Wallis (in collaboration with Leuchars, Collavo and Davies). She demonstrated that one could inject syngeneic chromosomally marked lymph node or spleen cells into unirradiated hosts, and that for periods up to one year these cells equilibrated with host lymphocytes in an additive, rather than substitutive relationship. Using specific T and B cell mitogens, she showed that these cells were retained in roughly the proportions of cell types injected, i.e. there is no detectable difference in the lifespan of lectin stimulatable T and B lymphocytes. Furthermore, antigenic stimulation results in proliferation of donor cells as well as host cells, in approximately their ratio predicted by lectin stimulation. Antibody responses in these "hyper-lymphoid" mice were 150-200% of injected littermates. These results with adoptive primary responses stand in sharp contrast to the findings in several labs that unirradiated hosts possess some radiosensitive barrier to the transfer of adoptive secondary re-sponses. It is clear that these findings require clarification in concomitant experiments to elucidate the nature of that "barrier". Perhaps it is related to a population of regulatory cells which are radiosensitive (as in the case of Nachtigal's breakdown of tolerance) and which are more efficient at regulating "memory" cells than "virgin" cells.

The events leading up to antigen recognition by cells capable of generating specific contact sensitivity were analyzed in the DNP model by Søeberg, Balfour and Sumerska. Following ear painting with DNFB, the afferent lymph contains free DNP, DNFB, DNP-proteins, and DNP-coated white blood cells. Each of these constituents is present in concentrations sufficient for sensitization if infused into an afferent lymphatic. Thus it seems likely that primary recognition of contact sensitizing antigens may occur in the draining lymph node, and not solely by peripheral sensitization. This brings out possible differences between the properties of antigen-specific cells res-ponding to this class of antigens by induction of antigen-specific effector cells, and the effector cells themselves; these latter cells apparently have the property of recognizing and reacting to antigens in situ, generating a local delayed hypersensitivity (or cytolytic) response. This is in direct parallel with EAE, in which case the antigen bearing targets are always present, but susceptibility to the cell-mediated demyelinization requires lymphoid tissue sensitization and generation of circulating cytotoxic effector cells. Perhaps as a class the cells responsible for primary recognition are non-recirculating, whereas the effector cells are recirculating. With the current ability to relate various T_1/T_2 cell activities to cell surface representation of Ly 1 vs Ly 2, 3 antigens, it shall be most interesting to characterize the cell lineages involved in primary recognition, recall, and lesion induction in the contact sensitivity system.

Further differences in the biological behaviour of cells in the afferent vs efferent lymph nodal lymph were reported by Scollay and Hall. They clearly demonstrated (using normal lymphocyte transfer reactions) that afferent lymph cells were greatly depleted of alloreactivity compared with efferent lymph cells. Further, that blood lymphocytes were also deficient compared to efferent lymph-ocytes, but were somewhat more reactive than afferent lymphocytes. All three classes were about equal in their capability to recirculate from blood to lymph, although the recirculation capacity of the alloreactive fraction of each cell population was not tested. The lack of reactivity was not due to the presence of suppressor cells, as cell mixtures were as effective as the component cells. These experiments raise questions concerning the function of lymphocytes capable of recirculating through the skin (and subsequently to enter afferent lymphatics). If they represent cells specifically reactive to antigens found in the skin, it would not be surprising that they lack reactivity as a population to an unrelated alloantigen. It would seem, then, that it will be necessary to test whether these cells differ from efferent duct lymphocytes as a general subclass unrelated to antigen specificity, or if they represent a subclass selected as to the repertoire of antigens to which they may respond.

Finally, Weissman (in collaboration with Gutman and Friedberg) reported data that stimulation with thymus dependent antigens leads to the early (3-4 days) development of large germinal centers in draining lymph nodes, and that these germinal centers inevitably contained cells bearing T cell surface antigens in high concentrations in the cortical pole of the germinal centers. Stimulation by thymus independent antigens did not result in the formation of germinal centers in concert with the generation of antibody formation. However, late development (8-10 days) of small germinal centers in follicles was an irregular but significant event following thymus independent antigenic stimulation. These, too, inevitably contained high con-centrations of T antigen positive cells in their cortical poles. One thymus independent antigen, DNP_{32}-lys-ficoll, gave contradictory responses; the first batch gave rise to a high frequency of early germinal centers, whereas the second batch behaved just like other thymus independent antigens. Although it is tempting to relate the time course of appearance of germinal centers to the generation of immunological memory and IgG responses, as well as the well known delayed appearance of radiolabeled antigen in follicular B cell domains, several antecedent questions remained to be answered: (1) Are these T antigen positive cells derived from precursor T cells? (2) Are they specific for the antigen which induces them? (3) Are they of a lymphocyte subclass known to be involved in helper (or suppressor) T cell functions? (4) Are the B cells entering blastogenesis in germinal centers the precursors of specific antibody forming cells, memory cells, both, or neither? (5) Do antigen specific B cells preferentially lodge in germinal centers induced by their complementary antigen? (6) Are the factors responsible for follicular antigen localization in the inductive phases of the immune response the products of antigen activated specific T or B cells? It is clear that we shall require the answer to several of these questions before we begin to understand the role of "Lymphatic Tissue and Germinal Centers in Immune Reactions".

Cell Interactions in Immune Responses

CELL INTERACTIONS IN IMMUNE RESPONSES: ROLE OF T LYMPHOCYTES

J.F.A.P. Miller

Walter and Eliza Hall Institute of Medical Research
Royal Melbourne Hospital P.O.
Melbourne 3050, Australia

It is well established that the thymus exerts a widespread influence, not only in the development of immune capacity, but also in the regulation of immune functions. Once differentiated, T cells may become involved in controlling a wide variety of cellular and humoral immune responses by producing quantitative as well as qualitative modifications. Collaboration between lymphocytes has now been documented in both cell-mediated and humoral immunity, i.e. between various subsets of T lymphocytes as well as between T and B cells, as will be evident from the various papers in this Symposium. The T cells can either promote or suppress the function of other lymphocytes, depending on the circumstances, and macrophages often play an essential role in the mediation of lymphocyte interactions.

T-CELL FACILITATION OF B-CELL ANTIBODY RESPONSES

In many humoral immune responses, T and B lymphocytes work together, not separately, as part of a network in which collaborative and feedback loops determine the outcome[1]. It has been suggested that specific B-cell triggering requires at least 2 signals: the binding of antigenic determinants to membrane immunoglobulin (Ig) receptors and another signal, which according to some is said to be derived from T cells[2]. Three experimental situations appear not to make it essential to postulate the existence of a second signal that must be delivered by T lymphocytes. First, not all humoral antibody responses are T-cell dependent. Those highly influenced by T cells are high-affinity antibody (e.g. secondary responses), IgE and IgG, whereas low-affinity antibody and IgM responses are marginally or not T-cell dependent. For example, antibody to human serum albumin (HSA) is found in all the Ig classes in mice injected with alum precipitated HSA. Neonatal thymectomy decreases anti-HSA antibody production, but this reduction occurs only in the IgG_1 class, not in the IgG_{2a}, IgG_{2b}, IgM or IgA[3]. If the second signal for B-cell triggering had to be delivered by the few residual T cells left after neonatal thymectomy, one might have anticipated the reduction in anti-HSA antibody to be represented in all the Ig classes, not solely in IgG_1. Secondly, it is clear that hypothymic nu/nu mice do produce IgM antibody in normal amounts in response to some antigens. If such an antibody response is claimed to be dependent on residual T cells, said to have been committed by having been primed to cross-reacting antigens in early life[4], one wonders why such T cells have never yet been able to reject skin grafted from many different mouse strains and even from rats. This is particularly relevant in view of the reports of cross-reactivity between some histocompatibility antigens and gut-associated bacteria[5]. Thirdly, turning away from nu/nu mice, there are experimental systems which show that, provided certain conditions of antigen dose and hapten density are fulfilled, B lymphocytes can be triggered to produce IgG antibody (and even high affinity antibody) in the absence of appropriate T cells (e.g. ref. 6 and paper by Doria and Agarossi in this Symposium).

The experimental finding of T-cell independent antibody responses allows the following conclusions. (1) B lymphocytes, including the precursors of IgG and high-affinity antibody producers, can be stimulated by antigen in the absence of appropriate T cells, provided certain conditions of antigen dose are fulfilled. (2) The effect of appropriately activated T cells on B-cell responsiveness to antigen cannot therefore be a sine qua non for B-cell triggering. On the contrary, it would seem more logical to assume the function of activated T cells in B-cell responses to be immunoregulatory[1].

A vast amount of in vitro work has been done in an attempt to determine the mechanism of T and B-cell collaboration. As a result, certain antigen-specific T-cell factors have been implicated as mediators. One such factor is claimed to be IgT, a T-cell derived Ig with a capacity to bind to macrophages[7]. Another is a non-Ig, antigen-specific product coded by genes which, in mice, lie close to the K end of the histocompatibility complex[8]. Although such factors must play an important role in T-cell physiology, it should be stressed that it is sometimes difficult to relate in vitro events to the in vivo situation. Thus, as mentioned above, IgG responses are much more T-cell dependent than IgM, and most investigators using in vitro

systems to generate such T-cell factors have generally confined
their observations to IgM responses. Furthermore, and especially
relevant to the topic of this Conference, germinal centre formation, which is a characteristic marker of effective T and B-
cell cooperation in vivo, has not yet been reproduced in vitro.
Other theories of T and B-cell cooperation have invoked the
operation of nonspecific T-cell factors. Since the fundamental
function of T cells is cellular immunity, and since nonspecific
factors are instrumental in many T-cell mediated responses, and
often act through macrophages, it is not unreasonable to assume
that similar nonspecific factors indirectly influence B-cell
responsiveness[1].

     The production of high-affinity antibodies is more easily
suppressed during tolerance induction than low-affinity antibodies, and likewise IgG antibodies are more easily suppressed
than IgM[9]. In keeping with these observations it is likely
that B cells with high intrinsic antigen-binding capacity will
be more susceptible to receptor blockade if antigen tends to
persist than B cells with lower antigen-binding potential. This
may be the reason why persistent, poorly degradable, antigen
generally elicit only IgM response, not IgG. On the other hand,
degradable, nonpersistent, antigens elicit both IgM and IgG
responses and it is the IgG and the high-affinity antibody
response which is diminished or abolished in the absence of T
cells, the IgM or low-affinity antibody response being unaffected or reduced but not abolished (e.g. ref. 10). These observations would appear to link (a) antigen persistence, (b) susceptibility of potential IgG producers to paralysis and (c) absence
of a T-cell influence[1,11]. Recent experiments by Graham
Mitchell[12] have further substantiated these correlations. A
conjugate of dinitrophenyl (DNP) on rabbit anti-pneumococcal
polysaccharide SIII could trigger DNP-primed B cells to produce
IgG anti-DNP antibody provided SIII was also given. It is
unlikely that this effect could be explained in terms of a
mitogenic signal to IgG precursor B cells by SIII since in other
experiments[13] DNP.SIII was highly tolerogenic for DNP-primed B
cells. Furthermore, dinitrophenylated normal rabbit Ig could
not substitute for the rabbit anti-SIII antibody, accessory cell
inactivation in the irradiated recipients reduced anti-DNP
responses and removal of T cells with anti-Thy-1 serum totally
abolished the response (this being restored by addition of
cortisone-resistant thymus cells). These results can be
accomodated by the hypothesis that the antigen-antibody complex,
(DNP-rabbit anti-SIII antibody)-SIII, may nonspecifically
activate the T-cell/macrophage axis and hence become readily
removed from the microenvironment of the relevant DNP-sensitive
IgG precursor B cells, thereby preventing paralysis.

T-CELL SUPPRESSION OF B-CELL ANTIBODY RESPONSES

The possibility of a suppressor effect of T cells on B-cell responsiveness became evident when it was found that cells from tolerant animals could be mixed with cells from normal animals and prevent these from producing antibody to the specific antigen[14]. Since then, other experimental systems (i.e. not involving specific tolerance) have been described in which reduction of antibody responses has been attributed to "suppressor T cells"[14]. It is not possible to discuss all T-cell dependent suppression systems nor their mechanism of action. I will therefore summarize some of the salient findings in the particular experimental model we have used: the adoptive transfer of anti-DNP antibody responses in irradiated recipients of DNP-primed B cells (spleen cells from DNP.Flagellin primed mice pretreated with anti-Thy-1 serum and complement), spleen cells from mice primed to human gammaglobulin (HGG) and spleen cells from mice tolerized to HGG[15]. Suppression of the anti-DNP response to DNP.HGG in irradiated recipients of HGG primed and DNP primed cells was observed when HGG tolerant spleen cells were added, the optimal ratio of HGG tolerant:HGG primed:DNP primed cells being 5 : 1 : 1. IgG responses were suppressed more markedly than IgM. Suppression by tolerant spleen cells was dependent on the presence of 2 cell types: a T cell and an adherent cell, probably a macrophage. The T cells mediating suppression were not present in the recirculating lymphocyte pool (thoracic duct lymphocytes from tolerant mice, unlike spleen cells, did not suppress), and may have been derived relatively recently from the thymus (spleen cells from HGG tolerant mice were less suppressive if the mice had been thymectomized, as adults, more than 4 weeks before). The site of action of the suppressor effect appeared to be at the post helper cell level (and probably at the B-cell level) since simultaneous challenge with DNP coupled to another carrier, as well as the inducing carrier (HGG) failed to induce the anti-hapten response. Thus, although suppression was specific in induction (presumably depending on activation of specific T cells), it was nonspecific in expression. We could distinguish the two phenomena, suppression and tolerance, on the following grounds. Thymus cells from tolerant mice, although unable to mediate suppression, were unresponsive on adoptive transfer with normal B cells. Tolerance could be induced with HGG deaggregated in an ultracentrifuge with either an angle or a swingout head; suppression only if HGG was deaggregated in the former. Adult thymectomy prolonged tolerance, but tended to diminish the extent of suppression. An absolute requirement for macrophages was essential for suppression; this contrasts with the conventional dogma that tolerance induction will occur only if the macrophage system is bypassed. Excellent suppression was obtained in BALB/c mice which are notoriously resistant (by virtue of hyperactive phagocytes) to tolerization with protein antigens, including HGG. Evidence is available that T cells become tolerant within a day and that the state of tolerance persists for over 100 days[16]. By contrast, T-cell dependent suppression was demonstrable only between day 3 and day 28 after tolerization. The mechanism of suppression operating in this particular model has not been elucidated. The requirement for macrophages from specifically tolerant mice and the observation that suppression was specific in induction though not in expression, implicate a role for antigen-antibody complexes operating within microclusters of T cells, B cells and macrophages. Thus, suppression, like help, is T-cell and macrophage dependent, nonspecific in expression and affects IgG more than IgM responses. Further experiments will determine whether or not the same basic mechanism can account for both phenomena.

INTERACTIONS AMONG SUBSETS OF T CELLS

Evidence for interactions between various T lymphocytes in cellular immunity has been observed and will be presented during this conference. The identification of different subsets of T cells has been placed on a sound basis by the elegant work of Boyse and his colleagues[17] who used antibodies directed against Ly differentiation antigens to distinguish between pre-helper (Ly-1) and pre-killer (Ly-2,3) T cells. Further work is required to clarify what subclasses of T cells interact in various cellular immune responses. A more controversial type of T-T interaction, that cannot be totally dismissed, may operate via transfer factor (TF). The TF phenomenon has been observed for 20 years in the human[18], but has not been reproduced unequivocally in any other animal species. Because of the reports of spectacular success with TF in the control of some infections, it seems imperative that the phenomenon should be reproduced in an animal model. This is not only to determine critically whether such a factor controlling T-cell mediated immunity may be universal, but also to establish precisely its mechanism of action.

CONCLUSIONS

I cannot offer a comprehensive mechanism of T and B-cell cooperation, nor do I think there can be only one way in which such cells interact. On the contrary, a diversity of mechanisms is likely to have evolved to allow a complex system of cells, with differing anatomical and physiological relationships, to cope with the introduction of antigens that differ widely in

physicochemical properties. It is evident that a deeper understanding of the mechanisms involved will pave the way for
practical methods of manipulating selectively different sets of
lymphocytes and their responses. We hope this may eventually
be applicable to clinical medicine for use in various infectious
diseases, notably parasitic diseases, in vaccinating procedures,
anergic states, immune deficiency diseases, allergic conditions,
autoimmune diseases, transplantation of tissues and organs, and
the cancer problem.

REFERENCES

1.   Miller, J.F.A.P. 1975. Ann. N.Y. Acad. Sci. 249, 9.
2.   Bretscher, P. 1972. Transplant. Rev. 11, 217.
3.   Hay, F.C. and Torrigiani, G. 1973. Europ. J. Immunol. 3, 657.
4.   Kirov, S.M. 1974. Europ. J. Immunol. 4, 739.
5.   Rapaport, F.T. and Chase, R.M. 1964. Science 165, 407.
6.   Klinman, N.R. and Doughty, R.A. 1973. J. Exp. Med. 138, 473.
7.   Marchalonis, J.J. 1974. J. Med. 5, 329.
8.   Munro, A.J., Taussig, M.J., Campbell, R., Williams, H. and
         Lawson, Y. 1974. J. Exp. Med. 140, 1579.
9.   Siskind, G.W. and Benacerraf, B. 1969. Adv. Immunol. 10, 1.
10.   Gershon, R.K. and Paul, W.E. 1971. J. Immunol. 106, 872.
11.   Mitchell, G.F. 1975. Transplant. Rev. 23, 119.
12.   Mitchell, G.F. 1975. Immunology 28, in press.
13.   Mitchell, G.F., Humphrey, J.H. and Williamson, A.R. 1972.
         Europ. J. Immunol. 2, 460.
14.   Gershon, R.K. 1974. Contemp. Topics Immunobiol. 3, 1.
15.   Basten, A., Miller, J.F.A.P. and Johnson, P. 1975.
         Transplant. Rev. 26, in press.
16.   Weigle, W.O., Chiller, J.M. and Habicht, G.S. 1972.
         Transplant. Rev. 8, 3.
17.   Cantor, H. and Boyse, E.A. 1975. J. Reticuloendoth. Soc.
         17, 115.
18.   Lawrence, H.S. 1974. Harvey Lectures 68, 239.

INDUCTION OF HAPTEN RECOGNIZING HELPER FUNCTION BY HEAVILY TRINITROPHENYLATED SHEEP ERYTHROCYTES

D. Naor, R. Berman-Goldman, M. Kahan, H. Goldfisher,
R. Laskov, E. Simon, and R. Tchakirov

Lautenberg Center for General and Tumor Immunology and
The Department of Experimental Medicine and Cancer
Research

Hebrew University - Hadassah Medical School, Jerusalem

Very important progress has been made over the last five years in the understanding of the regulation of the immune response (1), the genetic control of the immunological system (2) and the cellular cooperation of T and B cells for antibody production (3). However, the practical application of this increased understanding remains a major challenge of modern immunology. In attempting to apply the accumulated knowledge concerning cellular cooperation in the immune response, Mitchison has suggested the challenge of antigen sensitized animals with tumors coupled to the sensitizing antigen as a means of improving the anti tumor response. It was assumed that the sensitizing process would stimulate thymus influenced cells which might help tumor recognizing cells to reject the tumor (4). A few investigators have tested this approach and two groups have reported successful results (5,6). Our efforts have been focused on the developing of an immunological helping system with recognition capacity of both the hapten and the carrier of the inducer antigen. On obtaining a reliable and reproducible system, attempts were made to use the hapten recognizing helper cells to improve anti tumor responses to tumor cells coated with the homologous hapten. The materials and the methods which were tested in this work were described in detail in our previous papers (7,8).

CBA mice were injected with non lysable heavily trinitrophenylated sheep red cells. (In any designation of trinitrophenylated sheep red cells the final trinitrobenzene sulfonic acid (TNBS) concentration per ml in the conjugation mixture with sheep red cells is indicated, e.g. 128 mg TNBS per 1 ml red cells suspension = $TNP_{128}SRC$). Such $TNP_{128}SRC$ primed mice produced low anti SRC and

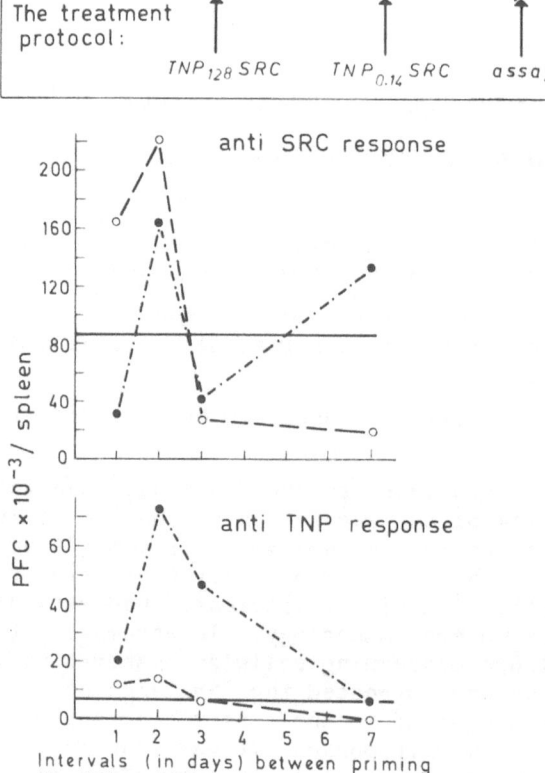

FIG. 1:   Development of immunological memory induced with $TNP_{128}SRC$.
Mice were injected at day 0 with $TNP_{128}SRC$. Half of these mice and
unprimed mice were challenged 1, 2, 3 and 7 days after the priming
with $TNP_{0.14}SRC$. The mice were killed 4 days after challenge and
the splenic anti TNP and SRC PFC responses were assayed.

----   Direct PFC/spleen of $TNP_{128}SRC$ primed mice which were
        challenged with $TNP_{0.14}SRC$.
-.-.-. Indirect PFC/spleen of $TNP_{128}SRC$ primed mice which were
        challenged with $TNP_{0.14}SRC$.
_____ The total number of PFC/spleen of unprimed mice which were
        challenged with $TNP_{0.14}SRC$.

TNP plaque forming cell (PFC) and haemagglutination (HA) responses, 4 days after immunization and negligable responses thereafter (9). However, mice which were primed with $TNP_{128}SRC$ and challenged two days later with lightly trinitrophenylated SRC, $TNP_{0.14}SRC$, produced, 4 days after the challenge, much stronger anti SRC and TNP PFC responses than unprimed mice which were injected with $TNP_{0.14}SRC$ only (Fig. 1). The highest secondary anti SRC and TNP PFC responses were obtained when $TNP_{128}SRC$ primed mice were challenged 2 days after the priming and assayed 4 days after the challenge. When the challenge antigen was injected 3 and 7 days after priming, and the immune response was recorded 4 days after the challenge, a gradual decrease of the secondary anti TNP PFC response was observed. The anti SRC PFC secondary response also decreased when the animals were challenged 3 days after priming, but a second wave of increased anti SRC PFC secondary response was observed when the animals were challenged 7 days after priming. It was found that humoral factors were responsible for the fall in the capacity to recall the secondary response later than 2 days after priming (9). Thus, $TNP_{128}SRC$ induced an immunological memory in mice to both SRC and TNP determinants. Our next series of experiments were performed in order to determine whether this immunological memory or helper function is mediated by SRC recognizing cells only, or by both SRC and TNP recognizing cells.

Different groups of mice were sacrificed 2, 4, 12 and 18 days after priming with $TNP_{128}SRC$. Spleen cells from these mice were tested for their ability to incorporate ^3H-thymidine after their in vitro stimulation with 5×10^7 SRC or 4 µg heavily trinitrophenylated human serum albumin, $TNP_{10}HSA$ (Ten moles of TNP were coupled with 1 mole of HSA). Non specific stimulators, concanavalin A (Con A) and E. coli lipopolysaccharide (LPS) and different doses of relatively lightly trinitrophenylated HSA (TNP_5HSA) were also included in the thymidine uptake assay system and their ability to stimulate the DNA synthesis was measured. The results in Table 1 are expressed as a stimulation index (see table footnote). Both SRC and $TNP_{10}HSA$ stimulated the ^3H-thymidine uptake by the primed spleen cells. However, the light conjugate TNP_5HSA was unable to stimulate DNA synthesis. The non specific stimulators, Con A and LPS elicited a high level of ^3H-thymidine uptake, as expected. This finding suggests therefore, that $TNP_{128}SRC$ induce immunological memory which could be recalled in vitro by stimulation of SRC and TNP recognizing cells. The fact that only the heavily trinitrophenylated HSA, $TNP_{10}HSA$, stimulated the DNA synthesis is not surprising since it is well known that a threshold of binding energy is needed for activating the receptor molecules and such energy could be provided only by high density conjugates. Since different doses of TNP_5HSA were unable to stimulate the ^3H thymidine uptake, the response was considered specific for SRC and $TNP_{10}HSA$.

These findings were further confirmed by measuring the number

Table 1: In vitro recall of the immunological memory induced
          with $TNP_{128}SRC$.

Exp.	Spleen cells stimulated with:	Stimulation index at day:			
		2	4	12	18
1	Con A	23.0	19.0	8.2	26.3
	LPS	17.6	11.0	5.0	17.3
	SRC	4.8	4.0	1.3	3.5
	$TNP_{10}HSA$ 4 μg	2.0	3.6	2.1	4.2
2	$TNP_{10}HSA$ 4 μg		4.2		
	TNP_5HSA 10 μg		1.0		

Mice were injected with $TNP_{128}SRC$ and 2, 4, 12 and 18 days later
spleens were removed and cell suspensions were prepared. ^3H
thymidine uptake was performed as described in ref. 10 and 11.
The trinitrophenylation of human serum albumin was prepared
according to ref. 12. Stimulation index: The average uptake of
^3H thymidine by cells in stimulated cultures over the average
uptake of ^3H thymidine by cells in the non stimulated cultures.

Table 2: In vitro recall of immunological memory. Existence of
          TNP and SRC recognizing thymus derived cells.

Spleen cells stimulated with:	Stimulation index of the following cell populations:			
	Untreated spleen cells	'T' cells	'B' cells	'T + B' cells
Con A	31.0	368.0	3.8	25.4
LPS	34.0	4.8	20.8	16.7
SRC	5.0	8.0	3.5	7.0
$TNP_{10}HSA$	3.0	6.0	2.6	2.0

Mice were injected with $TNP_{128}SRC$. 4 days later, spleen cells were
removed and cell suspensions were prepared. Enriched populations of
T and B cells were prepared as described in ref. 13, 14. The
cultures were prepared as described in ref. 10, 11. Stimulation
index: See table 1.

of antigen binding cells (15). Spleen cells from mice primed with
$TNP_{128}SRC$ were able to form rosettes with $TNP_{14}DRC$ (Trinitrophenylated donkey red cells), SRC, $TNP_{14}SRC$ but not with DRC. More
rosettes were formed with $TNP_{14}SRC$ than with SRC and $TNP_{14}DRC$.
Moreover, the rosettes which were formed with $TNP_{14}SRC$ were more
stable than those which were formed with SRC, since preincubation
of spleen cells at 37°C for 30' reduced the number of rosettes
formed with SRC by 85% as compared to 40% reduction for rosettes
formed with $TNP_{14}SRC$. Thus, $TNP_{128}SRC$ stimulate in mice the
appearance of TNP recognizing cells and SRC recognizing cells.
Subsequent experiments were performed to determine the cellular
origin of these SRC and TNP recognizing cell populations.

Mice were primed with $TNP_{128}SRC$ and sacrificed 4 days later.
The spleens of these mice were removed and cell suspensions were
prepared. An enriched population of T cells was obtained by
filtering the spleen cells suspension through an anti mouse γ
globulin coated column (13, 14). An enriched population of B cells
was obtained by killing thymus derived T cells with anti mouse brain
and complement (13). Untreated spleen cells, T cells, B cells and a
mixture of T and B cells were stimulated with SRC, $TNP_{10}HSA$, Con A
(T cells stimulator, 3) LPS (B cells stimulator, 3) and the ^3H
thymidine uptake capacity was determined and expressed as a stimulation
index. Table 3 shows that T cells after specific antigen stimulation
incorporated relatively more ^3H thymidine than untreated spleen cells, a
mixture of B + T cells or B cells alone. The efficiency of the
purification procedure was indicated in this experiment by the relative
capacity of Con A to selectively stimulate T cells, but not B cells,
and LPS to selectively stimulate B cells, but not T cells. It should
be pointed out that some difficulties have been encountered, recently,
in stimulating enriched T cell population by specific antigens in the
absence of additional peritoneal exudate cells. The detection of
thymus derived TNP recognizing cells in $TNP_{128}SRC$ primed mice raised
the question of whether TNP recognizing helper cells were present
in such animals. It was realized, however, that TNP recognizing cells
and TNP helper cells are not necessarily the same population of cells.

It is well known that carrier recognizing cells are able to help
the anti hapten response of the homologous hapten-carrier conjugage.
However, the existence of hapten recognizing cells which cooperate
with either anti hapten or anti carrier antibody precursor cells is
only rarely evident (16). The following experiment explores the
existence of hapten recognizing helper function in our system.

$TNP_{128}SRC$ primed mice when challenged with trinitrophenylated
mouse red cells ($TNP_{8.6}MRC$) produced a significant anti SRC PFC
response 4 days after the challenge. (Table 3 group A). This
experiment suggests that $TNP_{128}SRC$ stimulate in mice the appearance
of TNP recognizing cells which help the anti SRC response. These

Table 3:   Improved anti SRC response following induction of TNP recognizing helper function.

Mice were injected with		No. of PFC ($\times 10^{-3}$) per spleen at day 6 indicated with[a]			
Day	Day	SRC		TNP-DRC	
0	2	D	ID	D	ID
A TNP$_{128}$SRC	TNP$_{8.6}$MRC	66.9	35.7	10.3	0[b]
B	TNP$_{8.6}$MRC	0	0	10.8	0
C TNP$_{128}$SRC		0.3	0	0.2	0.7

Mice (3 per group) were treated as described in the footnote of table 1, with the difference that the challenge dose was TNP$_{8.6}$MRC. Similar results were obtained in 5 other experiments. The trinitrophenylation of SRC, DRC and MRC was done according to ref. 17. Jerne's haemolytic plaque assay was used (18). The anti DRC PFC response was 0 in all groups.

[a] Assayed against the various red cell types indicated and expressed as the mean number $\times 10^{-3}$.

[b] Zero <0.1 (i.e. <100 PFC/spleen).

cells were activated by the challenge dose of TNP-MRC, and cooperated with precursors of anti SRC antibody producing cells which, in the presence of residual priming antigen (TNP$_{128}$SRC), produced an anti SRC antibody response. An alternative possibility is that anti hapten antibodies mediate the helper function (19).

Thus, TNP$_{128}$SRC stimulate, in mice, the appearance of both TNP and SRC recognizing helper functions. The possibility of utilising this function to provide an anti tumor response to TNP coated tumor cells was examined in our last series of experiments. BALB/c mice were challenged with trinitrophenylated EL4 allogeneic tumor cells (originating in C57Bl mice) 4, 7, and 14 days after their priming with TNP$_{128}$SRC. 13 days following challenge the mice were sacrificed and their spleen cells were tested for their cytotoxicity to non modified ^{51}Cr labeled EL4 cells (20). Different control groups were included in this experiment as indicated below. As recorded in Fig. 2, spleen cells from mice, which were primed with TNP$_{128}$SRC at different times before challenge with TNP-EL4, were more cytotoxic than spleen cells from mice which were injected with TNP$_{128}$SRC, at the same time, but challenged with non modified tumor cells. Spleen cells from mice which were primed with TNP$_{128}$SRC but were not

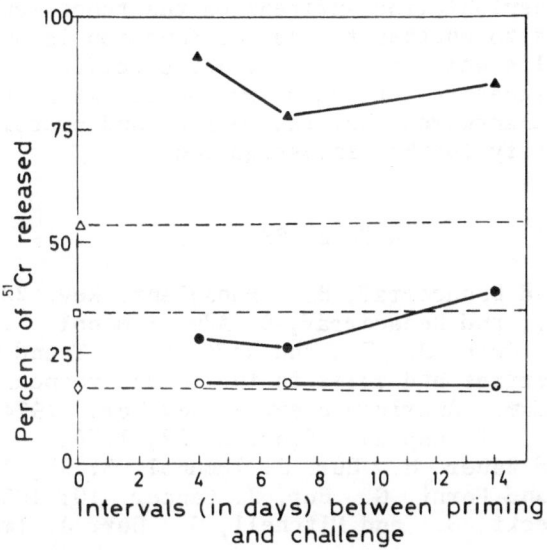

FIG.2: Improved allogeneic anti tumor response following induction of TNP recognizing helper function.

Mice were treated as described in the text and the immune response of the following groups was determined by the chromium release assay. (20).

▲————▲ Mice primed with $TNP_{128}SRC$ and challenged with TNP-EL4.
●————● Mice primed with $TNP_{128}SRC$ and challenged with EL4.
○————○ Mice primed with $TNP_{128}SRC$ and not challenged.
△   Mice not primed but challenged with TNP-EL4.
□   Mice not primed but challenged with EL4
○   Normal mice.

Trinitrophenylation of tumor cells was performed by incubating 80-150 x 10^6 EL4 cells in 10 ml of 10^{-5} M TNBS in RPMI at 37°C for 45'. 3 x 10^5 modified or unmodified tumor cells were injected per mouse.

challenged with tumor cells indicated the background cytotoxic response, characteristic of spleen cells from normal mice. Spleen cells from non primed mice which were injected with TNP-EL4 tumor cells were more cytotoxic than spleen cells from non primed mice which were injected with non modified tumor cells. However, spleen cells from non primed mice which were injected with TNP-EL4 tumor cells were less cytotoxic than spleen cells from mice which were primed with $TNP_{128}SRC$ and challenged with TNP-EL4. Thus, TNP recognizing helper function may cooperate with thymus derived cells for production of allogeneic anti tumor response. According to this interpretation the helper function cooperated with cells which recognize the transplantation antigens on the tumor membrane. The question arises as to whether the helper function is able to cooperate with cells which recognize tumor specific antigens in the production of a syngeneic anti tumor response. At present this question remains unanswered, but theoretical and practical consideration justify further investigation.

REFERENCES

1. Katz, D.H., and Benacerraf, B. Transplant. Rev. 22: 175, 1975.
2. McDevitt, H.O., and Benacerraf, B. Adv. Immunol. 11: 31, 1969.
3. Greaves, M.F., Owen, J.J.T., and Raff, M.C. T and B lymphocytes origins, properties and roles in the immune response. Excerpta Medica Amsterdam. American Elsevier New York, 1974.
4. Mitchison, N.A. Transplant. Proc. 2: 92, 1970.
5. Kurth, R., and Bauer, H. Eur. J. Immunol. 3: 95, 1973.
6. Cavallo, G., and Forni, G. Eur. J. Cancer. 10: 103, 1974.
7. Naor, D., Morecki, S., and Mitchell, G. Eur. J. Immunol. 4: 311, 1974.
8. Naor, D., Saltoun, R., and Falkenberg, F. Eur. J. Immunol. 5: 220, 1975.
9. Kahan, M., and Noar, D. Manuscript in preparation.
10. Mugraby, L., Gery, I., and Sulitzeanu, D. Eur. J. Immunol. 4: 402, 1974.
11. Mugraby, L., Gery, I., and Sulitzeanu, D. Immunology, 26: 787, 1974.
12. Williams, C.A., and Chase, M.W. Methods in Immunology and Immunochemistry. Vol. 1, p. 128. Academic Press, New York, 1967.
13. Wigzell, H., Sundqvist, K.G., and Yoshida, T.O. Scand J. Immunol. 1: 75, 1972.
14. Campbell, P.A., and Grey, H.M. Cell. Immunol. 5: 171, 1972.
15. Laskov, R., and Simon, E. Israel J. Med. Sci. 9: 175, 1973.
16. Mitchison, N.A. Eur. J. Immunol. 1: 68, 1971.
17. Rittenberg, M.B., and Pratt, K.L. Proc. Soc. Exp. Biol. Med. 132: 575, 1969.
18. Jerne, N.K., Nordin, A.A., and Henry, C. In: Cell bound antibodies. p. 109, Amos, B., and Koprowski, H., ed., Wistar Inst., Press, Philadelphia, 1963.
19. Janeway, C.A. Jr., and Paul, W.E. Eur. J. Immunol. 3: 340, 1973.
20. Berke, G., and Amos, D.B. Transplant. Rev. 17: 71, 1973.

IN VITRO PROLIFERATIVE REACTIONS BY LYMPHOCYTES FROM BOTH RESPONDER AND "LOW" RESPONDER MICE TO (T,G)-A--L

Joost J. Oppenheim, Edna Mozes and Michael Sela

Department of Chemical Immunology

Weizmann Institute of Science, Rehovot, Israel

The capacity to mount an antibody response to many immunogenic systems is under the control of immune response (Ir) genes which are linked to the major histocompatibility locus (H-2) of the mouse (1). Inbred mice of the H-2^b type manifest IgM and IgG antibody responses when immunized with a synthetic antigen such as poly(Tyr, Glu)-polyDLAla--polyLys ((T,G)-A--L) (2). In contrast, mice of the H-2^k or ^{s} type are "low" responders that ordinarily produce only low titers of both IgM and IgG antibodies to (T,G)-A--L (3). In addition, lymphocytes from sensitized responder mice have specific in vitro secondary proliferative reactions to (T,G)-A--L, whereas lymphocytes from sensitized low responders do not (4).

An antigen specific factor is produced by "educated" thymus cells of responder mice, which can replace the requirement for specific T cells in the antibody response of B cells to (T,G)-A--L (5). Although low responder C3H/He B cells fail to make antibody in response to factor plus antigen, their T cells are capable of making the factor indicating that they have defective B cells (5). In contrast, low responder SJL mice fail both to make and respond to the T cell factor indicating that both their T and B cells are defective (6). Crosses of low responder mice with T cell defects produces F1 hybrid responders (7). Thus at least 2 major histocompatibility linked genes determine the level of immune response to (T,G)-A--L.

We have compared the effect of T cell factors on the in vitro lymphoproliferative response of responder mice with low responders C3H/He and SJL mice with different genetic defects. In the course of these studies we made the unexpected observation that with increasing time after immunization the in vitro lymphoproliferative

response of low responders became as active as that of responder
lymphocytes.

Stimulants. The T cell mitogen phytohemagglutinin (PHA, Bur-
roughs Wellcome) and B cell mitogen lipopolysaccharide endotoxin
(LPS, Salmonella typhosa 0901 (Difco) were used. Antigens used included Purified Protein Derivative (PPD, Connaught Labs.), (T,G)-
A--L, and poly-L-(Phe,Glu)-polyD,L-Ala-poly-L-Lys (Phe,G)-A--L (6).
T cell factor was prepared (6). The resultant supernatant was centrifuged (17,650 G for 30 min), dialysed overnight to remove inhibitory aggregates and small molecules and sterilized with millipore
filters.

Cell cultures. The draining lymph nodes and occasionally the
spleens from 5-10 syngeneic mice were aseptically removed and pooled 3-13 weeks after immunization with 10 μgm (T,G)-A--L in CFA into
the footpads. The lymphocytes were gently teased from the organs,
washed twice and suspended in RPMI 1640 supplemented with antibio-
tics, 2 mM glutamine, 2.5×10^{-5}M 2 mercaptoethanol and 1% fresh heparinized mouse plasma or serum. Lymphocytes were fractionated using
glass beads and nylon columns to obtain nonadherent T enriched populations (8). These eluted cells required 5-10% filtered fetal calf
serum (FCS) in the medium in order to grow. Lymphocytes were treated with 1:5 dil. of rabbit antimouse thymocyte antisera (provided
by Drs. I. Gery & Y. Stupp, Hadassah Hosp.) which had been absorbed
twice with mouse kidney and liver cells. They were then washed and
exposed to 1:6 dil. guinea pig complement (absorbed with agarose).
This produces lymphocyte population enriched for immunoglobulin
bearing B cells.

Cultures gave maximal responses as reported (9,10) with 10^6
lymphocytes in 0.2 ml/well in tissue culture plates with flat bot-
toms (Microtiter II, Falcon #3040). They were incubated for 4 days
at 37°C in an atmosphere of 7% O_2, 10% CO_2 and 83% N_2. Cultures were
exposed to 0.5 μc tritiated thymidine (TdR^{3}H, spec. act. 2Ci/mM.
Amersham) for the final 6 hrs of incubation. They were processed
using an automatic harvester (MASH II, Microbiol. Assoc.).

RESULTS AND DISCUSSION

With increasing time after immunization the degree of "spontaneous" DNA synthesis by unstimulated cultures progressively decreased. This resulted in progressively better detection of TdR^{3}H incorporation by antigen stimulated cultures in mice tested 2-13 weeks
after immunization. Cultures of lymph node cells (LNC) from responder
mice immunized with (T,G)-A--L showed significant increases in vitro
proliferative responses to higher and less to lower doses of (T,G)-
A--L (Table 1). In contrast, responder spleen cells and low responder LNC showed low reactions only to higher doses of antigen. Concomitantly LNC from responders as well as low responders reacted equally well to PPD, PHA and LPS.

TABLE 1. In vitro lymphoproliferative response 3 weeks after immunization

Stimulant	Conc. µgm/ml	Responder C57BL/6	Low responders C3H/He	SJL
None	-	148*	426	304
(T,G)-A--L (H)**	100	1725	644	895
"	10	720	941	651
"	1	261	-	449
" (U)**	100	700	875	301
"	10	543	936	411
(Phe,G)-A--L (H)	100	996	801	640
" (U)	100	536	1085	334
PPD	10	645	2140	1748
PHA	0.5	4956	1129	2990
LPS (H)	50	5730	327	3696

*Mean cpm of TdR^{3}H incorporated by duplicate cultures. Underlined values were significantly elevated above the unstimulated cpm (p<.05).

**H - antigen boiled for 1-2 hrs; U - antigen not heated.

In general, heated (boiled for 1-2 hrs) preparations of the synthetic polypeptides, presumably due to aggregation, were some-what more effective in vitro stimulants than unheated antigens. The proliferative responder C57BL/6 mice immunized with (T,G)-A--L or DNP-BSA proliferated in vitro only in response to the immunizing antigen. However, LNC from responder mice sensitized with (T,G)-A--L showed considerable proliferative response to (Phe,G)-A--L. This parallels the high degree of cross-reaction between both antibodies and T cell factors to (T,G)-A--L and (Phe,G)-A--L (11). It suggests that the A--L component must be involved in lymphocyte activation.

The effect of adding serial 2 fold dilutions of supernatants containing T cell factors to cultured lymphocytes was tested. The supernatants were generally inhibitory at dilutions of 1:2 and 1:4. At higher dilutions they nonspecifically increased the TdR^{3}H incorporation by cultures from immune or normal responder spleen cells and LNC of sensitized low responders. The supernatants selectively suppressed the TdR^{3}H uptake of unstimulated cultures of lymphocytes enriched for B cells (by ATS+C'). This resulted in an apparent increase in the response of all stimulated cultures relative to the controls (E/C). However, equal suppression of TdR^{3}H uptake by un-stimulated cultures of (T,G)-A--L immunized responder mouse LNC with concomitant increases in E/C was obtained by supernatants containing T cell factors against noncrossreactive (T,G)-A--L or DNP-BSA (Table 2). Therefore, T cell factors do not specifically inhibit

TABLE 2. Effect of T cell factor on proliferation of LNL from C57BL/6
responder mice: 6 weeks after immunization

Stimulant	Conc. μgm/ml	+ medium only cpm	+1:8 dil. of factor vs. (T,G)-A--L cpm	+1:8 dil. of factor vs. DNP-BSA cpm
None	-	502	305	203
(T,G)-A--L (H)	100	1137	1153	962
"	10	691	703	847
DNP-BSA	100	732	887	533
PPD	10	2413	1802	1889
LPS (H)	50	1281	7510	6908
PHA	0.5	15350	407	407

suppressor cell activity and have only nonspecific relative enhancing effects on short-term in vitro lymphoproliferation.

In the course of these studies some of the mice were tested
only 2-3 months after immunization. We were surprised to obtain
equally significant lymphoproliferative responses to (T,G)-A--L by
low responders as by responder mice (Table 3). Similar observations
have been repeatedly made with CKB and C3H/He mice that are thought
to have B cell defects (5) as well as SJL mice whose B as well as T
cells are presumed to be defective (6). It is unlikely that these
unexpected observations are due to either mutations in the mouse colonies or mixups since LNC from low responders of the same batch of
immunized mice had had low proliferative reactions 3-6 wks after
immunization

TABLE 3. In vitro lymphoproliferative response 8 weeks after
immunization

Stimulant	Conc. μgm/ml	Responder C3H·SW	Low responders C3H/He	SJL
None	-	85	543	41
(T,G)-A--L (H)	100	2022	4130	3327
"	10	1024	4490	1275
"	1	1000	3082	2115
(T,G)-A--L (U)	100	553	770	3093
"	10	778	962	2648
PPD	10	229	2828	9291
LPS (H)	50	18312	2709	8816
PHA	1	4372	5250	493

There are a number of diverse situations in which the genetic
defect in the low responders has been overcome. Administering the antigen on an immunogenic carrier such as methylated BSA (12), or in
conjunction with an allogeneic reaction (13) will lead to normal
antibody production by low responders. Furthermore, the embryonic
lymphoid tissues of low responder mice proliferate as well as those
from responders (14) and tetraparental mice make antibody responses
of the low responder allotype (15). Thus the gene defect is not absolute and the Ir genes may control regulatory mechanisms governing
the rate or expression of an immune response. For example, there
may be differences in the degree of suppressor T cell activity between low and high responders. Alternatively there may be selective
defects in subpopulations of T cells in the low responders. Finally,
since the random (T,G)-A--L copolymer is not homogeneous, the delayed proliferative response may be to a minor antigenic configuration
to which low responders in time can respond, because a smaller clone
of reactive cells takes longer to become detectable.

We have tested the hypothesis that different classes of lymphocytes may be responsible for the in vitro proliferative response of
low and high responders. We also find that nonadherent responder
lymphocytes eluted from nylon columns enriched for T cells proliferate to a significant extent to (T,G)-A--L (4). Similarly T cell enriched lymphocytes from low responder SJL that fail to proliferate
in response to the B cell mitogen LPS, do respond to (T,G)-A--L
(Table 4). However, this does not rule out the possibility that B
cells also contribute to the proliferative response. Lymphocytes
that were treated with heterologous ATS or anti-θ plus complement,
which enriched their immunoglobulin positive B cell content, also
showed significant proliferative reactions to (T,G)-A--L. However,
these cells also still responded to PHA indicating that they were
not free of contaminant functioning T cells. Thus T cells contribute to the proliferative reactions of both high and low responders.

TABLE 4. Proliferation by SJL "low" responder T and B enriched LNL:
eleven weeks after immunization

Stimulants	Unfractionated LNL	Eluted off glass beads	Eluted off nylon	Treated with ATS+C'
None	638	400	146	549
(T,G)-A--L (H)	8349	6404	855	1991
" (U)	8251	6223	252	2168
PPD	12839	12987	555	2731
LPS (H)	8684	9729	76	8392
PHA	1245	1403	17253	13670

In summary (T,G)-A--L can induce specific in vitro lymphoproliferative reactions in LNC from immunized mice. From 3-8 weeks
after immunization lymphocytes from responder mice react to a much
greater degree than from low responders. These proliferative reactions are not specifically enhanced by supernatants of "educated"
T cells. However, 2 to 3 months after immunization the lymphoproliferative response of the low responders rises to the same level as
that of responder mice.

Supported in part by a grant 1RO1 AI 11405-03 from the National
Institutes of Health, U.S. Public Health Service. We appreciate
the expert technical assistance of Clauditte Rabinowitz, Molly
Dayan and Heide Zinger.

References

1. B. Benacerraf and H.O. McDevitt, Science 175:273, 1972.

2. H.O. McDevitt and M. Sela, J. Exp. Med. 122:517, 1965.

3. H.O. McDevitt, J. Immunol. 100:485, 1968.

4. P. Lonai and H.O. McDevitt, J. Exp. Med. 140:977, 1974.

5. M.J. Taussig, E. Mozes and R. Isac, J. Exp. Med. 140:301, 1974.

6. E. Mozes, R. Isac and M.J. Taussig, J. Exp. Med. 141:793, 1975.

7. A.J. Munro and M.J. Taussig, Nature (in press) 1975.

8. M.H. Julius, E. Simpson and L.A. Herzenberg, Eur. J. Immunol.
   3:645, 1973.

9. A.B. Peck, E. Katz-Heber and R.E. Click, Eur. J. Immunol. 3:516,
   1973.

10. A.B. Peck and F.H. Bach, J. Immunol. Meth. 3:147, 1973.

11. E. Mozes, R. Isac, D. Givol, R. Zakut and D. Beitsch in these
    proceedings.

12. J. Green, W.E. Paul and B. Benacerraf, J. Exp. Med. 123:859,
    1966.

13. J.C. Ordal and F.C. Grumet, J. Exp. Med. 136:1195, 1972.

14. M.L. Tyan, J. Immunol. 108:65, 1972.

15. K.B. Bechtold, T.G. Wegmann, J.H. Freed, F.C. Grumet, B.W.
    Chesebro, L.A. Herzenberg and H.O. McDevitt, Cell Immunol. 13:
    264, 1974.

EFFECT OF INTERACTION BETWEEN HAPTEN-SPECIFIC CELLS PRESELECTED FOR DIFFERENT RECEPTOR AFFINITIES AND CARRIER-PRIMED CELLS ON ANTIBODY AVIDITY *

G. Doria and G. Agarossi
CNEN-Euratom Immunogenetics Group
Laboratory of Radiopathology
C.S.N. Casaccia (Rome), Italy

Our previous studies, *in vivo* (1) and *in vitro* (2), have shown that carrier-priming enhances antibody response and avidity. Under optimal conditions for these carrier effects to occur, C3HeB/FeJ and (C57Bl/10xDBA/2)F1 mice either carrier-primed with HRBC or -unprimed were given the conjugate TNP-HRBC. Thereafter, spleen cells from the carrier-primed or -unprimed mice were daily pooled and assayed by the hemolytic plaque technique with TNP-SRBC to determine the number of direct PFC anti-TNP. Avidity of antibodies secreted by PFC was estimated from inhibition of PFC by soluble TNP-BSA (35 mols TNP/mol BSA). Aliquots of TNP-BSA dissolved in PBS at different concentrations and aliquots of spleen cells were plated in agar containing TNP-SRBC. The number of direct PFC developed after addition of guinea pig complement was decreased by TNP-BSA. Percent inhibitions of PFC were transformed to probits which appeared linearly related to the log dose of inhibitor. The reciprocal of the dose of inhibitor that suppressed 50% of the PFC was taken as an estimate of avidity: the higher the antibody avidity, the lower the inhibitor dose and the higher its reciprocal. The dose of inhibitor was referred to TNP-lysyl residues and calculated from spectrophotometric measurements of the TNP-BSA solution at λ max 348 nm by assuming 15,400 as the molar extinction coefficient for the TNP-lysyl residue. In each PFC inhibition assay, spleen cells were exposed to amounts of TNP-lysyl residues ranging from 10^{-5} to 10^{-1} mg. The conjugate preparations and the assays for direct PFC anti-TNP and for antibody avidity have been described in great detail elsewhere (3). The results of a tipical experiment, in which C3HeB/FeJ mice carrier-primed with 2×10^5 HRBC 3 days earlier or -unprimed were immunized with 4×10^6 TNP-HRBC, are reported in Table 1. It can be seen that carrier-priming increases both PFC response and antibody avidity. Analyses (not shown) of histogram distributions of PFC of different avidities revealed in carrier-primed mice a shift toward higher avidity values.

* Supported by CNEN-Euratom Association Contract. Publication No. 1209 of the Euratom Biology Division.

Table   1

EFFECT OF CARRIER PRIMING ON THE RESPONSE AGAINST TNP

HRBC-priming	Days after immunization with TNP-HRBC				
	1	2	3	4	5
	PFC $(\times 10^3)$/Spleen				
Yes	11	7	49	112	23
No	7	6	12	15	10
	Avidity (mg^{-1})				
Yes	106 (121–93)	305 (414–224)	1049 (1254–877)	791 (861–727)	302 (389–235)
No	43 (52–36)	69 (89–54)	61 (73–51)	40 (49–33)	81 (94–69)

Four mice/group. Numbers in parentheses are 95% confidence limits

Several experiments support the view that carrier-priming stimulates T cells that help B cells to produce antibodies against the hapten (4). The finding of Gershon and Paul (5) that T cells can increase antibody affinity suggests that cell cooperation is instrumental to the production of high affinity antibodies. How cell cooperation results in selection of high affinity antibody-producing cells has not been elucidated. According to the maturation theory of antibody affinity (6) it could be envisaged that carrier-stimulated T cells may favour antigen selection by expanding the B cell population on which antigen will exert its selective pressure (7). A variant of this view proposes that high affinity receptor B cells are first selected by antigen and then allowed to proliferate and differentiate into antibody-forming cells if an optimal number of T cells is present (8). Both hypotheses are supported by the observation that the carrier effect on antibody avidity was more pronounced when animals (unpublished data) or spleen cells *in vitro* (2) were stimulated with lower doses of TNP-HRBC. Indeed, the maturation theory predicts that lower antigen concentrations trigger cells with higher affinity receptors. An alternative mechanism, suggested by Mitchell (9), ascribes to T cells an antigen clearance function by phagocyte activation resulting in protection of high affinity receptor B cells which are very sensitive to "high dose" tolerance.

The mechanism of the carrier effect on antibody avidity was investigated by experiments in which hapten-specific cells preselected for high or low receptor affinity by different doses of hapten conjugated to one carrier were transferred into irradiated recipients preimmunized with another carrier, and then stimulated with the same hapten conjugated to the second carrier.

In one experiment, groups of donor (C57Bl/10xDBA/2)F1 mice were injected I.P. with a single dose (10^0 or $10^4 \mu g$) of TNP-BGG (61 mols TNP/mol BGG) in CFA or uninjected. After 49 days, 5 mice of each donor group were sacrificed and their spleen cells pooled, washed, and transferred (4×10^7 nucleated cells I.V.) into two groups of 900 R syngenic recipients, one of which had been carrier-primed with HRBC (2×10^6 I.V.) 3 days before irradiation. All recipients (8 mice/group) were then injected I.V. with TNP-HRBC (5×10^8 immediately after irradiation and on day 3) and sacrificed on day 6 to evaluate in pooled spleen cells of each group the number of PFC and avidity of antibodies against TNP.

The results of this experiment, reported in Table 2, are consistent with those of another similar experiment in which donors were sacrificed 28 days after injection of TNP-BGG. Carrier-priming of the recipients always increased the number of PFC. The carrier effect on avidity was dependent upon the TNP-BGG dose given to donors. Carrier-priming of the recipients produced an increase in antibody avidity when donors were given no TNP-BGG or a high dose of it, the increase being much greater in the latter case. The highest avidity values were obtained in carrier-primed recipients of cells from donors given $10^4 \mu g$ TNP-BGG. No carrier effect on avidity was ever observed when donor cells had been preselected by a very low dose of TNP-BGG.

Table 2

RESPONSE AGAINST TNP IN HRBC-PRIMED OR -UNPRIMED 900R-RECIPIENTS GIVEN SYNGENIC SPEEN CELLS AND TNP-HRBC

TNP-BGG (μg) in CFA given to donors 49 days prior to cell transfer	PFC ($\times 10^3$)/Spleen		Avidity (mg^{-1})	
	HRBC-primed	Unprimed	HRBC-primed	Unprimed
0	1008	43	3014 (3518–2583)	1400 (2031– 965)
10^0	2355	720	3514 (3976–3106)	3525 (4569–2719)
10^4	1024	75	5176 (6320–4329)	516 (605– 439)

Numbers in parentheses are 95% confidence limits

That cell selection occurred in the donor spleens is apparent from the numbers of PFC and avidity values in the carrier-unprimed recipients. These data indicate that both doses of TNP-BGG increased the numbers of PFC precursors, $10^0 \mu g$ selecting high affinity receptor cells while $10^4 \mu g$ selecting cells with average affinity below the value of unselected cells.

Histogram distributions of PFC of varying avidities (data not shown) revealed great heterogeneity in all cell populations from both carrier-primed and -unprimed recipients. However, when donors were given $10^4 \mu g$ TNP-BGG carrier-priming induced a shift of the PFC distribution toward higher avidity values. This carrier effect was less pronounced when donors were uninjected. No shift toward the high avidity side resulted from carrier-priming when donor cells were preselected by $10^0 \mu g$ TNP-BGG.

Based on the demonstration that precursor cell and secreted antibody avidities are correlated (10), the present findings can be explained by the following hypothesis. Carrier-primed T cells act selectively on hapten-specific B cells endowed with low density receptors of very high affinity.

This hypothesis implies that there are subpopulations of B cell precursors which differ not only in receptor affinity but also in receptor density. Evidence in favour of this possibility was provided by Willcox and McMichael (11). Two additional assumptions are made: a) low density receptor cells are stimulated only by high antigen concentrations, e.g. they require more than one hit to divide; b) low density receptors are of higher affinity than high density receptors. Thus, the antigen concentration following injection of $10^4 \mu g$ TNP-BGG could expand precursor B cells with low density receptors of very high affinity and paralyse cells with high density and high affinity receptors. A much smaller antigen concentration following injection of $10^0 \mu g$ TNP-BGG could select only high density receptor cells of high affinity.

When precursor B cells are triggered by TNP-HRBC into PFC anti-TNP, T cells anti-HRBC could help cell differentiation by orienting and concentrating the conjugate on TNP-specific B cells (12). Macrophages could partecipate in this process (13). Low density receptor B cells require T cell cooperation to start differentiating into antibody-forming cells. High density receptor B cells do not require any antigen concentrating device. Hence, HRBC-primed T cells selected TNP-specific B cells with low density receptors of very high affinity, a cell subpopulation present in unselected spleen cells, less frequent in spleen cells from donors given $10^0 \mu g$ TNP-BGG, and abundant in spleen cells from donors given $10^4 \mu g$ TNP-BGG. Stimulation of HRBC-primed T cells by TNP-HRBC could induce T cell liberation of mitogenic factors that may account for the larger numbers of PFC observed in all groups of carrier-primed recipients.

Under alternative hypotheses (7-9), the carrier effect on avidity should have been most evident when donor cells were preselected for high affinity receptors by $10^0 \mu g$ TNP-BGG, unless donor cell affinity were very homogeneous or at the maximum level. In fact, the present results showed no carrier effect on avidity when donor cells were preselected by $10^0 \mu g$ TNP-BGG, although in unprimed recipients the heterogeneity of the histogram distribution of PFC of different avidities was large and the average avidity value was below the level reached in carrier-primed recipients of cells from donors given $10^4 \mu g$ TNP-BGG.

References

1. Doria G. and Agarossi G., Fed. Proc. 32:993 Abs, 1973.

2. Doria G., Agarossi G., Di Pietro S., Garavini M., and Mancini C., in Lymphocyte Recognition and Effector Mechanisms, Ed. Lindahl-Kiessling K. and Osoba D., Acad. Press, p. 163, 1974.

3. Doria G., Schiaffini G., Garavini M., and Mancini C., J. Immun. 109: 1245, 1972.

4. Mitchison N.A., Eur. J. Immun., 1: 18, 1971.

5. Gershon R.K. and Paul W. E., J. Immun. 106: 872, 1971.

6. Siskind G. W. and Benacerraf B., Adv. Immun. 10: 1, 1969.

7. Katz, D. H. and Benacerraf B., Adv. Immun. 15: 1, 1972.

8. Taniguchi T. and Tada T., J. Exp. Med., 139: 108, 1974.

9. Mitchell G.F., in Progress in Immunology II, Ed. Brent L. and Holborow J., North-Holland, vol. 3, p. 89, 1974.

10. Julius M.H. and Herzenberg L.A., J. Exp. Med., 140: 904, 1974.

11. Willcox H.N.A. and McMichael A.J., Eur. J. Immun., 5: 131, 1975.

12. Mitchison N.A., Taylor R.B., and Rajewsky K., in Developmental Aspects of Antibody Formation and Structure, Ed. Sterzl J., Czech. Acad. Sci., p. 547, 1970.

13. Feldmann M. and Nossal G.J.V., Transplantation Rev. 13: 3, 1972.

CELL INTERACTION IN B/W MICE: A REVERSIBLE DEFECT AT THE T-CELL LEVEL

John C. Roder, David A. Bell and Sharwan K. Singhal

Depts. of Medicine, and Bacteriology and Immunology
University of Western Ontario
London, Ontario, Canada N6A 5C1

INTRODUCTION

There is abundant evidence showing that many T cell functions are impaired in overtly autoimmune New Zealand mice (reviewed in 1). An example of this is the age dependent decline in antibody responses to T dependent, but not T independent antigens which accompanies the spontaneous rise in auto antibody formation. It has been suggested (2, 3) that the antibody mediated autoimmune phenomena occurring in these mice may reflect an early loss of suppressor T cells and it would be expected that the increase in thymocytotoxic auto-antibody (4) would cause a reduction in T cells and hence a decline in T dependent antibody responses. Our studies examine the nature of the defect leading to a loss of responsiveness to SRBC and the results support our hypothesis (5) that in aging B/W mice there arises a suppressor of T cell activation which prevents the induction of T cell help and possibly T cell tolerance to self antigens.

MATERIALS AND METHODS

Young (4-6 wk) and old (6-8 month) NZBxNZW F_1 mice (B/W) were bred in our laboratory from parental stock obtained from the University of Alberta. Spleen cells from female mice were cultured under standard Mishell-Dutton conditions with SRBC unless specified otherwise. Antibody formation was measured by enumerating direct (IgM) hemolytic plaque forming cells (PFC). Treatment of cell populations with anti-θ or anti Ig serum and complement has been described previously (6).

RESULTS

The Immunocompetence of B and T Cells in Old B/W Mice

We have previously shown (7) as have others (8, 9) that old
B/W mice have a markedly deficient primary response to SRBC whereas young B/W mice respond normally. Cell transfer experiments
were performed in lethally irradiated (1000R) old syngeneic recipients. As shown in Table 1, combinations of old B/W bone marrow
and thymus cells attained the same level (p$>$0.05) of PFC response
as did young B/W donor bone marrow cells and thymocytes. The
level of PFC response by B and T cells in both young and old B/W
mice was higher than that observed in normal strain BDF mice
(p$<$0.01). These results indicated that intact old B/W mice which
do not respond to a single injection of SRBC do possess immunocompetent lymphoid cells potentially capable of cooperating upon transfer into lethally irradiated old B/W mice. The next series of
experiments were designed to identify the cellular defect in the
intact animal.

TABLE I

PFC RESPONSE OF CELLS TRANSFERRED INTO IRRADIATED OLD MICE

Cells Transferred	Route Antigen Injected	Adoptive Transfer (PFC/spleen*)		
		B/W Old into old	B/W Yo. into old	BDF yo into old
B + T	i.v.	a17819+2679	b12905+1963	c4516+620
B	i.v.	1083+ 537	342+ 8	62+ 33
T	i.v.	416+ 214	344+ 135	12+ 6
spleen	i.v.	d7798+ 978	-----	8433+410
B + T	i.p.	6479+ 317	-----	-----

30 x 10^6 B and/or 120 x 10^6 T cells, or 10^8 spleen cells were
transferred together with 4 x 10^8 SRBC into groups of lethally
irradiated old syngeneic recipients.
*Values represent the mean direct PFC/spleen $\pm$ standard error, 7
days after cell transfer.
a vs. b, ns
a and b vs. c, p$<$.01
d vs. e, ns

Enhancement of the Anti-SRBC PFC Response in Old B/W Mice with LPS

As shown in Table II the anti-SRBC response in old B/W mice was low when either SRBC or various doses of E. coli lipopoly-saccharide (LPS) were injected alone. However when LPS and SRBC were injected simultaneously a 20 fold enhancement of the response was observed.

TABLE II

THE ENHANCING EFFECT OF LPS ON ANTI-SRBC
RESPONSE IN OLD B/W MICE

Injection[a]		Direct PFC/10^6
LPS (ug.)	SRBC	
5	−	56 ± 18
50	−	110 ± 24
250	−	88 ± 8
0	+	40 ± 6
5	+	474 ± 32
50	+	1876 ± 70
250	+	1115 ± 100

[a]E. coli (055:B5) LPS and/or 4×10^8 SRBC were injected i.v.
[b]Values represent the mean PFC/10^6 ± standard error 4 days after injection

Cell Synergism Between Primed T Cells and Non-primed Spleen
Cells in B/W Mice

Although old B/W mice do not mount a primary response to SRBC they do respond to a second injection of antigen (7-9). As shown in Fig. 1 when low dose primed (2×10^7 SRBC) old spleen cells were mixed in various ratios with non-primed spleen cells and SRBC in vitro, a marked cooperative effect was observed. The cooper-ating cells in the primed population were θ positive. Further experiments (6) revealed that θ positive, Ig negative, radiore-sistant T cells in the primed population were capable of cooper-ating with θ negative, Ig positive, radiosensitive B cells in the non-primed population.

Restoration of the Response of Old B/W Mice with Activated T Cells

Young or old B/W thymocytes (75×10^6) and SRBC were injected into lethally irradiated old syngeneic recipients and 7 days later recipient spleens were used as a source of ATC. As shown

in Fig. 2 when graded doses of ATC were added to 15 x 10^6 old B/W
spleen cells in vitro a marked restoration of the response was
observed. It was further revealed that θ positive, Ig negative
cells in the ATC population were cooperating with θ negative cells
in the old spleen. Recipient spleens from mice injected with
thymocytes or SRBC alone did not restore the response and ATC
cultured alone produced only minimal numbers of PFC. In addition
ATC added to anti θ treated old spleen cells resulted in a greater
(p < 0.02) enhancement than when added to normal mouse serum (NMS)
treated old spleen cells as shown in Fig. 3. This suggested that T
cells in the old B/W spleen might be responsible for blocking B cell
interaction with ATC.

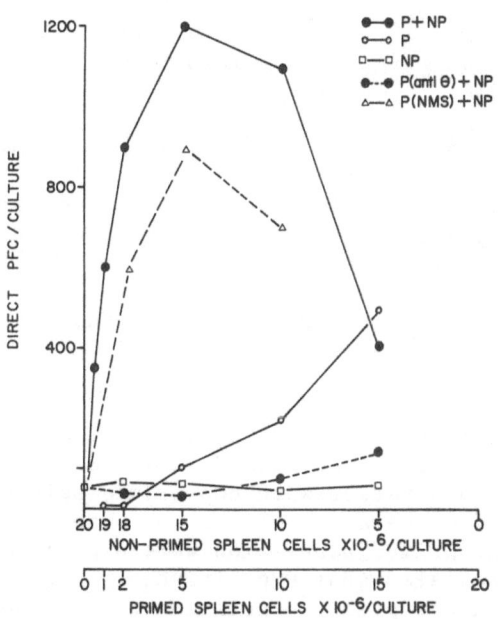

Fig. 1: Cell synergism between primed T-cells and non-primed
spleen cells in old B/W mice. Mice were primed by injecting
iv, 2 x 10^7 SRBC 2 days before sacrifice. Varying numbers of
anti-serum treated or untreated primed (P) or non-primed (NP)
spleen cells were cultured separately or were mixed together to
yield 20 x 10^6 spleen cells/culture.

Suppression of the Anti-SRBC Response of Young B/W Spleen Cells by Old B/W Spleen Cells and Thymocytes in Vitro

As shown in Table III when 10^7 non-responsive old B/W spleen cells or thymocytes were added to 15×10^6 young B/W spleen cells in culture, the anti-SRBC PFC response was suppressed by 85 and 68% respectively. This suppression was not due to cytotoxic effects and was not due to cell crowding or simply diluting out responding young cells, since the addition of equal numbers of intact or irradiated young spleen cells did not suppress the response. The suppression was unique to old B/W mice in that it could not be demonstrated in age-matched normal strain BDF mice (unpublished observation).

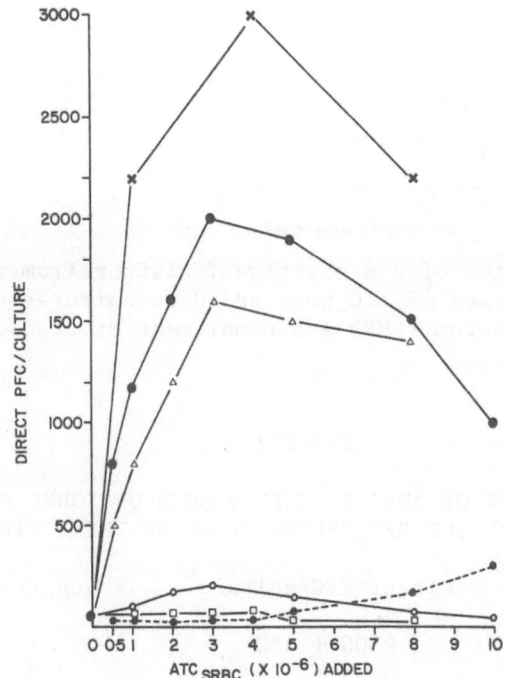

Fig. 2: Restoration of the old B/W spleen cell response by activated T cells. Graded doses of ATC (●—●), anti θ serum and complement treated ATC (O), anti Ig serum and complement treated ATC (Δ) or spleen cells from recipients injected with thymocytes or SRBC alone (□) were added to 15×10^6 old B/W spleen cells cultured with SRBC. ATC were also cultured alone (●--●)and anti Ig serum and complement treated ATC were added to anti θ serum and complement treated old spleen cells (×).

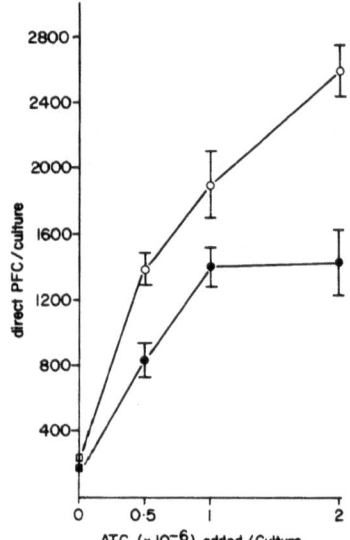

■ old spl. (NMS)
□ old spl. (anti Θ)
● old spl. (NMS) + ATC
○ old spl. (anti Θ) + ATC

Fig. 3: Elimination of a θ positive inhibitor from old B/W spleen
cells. Graded doses of ATC were added to cultures of anti θ
or normal mouse serum (NMS) and complement treated old B/W spleen
cells.

TABLE III

SUPPRESSION OF ANTI–SRBC RESPONSES OF YOUNG SPLEEN
CELLS BY OLD B/W SPLEEN CELLS OR THYMOCYTES

Cells Added[a]	Direct PFC/culture[b]	% Suppression
none	4800 $\pm$ 450	–
yo. spl.	6525 $\pm$ 125	0
old spl.	748 $\pm$ 13	85
yo. thymus	4560 $\pm$ 22	5
old thymus	1536 $\pm$ 624	68
yo. spl.	4450 $\pm$ 275	7

[a]10^7 cells were added on day 0 to 15×10^6 young spleen cells.
  The response of 10^7 old spleen cells alone was 25 ± 8 PFC/
  culture.
[b]Values represent the mean PFC $\pm$ standard error determined on
  day 5

DISCUSSION

The antibody response of SRBC is dependent upon complex cellular interaction between T and B derived cells and macrophages (10) and an intrinsic defect or quantitative deficiency of any one or more of these cells could potentially result in the age dependent decline in the anti-SRBC response in B/W mice. It was possible that the deficient anti-SRBC response in old B/W mice (7-9) was due to a decline in helper T cells, since many T cell functions are deficient (1) and there is a slight age dependent decline in numbers of theta positive cells (11). We have investigated these possibilities and attempted to characterize the nature of the defect in these mice. The failure of syngeneic young spleen, thymus, bone marrow (7) or peritoneal exudate cells (7, 12) to restore the response of old B/W spleen cells argues against any simple lack of a cell type as a mechanism of non-responsiveness in these mice. Furthermore these findings and those of others showing the ability of syngeneic thymocytes to restore the defective SRBC response in nude (13, 14) or thymectomized mice and mice undergoing antigenic competition (15) argue against (i) a quantitative deficiency in helper T cells which could arise due to a thymocytotoxic auto-antibody (16) and (ii) a relative T cell deficiency arising due to competition with auto antigens for available T cells or their products.

The question of the intrinsic immunocompetence of B and T cells was investigated by adoptively transferring lymphoid cells from old non-responsive B/W mice, young responsive B/W mice or normal strain mice into lethally irradiated old syngeneic recipients. It was found that combinations of old B/W bone marrow and thymocytes resulted in marked synergism and the level of response obtained was similar to that of young B/W or normal strain donor cells. These results indicated that intact old B/W mice which do not respond to SRBC do however have immunocompetent lymphoid cells potentially capable of cooperating fully in an immune response and suggested that these cells might be suppressed in some way.

Further experiments revealed that the defect or block in the intact animal involved the process of T cell activation. First, the simultaneous injection of SRBC and LPS (B cell mitogen) into old B/W mice restored the response presumably by circumventing the T cell requirement as it does in nude (17, 18) and T deprived mice (19). Secondly, the addition of θ positive, Ig negative, radio-resistant spleen cells from primed old B/W mice to θ negative, Ig positive, radiosensitive non-primed old B/W spleen cells in vitro resulted in a marked cooperative response, also observed by others in normal strain mice (20). This suggested that (i) old B/W splenic T cells could be primed for immunologic memory even though an immune response was not mounted and (ii) these primed T memory

cells could be converted to T helper cells upon a second exposure
to antigen and restore the response of old non-primed B/W spleen
cells by a cooperative interaction witn B cells. Thirdly, the
in vitro response of old B/W spleen cells was restored in a dose
dependent manner by adding young or old θ positive, Ig negative ATC.
This restoration has been shown to be specific in experiments
utilizing ATC against horse, burro and sheep erythrocytes (6).
Further, experiments revealed that an even greater degree of restoration was possible if ATC were added to anti-θ treated old spleen
cells suggesting the existence of a θ positive suppressor cell in
old B/W spleens. More direct evidence was obtained by showing that
old but not young spleen and thymus cells markedly suppressed the
PFC response of young B/W spleen cells in vitro. Splenic suppressor
cells were found to be small, radioresistant non-adherent cells
that may act on early events in T cell triggering (5). It is not
yet known whether this spleen cell is a B cell or a T cell but it
appears with age before the decline in T cell mitogen and helper
responses and preceeds the rise in auto antibody production. It has
been shown that the increasing resistance to tolerance induction
in aging B/W mice is a T cell (21, 22) and not a B cell defect
(22, 23) and it is quite conceivable that a suppressor interferring
with the activation of T helper cells might also be involved in
inhibiting T cell activation for self-tolerance.

With age in B/W mice some suppressor cell function may decline
(2), and as we have shown others may increase. The relationship
between these two findings is unclear but we would like to suggest
that the presence of suppressor cells as a cause of autoimmunity
is a viable alternative to the prevalent hypothesis that a loss
of suppressor T cells allows self-reactive B cells to escape normal
regulatory mechanisms.

SUMMARY

The anti-SRBC PFC response of old B/W mice can be restored
by adding specifically activated T cells or primed spleen cells
in vitro as well as by injecting LPS and SRBC in vivo. Since non-
responsive old B/W bone marrow and thymocytes cooperated in a
normal manner upon adoptive transfer, this suggested that the lack
of response to SRBC in the intact animal was due to a block in T
cell activation and not due to intrinsic defects in lymphoid cells
necessary to initiate a response. The block in T cell activation
might be mediated by a suppressor cell found in old B/W spleens
and it was hypothesized that this suppressor might also lead to a
loss of self-tolerance.

ACKNOWLEDGEMENTS

The authors wish to thank Marilyn McCann for excellent technical assistance and Sue Melanson, Judy Verge and Phyllis Hobson for typing the manuscript. This work was supported by the Medical Research Council of Canada.

REFERENCES

1. Talal, N., and Steinberg, A.D.: In: Current Topics Microbiol. and Immunol., Springer-Verlag, New York 64: 79, 1974.

2. Steinberg, A.D., Gerber, N.L., Gershwin, M.E., Morton, R., Goodman, D., Chused, T.M., Hardin, J.A. and Barthold, D.R.: Suppressor Cells in Immunity, edited by S.K. Singhal and N. R. Sinclair, University of Western Ontario Press, London, Canada, 1975.

3. Allison, A.C.: In: Contemporary Topics in Immunobiology, Vol. 3, eds. M.D. Cooper and N. Warner: Plenum Press, N.Y., p. 227, 1974.

4. Shirai, T., Yoshiki, T. and Mellors, R.C.: Clin. Exp. Immunol. 12: 455, 1972.

5. Roder, J.C., Bell, D.A., and Singhal, S.K.: In: Suppressor Cells in Immunity ed. by S.K. Singhal and N.R. Sinclair, University of Western Ontario Press, London, Canada, 1975.

6. Roder, J.C., Bell, D.A. and Singhal, S.K., J. Immunol., 1975, in press.

7. Roder, J.C., McCann, M.J. and Bell, D.A.: Proc. Fed. Am. Soc. Exp. Biol., 33: 732, 1974.

8. Salomon, J.C. and Benveniste, J.: Clin Exp. Immunol., 16, 481, 1969.

9. Morton, J.I. and Siegel, B.V.: Immunol., 16: 481, 1969.

10. Claman, H.N. and Mosier, D.E.: Progr. Allergy, 30: 120, 1966.

11. Stutman, O.: J. Immunol., 109: 602, 1972.

12. Chused, T. and Kassan, S.: Proc. Fed. Am. Soc. Exp. Biol., 34: 949, 1975.

13. Aden, D.P., Reed, N.D. and Jutila, J.A.: Proc. Soc. Exp.

Biol. Med., 140: 548, 1972.

14. Adams, P.B.: Austral. J. Exp. Biol. Med., 665, 1972.

15. Pross, H.F. and Eidinger, D.: Immunol., 25: 269, 1973.

16. Shirai, T. and Mellors, R.C.: Proc. Natl. Acad. Sci., USA, 68: 455, 1971.

17. Watson, J., Trenkner, E. and Cohn, M.: J. Exp. Med., 138: 699, 1973.

18. Sjoberg, O., Andersson, J. and Moller, G.: Eur. J. Immunol., 2: 326, 1972.

19. Jones, J., and Kind, P.D.: J. Immunol., 108: 1453, 1972.

20. Kettman, J. and Dutton, R.W., Proc. Natl. Acad. Sci. USA, 68: 699, 1971.

21. Playfair, J.H.L.: Immunology, 21: 1037, 1971.

22. Jacobs, M.E., Gordon, J.K. and Talal, N.J.: Immunol., 107: 359, 1971.

23. Purves, E.C. and Playfair, J.H.L., Clin. Exp. Immunol., 15: 113, 1973.

T-CELL DEPENDENCY OF THE RESPONSE TO PVP IS DEPENDENT ON MATURITY OF B-CELLS

Birger Andersson and Henric Blomgren

Department of Tumor Biology

Karolinska Institutet, Stockholm, Sweden

Polyvinyl pyrrolidone (PVP) belongs to the group of thymus independent (TI) antigens. Among those antigens are various polymeric molecules such as bacterial polysaccharides and their respective hapten derivatives (1-4, 6), poly-D-aminoacids (5) and, as mentioned, PVP (7). In contrast to the thymus dependent (TD) antigens (8) the TI ones seem capable of eliciting humoral antibody responses without the aid of helper T-cells. The response to many of the TI antigens consists exclusively of IgM, and therefore T-lymphocytes have been postulated as necessary for normal IgG responses. This concept however seems uncorrect, since PVP (9 and Tables 1, 2) and DNP-lys-Ficoll (6) elicit IgM and IgG responses, which both are TI.

Among other features of the anti-PVP response can be mentioned that no maturation of affinity with time after immunization can be observed in the IgG production.

NVP, the monomer of PVP, is immunogenic first after coupling to a carrier protein molecule, and the antibody response is TD in contrast to the TI response to PVP in the same experimental model.

Another interesting feature of the anti-PVP response is that high humoral antibody response in mice is genetically determined by one dominant gene (Table 3). All mice on an A/Sn genetic background seem to possess this gene and all other strains so far tested are low responders. The genetic analysis is not yet completed, but in preliminary experiments linkage to H-2, C5 deficiency, coat colour or the X chromosome was not demonstrated. The gene might be linked to the allotype locus of the Ig, but here the analysis is not yet finished.

Table 1. Cells Forming Antibody to PVP in Thymectomized, Irradiated and Bone Marrow Reconstituted Mice

	No Mice	PFC[xx]/Spleen IgM	IgG
TX 800R:BM[x]	5	2.13±0.06	2.45±0.07
TX 800R:BM + 5 × 10⁷ Thymus	6	1.89±0.19	2.54±0.08

x) Adult (A/Sn × C57BL) F_1 mice were thymectomized, two weeks later irradiated with 800R and given 10^7 bone marrow cells, two weeks later injected with 1 μg of PVP or 1 μg of PVP together with thymus cells.

xx) One week after immunization the number of cells forming plaques against NVP-BSA coated SRBC were determined. IgM-PFC were developed with complement only. IgG-PFC represents the increase after developing with anti-Ig followed by complement.

Table 2. Distribution of Antibodies in Sera from Mice Immmunized with 1 μg of PVP (MW 360,000) 10 Days Earlier.

Mouse strain	Antigen Binding Capacity[x] serum[xx]	IgM[xx]	IgG[xx]
A/Sn	1216	450	214
C57BL	242	67	43
CBA	116	72	43

x) Nanogram of radio-iodinated PVP bound per ml of serum as determined by a modification of the Farr assay.

xx) Sera from 10 immune mice in each group were pooled and fractionated on Sephadex G 200. The first and second eluted peak was concentrated back to the original serum volume and tested. From (9).

Table 3. Genetics of the Antibody Response of Mice to PVP.

Strain	Antibody response[x] High[xx]	Low[xx]	Low responder %
A/Sn	32	0	0
C57BL	0	24	100
(A/SnxC57BL)F_1	22	0	0
(A/SnxC57BL)F_2	49	16	25

x) Hemolytic titer day 10-12 after 1 μg of antigen

xx) High responders showed titers $\geqslant 3^4$, and low were $\leqslant 3^3$.

Having presented some background information of the anti-PVP system we now turn to the main topic of this presentation. As briefly mentioned above, TI antibody responses can be obtained with this antigen (7). We report here that the TI response occurs only with mature B-cells, and that when immature B-cells used TD responses are instead observed. Some of the data have been reported elsewhere recently (10).

The main finding is described in Table 4. It can be seen that spleen B-cells from adult mice are able to respond optimally by themselves to PVP when transferred to irradiated recipients, whereas young spleen B-cells need the addition of helper T-cells in order to respond optimally. It is further demonstrated in Table 7 that T-cells specific for PVP are responsible for the helper effect.

The observation made in Table 4 that T-cells actually suppress the antibody response of adult B-cells is in line with numerous reports on suppressor T-cells during the past few years (11).

In some experiments with similar design as those described in Table 4 we were able to show that the cortisone resistant fraction of the thymus contains the active suppressor and helper cells in the anti-PVP system. Thymus cells passed over anti-Ig columns were still active, and this strongly indicates that the

Table 4. Helper or Suppressor Effect of Thymus Cells Exerted on Young or Adult Spleen B-cells in their Response to PVP.

Spleen	Thymus[x]	Antibody response[xx]
2 months, 2×10^7	-	3.9 ± 0.5
2 months, 2×10^7	10^7	1.8 ± 0.5
2 weeks, 2×10^7	-	2.2 ± 0.5
2 weeks, 2×10^7	10^7	4.1 ± 0.3

x) Normal, 2 month old mice used as thymus cell donors.

xx) Antibody titre ($\log_2$) 2 weeks after 750 rad and intravenous infusion of cells. From (10).

active cells in the thymus are T-cells and not contaminating B-cells.

Comparing spleen B-cells from young and adult mice we found that the immature B-cells have less cells bearing the C3 receptor. Further, as shown in Table 5, it was possible to correlate the TI and TD behaviour respectively with the physical presence or absence of C3 receptor bearing cells using EAC columns to deplete those cells.

Table 5. Effect of C3 Receptor Lymphocyte Depletion on Thymus Dependency of the anti-PVP Response of Mice.

Cells	Ig positive %	EAC positive %	Antibody response $\log_2$ hemolytic titer
Control	38	46	2.83
Control + Thymus	-	-	1.33
EAC column passed	29	3	3.17
EAC column passed + thymus	-	-	5.00

Whether the C3 receptor is essential for the TI triggering of the B-lymphocytes in the anti-PVP response remains to be settled. Here should only be mentioned (12) that PVP is very efficient in activating complement on cell surfaces and as seen in Table 6 incubation of spleen cells with PVP and GPC inactivates the PVP specific precursors.

Table 6. Specific Inactivation of PVP Specific B-cells by Treatment with Antigen and Complement.

Treatment of cells in vitro			Injection to recipients	Antibody response in irradiated recipients	
				Log$_2$ hemolytic titer	
PVP	GPC	GPC 56°	GPC	PVP	HRBC
+	-	+	-	4.17	5.3
+	+	-	-	< 1.0	5.7
-	-	+	-	5.3	5.8
-	+	-	-	5.0	6.0
+	-	-	+	< 1.0	5.0

5-6 mice per group.

Table 7. Helper and Suppressor Effects of Normal, Immune or Tolerant Thymus Cells.

Thymus	Antibody Response	
	Adult Spleen	Young Spleen
-	5.6$\pm$0.3	1.8$\pm$0.8
Normal	1.2$\pm$1.2	4.5$\pm$0.3
Immune	1.9$\pm$o.7	3.3$\pm$0.4
Tolerant	5.6$\pm$0.2	1.8$\pm$0.9

Experimental conditions as in Table 4. From (10).

REFERENCES

1. Feldmann, M. and Basten, A. J. Exp. Med. 134:103, 1971.

2. Möller, G. and Michael, G. Cell. Immunol. 2:309, 1971.

3. Howard, J. G. et al. Cell. Immunol. 2:614, 1971.

4. Miranda, J. J. Immunology 23:829, 1972.

5. Sela, M., Mozes, E., and Shearer, G.M. Proc. Nat. Acad. Sci. U.S.A. 69:2696, 1972.

6. Sharon, R. et al. J. Immunol. 114:1585, 1975.

7. Andersson, B. and Blomgren, H. Cell. Immunol. 2:411, 1971.

8. Transplantation Reviews. Vol. 1. Antigen Sensitive Cells. Their Source and Differentiation (Ed. G. Möller). Munksgaard, Copenhagen, p 1-149, 1969.

9. Andersson, B. Doctoral Thesis, Karolinska Institute, Stockholm, Sweden. 1972.

10. Andersson, B. and Blomgren, H. Nature 253:5491, 1975.

11. Gershon, R. K. in Contemporary Topics in Immunobiology (Ed. M. Cooper) Plenum, New York p 1-40, 1974.

12. Kabat, E. A. and Mayer, M. M. Experimental Immunochemistry. Charles Thomas, Springfield, Ill. U.S.A. p 168, 1961.

This work was supported by the Swedish Cancer Society, the Karolinska Institute and by NIH contract No. NO1 -CB-33866 and contract No. NO1-CB-33868.

DIFFERENTIATION OF CYTOTOXIC T LYMPHOCYTES ENHANCED BY T CELL FACTORS PRODUCED DURING MIXED LYMPHOCYTE INTERACTIONS

A. Altman and I.R. Cohen

Department of Cell Biology, The Weizmann Institute of

Science, Rehovot, Israel

Cooperation between subpopulations of T lymphocytes was demonstrated in graft-vs.-host (1) and in recruitment (2) reactions in vivo and in the mixed lymphocyte culture (MLC) in vitro (3-5). It was hypothesized that such cooperation is mediated by soluble factor(s) generated during allogeneic mixed lymphocyte interactions (4-6). We found (7) that the addition of allogeneic stimulator lymphocytes to the sensitization phase of an in vitro T cell mediated anti-fibroblast reaction (AFR) enhanced sensitization as evidenced by an increased cytolytic capacity of the sensitized T lymphocytes. In addition we found that the same effect could also be produced by T-cell soluble factors generated in the MLC (8). In the present study we investigated at what stage of the sensitiz-ation phase the MLC active factor(s) exert their effect, and whether the factors can be produced by thymocytes.

MATERIALS AND METHODS

Anti Fibroblast Reaction (AFR)

Mouse lymph node cell (LNC) suspensions were prepared and sensitized on allogeneic fibroblast monolayers as described previously (7,8). Briefly 30 x 10^6 LNC were cultured for 4 days on allogeneic embryonic fibroblast monolayers, and then assayed for cytolytic capacity by transfering them to monolayers of ^{51}Cr-labelled target fibroblasts (20:1 ratio) for 24 hours.

Preparation of MLC Supernatants

Spleen or thymus cell suspensions were cultured for 48 hours with 1000 r irradiated syngeneic (control) or allogeneic (experimental) spleen cells. The culture supernatants were collected by centrifugation, and added to the sensitization phase of the AFR at a 1:4 final dilution.

RESULTS

Augmentation of AFR by MLC Supernatants

MLC (or control) supernatants were added to the sensitization phase of the AFR, and their effects on the development of cytotoxic T lymphocytes (CTL) was studied. We found (Fig. 1) that the presence of MLC supernatants augmented sensitization as evidenced by a marked increase in target cell lysis. This helper effect (HE) was produced even when the MLC-stimulator lymphocytes were unrelated (allogeneic) to the sensitizing fibroblasts in the AFR. However, we found previously that these supernatants only increased cytolysis of specific target cells (8). Thus the relative specificity of lysis was retained when the lymphocytes were sensitized in the presence of MLC supernatants.

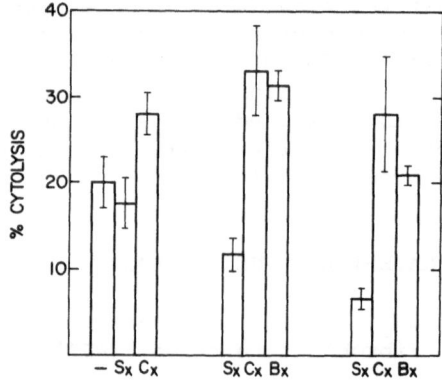

Fig. 1. The effect of MLC supernatants on the AFR. SWR lymphocytes were sensitized against C3H (AFR) in the absence (-) or presence of supernatants of MLC of SWR spleen cells against different strains (S-SWR, C-C3H, B-C57BL).

Effect of MLC Supernatants on CTL Differentiation

In order to find out in what way the MLC factor(s) affect the differentiation of CTL, we assayed the cytolytic capacity of sensitized lymphocytes after 3, 4 or 5 days of sensitization to allogeneic fibroblasts in the presence of control or MLC supernatants. It was found (Table 1) that in the presence of MLC supernatants, the development of CTL was faster, and the peak of the cytolytic response was reached one day earlier. To find out at what stage of the sensitization phase of the AFR the MLC factor(s) exert their effect, we added the MLC supernatants at various stages of the sensitization phase. We found (Table 2) that the presence of the active supernatant during the second day (24-48 hours) of sensitization was necessary and sufficient to produce a helper effect. We found previously (8) that the presence of the MLC supernatant during the cytolytic effector phase of the AFR had no effect whatsoever. Thus, the MLC active factor(s) seem to act by promoting the differentiation of specifically sensitized T lymphocytes into effector cells.

Table 1.   The effect of MLC supernatants on the development of effector lymphocytes with time in the AFR.

Days of sensitiz- ation	% Cytolysis following sensitization in:		Helper* index
	Control medium	MLC medium	
3	12.7 $\pm$ 1.4	22.3 $\pm$ 1.1	1.8
4	21.9 $\pm$ 0.4	34.1 $\pm$ 0.6	1.6
5	29.2 $\pm$ 3.3	34.1 $\pm$ 6.0	1.2

SWR lymphocytes sensitized against C3H fibroblasts in the presence of control (C57BL) or MLC(C57BL + C3H) spleen cell free-medium for 3, 4 or 5 days. Cytolysis measured after 24 hours (Effector : target cell ratio 10:1).

* helper index = ratio of cytolysis following sensitization in:

MLC medium
control medium

Table 2. The effect of MLC cell-free supernatants present during
          different stages of the sensitization phase of the AFR*

Exp. No.	Sensitization phase Time of presence of spleen culture medium (hours)	Cytolytic-effector phase % cytolysis control medium	MLC medium	P <	helper index
1	0 - 80	35.9+3.1	49.8+4.3	0.001	1.4
	0 - 24	25.3+1.9	23.7+2.7	0.10	0.9
	24 - 80	31.9+5.5	47.9+3.6	0.01	1.5
	48 - 80	21.6+2.2	21.0+3.2	0.10	1.0
2	0 - 72	25.4+0.9	32.2+2.1	0.001	1.3
	0 - 24	20.0+2.1	21.8+2.0	0.10	1.1
	24 - 48	23.1+1.0	31.5+3.2	0.002	1.4

*In both experiments, SWR LNC were sensitized against C3H
 fibroblasts.
  Exp. 1: 37.5% fresh spleen culture medium - SWR (Control) or
           SWR + Balb/c (MLC)
  Exp. 2: 5% lyophilized, x3 concentrated, culture medium -
           SWR (Control) or SWR + C57Bl/6 (MLC).

Generation of Helper Activity by Thymocytes

        To find out which lymphocytes are responsible for the produc-
tion of MLC helper factor(s), and what is their relation to those T
lymphocytes which undergo sensitization in the AFR, we tested the
ability of thymocytes to generate these factor(s) in the MLC. We
found (Fig. 2) that the active soluble factor(s) were produced
efficiently when thymocytes served as MLC-responder cells. That
the active factor(s) were generated by the responding thymocytes,
and not by the irradiated stimulator spleen cells, is evident from
our previous findings (8) that irradiated lymphocytes are unable to
generate these factors. These results support our previous finding
(8) that the generation of helper factors in the MLC depends on T
lymphocytes. In our experiments we consistently failed to achieve
sensitization in vitro of thymocytes against allogeneic fibroblasts.
Thus, thymocytes which by themselves cannot differentiate into CTL
in the AFR, can generate MLC helper factor(s).

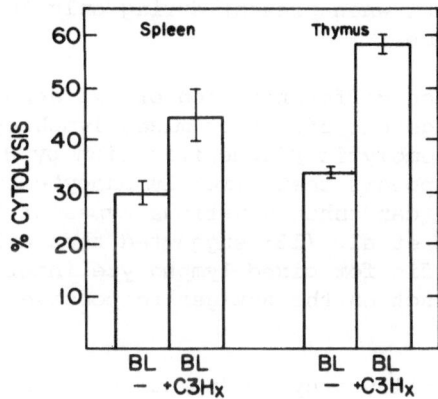

Fig. 2. The effect on the AFR of supernatants derived from MLC's of responder thymocytes or spleen cells. SWR lymphocytes sensitized against C3H fibroblasts in the presence of supernatants derived from control cultures (C57BL spleen or thymus cells) or MLC's (C57BL spleen or thymus cells plus 1000 r irradiated C3H spleen cells).

DISCUSSION AND SUMMARY

Recently we studied the effect of the stimulus provided by mixed lymphocyte interactions on the development of cytotoxic lymphocytes in a T cell-mediated anti fibroblast reaction (AFR). We found that the addition of allogeneic stimulator lymphocytes (7) or of MLC-generated, T cell derived soluble factors (8) to the sensitization phase of the AFR augmented sensitization as evidenced by a significantly increased target cell lysis. Two questions were investigated in the present study. First, at precisely what stage of the AFR sensitization phase the helper effect of the MLC stimulus is exerted. Secondly, in what way the T lymphocytes which generate the MLC helper factor(s) and those T lymphocytes which become sensitized against allogeneic fibroblasts, are related to each other.

Our findings (8, see also Table 2) that the MLC supernatants have no effect when present during the first 24 hours of the sensitization phase, or during the whole cytolytic phase demonstrate that the active factor(s) do not affect primary recognition events which occur during the first hours of sensitization (9, 10), nor do they affect fully differentiated effector lymphocytes. Rather, they seem to affect specifically sensitized lymphocytes by enhancing their differentiation into CTL, as evidenced by the positive helper effect of the MLC supernatants when present during only the second day of the sensitization phase.

This effect on the differentiation of CTL appears to be analogous to the allogeneic effect of mixed lymphocyte interactions on the induction of hemolytic plaque formation by B lymphocytes (11, 12). Thus, it appears that mixed lymphocyte interactions, both in vitro and in vivo, can enhance various types of immune reactions. Accordingly, Lafferty et al. (13) suggested that allogeneic stimulation, an event specific for mixed lymphocyte interactions, can have a marked adjuvant effect on the antigen-responsive capacity of the immune system.

By using congenitally athymic (nu/nu) mice on two different genetic backgrounds we found previously (8) that the generation of helper activity in MLC media depended upon T lymphocytes capable of proliferation. Thus, when spleen cells of nude mice served as MLC "responders", no helper activity was demonstrable in the medium. In accordance with this we found here (Fig. 2) that thymocytes are capable of generating the active helper factor(s) in the MLC. However, such cells are by themselves unable to undergo sensitization against allogeneic fibroblasts and to develop cytotoxic capacity. It is possible, therefore, that T lymphocytes which produce helper factor(s) in the MLC are distinct from those T lymphocytes which undergo sensitization in response to allogeneic fibroblasts.

REFERENCES

1. Asofsky, R., Cantor, H. and Tigelaar, R.E., Progr. Immunol., 1:369, 1971.
2. Cohen, I.R., Eur. J. Immunol., 3:829, 1973.
3. Bach, F.H., Segall, M., Stouber-Zier, K., Sondel, P.M., Alter, B.J. and Bach, M.L., Science (Wash. D.C.), 180:403, 1973.
4. Wagner, H., J. Exp. Med., 138:1379, 1973.
5. Wagner, H., Rollinghoff, M. and Nossal, G.J.V., Transplant. Rev., 17:3, 1973.
6. Nabholz, M., Vives, J., Young, H.M., Meo, T., Miggiano, V., Rijnbeek, A. and Shreffler, D.C., Eur. J. Immunol., 4:378, 1974.
7. Altman, A. and Cohen, I.R., Eur. J. Immunol., 4:577, 1974.
8. Altman, A. and Cohen, I.R., Eur. J. Immunol., in press, 1975.
9. Altman, A., Cohen, I.R. and Feldman, M., Cell Immunol., 7:134, 1973.
10. Feldman, M., Cohen, I.R. and Wekerle, H., Transplant. Rev., 12:57, 1972.
11. Schimpl, A. and Wecker, E., Nature, New Biol., 237:15, 1972.
12. Katz, D.H., Transplant. Rev., 12:141, 1972.
13. Lafferty, K.J., Walker, K.J., Scollay, R.G. and Killby, V.A.A., Transplant. Rev., 12:198, 1972.

ENHANCING EFFECT OF RADIORESISTANT SPLEEN CELLS ON THE PRIMARY

IMMUNE RESPONSE AGAINST SHEEP RBC BY MOUSE SPLEEN CELLS IN VITRO

F.H. Lubbe and O.B. Zaalberg

Medical Biological Laboratory TNO

139, Lange Kleiweg, Rijswijk Z.H., The Netherlands

The requirement of three cell types for the immune response against sheep RBC, both in vivo and in vitro, has been recognized for some time. Two of these cell types were found to be radio-sensitive, one to be radioresistant (1,2,3,4). Their tendency to adhere to a substrate has been used to separate the radio-resistant cells from the radiosensitive ones. The macrophage was considered to be the most likely candidate for the radioresistant cell.

In our experiments on the in vitro education of thymus derived cells to helper cells, T-cells from normal spleens were added to irradiated spleen cells (800 rads) together with sheep RBC and incubated during several days. Thereafter the cells were collected and different numbers added to normal spleen cell cultures to test for a stimulating effect on the immune response. The control cultures, containing irradiated spleen cells and sheep RBC only, were however found to stimulate the immune response also. Both the supernatant and adherent cells from these cultures were active in this respect. The supernatant population of the irra-diated spleen cell culture contained, beside numerous dead cells, significant quantities of mononuclear cells which had phagocytized sheep RBC and dead cells, lymphoid cells which according to the binding of specific antibodies were thymus derived, cells carrying immune globulins at the cell surface, a few plasma cells and cells of the hemopoietic system. The adherent cells consisted of phago-cytizing cells and lymphoid cells. In order to determine which of all these cell types were responsible for the enhancing effect of the immune response,the cells were separated by velocity sedimen-tation and the fractions tested for activity. We speculated that perhaps the surviving thymus derived cells were guilty of this effect.

Material and Methods. (CBA/Rij X C57B1/Rij) female F 1 hybrids 10 to 12 weeks of age were used. These comprised specific pathogen free (SPF) mice and mice reared under conventional conditions. Our modification of the Mishell and Dutton in vitro culture technique is described in previous publications (5,6). For the primary immune response, normal spleen cells from SPF mice were used. Ten million spleen cells per culture dish gave an suboptimal immune response in vitro. This number was chosen to augment the enhancing effect by the added irradiated spleen cells.

For the culturing of the irradiated spleen cells, culture dishes were filled with spleen cells from mice irradiated 15 to 30 minutes earlier with 800 rads. In most experiments sheep RBC were added and the dishes incubated on a rocking platform during one to three days. Thereafter the supernatant cells were washed of with a pasteur pipet and added to the normal spleen cell cultures. When the adherent cells were tested, they were removed with a rubber scraper. The irradiation conditions and dosimetry have been described in another publication (7).

The velocity sedimentation was executed as described by E.A. Peterson (8) with the modifications by R.G. Miller (9). The diameter of the chamber was 9 cm and the volume 650 ml. The loading of the chamber was always kept below the "streaming limit". The cells were sedimented for four hours and collected in 16 fractions of 40 ml. Then the cells were washed in tissue culture medium, counted and known numbers of surviving cells (dye exclusion) added to the normal spleen cell cultures.

T- and B-cells were detected by incubating cell samples with rabbit anti mouse thymocyte serum (absorbed with normal bone marrow cells or with cells from an immunoglobulin producing mouse myeloma tumor). This was followed by incubation with a FITC conjugated pig anti rabbit Ig serum and a TRITC conjugated rabbit anti mouse Ig serum. Both conjugated sera were obtained from "Nordic Pharmaceuticals and Diagnostics" in Tilburg, The Netherlands. The samples were observed with a Zeiss photomicroscope provided with a Ploem type illuminator. The significance of the experimental results was determined with the Wilcoxon-Mann-Whitney test.

Results and Discussion. The first ten fractions from the sedimentation chamber, comprising about 25 % of the recovered cells, were pooled because they contained chiefly cells which had phagocytized great numbers of erythrocytes and dead cells. To all the available criteria (10), these cells were classified as macrophages. The other cell types in these pooled fractions were hemopoietic cells, many with degenerative changes (multinucleated and giant cells). The fractions 11 and 12, comprising about 50 % of the recovered cells consisted of hemopoietic cells, granulocytes, lymphoid cells (approx. 20 %), erythrocytes and macrophages (approx. 10 %). Many lymphoid cells in these two fractions showed immunofluorescence with conjugated anti T-cell serum. The cell composition of the fractions 13 and 14 did not differ much from that of the fractions 11 and 12. In table 1 the immune response by normal spleen cells combined with cells from the different fractions is presented.

TABLE 1: THE EFFECT OF IRRADIATED SPLEEN CELLS, PRECULTURED IN VITRO, ON THE PFC RESPONSE AGAINST SHEEP RBC BY NON IRRADIATED SPLEEN CELLS IN VITRO

Culture conditions of the irradiated spleen cells (800 rads)			Number of irradiated spleen cells added to normal spleen cells (x 10^6)	PFC/dish, fraction of control
Number of spleen cells per dish (x 10^6)	Number of SRBC per dish (x 10^6)	Incubation time (days)		
--	--	--	--	1.00 (548)** ***
20	20	1	0.5	0.65 sign.
			0.25	0.96
20	20	3	0.25	1.62 sign.
			MF 0.15*	1.64 sign.
			LF 0.15	1.23
--	--	--	--	1.00 (570)
20	20	3	0.25	1.56 sign.
			MF 0.15	1.92 sign.
			LF 0.15	0.88
--	--	--	--	1.00 (1168)
20	20	3	0.25	1.53 sign.
			MF 0.125	1.77 sign.
			LF 0.25	1.14
			0.125	1.08

* The macrophage rich fraction (MF) contained for the three experiments respectively 78 %, 73 % and 76 % macrophages, the other cells were hemopoietic cells. The fractions rich in lymphoid cells (LF) were contaminated with respectively 6 %, 16 % and 9 % macrophages.

** Number of PFC/dish of control cultures.

*** Significance level < 0.05.

Only the fractions rich in macrophages caused some enhancement. The conditions during the incubation of the irradiated spleen cells was further varied as to number of irradiated spleen cells (10 - 60 x 10^6 cells/dish) and sheep RBC (0, 5, 10, 20, 50 and

100×10^6 SRBC/dish), duration of incubation and choice of donor
mice. Only the shortening of the incubation time had effect. Inhibition instead of enhancement by the irradiated spleen cells was
observed. The same population of irradiated spleen cells cultured
for 3 days caused stimulation of the immune response (table 1).
However, when the irradiated spleen cells immediately after irradiation were added to the normal spleen cells, the immune response
was stimulated (8×10^6 cells/dish was found to be optimal).
The irradiated spleen cells from SPF mice did not stimulate the
immune response (table 2). Increasing the number of irradiated
spleen cells, occasionally gave some improvement.

TABLE 2: THE EFFECT OF IRRADIATED SPLEEN CELLS, PRECULTURED IN
VITRO, ON THE PFC RESPONSE AGAINST SHEEP RBC BY NON IRRADIATED
SPLEEN CELLS IN VITRO

Culture conditions of the irradiated spleen cells (800 rads)			Number of irradiated spleen cells added to normal spleen cells ($\times 10^6$)	PFC/dish,[*] fraction of control
Number of spleen cells per dish ($\times 10^6$)	Number of SRBC per dish ($\times 10^6$)	Incubation time (days)		
--	--	--	--	1.00 (755)[**]
SPF mice				
20	20	3	1.6	1.02
			0.8	1.13
			0.4	1.09
Conv. mice				
20	20	3	0.4	1.53 sign.[***]
			0.2	1.65 sign.

[*]   In all these experiments the normal spleen cells were taken
      from SPF mice.
[**] Number of PFC/dish in control cultures.
[***] Significance level < 0.05.

However, the number of phagocytizing cells that could be recovered
from the spleens of SPF mice was about a third of the numbers
recovered from the conventional mice.

Summary. Irradiated spleen cells cultured for 3 days, caused a stimulation of the primary in vitro immune response by normal spleen cells. These irradiated spleen cells were fractionated by velocity sedimentation and the fractions were tested for their stimulating activity. Only the macrophage enriched fractions were found to cause stimulation. The macrophages in these fractions were stuffed with erythrocytes and dead cells. The fractions enriched in thymus derived cells, had no effect on the immune response.

Irradiated spleen cells cultured for 24 hours caused inhibition. It has not yet been determined whether this inhibition was due to some transient change in the macrophage population during incubation. The stimulating effect by the irradiated spleen cells from SPF mice was strongly reduced, which at least partly could be ascribed to the naturally occurring low number of macrophages in the spleens of these mice.

References

1. D.E. Mosier and L.W. Coppleson. Proc. N.A.S., 61: 542 (1968).

2. K.U. Hartmann, R.W. Dutton, M.M. McCarthy and R.I. Mishell. Cellular Immunol., 1: 182 (1970).

3. H. Cosenza, L.P. Leserman and D.A. Rowley. J. Immunol., 107: 414 (1971).

4. R.M. Cgorczinski, R.G. Miller and R.A. Phillips. J. Exp. Med., 134: 1201 (1971).

5. G. Rossi and O.B. Zaalberg. J. Immunol., 113: 424 (1974).

6. O.B. Zaalberg, V.A. van der Meul and M.J. van Twisk. J. Immunol., 100: 451 (1968).

7. O.B. Zaalberg, V.A. van der Meul and G. Rossi. Eur. J. Immunol., 3: 698 (1973).

8. E.A. Peterson and W.H. Evans. Nature (London), 214: 824 (1967).

9. Personal communication.

10. R. van Furth, Z.A. Cohn, J.G. Hirsch, J.H. Humphrey, W.G. Spector and H.L. Langevoort. Bulletin W.H.O., 46: 845 (1972).

EFFECTOR CELL REQUIREMENTS FOR ANTIBODY-DEPENDENT AND MITOGEN-INDUCED CYTOTOXICITY

Erwin W. Gelfand

Department of Immunology

The Hospital For Sick Children, Toronto, Canada

The generation and characterization of cytotoxic effector cells has been studied in several laboratories using a variety of xenogeneic, allogeneic and syngeneic systems (1-3). We have attempted to characterize the cell requirements for cytotoxic effector function in man in two independent assays, cytotoxic activity of non-immune effector cells for antibody-coated target cells and cytotoxic activity for target cells in the presence of mitogen. It has been suggested by several groups that antibody-dependent cytotoxicity (ADC) reflects the functional activity of B-lymphocytes whereas T-lymphocytes are active in mitogen-induced cytotoxicity (MIC) (1-4). Our earlier studies in rabbit suggested that the predominant effector cell in ADC was of monocyte-macrophage origin rather than a B-cell (5-7) and this has also been shown to be the case in mouse (8).

Human cells offer several distinct advantages as effector cells since they are very active in these assays, they are readily available and they are highly suitable for studying various cell populations with currently available surface marker techniques. In many animal studies a variety of cell separation techniques have been utilized in an attempt to enrich or deplete subpopulations of cells. In order to circumvent the hazards of interpretation of cell separation procedures in achieving "pure" B and T-cell populations, we have taken advantage of available normal human tissues selected for differences in cell types as well as studying the functional activity of cells obtained from the peripheral blood of patients with various immunodeficiency disorders involving the absence of demonstrable B, T, or both B and T lymphocytes.

Cytotoxicity was measured in a chromium release assay with chicken red blood cells (CRBC) and Chang human liver cells serving as target cells. For ADC, effector cells were added to antibody (rabbit)-coated target cells at an effector-target cell ratio of 1:1 to 50:1. Cultures were terminated at 4 hours. In MIC, 10-20 µgm/ml PHA-P (Difco) was added to the incubation mixture of non-antibody coated but ^{51}Cr-labeled CRBC and effector cells at similar effector cell-target cell ratios and cultures terminated after 20 hours. Effector cell suspensions were obtained from peripheral blood (PBL), tonsil (TLN), thymus (THY), and cultured human lymphocyte lines (CHL). These cell suspensions were initially fractionated on isopaque-ficoll gradients to obtain mononuclear cells free of contaminating red cells or granulocytes (less than 3% contamination). Polymorphonuclear or eosinophil-enriched suspensions (more than 80%) were obtained by dextran sedimentation of peripheral blood from normal individuals or 2 patients with eosinophilia. In some experiments cells suspensions were incubated on plastic petri

Table 1

CYTOTOXIC ACTIVITY AND CELL SURFACE MARKERS IN VARIOUS TISSUES*

	PBL	TLN	THY	CHL
E(%)	45-60	15-25	90-95	0
EA(%)	10-20	0-2	0	0
EAC(%)	5-15	50-65	0-1	20-80
sIg(%)	5-12	60-70	0	15-65
^{3}H(cpm x 10^3)	20-50	8-12	12-25	ND
CRBC + ADC	42.2 ± 2.0	6.2 ± 1.7	2.3 ± 0.4	2.0 ± 0.6
CRBC MIC	42.5 ± 2.1	28.4 ± 5.3	2.3 ± 0.6	2.3 ± 1.0
CHANG$^+$ ADC	21.0 ± 1.5	1.8 ± 0.6	0.8 ± 0.3	0.9 ± 0.2

*Ranges for PBL: peripheral blood, 27 normals. TLN: tonsillar cells, 9 tonsils. THY: thymus cells, 3 thymuses. CHL: cultured human lymphocyte lines, 9 lines. $^+$Cytotoxicity assay was carried out using 2.5 x 10^5 PBL effector cells or 5 x 10^6 TLN, THY or CHL and 5 x 10^4 target cells. Cytotoxicity is expressed as % specific ^{51}Cr release $\pm$ SEM. ND: not done because of high spontaneous incorporations.

TABLE 2

CYTOTOXIC ACTIVITY IN IMMUNODEFICIENCY

	PBL	SCID	AG	CVID	WA	AT
E(%)*	45-60	0-10	N	N	3-8	N
EAC(%)*	5-15	0-60	0	1-33	N	N
sIg(%)*	5-12	0-65	0	0-28	N	N
^{3}H(cpm x 10^3)*	20-50	<1	N	N	6-9	N
CRBC$^+$ ADC	42.2$\pm$2.0	50.9$\pm$2.8	40.6$\pm$2.5	49.0$\pm$4.4	58.0$\pm$2.0	58.6$\pm$8.2
MIC	42.5$\pm$2.1	48.9$\pm$4.4	49.3$\pm$3.9	46.6$\pm$5.1	55.0$\pm$2.0	34.2$\pm$6.0
CHANG$^+$ ADC	21.0$\pm$1.5	ND	19.8$\pm$3.0 (5.3$\pm$0.6)	16.9$\pm$2.9	31.9$\pm$1.6	27.4$\pm$7.4

*Range for PBL: peripheral blood, 27 normals. SCID: severe combined immunodeficiency disease, 3 patients. AG: agammaglobulinemia, results with CRBC 4 patients, with Chang 3 patients. The single AG patient with abnormal results is shown in parentheses. CVID: common variable immuno-deficiency disease, 9 WA: Wiskott-Aldrich, 1 patient. AT: ataxia-telingiectasia, 4 patients.

$^+$Cytotoxicity assay was carried out using 2.5 x 10^5 effector cells and 5 x 10^4 target cells.

N: Normal. 0: no rosettes or fluorescence seen. ND: not done.

dishes and were treated with iron plus magnet prior to their use in
the assay. E, EA and EAC rosettes were performed as previously
described (9).

The results of the studies of cell surface markers and cytotoxic activity of non-immune effector cells, obtained from several
tissues, using CRBC and Chang as target cells are compared in
Table 1. As previously discussed, E-rosettes and PHA-induced ^{3}H-
thymidine incorporation are a marker of functional T-cells; EAC,
where A is a 19S (IgM) antibody and C3 is in the C3d state and
surface immunoglobulin (sIg) are markers of B-lymphocytes; and EA
where A is a 7S (IgG) antibody is a marker for monocytes or macrophages (10, 11). As shown in Table 1, there is no correlation between numbers of B or T cells and ADC or MIC. PBL showed the greatest activity in either assay (even at effector-target ratios of 1:1),
whereas TLN, which are predominantly B cells, showed little activity in both assays. At effector cell concentrations 50 times
greater than PBL, some TLN activity could be observed and may
simply reflect the contribution of contaminating non-lymphoid cells,
i.e. monocytes-macrophages. Thymocytes, despite their high T-cell
numbers and PHA-induced proliferation failed to mediate MIC even
at 50-fold higher cell concentrations compared to PBL. CHL from 9
different B cell lines failed to react in either assay. Only PBL
demonstrated cytotoxic activity against antibody-coated Chang cells.
The removal of adherent and iron ingesting cells from PBL did not
significantly alter the results when compared to untreated cells.

The failure to demonstrate a correlation between B and/or T-
cells in ADC and MIC was further strengthened by our findings in
patients with various immunodeficiency diseases taking advantage
of their "inborn" lack of various cell populations without relying
on cell separation techniques (Table 2). The three patients with
severe combined immunodeficiency disease (SCID) in the absence of
functional T or B cells (one patient had 10% E-rosettes but no EAC,
one patient 60-65% EAC and no E, one without E or EAC-rosettes)
demonstrated normal activity in ADC or MIC for CRBC. Despite the
absence of B cells, the four male patients with congenital agammaglobulinemia demonstrated normal ADC and MIC for CRBC and three
out of four had normal ADC against Chang cells. Patients with
common variable immunodeficiency had variable numbers of B lymphocytes (10) and a wide range of serum immunoglobulin levels but there
were no significant differences from normals in their cytotoxic
activities. One patient with the Wiskott-Aldrich syndrome (and
low T-cell numbers) and several patients with ataxia-telangiectasia
also demonstrated normal ADC and MIC.

As neither ADC nor MIC could be correlated with functional B
or T cells, populations of non-lymphoid cells were tested in both
assays. As illustrated in Table 3 both polymorphonuclear leukocytes

Table 3

CYTOTOXIC ACTIVITY OF NON-LYMPHOID CELLS

	CRBC[+]		CHANG[+]
	ADC	MIC	ADC
PBL	42.2$\pm$2.0	42.5$\pm$2.1*	21.0$\pm$1.5
PMN	34.9$\pm$1.0	41.1$\pm$3.6*	1.7$\pm$0.3
EOS	30.9$\pm$1.1	27.3$\pm$1.0*	1.2$\pm$0.2
MØ PEC	23.2$\pm$0.8	46.9$\pm$4.2*	2.0$\pm$0.9
MØ CULTURED	33.5$\pm$8.1	42.3$\pm$3.6*	1.4$\pm$0.2

[+]Cytotoxicity assay was carried out using 2.5 x 10^5 PBL or MØ or 1.0 x 10^5 PMN or EOS and 5 x 10^4 target cells. Cytotoxicity is expressed as % specific ^{51}Cr release $\pm$ SEM. PBL: peripheral blood, 27 normals. PMN: polymorphonuclear leukocytes, 3 normals. EOS: eosinophils, 2 patients. MØ: macrophages: PEC: peritoneal exudate cells, 2 patients. Cultured: 4 cultures. *20 hour incubation *4 hour incubation.

and eosinophils were active in ADC and MIC for CRBC but not for Chang cells. MIC activity was rapid with substantial lysis observed by 4 hours; at this time PBL demonstrated little if any lysis. Peritoneal exudate cells (from 2 patients with nephrosis) containing more than 40% EA cells, lysed CRBC but failed to lyse Chang cells. Similarly plastic adherent PBL cells, maintained in culture for 10-14 days and containing more than 50% EA cells failed to lyse antibody-coated Chang cells, even at higher effector cell-target cell ratios (up to 20:1), but were able to lyse CRBC.

These results therefore suggest that there may be several potential effector cell populations in man and that effector cell requirements may be different depending on the target cell chosen. The studies utilizing cells from the patients with various forms of immunodeficiency indicate that functional T or B cells are not required for ADC or MIC against CRBC. Granulocytes (polymorphonuclear and eosinophils) were also effective for CRBC in ADC or MIC. Despite the large numbers of B cells, TLN was relatively inactive in ADC while THY, rich in T cells, was inactive in MIC. Chang cells were not susceptible to significant lysis by other than isopaque-ficoll separated PBL; granulocytes, macrophages, B cells (TLN and CHL) and T cells (THY) were inactive. The exact nature of the effector cell for antibody-coated Chang cells remains uncertain but were present

in 3/4 patients with congenital agammaglobulinemia without B cells
as can best be determined by conventional surface markers.

The cytotoxic effector cell may therefore represent a lymphoid
cell which has not acquired specific cell markers other than the
Fc receptor or we feel may be a cell of monocyte origin but with
different properties from monocytes/macrophages which are active
against CRBC. (Either possibility is in keeping with the K cell
concept) (12). Supporting evidence for this distinction has been
obtained in cell fractionation studies of PBL on discontinuous
bovine serum albumin gradients. In these experiments effector
cells cytotoxic for antibody-coated CRBC were enriched in the
upper less dense fractions while a slightly denser fraction of
cells were active against Chang.

REFERENCES

1. Perlmann, P. and Holm, G., Adv. Immunol. 11: 117, 1969.
2. MacLennan, I.C.M., Transpl. Rev. 13: 67, 1972.
3. Perlmann, P., Perlmann, H. and Wigzell, H., Transpl. Rev.
    13: 91, 1972.
4. VanBoxel, J.A., Paul, W.E., Frank, M.M. and Green, I.,
    J. Immunol. 110: 1027, 1973.
5. Gelfand, E.W., Resch, K. and Prester, M., Europ. J. Immunol.
    2: 419, 1972.
6. Resch, K., Gelfand, E.W. and Prester, M., J. Immunol., 112:
    792, 1974.
7. Gelfand, E.W., Morris, S.A. and Resch, K., J. Immunol. 114:
    919, 1975.
8. Greenberg, A.H., Hudson, L., Shen, L. and Roitt, I.M., Nature
    242: 111, 1973.
9. Gelfand, E.W., Baumal, R., Huber, J., Crookston, M.C. and
    Shumak, K., New Eng. J. Med. 289: 1385, 1973.
10. Gelfand, E.W., Biggar, W.D. and Orange, R.P. Ped. Clin. N.
    Amer. 21: 745, 1974.
11. Abramson, N., Gelfand, E.W., Jandl, J.H. and Posen, F.S., J.
    Exp. Med. 132: 1207, 1970.
12. Perlmann, P. and MacLennan, I.C.M., Progress in Immunology II,
    3: 347, 1947.

Supported by a grant (MA 4875) from the Medical Research Council
of Canada

RECRUITMENT OF EFFECTOR LYMPHOCYTES BY INITIATOR LYMPHOCYTES:

RECRUITED LYMPHOCYTES ARE IMMUNOSPECIFIC

S. Livnat and I.R. Cohen

Department of Cell Biology
The Weizmann Institute of Science
Rehovot, Israel

INTRODUCTION

We have been investigating T lymphocyte interactions in the development of effector lymphocytes in a cell-mediated immune response (1-3). We found that mouse or rat initiator lymphocytes, sensitized in vitro against allogeneic fibroblasts, recruit syngeneic effector T lymphocytes. This recruitment reaction can be triggered in the draining popliteal lymph nodes (PLN) of animals by injecting their hind footpads with in vitro sensitized initiator T lymphocytes. The initiator lymphocytes do not themselves proliferate or differentiate into effector cells. Instead, T lymphocytes of the recipient accumulate in the enlarging PLN. These recruited T lymphocytes were found to mediate immunospecific cytotoxicity in vitro, or allograft rejection in vivo, against the same antigens which induced sensitization of the initiator lymphocytes.

The origin of the recruited T lymphocytes, and the basis of their immunospecificity are central questions. We found that T lymphocytes labeled with radioactive ^{51}Cr were trapped in the recruiting PLN after injecting them intravenously (iv). Hence, trapping of circulating lymphocytes appears to play a role in the enlargement of the PLN following injection of initiator lymphocytes.

What is the basis of the immunospecificity of the recruited lymphocytes? Are they immunologically committed before they are recruited, or do they acquire specificity from the initiator T lymphocytes? To investigate this, we tested the Graft-versus-Host (GvH) - inducing capacity of lymphocytes recruited in the PLN compared to lymphocytes located elsewhere in the same recipients. We

found that precursors of immunospecific GvH-reactive lymphocytes
were depleted from the spleen and distal lymph nodes (LN), and were
sequestered in the PLN during the recruitment response. Thus it
appears that T lymphocytes trapped in the PLN during recruitment
are already committed to the specific antigens used to sensitize
the initiator T lymphocytes in vitro. Furthermore, these recruited
lymphocytes include the precursors of specific GvH-reactive
lymphocytes.

MATERIALS AND METHODS

Sensitization of Initiator Lymphocytes

BALB/c spleen cells were sensitized for 16-24 hours against
allogeneic C57BL/6 or C3H/eb fibroblasts in Eagle's medium. The
incubation was at 37° in 10% CO_2 in moist air (1-3).

Recruitment Response

10^7 viable sensitized initiator lymphocytes in 0.05 ml phosphate-buffered saline (PBS) were injected into left hind footpads of
BALB/c recipients. This induces a response in the draining left
politeal lymph node (PLN), in which the PLN enlarges, circulating
lymphocytes are trapped, and effector cells develop (1-3).

GvH Assay

At various intervals after injection of initiator lymphocytes,
the PLN's, brachial and axial LN's, and spleens were removed, and
cell suspensions in PBS were prepared. Volumes of 0.05 ml containing
5×10^6 nucleated cells were injected into left footpads of
$(BALB/c \times C57BL/6)F_1$ hybrid recipients to induce a local GvH response. Five days later, PLN's of the F_1 recipients were removed and
weighed. GvH reactivity was expressed as a PLN enlargement Index:
weight of left (exp.) PLN/weight of right (control) PLN $\pm$ standard
deviation.

RESULTS

In previous experiments (1,3) we showed that during recruitment,
the responding PLN's enlarged between days 2 and 6, and thereafter
returned to normal size after about 8 days. Circulating lymphocytes

were trapped in the PLN. The kinetics of trapping closely paralelled
enlargement. To see if the trapped lymphocytes were immunospecific,
we tested the capacity of lymphocytes from the recruiting PLN, from
distal LN's (pool of contralateral PLN, and brachial and axillary
LN's), and from the spleen to induce a GvH response against the
specific alloantigens against which the recruitment response was
initiated. In BALB/c mice injected with initiator lymphocytes
sensitized against C57BL fibroblasts, spleens and distal LN's were
significantly depleted of specific GvH-reactive cells on day 6
(Fig. 1). PLN lymphocytes had normal GvH reactivity. However,
when the recruitment was directed against C3H alloantigens, or when
there was no recruitment induced, the anti-C57BL GvH response was
equivalent in PLN's, distal LN's, and spleens.

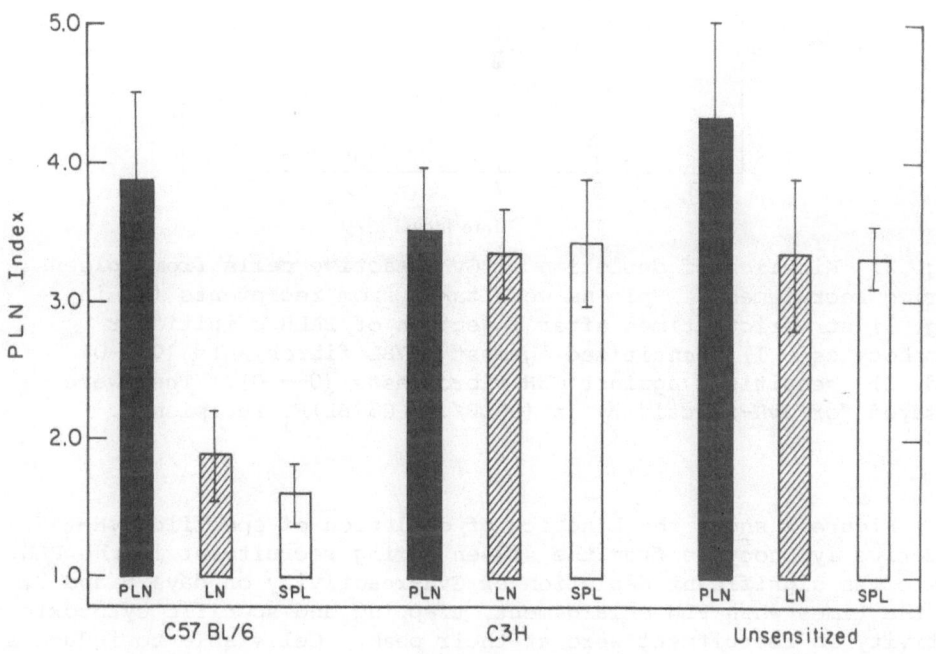

Fig. 1. Depletion of specific GvH-reactive cells during recruitment.
On day 6 after injection into footpads of BALB/c initiator lymphocytes sensitized against: 1) C57BL fibroblasts, 2) C3H fibroblasts,
or 3) unsensitized, recipient lymphocytes from reacting left politeal
lymph nodes (PLN), distal LN's (LN) or spleens (SPL) were tested for
local GvH reactivity in (BALB/c x C57BL/6)F$_1$ hosts. Vertical bars
indicate standard deviation.

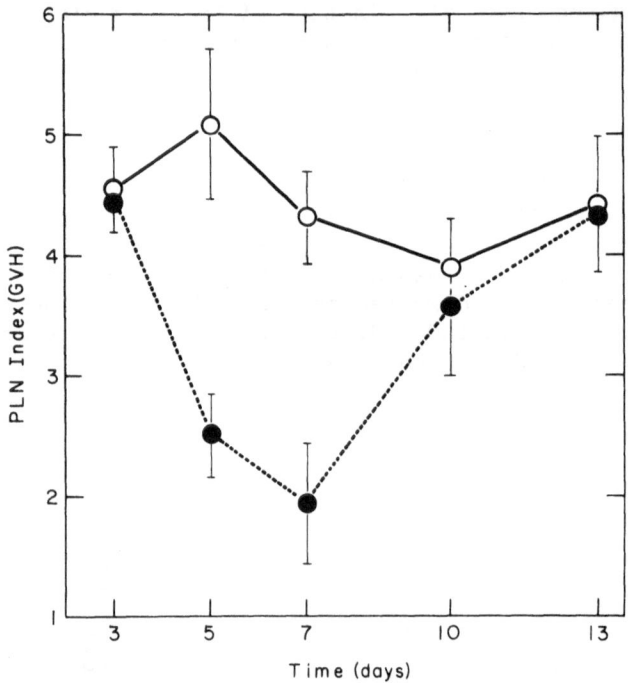

Fig. 2.   Kinetics of depletion of GvH-reactive cells from spleens
during recruitment.   Spleens were taken from recipients (as in
Fig. 1) at various times after injection of BALB/c initiator
lymphocytes: 1)   sensitized against C57BL fibroblasts (O---O)
and   2)   sensitized against C3H fibroblasts (O——O).   They were
assayed for GvH-reactivity in (BALB/c x C57BL)F$_1$ recipients.

     Figure 2 shows the kinetics of depletion of specific GvH-
reactive lymphocytes from the spleen during recruitment in the PLN.
There was significant depletion of GvH-reactivity on days 5 and 7,
at the times when PLN enlargement, trapping and specific cytotoxic
activity in recruitment were at their peak.   Cells able to induce a
GvH-reaction were again demonstrable in the spleens of these animals
by days 10-13.   Thus there appears to be an association between
depletion of GvH-reactive lymphocytes from distal lymphoid organs
and PLN enlargement and trapping.

     Allogeneic fibroblasts which may have detached from the
sensitization cultures and contaminated the initiator lymphocyte
population were not responsible for the depletion of GvH-reactive
cells.   We found (data not shown) that 10^6 C57BL fibroblasts
(20-fold more than the maximal contamination) injected directly
into footpads, could not induce such depletion.

DISCUSSION

Recruitment of effector T lymphocytes involves the trapping of circulating lymphocytes in the responding lymph node. The above results indicate that the recruited cells appear to be committed, before their recruitment, to the antigen against which the initiator T lymphocytes were sensitized. Specific, alloantigen-reactive GvH precursor lymphocytes are depleted temporarily from spleens and distal LN's and sequestered in the recruiting PLN in the course of the recruitment response.

Studies by other investigators (4-7) have shown that antigen could induce a sequestration of specifically reactive lymphocytes into the responding lymphoid organ. This resulted in their depletion from the recirculating pool. A major difference is, however, that in our studies initiator T lymphocytes triggered by antigen, and not antigen itself, induced such depletion of reactive cells from distal lymphoid organs and their sequestration in the reacting organ.

The finding that recruited lymphocytes are immunospecific suggests possible mechanisms for the initiator lymphocyte-recruited lymphocyte interaction leading to the development of effector T lymphocytes. The fact that the two interacting lymphocyte classes belong to different T subsets (Livnat and Cohen, in preparation), but that both bear specific antigen receptors, indicates that the alloantigen in some form may have a role in the interaction. The recruitable T lymphocyte, which also appears to be the GvH precursor cell, could be the precursor of the effector T lymphocyte, or a regulatory T lymphocyte (8).

REFERENCES

1. Cohen, I.R. Cell. Immunol. 8:209, 1973.
2. Treves, A.J. and Cohen, I.R. J. Nat. Canc. Inst. 51:1919, 1973.
3. Livnat, S. and Cohen, I.R. Eur. J. Immunol., 1975, in press.
4. Ford, W.L. Clin. Exp. Immunol. 12:243, 1972.
5. Rowley, D.A., Gowans, J.G., Atkins, R.L., Ford, W.L., and Smith, M.E. J. Exp. Med. 136:499, 1972.
6. Sprent, J., Miller, J.F.A.P., and Mitchell, G.F. Cell Immunol. 2:171, 1971.
7. Sprent, J. and Miller, J.F.A.P., J. Exp. Med. 138:143, 1973.
8. Katz, D.H. and Benacerraf, B., Transpl. Rev. 12:14, 1972.

HISTOPHYSIOLOGY OF THE HELPER T CELL SYSTEM IN RABBITS

G.H. Blijham

Department of Histology, University of Groningen

Oostersingel 69^{I}, Groningen, The Netherlands

INTRODUCTION

In rabbits antibody formation to sheep erythrocytes (SRBC) is dependent on the presence of thymus derived antigen reactive (T) cells (1,2). Little firm evidence is available, especially in this species, on the properties of these virginal precursors of helper T cells (pre-HTL) and the cells resulting from their interaction with antigen: helper T cells (HTL) and memory T cells (imm-HTL)(3,4). The results to be presented here deal with the characteristics of helper memory development in rabbits.

In preliminary studies transfer experiments were found to be unsatisfactory due to allogeneic interactions ("allogeneic effect") interfering with the expression of specific helper memory. To avoid these complications a totally autologous system was developed, making use of two observations made in mice. Firstly the development of T memory was found to be an early event after immunization, preceding the occurence of B memory (5). Secondly there is some evidence that T cell priming might lead to acceleration, rather than heightening, of the anti-SRBC response (6,7). On the basis of these findings we studied the effects of intravenous (i.v.) priming with SRBC on the kinetics of the plaque-forming-cells (PFC) response of popliteal lymph nodes (PLN) stimulated 3 or 4 days later with SRBC subcutaneously (s.c.)

MATERIALS AND METHODS

Adult rabbits (Gold-Agouti (GA) or Hollander (H)) weighing 1.5-3 kg. were used. SRBC used for immunization and plaque assay were freshly obtained each fortnight, and stored in Alsever's solution at 4°C. Cell-suspensions from spleen, lymph node, bone marrow, or thymus were always prepared in Medium 199 (Gibco) buffered with bicarbonate, and kept at 4°C untill being plaqued. Operations were performed under aseptical conditions using pentobarbital anaesthesia. Cell-suspensions were tested for anti-SRBC and anti-ChRBC PFC according to the method of Cunningham and Szenberg (8). To develop IgG-PFC a sheep-anti-rabbit-IgG serum prepared in our laboratory was used.

RESULTS AND DISCUSSION

The Acceleration Effect

Rabbits were stimulated with SRBC (2×10^9) s.c., and numbers of anti-SRBC DPFC (IgM producing cells) in draining PLN were determined 1 to 5 days later. Some animals (experimentals) were preimmunized 4 days earlier with SRBC i.v. (2×10^9), others (controls) were not preimmunized. In earlier experiments it was found that i.v. immunization as such does not lead, at the dose used here, to the appearance of PFC in PLN; the two groups of the present experiment (with or without i.v. priming) therefore are comparable in that both PFC-reactions in the lymph nodes are elicited by the s.c. immunization.

Results are shown in table 1. The most important effect of i.v. priming appears to be a significant acceleration of the PLN PFC reaction; the latent phase is shorter, peak PFC-numbers (which are only about 2 times higher as compared to controls) are reached about 24 hrs. earlier (around day 3 after stimulation). This phenomenon

TABLE 1. EFFECTS OF I.V. PRIMING ON THE ANTI-SRBC RESPONSE
IN LYMPH NODES CHALLENGED 4 DAYS LATER S.C.

Days after SRBC s.c.	Rabbits	Controls:DPFC (no SRBC i.v.)	Number Rabbits	Experimentals:DPFC (SRBC i.v. day -4)
1	GA. 4x	1 (0-2)	GA. 4 x	38 (7-53)
2	GA. 5x	15 (7-24)	GA. 5x	189 (65-293)
3	GA. 5x	51 (35-66)	GA. 5x	1321 (327-2854)
4	GA. 4x	743 (399-1080)	GA. 4x	1521 (624-2705)
5	GA. 2x	790 (623-956)	N.D.	N.D.

arithmetic mean and range of numbers of DPFC/10^6 LNC are given
N.D.: not done

TABLE 2. EFFECTS OF I.V. PRIMING ON THE KINETICS OF THE
LYMPH NODE ANTI-SRBC RESPONSE

Ratio	Rabbits	Controls (no SRBC i.v.)	Experimentals (SRBC i.v. day -4)
2/1	GA. 4x	--	12.3
3/2	GA. 4x	3.4	9.2
4/3	GA. 4x	14.6	1.2
5/4	GA. 2x	1.1	N.D.
4/3	H. 12x	15.0 (5.3-43.0)	0.9 (0.2-2.5)

ratio x/y: number $DPFC/10^6LNC$ at day x // number $DPFC/10^6LNC$ at
day y after s.c. immunization with SRBC.

has been called "acceleration effect" (6): already 4 days after
immunization a state of memory has developed, which enables lymph
nodes to react in a "secondary way" with respect to the speed of
antibody formation.

Next we looked for a simple parameter to describe PLN reactions
as fast or slow. For that reason ratio's between PFC-numbers obtained
at two successive days of the PLN-reaction were calculated. Results,
shown in table 2,make clear that both primary and accelerated
reactions consist of two days of increase (ratio's about 10) followed
by a plateau (ratio about 1). Moreover, it appears that primary and
accelerated reactions are most easily distinguished from each other
by using the ratio 4/3; in primary reactions this ratio is about 15,
in accelerated responses about 1. By using, in one individual rabbit,
the right PLN for detection of third day, and the left PLN for
detecting fourth day PFC-numbers, individual ratio's 4/3 could be
calculated. Results (table 2,H) indicate that the acceleration effect is characterized by the occurence of a ratio 4/3 lower than 2.5.

We like to interpret the acceleration effect as the expression
of T memory (which itself is defined here as changes in the T cell
population leading to "better" (higher or faster) humoral immune
responses). It appears early after immunization, which is a property
of T memory (5), and was shown in mice to be an expression of carrier
memory (7). However, according to some theories B cells might undergo
some changes early after immunization without being induced to become
antibody forming cells (9). These memory B cells would be able to
transform into AFC much faster after new antigenic stimulation.
We designed the following experiments to test wether these cells
play a role in our experimental system.

The Acceleration Effect Does
Not Depend on B Memory

Ch(icken)RBC and SRBC cross-react at the antibody level, presumably since both erythrocytes carry the Forssman determinant (10.)For instance 8 days after immunization with ChRBC 1277 anti-ChRBC DPFC/10^6 spleen cells could be detected, and in the same spleen 1175 anti-SRBC DPFC/10^{6}SC were found. When these spleen cells were assayed in a mixture of ChRBC and SRBC 90% of the plaques were clear i.e.both erythrocytes were lysed. Interestingly, all these plaques were only clear in the centre, while at the periphery a rim of partial (only SRBC) lysis could be seen. These sombrero's (11) obviously are the result of differences in lysis susceptibility between ChRBC and SRBC.

On the basis of these results a high degree of cross-reactivity between ChRBC and SRBC at the B cell level should be expected; it was tested wether this cross-reactivity also occurs at the level of the acceleration effect.

Rabbits were primed with ChRBC i.v., and given ChRBC and SRBC s.c. 4 days or 4 weeks later. Three and 4 days thereafter numbers of DPFC and IPFC in draining PLN were determined. Results (table 3) are expressed in two ways: (i) the ratio 4/3 indicating the fastness of the reaction, and (ii) the ratio (I-D)/D (numbers IPFC minus DPFC at D.4/ numbers DPFC at day 4) indicating the relation between IgG and IgM production in these nodes. It is important to note that only numbers of anti-SRBC PFC are used, also in ChRBC stimulated PLN (group III). Two conclusions can be drawn from table 3.
(i). The occurence of cross-reactivity at the B cell level is con-

TABLE 3. EFFECTS OF I.V. PRIMING WITH CHRBC ON THE ANTI-SRBC
LYMPH NODE RESPONSE

Group	Ag^I- int. -Ag^{II}	Rabbits	Ratio 4/3	Ratio (I-D)/D
I	-- --- - S	H.12x	15.0 (5.3-43.0)	0.10 (0-0-29)
II	Ch - 4 d. - S	H. 2x	20.6	1.45 (1.9;1.0)
III	Ch - 4 d. - Ch	H. 2x	0.5	0.62 (0.38;0.87)
IV	Ch - 4 w. - S	H. 4x	8.3	5.4 (2.6-8.0)

ratio 4/3: number anti-SRBC DPFC/10^{6}LNC at day 4/ibidem day 3
ratio (I-D)/D: number anti-SRBC (I-DPFC)/DPFC, both per 10^{6}LNC and
both determined at day 4 after Ag^{II}. Ag^I:i.v.; Ag^{II}: s.c..

firmed. In ChRBC- primed rabbits challenged with SRBC, much more anti-
SRBC IgG is produced than in controls (compare group I en IV) and
about as much as in "true" secondary reactions. Therefore we can
conclude that SRBC can stimulate ChRBC-specific memory B cells.
(ii). Despite this cross-reactivity at B cell level no acceleration
effect is observed in SRBC-stimulated PLN after ChRBC priming
(group II), although this antigen as such is perfectly able to prime
for accelerated reactions against cross-reactive determinants
(group III).

These results are imcompatible with a model of B memory being
responsible for the acceleration effect and point to a central role
for T cells. Interestingly, in contrast to findings in mice (12,13)
in these experiments cross-reactivity at the T cell level appeared
to be more restricted than with B cells.

Some Characteristics of T Memory

Sofar it can be concluded that within 4 days after i.v. priming,
memory T cells have appeared which enable lymph nodes to perform,
upon challenge, an accelerated humoral immune response. This
acceleration most likely is the expression of a qualitative change
within the T cell population.

We next investigated wether the capacity to accelerate lymph
node reactions is also carried by cells present several weeks after
priming. Results are shown in the upper part of table 4. Accelerated
reactions (ratio 4/3 less than 2,5) indistinguishable from those
obtained at intervals of 4 days were found with longer intervals
(2 or 4 weeks). Intermediate types of reaction were found when s.c.
challenge was given 5 month after priming. It is concluded that during

TABLE 4. T MEMORY IN RABBITS: PERSISTENCE AND EFFECT OF SPLENECTOMY

Experiment	Rabbits	Ratio 4/3
- - - - - S s.c.(1)	H. 12x	15.0 (5.3-43.0)
S i.v.-4d-S s.c.(2)	H. 12x	0.9 (0.2- 2.5)
S i.v.-2w-S s.c.(3)	H. 2x	1.6 (0.8; 2.4)
S i.v.-4w-S s.c.(4)	H. 4x	0.7 (0.3- 1.1)
S i.v.-5m-S s.c.(5)	GA. 4x	3.9 (2.6- 5.7)
Sx-4w-S i.v.-4d-S s.c.(6)	H. 3x	0.7 (0.5- 1.0)
S i.v.-2d-Sx-2d-S s.c.(7)	H. 2x	0.7 (0.6; 0.7)

for explanation of ratio 4/3 see table 3. S:SRBC Sx:Splectomy
arithmetic mean and range are given.

(at least) 4 weeks after immunization no return to a primary reaction
pattern can be seen, suggesting that the acceleration effect is not
(only) the expression of the persistence of effector cells (HTL),but
(also) of the presence of a new class of memory T cells (imm-HTL).

Finally some experiments on the importance of the spleen for
the development of helper memory after i.v. immunization were
performed; results are shown in the lower part of table 4.
Splenectomy done before (group 6) or during (group 7) i.v. priming
does not prevent the development of memory T cells. It can be added
that also the height of the PFC reaction in these PLN is not
significantly altered as compared to controls.

These results suggest that the T cell reaction leading to the
development of helper memory after i.v. priming takes place, at least
for the greater part, outside the spleen. Experiments not presented
here showed that (i)moreover thymus nor bone marrow are important
breeding sites for T memory after i.v. immunization, and that (ii)
after i.v. injection SRBC readily reach rabbit lymph nodes. We
therefore suggest that following i.v. SRBC administration T cell
reactions leading to T memory especially occur in peripheral lymph
nodes; this explains the antigen induced depletion of SRBC-reactive
cells in rabbit bone marrow found earlier (1) but it is in contrast
to the situation in mice where T cells are said to be recruited in
the spleen after i.v. immunization (14).

ACKNOWLEDGEMENTS

F.J. Keuning, P. Nieuwenhuis, A.W. Polman and J.F Prins are
gratefully acknowledged for helpfull discussions and technical
assistance. This work was supported by a grant from the Dutch
Foundation for Basic Medical Research (FunGo).

REFERENCES

1. Abdou, N.I. and M. Richter. Adv. Immunol. 11. 202. 1969.
2. Ozer, H. and B.H. Waksman. Adv. Exp. Med. and Biol. 29. 167. 1973.
3. Miller, J.F.A.P. Cont. Top. Immunobiol. 2. 151. 1973.
4. Hartmann, K.U.J. Exp. Med. 132. 1267. 1970.
5. Cunningham, A.J. and E.E. Sercarz. Eur.J. Immunol. 1. 413. 1972.
6. Golub, E.S. Cell. Immunol. 3. 62. 1972.
7. Fidler, J.M., E.M. McDaniel and E.S. Golub. Cell. Immunol. 4.29.'72.
8. Cunningham, A.J. and A. Szenberg. Immunol. 14. 599. 1968.
9. Askonas,B.A.,A.Schimpl and E. Wecker. Eur.J. Immunol. 4. 164. 1974.
10.Springer, G.F. Progr. Allergy. 15. 9. 1971.
11.Cunningham, A.J. and L.M.Pilarski. Eur.J.Immunol. 4. 319. 1974.
12.Hoffman, M. and J.W. Kappler. J. Immunol. 108. 261. 1972.
13.Plaïfair,J.H.L. and S. Marshall-Clarke.Immunol. 24. 579. 1973.
14.Sprent, J. and J.F.A.P. Miller. J.Exp. Med. 139. 1. 1974.

INTERFERENCE OF CYCLOPHOSPHAMIDE WITH THE DEVELOPMENT OF T HELPER ACTIVITY IN RABBITS

A.A. van den Broek and G.H. Blijham

Department of Histology, University of Groningen

Oostersingel 69/1, Groningen, The Netherlands

INTRODUCTION

In rats antibody formation against Brucella was suppressed by a single injection of cyclophosphamide given between 1 day before and 4 days after antigenic stimulation (1). A selective suppression of 7S antibody synthesis was described in rats immunized with Sheep Red Blood Cells (SRBC) after treatment with a course of 5 daily injections of cyclophosphamide, started 2 days after antigen injection (2). In mice a cyclophosphamide induced immunological tolerance to SRBC was found when the drug was given simultaneously with or 2 days after antigen injection (3.4). In most of these systems, coöperation between T and B cells is required for antibody production. In rats (5), guinea pigs (6) and rabbits (7) the histological changes caused by a single injection of cyclophosphamide were described. In all species cells homing in the non-thymus-dependent area's of spleen and lymph nodes proved to be sensitive to the drug.

The experiments to be presented were conceived to investigate the effects of a single injection of cyclophosphamide (100 mg/kg b.w.) on B- and T-cells of rabbits, which were immunized with either a thymus-independent antigen (Salmonella java (F1a); 5×10^5 formol killed organisms applied intravenously) or a thymus-dependent antigen (Sheep Red Blood Cells (SRBC) given subcutaneously in the hindlegs). In the latter case some of the animals were preimmunized intravenously with SRBC. This i.v. antigen injection induces a production of T memory cells. These cells together with unprimed B cells seem to be responsible for the accelerated response found in the lymph nodes of these animals, after the s.c. SRBC injection given 4 days after preimmunisation (8). This finds its expression in the high number of PFC on day 3 after the s.c. antigen injection and the absence of increase in PFC's between day 3 and 4.

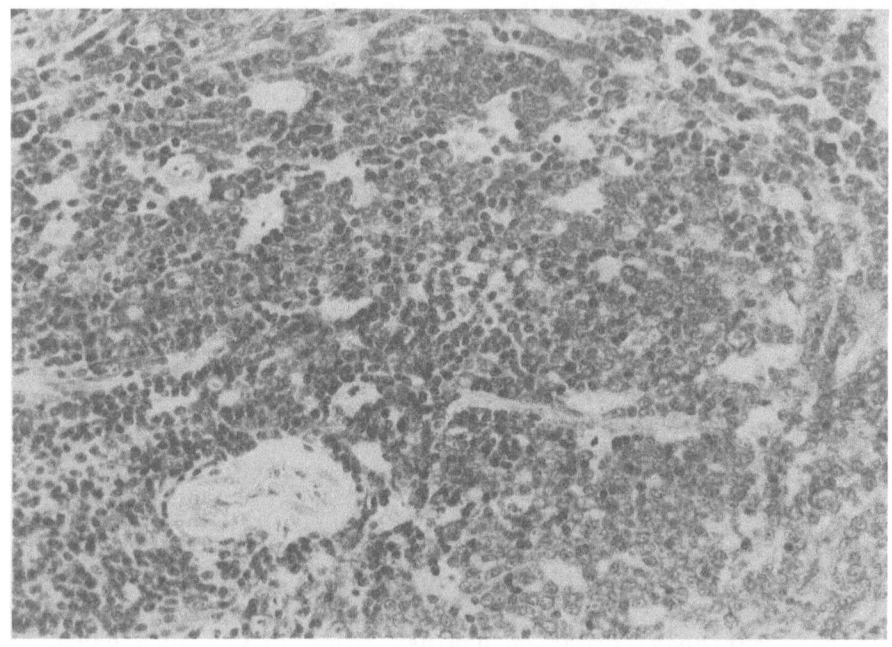

Fig. 1. Spleen, 12 hrs. after cyclophosphamide injection:
- follicle with activated macrofages and intact follicular lymphocytes and marginal zone cells;
- periarteriolar lymphocyte sheath is intact.

Table 1

The mean H-Agglutinin titers on day 6, 8, 10, 15 and 20 after the
i.v. injection with Salmonella java antigen.

day	6	8	10	15	20
controle	8	8.5	8	8(3)	8.5(6)
Ag/Cy	8	7.5	6.7	5	4.7(2)
Ag - 1½d - Cy	0	0	0	0	2
Ag - 2d - Cy	0	0	0	0	2
Ag - 3d - Cy	3	3	2	0	-

( )= titer after treatment of the serum with mercaptoethanol.

RESULTS

The morphological picture of a spleen section 12 hrs. after treatment with cyclophosphamide is demonstrated in figure 1. From this figure it can be seen, that during these 12 hours only a moderate destruction of both follicular lymphocytes and marginal zone cells occured. Macrophages with engulfed nuclear debris could be distinguished, between the majority of small lymphocytes and marginal zone cells, which had survived. The peri-arteriolar lympho-cyte sheath seemed to be unaffected. Twenty-four hours after cyclo-phosphamide treatment no signs of destruction where present anymore. Cyclophosphamide caused an evident cell destruction in active germi-nal center if present. Many so called "tingible Körper" macrophages could be distinguished. Within 4 days germinal centre activity had restored. Signs of mitotic death or mitotic arrest were never seen.

Cyclophosphamide given simultaneously with or after antigenic stimulation resulted in characteristic cytological changes of the differentiating elements of the plasmacellular reaction. Within 12 hours after application of cyclophosphamide plasmablast with large pale vacuoles in their strongly basophilic cytoplasm (i) and a con-spicuous fading of nuclear chromatin (ii) were found.

Histologically comparable effects were also observed in lymph nodes. Twelve hours after cyclophosphamide a moderate cell destruc-tion was found in the outer cortex, which had disappeared in the following 12 hours. No damage was found in the thymus-dependent area's.

In table 1 the mean H-agglutinin titers on day 6, 8, 10 and 15 after stimulation of 6 control rabbits are presented.

The titers show that IgM antibody production reaches its maxi-mum at about the 6th day after antigenic stimulation and that the first IgG antibodies could be shown at about day 10. In table 1, also the effects of cyclophosphamide on the antibody production is presented when cyclophosphamide was given at different moments with regard to antigen injection. It can be seen that neither IgM nor IgG could be found when cyclophosphamide was given at $1\frac{1}{2}$, 2 or 3 days after stimulation. However, a normal IgM response and a suppression of the IgG response was observed when cyclophosphamide was administered simultaneously with the antigen. IgG production was delayed till day 20.

The results obtained when cyclophosphamide was given, before (group A, B) simultaneously with or after (group C,) the s.c. injection of SRBC without (group A) or with (group B, C) an i.v. preimmunisation of the animals, are summarized in table 2. The number of direct P.F.C. on day 3 after s.c. antigen injection and the ratio between the number on day 4 and day 3 are presented as a parameter for the speed of the antibody production in the lymph node. It was found that cyclophosphamide given before the s.c. SRBC injection did not influence the response; the numbers of PFC's at day 3 and the 4/3 ratio's are identical to these obtained in

Table 2

The effect of cyclophosphamide on the direct P.F.C. response in lymph nodes without and with preimmunisation i.v. .

3 = the number of direct P.F.C.'s 3 days after the s.c. SRBC injection;

4/3= the ratio between the number of direct P.F.C.'s on day 4 and 3 after the s.c. SRBC injection.

A.   Cy. - x days - SRBC s.c. - 3/4 days Direct PFC

x = 4		x = 2		x = 1		x = 0				Controls	
3	4/3	3	4/3	3	4/3	3	4/3			3	4/3
35	8.5	63	3.2	2	40	14	16			66	2.0
4	21.5	23	20.4	48	9.3	170	2.1			8	24
28	3.4			100	7.8	34	1.2			23	30.4
23	33.3					24	2.1			63	13.3
						3	114.3			23	33.9
						3	66.7				
						21	3.1				
						6	16.3				
★ 22.5	16.7	43	11.8	50	19.0	31.7	27.7			36.6	20.7

B.   SRBC i.v.- (x days - Cy) - 4 days - SRBC s.c. - 3/4 Direct PFC

x = 0		x = 1		x = 2		x = 3		x = 4		Controls	
3	4/3	3	4/3	3	4/3	3	4/3	3	4/3	3	4/3
866	0.9	1450	1.4	65	12.8	30	6.8	1813	0.8	2134	0.3
2392	0.1	1562	0.5	75	8.6	55	2.7	165	5.6	2400	0.2
						122	6.8	837	1.1	2184	0.2
								143	2.4		
★ 1692	0.5	1506	1.2	70	10.7	60	5.5	739.5	2.5	2239	0.2

C.   SRBC i.v.- (x days - Cy) - 5 days - SRBC s.c. - 3/4 Direct PFC

x = 5		Control	
3	4/3	3	4/3
3078	0.6	1200	0.4
2140	0.9	3445	0.2
500	0.9		
389	2.0		
★ 1527	1.1	2322.5	0.3

★= mean number PFC day 3
mean 4/3 ratio's.

controls. Cyclophosphamide given simultaneously with or after the i.v. preimmunisation (group B) affects the P.F.C. response in the stimulated lymph node, most pronounced when the drug was given 2 or 3 days after the i.v. SRBC injection. The results obtained in this system when cyclophosphamide was given together with the s.c. antigen administration are ambiguous. However, a lengthening of the period between the i.v. and the s.c. antigen injection (group C) upto 5 days clearly indicates that cyclophosphamide given together with the s.c. challenge does not affect the accelerated P.F.C. response.

In accordance with these last findings are the results obtained with the secondary response to Horse Gamma Globulin. The secondary response was not affected when the drug was given simultaneously with the secondary antigen injection.

CONCLUSIONS AND DISCUSSION

From the observations described it is concluded that cyclophosphamide affects differentiating B- and T cells and not the precursors of these cells nor the end cells of the helper T cell response. This is sustained by the fact that the anti-Fla IgM response is suppressed only when the drug is given during a very restricted period of $1\frac{1}{2}$ to 3 days after antigenic stimulation; indicating that only the differentiating and multiplicating plasmacells responsible for IgM production are affected. The specific susceptibility of the IgG response when cyclophosphamide was given simultaneously with the antigen is most likely to be due to an effect on T helper cell response. In rabbit both T and B cells are necessary for IgG production. The IgG producing B cells probably are formed in active germinal centers (9, 10). An effect of cyclophosphamide on germinal centers was only found, when the drug was given during evident activity. Moreover this type of damage was never combined with a depression of IgG production (5).

The results obtained after immunisation with SRBC also indicate that differentiating T cells are susceptible for cyclophosphamide. The normal PFC response found when the drug was given before the s.c. - antigen injection point to normal functioning precursor B and T cells. The absence of the accelerated response found in lymph nodes after the s.c. antigen injection, when cyclophosphamide was given 2 or 3 days after the i.v. SRBC injection point to an effect on differentiating T cells. It was suggested that the i.v. injection of SRBC evokes a T cell response giving rise to T memory cells, which are responsible for the fastened PFC response found in lymph nodes after the s.c. challenge (8). Therefore, the last described effects of cyclophosphamide must be due to an influence on the process of differentiation and proliferation leading to the development of T memory cells. The results obtained with group C (cyclophosphamide given 5 days after pre-immunisation) indicate that the end cells of this response (T memory cells) are not affected by cyclophosphamide which is in accordance with the observed normal secondary response against Horse Gamma Globulin, when the drug was administered simultaneously with the second antigen injection.

Experiments to analyse the effect of cyclophosphamide on stimulated memory cells are in progress.

ACKNOWLEDGEMENTS

This investigation was supported by a grant of the foundation of Basic Medical Research (FUNGO).

The skilful help of Miss A.S. Wubbena and Mrs. M.B.O. van Amstel-Stikker and Mrs. N. Bergman-Visser is gratifully acknowledged.

REFERENCES

1. Stender, H., D. Strauch and H. Winter, Strahlentherapie 115: 175, 1961.
2. Santos, G.W. and A.H. Owens, Nature 209: 622, 1966.
3. Aisenberg, A.C., J.Exp.Med. 125: 833, 1967.
4. Dietrich, F.M. and P. Dukor, Path.Microbiol. 30: 909, 1967.
5. Kool, G.A., in B.D. Jankovic and K. Isakovic, Eds., Microenvironmental Aspects of Immunity, p. 399. Plenum Press New York - London, 1973.
6. Turk, J.L., P.D. Parker and L.W. Poulter, Immunology 23: 493, 1972.
7. Broek, A.A. van den, Immune Suppression and Histophysiology of the Immune Response (Thesis), Groningen, The Netherlands, 1971.
8. Blijham, G.H., This symposium.
9. Mulder, N.H., Thymus dependency of the antibody response (Thesis), Groningen, The Netherlands, 1973.
10. Keuning, F.J., in Proceedings of the Eighth meeting of F.E.B.S., 26, p. 1. North-Holland / American Elsevier, 1972.

ENHANCED IN VITRO IMMUNOGENICITY OF H-2 ANTIGENS IN THE PRESENCE OF Ia ANTIGENS

H.WAGNER and M.RÖLLINGHOFF

Institute of Medical Microbiology

65 Mainz/Germany, Augustusplatz

SUMMARY

In a primary and secondary MLC the in vitro immunogenicity of allogeneic PHA induced blast cells (which lack I region coded determinants) was compared to that of LPS induced blast cells. Unlike LPS induced blast lymphocytes (stimulator cells) which induced high cytotoxic activity, PHA induced blast cells were found to be poor stimulator cells in a primary MLC. Yet in a secondary MLC both types of stimulator cells induced cytotoxic activity equally well.

Using one type of responder cells the relative immunogenicity of various stimulator cells incompatible on either the H-2K and H-2D region or on the I region, or on the complete H-2 complex, was compared. The magnitude of cytotoxic response induced in a strain combination differing at the complete H-2 complex exceeded by far the sum of separate responses obtained against the H-2D region, H-2K region and the I region coded determinants respectively. These results suggest that the presence of I region coded determinants on allogeneic stimulator cells enhance the in vitro immunogenicity of H-2K and H-2D region coded transplantation antigens.

Abbreviations: PHA=Phytohemagglutinin, LPS=Lipopolysaccharide, MLC=Mixed lymphocyte culture, CML=Cell mediated lysis, LAD=Lymphocyte activating determinants.

INTRODUCTION

We and others have proposed that T_1-T_2 cell interactions during in vitro cytotoxic allograft responses may be a reflection of the antigenic dichotomy required for the induction of a MLC-CML (1-3). This concept implies that the proliferative response of T_1 cells as triggered by allogeneic I region controlled surface determinants (LAD) of the stimulator cells will not result in cytotoxic effector cells, but in an amplification of the capacity of anti H-2 reactive T_2 cells to differentiate into cytotoxic T cells. Therefore H-2 different and I region (LAD) positive stimulator cells ought to provoke a strong cytotoxic allograft response compared to I region negative stimulator cells. The present paper deals with experiments performed to test this prediction.

MATERIAL AND METHODS

Mice: The mice used were either kindly provided by Dr. Götze, Munich or purchased from Jackson Laboratories, Bar Harbour, Main, USA.

In vitro allograft system: The system used is based on a "one way" MLC and has been described in detail (1,4,5).

Cytotoxic assay: The method developed by Brunner et al. (6) has been used in a modified form (4). Either PHA or LPS induced blast lymphocytes (5,7) were used as targets. In selected experiments purified (velocity sedimentation technique at 1 g (8)) mitogen induced blast lymphocytes, prepared as described (5,7), were used either as stimulator cells (in the MLC) or as target cells (in the cytotoxicity assay). Percent lysis was calculated as described (7).

RESULTS

In Vitro Immunogenicity of Ia Positive and Ia Negative Stimulator Cells

Using Ia antigens as serological detectable marker for I region dependent surface structures we and others have reported that LPS induced blast lymphocytes do carry I region controlled determinants, whereas PHA induced blast cells, or fibroblasts, are negative (7,9). In the present experiments these cells were tested for their stimulating capacity in both a primary and secondary MLC. The splenic responder cells for the secondary MLC were derived from mice which had been immunised (6-8 weeks before) by i.p. injection of 30×10^6 of appropriate stimulator cells. The results of a representative experiment are given in Table 1 and indicate that in a primary MLC there exists a positive correlation between the

Table 1: Primary and secondary cytotoxic allograft responses of C57Bl/6 responder cells. Comparison of the stimulating capacity of various CBA strain derived cell types.

Stimulator cells (CBA/H, H-2^k	No of stimulator cells/culture	Primary MLC		Secondary MLC	
		% specific lysis of ^{51}Cr labelled LPS induced blast-target cells			
		(R) 20 : 1	2 : 1	10 : 1	2 : 1
spleen	5 x 10^5	84	32	90	47
LPS-blast^P	0	1	0	2	0
	5 x 10^4	32	11	76	39
	5 x 10^5	74	31	85	47
	2 x 10^6	40	19	53	-
PHA-blast^P	5 x 10^4	4	2	64	26
	5 x 10^5	19	7	88	51
	2 x 10^6	3	1	44	19
fibroblasts	5 x 10^4	5	0	73	35
	5 x 10^5	12	4	62	32

P = blast cells purified by the velocity sedimentation technique (8)
R = ratio effector cells to target cells

Legend: C57Bl/6 mouse derived splenic responder cells were cocultivated with graded numbers of x-irradiated H-2^k stimulator cells. In vitro generated cytotoxic activity was compared on a per "culture basis" (7) relative to that obtained with 5 x 10^5 splenic stimulator cells. Background lysis of LPS-blast target cells (3 hours assay) was 27%.

stimulating capacity of allogeneic cells and the presence of Ia antigens on the stimulator cells used.

Thus purified LPS-blast elicited far greater cytotoxic responses when compared to fibroblasts or PHA induced blast cells. The observation, that in a secondary MLC in contrast to a primary MLC the immunogenicity

of the cell types tested was almost equal suggested that the positive
correlation between immunogenicity and the presence of I region coded
determinants appeared to be restricted to primary in vitro allograft
responses.

Immunogenicity of the H-2 Complex Compared to H-2K and H-2D Region,
and I Region Coded Determinants

There is evidence that T cell mediated lysis against either I region
coded determinants or H-2K and H-2D coded determinants can be detected
in vitro by using LPS induced blasts as target cells (7). Therefore we attempted to compare the relative immunogenicity of determinants controlled
by the peripheral and central region of the H-2 complex to that caused
by a complete H-2 complex difference. Thus (A.SWxB10D2)F1 mouse derived responder cells were cocultured either with C57B1/6 stimulator cells
(anti H-2^b haplotype stimulation), or with B10BR mouse derived stimulator
cells (H-2K and H-2D region stimulation), or with ATL mouse derived
stimulator cells (I region stimulation). After 5 day of culture, the cells
were harvested and assayed for cytotoxicity against LPS-induced blast cells
carrying the haplotype used for immunisation (Table 2).
    The results given in Table 2 indicate that both, I region incompatibility
and H-2K/H-2D region incompatibility are capable to trigger in vitro the
generation of cytotoxic lymphocytes. However the magnitude of cytotoxic
responses obtained against the complete H-2 complex is much stronger than
the sum of the responses against the individual regions.

Table 2: Primary cytotoxic in vitro responses against determinants coded
         by different regions of the H-2 complex.

Responder cells	Stimulator cells	Stimulating region	% specific lysis of LPS target cells		
			(R) 50:1	10:1	2:1
(ASW x B10D2)F1	C57B1/6	H-2^b complex	100	90	32
	B10BR	H-2D, H-2K region	44	19	3
	ATL	I region	27	4	1

(R) Ratio effector cells to target cells.
    Background lysis of LPS blasts was less than 31 %.

DISCUSSION

The experiments reported support the concept that the allogeneic stimulus provided by I region controlled determinants results in an amplification of the capacity of T responder cells to differentiate into cytotoxic T effector cells (CTL). The data also provide evidence that I region controlled determinants can trigger the generation of CTL and represent the target of CTL. Therefore we may be confronted with the situation that within the I region of the H-2 complex loci are scattered controlling for either LAD's or/and for target determinants in CML. Our data clearly indicate that there exists no qualitative differences between peripheral (K, D) and central (I) regions of the H-2 complex in their capacity to provoke CTL during allogeneic cell interactions. However they further strengthen our original view that in the cytotoxic effector phase against allogeneic stimulator cells the majority of cytotoxic activity is directed primarily against determinants coded by the peripheral (K, D) region of the H-2 complex and that I region controlled determinants play a central role in the induction phase of CTL reactive against classical transplantation antigens (1). We consider the induction of T_1-T_2 cell interactions which result in enhancement of cytotoxic T cell responses as one of their biological functions.

LITERATURE

1. Wagner, H., Röllinghoff, M., and Nossal, G.J.V., Transplant.Rev. 17 : 3, 1973

2. Bach, F.H., Segall, M., Zier, K.S., Sondel, P.M., Alter, B.J., and Bach, M.L., Science (Wash. D.C.) 180 : 403, 1973

3. Häyry, P., and Andersson, L.C., Eur. J. Immunol. 4 : 145, 1974

4. Wagner, H., and Röllinghoff, M., Eur. J. Immunol. 4 : 745, 1974

5. Röllinghoff, M., Pfizenmeier, K., Trostmann, H., and Wagner, H., Eur. J. Immunol., 1975 (in press)

6. Brunner, K.T., Mauel, J., Cerottini, J.-C, and Chapuis, B., Immunology 14 : 181, 1968

7. Wagner, H., Hämmerling, G., and Röllinghoff, M., Immunogenetics 2 : 257, 1975

8. Miller, R.G., and Phillips   J.Cell.Physiol. 73 : 191, 1969

9. Hämmerling, G.J., Deak, B.D., Mauve, D., Hämmerling, U., and McDevitt, H.O., Immunogenetics 1 : 68, 1974

CO-OPERATION IS THE THING

A.J.S. Davies

Chester Beatty Research Institute, Institute of Cancer

Research, Fulham Road, London SW3 6JB England

Experimental immunology is in danger of becoming an intellectual game played by immunologists for the entertainment of immunologists. The rules for this game are based on the capacity of vertebrate organisms to make various responses to a variety of stimuli. The stimuli are characterized as antigens, which are innumerable but often proteins or polysaccharides, with or without other smaller determinants of specificity. The responses are similarly innumerable but often characterized as either humoral or cell-mediated. As with many other games, it is difficult to discern the present-day objectives of experimental immunology. In the past, the art of playing immunology related to the possibility that the immune responses of the organisms used in the games was some kind of defence mechanism, against invading pathogenic organisms. More recently this notion has not been popular, but other possibilities, such as that immune processes are manifestations of an autoregulatory morphostatic device, or that there is an immune surveillance mechanism operative against neoplastic cells, have found some favour.

I enjoy the infinite variety that the analytical approach has introduced into the immunological stimulus response paradigm. The substitution of whole responding organisms by cells in tissue culture and the demonstration of immune responses in irradiated animals, used as tissue culture vessels for introduced cells, seem to me perfectly legitimate. But I feel that this process of analysis must be followed closely by resynthesis in order that we maintain the original objectives of the game, namely, the disclosure of immunological mechanisms in metazoan organisms and particularly man in such a manner that we can regulate those diseases which may have an immunological basis.

It is against this rather moralistic background that I viewed the
papers in the session of cooperation between B and T lymphocytes in
the immune response.

Kahan and his colleagues sought to regulate the immune response
in order to bring about the better destruction of a tumour cell
population. They used initially heavily TNP-ilated SRBC, followed
later by TNP-ilated tumour cells. The results seemed to them to indicate that this method of treatment of the SRBC was compatible with
the development of a good T cell memory against TNP without the
development of much antibody during the course of the primary immune
response. The later challenge with tumour cells induced a good "T"
cell cytotoxic response against tumour cells.

Oppenheim et al. sought an _in vitro_ assay system for anti-(T,G)-A-L
cells taken from the lymph nodes of previously primed mice. They
adopted two criteria of response: firstly, incorporation of tritiated
thymidine, and secondly, production of PFC. The late 'proliferative'
response of cells from both responder and non-responder mice was
equivalent. This is compatible with the notion that in non-responder
strains some constraint on reaction to antigen exists which is itself
relatively short-lived.

Doria and Agarossi in their experiments explored the notion that
when high doses of antigens are injected into mice a population of B
cells is selected which has a low density of high affinity receptors.
These selected B cells react with carrier-primed T cells in such a
manner as to promote the production of high avidity antibodies. The
experiments, and their explanation are ingenious but I feel that in
transfer systems such as these the use of independent markers of which
cell is producing the antibody could be helpful.

The immune status of old NZW mice was revealed by Roder et al.
to include a marked deficiency in the capacity to respond to various
thymus dependent antigens. Roder showed in a variety of ways that the
T and B cells of these old and autoimmune mice were capable of reacting
to antigen _in vitro_ or on transfer to irradiated old or young syngeneic
recipients. It is possible to explain these findings in terms of suppressor "T" cells and indeed Roder presented evidence compatible with
this interpretation. However, as anti-DNA antibodies are present it
is tempting to wonder whether in any way they could interfere with
immune processes. Could any virus in these mice bring about the
impairment of immunological function?

PVP is an antigen to which the immune response can be thymus
dependent in young mice but relatively less so in older mice. This
conclusion is my extrapolation from the findings of Andersson and
Blomgren that young B cells required T cell help in a transfer system,
whereas old B cells were sometimes hindered thereby in responding to

PVP. This finding was associated with the development of a C3 receptor during the transition from thymus dependent to thymus independent immunological status. This link of C3 receptors, and thus by inference C3, with an immunological process has been made before in relation to 'thymus dependent' immune responses. The fuller description of the exact significance of C3 receptors should prove interesting, particularly as other accessory cells in the lymphoreticular complex, such as neutrophils and macrophages, may have them. From a situation a few years ago when receptors were few on the ground there seems now to have arisen an abundance of them. A simple example, perhaps, of the old adage, seek and ye shall find.

Altman and Cohen found that in their in vitro system in which T lymphocytes attack and kill foreign fibroblasts the addition of different foreign stimulator lymphocytes, or of supernatants from a mixed lymphocyte culture, enhances the lethal effects. I wonder whether the effect of blocked stimulator cells is necessarily due to the same mechanism as that operative when supernatants are added. Perhaps revelation of the nature of the "T" derived supernatant helper substance will help to answer this question.

Lubbe and Zaalberg thought initially, in their in vitro studies of the immune response, that an unusual radioresistant "T" lymphocyte was required. Happily it turned out that the third cell was a macrophage. This serves to emphasize that most immune responses in intact organisms probably involve not only T and B lymphocytes but also macrophages and various other cells such as mast cells, neutrophils, eosinophils and reticulum cells. The possibilities for cooperation in this "immunological orchestra" are extensive, whoever the conductor.

Lymphoid Cell Receptors
and Antigen Recognition

LYMPHOID CELL RECEPTORS AND ANTIGEN RECOGNITION

G.L. Ada and R.V. Blanden

Department of Microbiology, The John Curtin School of
Medical Research, Australian National University
Canberra, Australia

The subject of this session is at the very heart of immunology –
what the lymphocyte recognizes, what is the nature of the cell receptors whereby recognition occurs and what might happen to the
lymphocyte after the recognition event. In one sense, we are for-
tunate that these are topics which include controversial opinions
and data and at this meeting and among the speakers we have pro-
tagonists for different view points. So we are likely to have a
lively and enjoyable session. I doubt whether we will settle many
of the more controversial issues but we may well have some clarification.

Let's start with one aspect, the question of receptors for
antigen on the lymphocyte surface. Most of us use the term recept-
or in an operational sense and probably would not use the term if
we did not believe that an element of specificity was involved. For
some, that may be the only criterion. In the case of lymphocytes
especially, many would agree that binding of the antigen (or what
the receptor recognizes) should be a necessary, but not necessarily
sufficient step, in the pathway of events which leads to other
changes in the cell. These might be intracellular changes which
could result in differentiation, proliferation and so forth. Finally,
a more controversial aspect would be the origin of the receptor
molecule or complex. If it can be demonstrated that it is synthesized by the lymphocyte itself, this strengthens the argument but
we probably cannot rule out the possibility that a component produced
by another cell but cytophilic for the cell under discussion may
act as receptors on the latter, in terms of the first two points
made.

B lymphocytes

We come close to these criteria for B lymphocytes as there is
only one serious candidate - Ig - for the role of receptor for antigen. Much of the evidence has been summarized elsewhere (Ada and Ey,
1975). On "virgin" lymphocytes, probably both IgMs and IgD can act
as receptors, though to our knowledge, no one has isolated from B
cells antigen-IgMs complexes formed under conditions which would have
resulted in cell stimulation.

The evidence in favour of an individual lymphocyte or antibody secreting cell producing Ig of a single antigen-binding specificity is quite substantial. The findings of Dr. Miller and his
group that a small minority of B lymphocytes bind many molecules
of different antigenic specificities suggests that such cells have
receptors of different antigenic specificities. They consider
these cells might be progenitors of the mature B lymphocyte. One
of us (G.L.A.) has resisted this interpretation for some time.
It seems we need to know whether these multiple antigen binding
cells have any biological function and whether indeed they are
lymphocytes! It would be most useful if this information were
forthcoming.

Dr. Liacopoulos will present evidence which, contrary to almost
all workers' experience, suggests that a single antibody secreting
cell can produce antibodies of two different specificities. The
evidence for this is based upon inhibition studies at the single
cell level. With a reagent such as the red cell where the nature
of the antigenic structures is virtually unknown, the data bears
close scrutiny.

T lymphocytes

Few would deny that T lymphocytes possess receptors for antigens. There are reports which indicate that for certain antigens
the specificity of the T cell response is at least as great as
that of the B cell response; other reports suggest that substances
distinguished by B cells may not always be distinguished by T cells.
When we come to the question of the nature of the T cell receptor
there are great differences of opinion. Until very recently, this
has been examined mainly in two ways. The first is by direct
isolation. Usually the cell membrane is iodinated, then dissolved
in detergent, the component co-precipitated immunologically and the
precipitation examined by gel electrophoresis. When some thymomas
are examined in this way, the evidence is convincing that IgMs is
present on the surface of the cell and bio-synthetic labelling
confirms that this material is synthesized by the cell itself.
When this approach is used, either on cells in the thymus or on T

cells in the periphery, widely different results are found (Ada and
Ey, 1975). Some claim the recovery of IgMs; others have been
unable to detect any Ig. The second procedure is to label cells with
radioactive antigen and to see whether anti-immunoglobulin inhibits
the binding. This generally is a satisfactory approach for B cells
but again controversial results have been obtained for T cells.
Even the technique of labelling B cells with radioactive antigen can
give very variable results. For example, iodination of J. lalandii
haemocyanin with a slight excess of the oxidising agent chloramine
T partly denatures the protein. The use of such material in the
reaction with B lymphocytes gives unduly large numbers of cells
binding the antigen. There are detailed reports (e.g. Roelants and
Ryden, 1974; Hämmerling and McDevitt, 1974) that T cells bind some
antigens. However, of a number of antigens tested, only TGAL was
found to bind to leucocytes from bursectomised chickens and this
binding could be inhibited by normal rabbit globulin (Jensenius,
Crone and Kock, 1975). Furthermore, it has not been possible so far
to demonstrate in CBA mice T cells which bind J. lalandii haemocyanin
(J. -P. Lamelin and G.L. Ada, unpublished) despite the fact that such
mice mount T cell responses to these antigens. These results,
together with the failure to "suicide" T cells with highly labelled
antigen in the absence of B cells and/or macrophages (Basten, Miller
and Abraham, 1975) suggest that in vivo, other cells may present
antigen to the T cells in a special way. This brings in the question
of antigen recognition by T cells.

What does the T cell recognize?

Papers in the last session of the morning are concerned with
the recognition of antigen by T cells. Interest in this topic has
recently been enhanced particularly by the findings of Zinkernagel,
Doherty, Blanden and their colleagues (for review, see Doherty and
Zinkernagel, 1975) and of Shearer (1974) that cytotoxic T cells
appear to recognise specifically "altered self". This, together
with the findings of J.F.A.P. Miller (this conference) on the requirements for stimulation of T cells for DTH activity and the
results of Erb and Feldmann (personal communication) on the nature
of the macrophage-derived factor which stimulated T cells, allows
the development of a concept which it will be useful to keep in
mind during our discussions. Some essential points are (R.V.
Blanden, in preparation):

1. There are two main subsets of T lymphocytes which can be defined
both serologically and by functional tests. These are effector T
cells (T^E) which are cytotoxic and helper T cells (T^H) which may
help B cells or activate monocytes. Whether these latter activities
are shown by different cell populations within the T^H subset (Liew
and Parish, 1974) or by T cells of one lineage but at different

stages of differentiation (Gordon and Yu, 1973) is unknown. It is
possible that T^H cells may be required both for optimal T^E and B
cell responses.

2. The antigen-receptor dictionaries of these subsets differ from
each other and from the B cell dictionary in the following way. B
cells appear to recognize foreign antigenic patterns in a (relatively) simple, uncomplicated fashion. With (mouse) T cells however,
the dictionaries appear to be restricted so that they only recognize
foreign antigenic patterns associated in some way with products of
the H2 gene complex. Thus, antigens coded by genes in K or D
regions, modified as a result of viral infection, are recognized
by T^E cells (Doherty and Zinkernagel, 1975). Antigens coded in the
I region and associated with foreign antigens are recognized by T^H
cells. This has been shown for helper T cell activity (Erb and
Feldmann, 1975, and personal communication) and for DTH activity by
Miller (J.F.A.P. Miller).

3. As a consequence, T cell responses (in vivo) are triggered only
by allogeneic cell surface antigens (or certain similar xenogeneic
antigens) by alterations in configuration or arrangement of self
gene products caused by foreign antigens (termed "altered-self"
antigens).

4. The display or production of "altered-self" antigens is the
province of stimulator cells and the most appropriate candidates
for these are monocytes or macrophages. After infection of the
target cell by virus (in this case, ectromelia), active protein
synthesis must take place in the cell before it becomes susceptible
to lysis by the cytotoxic T cell. Presumably, this is also the case
of T^H cells, the antigen may need to be "processed" by the macrophage
in order to become integrated into the membrane.

5. Finally, Ir genes may operate in part by producing (in association with foreign antigens) antigenic complexes (altered self
antigens) which determine the amount of T^H cell induction and thus
the magnitude of the T^E cell and B cell responses. Thus, in the
case of low responders (in terms of IgG responses) to certain foreign
antigens, the defect may be an inadequate repertoire of either Ir
gene products expressed in stimulator cells or in the receptor
dictionary.

References

Ada, G.L. and Ey, P.L. The Antigens, ed. M. Sela, Academic Press,
    N.Y., 4 (1975). In the press.
Basten, A., Miller, J.F.A.P. and Abraham, R. J. exp. Med., 141
    (1975) 547.
Doherty, P.L. and Zinkernagel, R. Lancet (1975) In the press.

Erb, P. and Feldmann, M. Nature, 254 (1975), 352.

Gordon, J. and Yu, H. Nature New Biol., 244 (1973), 21.

Hämmerling, G.J. and McDevitt, H.O., J. Immunol., 112 (1974), 1726.

Jensenius, J.C., Crone, M. and Kock, C. Scand. J. Immunol., 4 (1975), 151.

Kirov, S.M. and Parish, C.R. (1975), submitted for publication.

Liew, F.Y. and Parish, C.R. J. exp. Med., 139 (1974), 779.

Roelants, G.E. and Ryden, A. Nature, 247 (1974), 104.

Shearer, G.M. Eur. J. Immunol. 4 (1974), 257.

PATTERNED ANTIGEN-BINDING CELLS OF MULTIPLE SPECIFICITY

Alexander Miller, Dominick DeLuca, Franco Celada, and

Eli Sercarz. Department of Bacteriology, University of

California, Los Angeles, California 90024, U.S.A.

In previous papers (1,2) and papers now in press (3), we have shown that there exists in all lymphoid tissue of the mouse (and other vertebrates) a subpopulation of cells which bind fluoro-chrome-labeled anti-Ig and protein antigens in a characteristic pattern. These patterned antigen-binding cells (ABC) bind large, multideterminant proteins at a very high frequency: in mouse tissues, 30-50% of these cells bear Ig receptors for any of five different proteins. On cells which bind two proteins, each is bound independently of the other. The observations that such multiple ABC appear very early in ontogeny (4,5), and that after antigen-induced shedding, reappearance of receptors on patterned ABC occurs (but only under conditions of protein synthesis), are consistent with models in which single patterned ABC synthesize (rather than acquire) many different receptors. The evidence is reviewed in some greater detail below. In addition, some new data which also tend to support the idea of multiple receptor synthe-sis by single cells are presented.

PREVIOUS STUDIES

Conditions of Assay. Because unfixed patterned ABC rapidly undergo antigen-induced stripping, we routinely employ aldehyde-fixed cells. It is important to note that fixation can be carried out after exposure to antigen without change in frequency of binding cells. Binding of enzyme antigens (beta-galactosidase, horseradish peroxidase) has been determined by use of a chromo-genic substrate. A more general method has been to use protein antigens conjugated with fluorescein (FITC) or tetramethylrhoda-mine (TRITC) at low F/P ratios. Detection was made possible by use of the Ploem epiillumination system. To assure plateau values for

frequencies of patterned ABC, fluorochrome-conjugated protein antigens were used at a concentration of 500 μg/ml/10^7 cells. Preincubation with unconjugated antigen gave essentially complete inhibition of observable binding by that protein but not of others.

Characteristics of Patterned ABC. Among the fixed cells which
bind anti-Ig, a small proportion in spleen and roughly half in
bone marrow show binding of anti-Ig in a complex pattern of "spots"
which have a circumscribed distribution over the cell surface, such
that in most focal planes of the microscope, two large, roughly
circular areas free of staining can be seen. When FITC- or TRITC-
protein is used as the stain, the majority of ABC are those with
patterned anti-Ig binding and the binding pattern is very similar.

Patterned ABC with T Markers. When fixed splenic T-cells
(prepared with nylon-wool columns) or cortisone resistant T-cells
are reacted with fluorochrome-antigens, about the same frequency
of patterned ABC is found as in whole spleen cell populations.
These ABC are a substantial subclass of T-cells binding anti-Ig
in a patterned manner. On all T-cells, a well-characterized rabbit
anti-T serum (as detected with FITC-goat anti-rabbit immunoglobulin)
is bound smoothly over the entire surface and differently than
anti-Ig or antigen.

Morphology and Eosinophilia. Patterned ABC superficially
appear to be medium to large lymphocytes with regard to size and
nucleus to cytoplasm ratio. However, their nuclei appear somewhat
more lobar and there are granules present in the cytoplasm (by
phase microscopy) which are eosinophilic. One of us (D. DeLuca)
is currently making a detailed study of the morphology of
patterned ABC at the light and electron microscope level.

Inhibition by Anti-μ Serum. A goat anti-μ prepared against
MOPC 104E IgM and absorbed with germ-free serum and 104E urinary
protein (the gift of R. Asofsky) was found to strongly inhibit
binding of protein antigens by patterned ABC, irrespective of
whether or not the cells were positive for anti-T binding.

Frequency of Single Patterned ABC and Double ABC. Among the
patterned ABC, a second fluorescent protein antigen was found to
bind to 30-50% of all cells capable of binding a single fluorescent
protein. Double ABC were as inhibitable with anti-μ or homologous
non-conjugated protein as single binding cells. Binding of both
antigens were in islands but individual islands varied widely in
relative amounts of each antigen bound.

Stripping and Reappearance of Receptors. When protein antigens are incubated with lymphoid populations, patterned ABC, specific for those antigens are lost. However, if B-cells (bone marrow

or spleen cells) or T-cells (splenic T-cells or cortisone-resistant thymus cells) are then incubated in absence of antigen under conditions which allow protein synthesis, multispecific ABC are regenerated to a frequency found prior to incubation.

AMEF EXPERIMENTS

Our data are consistent with a model in which patterned ABC present on their surface a set of receptors with different specificities. The limits of these sets is such that for a complex antigen such as a large protein, about half the ABC will have a receptor type specific for that antigen. It follows that for simpler antigens or antigens for which detection of binding is restricted, our model predicts a much lower frequency of ABC rather than a general lowering of detectability of ABC.

To test this idea, we have employed AMEF, a mutant protein of $\underline{E}$. $\underline{coli}$ β-galactosidase. AMEF is enzymatically active only when combined with antibody which has a specificity directed against a particular antigenic determinant on the molecule (6). As can be seen in Table 1, the substitution of AMEF for β-galactosidase in a typical chromogenic assay (2), leads to approximately a six-fold decrease in apparent ABC. However, if rabbit anti-galactosidase (which contains activating antibodies) is added to the AMEF-treated cells prior to assay with the chromogenic galactoside, then the same value is found for frequency of ABC as with β-galactosidase, indicating that the molecules had bound to the surface.

In Figure 1, the kinetics of appearance of ABC after treatment with native enzyme, AMEF, or AMEF and anti-galactosidase are shown. Although the plateau frequency of ABC is much lowered when AMEF alone is used, these ABC become detectable and darken at the

TABLE 1

APPARENT ABC IN CBA SPLEENS

$ABC/10^3$ CELLS

Addition	Expt. 1	Expt. 2
GZ	9.0	37.0
AMEF	1.4	6.6
AMEF + x-GZ	8.9	42.5
NONE	< 0.2	< 0.03

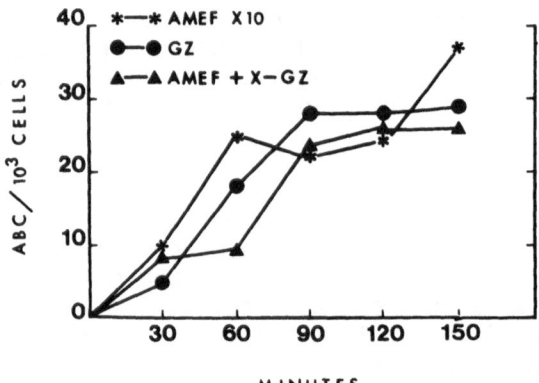

MINUTES

Figure 1. Kinetics of appearance of chromogen on ABC. Glutaraldehyde-fixed CBA spleen cells were incubated with 50 µg/ml galactosidase (GZ), 350 µg/ml AMEF or AMEF followed by rabbit anti-GZ.
After removal of excess antigen, the cells were incubated with the
chromogenic substrate, bromochloroindoxylgalactoside as described
previously (2).

same rate as is found with β-galactosidase. Thus, it appears that
AMEF on any one cell is either fully activated or not activated
at all (in the absence of added antibody).

In Table 2, it may be seen that for cells from different
individuals and from different lymphoid organs and for separated
B and T cells, there is little difference in the ratio of apparent
ABC for β-galactosidase and AMEF. These experiments were done
with CBA mice. In a preliminary survey, there was a suggestion
that some strains of mice may show markedly higher galactosidase to
AMEF ratios, especially in certain organs. However, these experiments have not yet been repeated.

IMPLICATIONS OF MULTISPECIFIC BINDING

Although our data do not formally preclude a model in which
multispecific patterned ABC arise by direct cell-to-cell transfer
of membrane components, the shedding and reappearance experiments
on cells in suspension make such a model unlikely. Other, less
directed transfer models are incompatible with the AMEF results.

TABLE 2

RATIO OF GALACTOSIDASE (GZ) TO AMEF ABC

Cell Source	GZ/AMEF			
Bone Marrow	12.7	6.7	7.7	
Thymus	2.5	5.8	-	
Lymph Nodes	2.0	3.7	6.0	
Spleen	4.7	8.5	9.3	9.0
Splenic B				6.6
Splenic T				8.6

We, therefore, assume at present, that multispecific ABC arise directly through intrinsic synthesis by each ABC. As we have discussed previously (3), such a model requires either that a single c region serve for transcription of many "v-c" messengers of varying v specificity (copy choice); or that the gene for a single c region be greatly expanded and then combined with different v regions. The latter possibility could result from intrinsic expansion or from cell-to-cell transfer of episomal elements containing "v-c" cistrons with different v regions.

The function of patterned ABC remains to be elucidated. We do, of course, consider the possibility that these cells are precursors of more restricted B and T cells. Another possibility, in light of the facile shedding observed in vitro, is that patterned ABC act in a regulatory manner, tending to dampen cellular interaction by interference. This interference may be nonspecific and prevent attachment of receptors to binding sites, or specific through provision of idiotypes (anti-idiotypes) which compete for receptors with antigen.

ACKNOWLEDGMENTS

Supported in part by a grant from the National Institutes of Health (AI 11183), a grant from the Damon Runyon-Walter Winchell Cancer Fund (Grant DRG-1077) and a grant from NATO (#606).

REFERENCES

1. Miller, A., DeLuca, D., Decker, J., Ezzell, R., and Sercarz, E.E. Amer. J. Pathol. 65:541 (1971).

2. DeLuca, D., Decker, J., Miller, A., and Sercarz, E.E. Cell. Immunol. 16:1 (1974).

3 a, b, c. DeLuca, D., Miller, A., and Sercarz, E.E. Cell. Immunol. 18 (1975), in press.

4. Decker, J., Clarke, J., MacPherson, L., Miller, A., and Sercarz, E.E. J. Immunol. 113:1823 (1974).

5. Decker, J. and Sercarz, E.E. Nature 252:416 (1974).

6. Celada, F., Ellis, J., Bodland, K., and Rotman, B. J. Exptl. Med. 134:751 (1971).

EVIDENCE FOR TWO ANTIBODY MOLECULES OF DIFFERENT SPECIFICITY

SECRETED BY BISPECIFIC MOUSE SPLEEN PFC MICROMANIPULATED "IN VITRO"

P. LIACOPOULOS, J. COUDERC and C. BLEUX

Institute of Immunobiology, Hôpital Broussais

96, rue Didot, 75674 PARIS CEDEX 14, France

Previous work of this laboratory showed the transient appearance of cells simultaneously reacting against two unrelated antigens, during an early period after double immunization (1, 2). The main problem about these double PFC, is the possibility of some low cross-reactivity between antigens of the pairs used. Previous investigation on this problem did not support the hypothesis that bispecific PFC are simply cross-reacting cells. However, since these cells are only 1-3 per cent of total PFC, the possibility remains that these cells produce either, one antibody reacting to a structurally similar area of different epitopes or one polyfunctional antibody reacting to structurally different determinants (3). The present study has been undertaken in order to see whether a bispecific PFC micromanipulated in a medium containing both indicator erythrocytes plus soluble antigen, continues to lyse the unrelated erythrocyte when lysis of the homologous erythrocyte was entirely inhibited.

For these experiments adult Swiss mice were given intravenously on day O, 2×10^8 highly dinitrophenylated sheep erythrocytes (TNP-SRBC). On day 4, the spleens cells of these mice were harvested, washed in Hank's medium and used for hemolytic plaque formation assay against native SRBC and TNP conjugated horse erythrocytes (TNP-HoRBC). For the detection of PFC, 10^7 spleen cells were mixed with 10^9 SRBC and/or 0.75×10^9 TNP-HoRBC in tris-buffered Eagle's medium supplemented with 10 percent guinea pig complement and sodium carboxy-methyl-cellulose to a final volume of 1 ml (4). Of the final suspension 0.2ml were deposited on a 24x50mm coverslip and then the drop was flattened out with another coverslip and both coverslips were set on a container which was then filled with paraffin oil and placed in the incubator of the micromanipulator. The spleen cells put in these monolayers developed hemolytic plaques

within 30 to 40 minutes. The majority of them were turbid as only
one erythrocyte type was lysed (monospecific PFC) but some (2-4%)
were clear indicating that both erythrocyte types were lysed
(bispecific PFC). The PFC were drawn into a micropipette and then
transferred and expelled into a second monolayer and 30 min. later
into a third monolayer. Receptor monolayers contained all the
constituents of the first monolayer except spleen cells. In the
experimental series, the second monolayer contained an excess of
specific soluble inhibitor (either TNP-BSA or soluble SRBC antigen)
in order to inhibit the corresponding specific lysis.

   The first series of cell transfers aimed to ascertain the
functional capacity of the micromanipulated PFC in three successive
media. It is shown in Table 1 that out of 72 monospecific PFC

TABLE 1 - Activity of individual monospecific or bispecific PFC of
          the 4th day after immunization with TNP-SRBC during
          transfer from the initial revealing medium into two
          successive media containing native SRBC and TNP-HoRBC.

Initial medium (SRBC+TNP-HoRBC) N° of PFC taken	2nd medium (SRBC+TNP-HoRBC) RBC lysis			N° of PFC transferred to the 3rd medium	3rd medium (SRBC+TNP-HoRBC) RBC lysis		
	Sple[1]	Dble[2]	None[3]		Sple[1]	Dble[2]	None[3]
Mono-specific	72	68	3	1	67	57	0	10
	100%	94.6	4.1	1.3	100%	84.6	0	15.4
Bispe-cific	103	9	92	2	92	18	54	20
	100%	9	89	2	100%	19	58	23

[1] Producing simple or turbid haemolytic plaques
[2] Producing double or clear haemolytic plaques
[3] Cells no more lysing erythrocytes

picked up from the original monolayers 71 remained functional in
the second monolayer (in which 3 became doubles) as did 57 (85%)
out of 67 successfully transferred into the third monolayer. About
the same rate of survival was found among bispecific PFC ; out of
103 transferred to the second monolayer 101 remained functional and
out of 92 transferred into the third monolayer, 72 (77%) still lysed
surrounding erythrocytes. However, deletion of double lyse has occurred in 9% in the second and in 19% of them in the third monolayer.

   In the following series micromanipulated cells were transferred
from the original monolayer to a second monolayer containing native
SRBC, TNP-HoRBC and soluble TNP-BSA (150 µg/ml) and then into the
third monolayer containing the erythrocytes alone. As reported
in Table 2, among 156 bispecific PFC transferred in the

TABLE 2 - Activity of individual bispecific PFC of the 4th day after immunization with TNP-SRBC during transfer from the initial revealing medium into successive media containing native SRBC and TNP-HoRBC. In the second medium soluble TNP-BSA inhibitor was added.

Initial medium (SRBC+TNP-HoRBC) N° of PFC taken (Bispecific)	2nd medium (SRBC+TNP-HoRBC+ TNP-BSA) RBC lysis Dble[1] sple[2] None[3]			N° of PFC transferred to the 3rd medium	3rd medium (SRBC+TNP-HoRBC) RBC lysis Dble[1] sple[2] None[3]		
156	19	125	12	136	65	49	22
100 %	12	80	8	100%	48	36	16

Behaviour in the three successive media of the 65 PFC producing a double lysis in the 3rd medium (second panel).
Double-Simple-Double lysis 50 (77%)
Double-Double-Double lysis 15 (23%)

[1] producing clear haemolytic plaques
[2] producing turbid haemolytic plaques
[3] Cells no more lysing erythrocytes

second medium containing soluble TNP-BSA, 125 i.e. 80% became mono-specific, versus only 9% in the absence of soluble inhibitor (Table 1) In the third monolayer where no inhibitor was present, out of 136 transferred cells 65 (48%) became again bispecific 49 (36 %) remai-ned monospecific and 22 (16%) ceased to lyse the erythrocytes. Among the 65 bispecific PFC fully functional in the three successive monolayers 50 (77%) lysed only one erythrocyte type (presumably SRBC) when TNP-BSA was present into the medium.

Morphological distinction between SRBC and HoRBC is not easy and therefore it was not possible to ascertain whether in the second monolayer containing soluble TNP-BSA only SRBC were lysed when par-tial lysis was observed. For this reason in a new series of experi-ments the second and third monolayers contained only TNP-HoRBC + TNP-BSA and SRBC + TNP-BSA respectively or SRBC + soluble SRBC antigen and TNP-HoRBC + soluble SRBC antigen. In the first of these series out of 77 bispecific PFC transferred, 16 still lysed TNP-HoRBC but 61 (79%) were inhibited by the presence of TNP-BSA in the second monolayer. Among 74 of these cells successfully transferred to the third monolayer (SRBC+TNP-BSA) 48 (65%) lysed SRBC in spite of the presence of TNP-BSA and 26 (35%) were inhibited or ceased to function (Table 3).

Back examination of the 48 PFC which lysed SRBC in the third medium showed that 37 (77%) of them could not lyse TNP-HoRBC in the pre-sence of TNP-BSA in the second medium whereas in the first medium

TABLE 3 - Activity of individual bispecific PFC during transfer
from the initial revealing medium into two successive
media containing either (2nd medium) only TNP-HoRBC
and TNP-BSA or (3rd medium) SRBC and TNP-BSA

Initial medium (SRBC+TNP-HoRBC) N° of bispecific PFC taken	2nd medium (TNP-HoRBC+TNP-BSA)		N° of PFC trans-ferred into the the 3rd medium	3rd medium (SRBC+TNP-BSA)	
	Lysis	No lysis		Lysis	No lysis
77	16	61	74	48	26
100%	21	79	100%	65	35

Behaviour in the three successive media of the 48 PFC active in the
3 rd medium :

Lysis - no lysis - lysis 37 (77%)
Lysis - lysis - lysis 11 (23%)

TABLE 4 - Activity of individual bispecific PFC during transfer from
the initial revealing medium into two successive media
containing either (2nd medium) only SRBC and soluble SRBC
antigen, or (3rd medium) TNP-HoRBC and soluble SRBC antigen

Initial medium (SRBC+TNP-HoRBC) N° of bispecific PFC taken	2nd medium (SRBC+S.SRBC Ag)°		N° of PFC trans-ferred into the 3rd medium	3rd medium (TNP-HoRBC + S.SRBC Ag)°	
	Lysis	No lysis		Lysis	No lysis
109	23	86	102	69	33
100%	21	79	100%	68	32

Behaviour in the three successive media of the 69 PFC active in the
3rd medium :

Lysis - no lysis - lysis 49 (71%)
Lysis - Lysis - Lysis 20 (29%)

° S.SRBC Ag : Soluble SRBC antigen

not containing TNP-BSA they lysed both SRBC and TNP-HoRBC. Similar
results were obtained when soluble SRBC antigen was used as specific inhibitor (Table 4). Among 109 bispecific PFC transferred into
the second medium, 86 (79%) were inhibited by the soluble SRBC
antigen. Of the 102 transferred into the third monolayer, 69 (68%)
readily lysed TNP-HoRBC in spite of the presence of soluble SRBC
antigen. These 69 PFC, fully functional in the third medium were
incapable, in their vast majority (71%) of lysing SRBC when soluble
SRBC antigen was present (second monolayer), whereas they did so

in the absence of the inhibitor (first monolayer).

In previous studies (1, 2, 5) it was found that immunization of mice with one erythrocyte of the pairs used, resulted in
the appearance of bispecific PFC in numbers that were 50 to 100
times less than those found after double immunization. It was
therefore inferred that the vast majority of the later bispecific
PFC might produce antibody of two different specificities. The
present results showed that in 70-80% of bispecific cells inhibition of one activity by soluble inhibitor does not interfere with
the other activity. The persistence of the unrelated lytic activity in the presence of soluble inhibitor shows that the inhibition
is not competitive as in the studies of Varga et al. (3). The
strictly specific inhibition of the lytic activity observed in
this study, proved that 70-80% of the bispecific PFC do not produce one type of cross-reacting or polyfunctional antibody but
two separate antibody molecules of different specificity.

REFERENCES

1. - Couderc, J., Bleux, C., Birrien, J.L. and Liacopoulos P
     J. Immunol., 111, 1155 (1973)
2. - Couderc, J., Birrien J.L., Oriol, R., Bleux C. and
     Liacopoulos P.
     Europ. J. Immunol., 5, 140 (1975)
3. - Varga, J.M., Koningsberg W.H. and Richards F.F.
     Proc. Nat. Acad. Sci. (Wash) 72, 3269 (1973)
4. - NOSSAL G.J.V., Warner N.L. and Lewis H.
     Cell. Immunol., 2, 41 (1971)
5. - Couderc J., Bleux C., Birrien J.L. and Liacopoulos P.
     Immunology, In the press (1975)

EARLY EVENTS IN THE GENERATION OF ANTIGEN-SPECIFIC CYTOTOXICITY IN MLC

W. Clark, J. Nedrud, M. Touton and L. Knoeber

Dept. of Biology and Molecular Biology Institute

University of California, Los Angeles, Calif. 90024

The generation of cytotoxicity in vitro has been shown to be accompanied by proliferation of the responding lymphocytes. Interference with the proliferative phase of the reaction has been shown to decrease the magnitude of the cytotoxic response as measured several days later (1-3); moreover, proliferation can occur in MLC without leading to cytotoxic effector cells (4,5). Two key points yet to be established, however, are whether or not one or more rounds of cell division are absolutely required for the initial expression of cytotoxicity in response to alloantigens, and whether or not appearance of cytotoxic function in responding cells requires expression of new genetic information.

We have examined these questions in both the primary and secondary MLC reactions. Since inhibitors of mitosis can interfere with the expression of cytotoxicity in the ^{51}Cr-release assay (6), we have used hydroxyurea (HU), an inhibitor of DNA synthesis, to block cell division. We used the inhibitor bromodeoxyuridine (BUdR) to block expression of any new cell-specific genes expressed during sensitization. BUdR has been found to differentially block new gene expression in eukaryotes without affecting normal cell functions, including mitosis (see review in ref. 7).

Primary MLCs were initiated using C57BL/6 mouse lymphocytes as responding cells, and irradiated DBA/2 mouse lymphocytes as stimulating cells. Final cell concentration was $2 - 3 \times 10^6$ lymphocytes/ml. in Dulbecco's Modified Eagle's Medium supplemented with amino acids and 2-ME as suggested by Cerrotini (8). Secondary MLCs (8,9) were initiated using immune C57BL/6 anti-DBA/2 lymphocytes from primary MLC (day 11-13) as responding cells, and irradiated

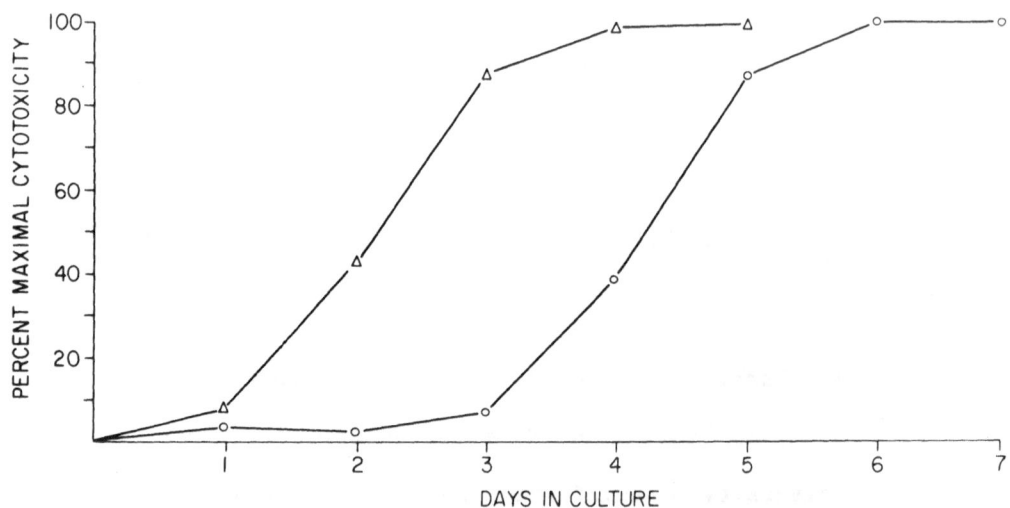

Figure 1.   Length of exposure to alloantigen required for development of cytotoxicity in MLC.   MLCs were initiated using
C57BL/6 lymph node cells and (C57BL/6 X DBA/2)Fl lymphocytes.
At various times the Fl cells were removed by treatment with
C57BL/6 anti-DBA/2 antiserum plus rabbit complement followed
by enzyme treatment to digest dead cells. ▲——▲ : per cent
maximal (normal serum treated) cytotoxicity developed at day
6 in MLC when cultures were treated with antiserum at times
indicated. ⊖——⊖ : normal pattern of generation of cytotoxicity as measured in a 4-hour assay.

DBA/2 lymphocytes as stimulating cells.   In the primary MLC, the
cytotoxicity was assayed against ^{51}Cr-labeled P815 mastocytoma cells
(maintained in DBA/2 mice) after 48 hours of culture.   In the
secondary MLC cytotoxicity was measured against the same target 24
hours after restimulation.

The length of exposure to alloantigen required for generation
of cytotoxicity in primary MLC is shown in Figure 1.   Cultures were
set up and the stimulating cells lysed with cytotoxic alloantiserum
plus complement at various time periods, and the effect of this
treatment on the generation of cytotoxicity was determined by
measuring ^{51}Cr release on day 6 of culture.   In these experiments,
cultures were set up using the lowest possible number of stimula-

ting cells consistent with full generation of cytotoxicity, to
facilitate complete removal of stimulating cells by antiserum
treatment. As can be seen from the data, stimulating cells were
absolutely required for the first 24 hours of culture, and removal
of stimulating cells had a depressive effect on the development of
cytotoxicity (expressed on a per cell basis) up to at least 48 hours
of culture. At 72 hours, removal of stimulating cells had essentially no effect on subsequent development of cytotoxicity.

One of the earliest responses to alloantigenic stimulus is DNA
synthesis. The effect of HU on DNA synthesis in C57BL/6 lymphocytes is shown in Figure 2. At doses of 0.5 mM or greater, HU can
shut down DNA synthesis in Con A-stimulated lymphocytes more than
90%. This effect is at least 75% reversible after 24 hours exposure at 0.5 mM, with very little loss of cell viability. There
also is little if any depressive effect of HU on the number of
blast cells produced in response to Con A.

The effect of HU on the generation of cytotoxicity in primary
and secondary MLC is shown in Figure 3. Because of non-specific

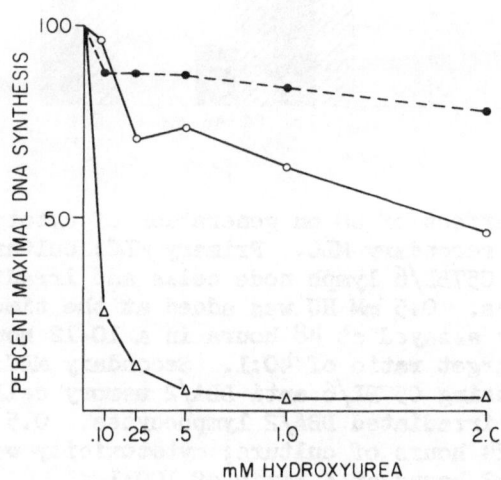

Figure 2. Effect of HU on DNA synthesis in C57BL/6 lymphocytes.
C57BL/6 lymph node cells were incubated 48 hours with 5 µg/ml
Con A. HU was added at various concentrations from 24-48 hours,
and the cells were labeled from 48-51 hours with 2 µCi ^{3}H-TdR.
△——△ : per cent maximal (no HU treatment) cpm incorporated
in the continued presence of HU. ○——○ : per cent maximal
cpm incorporated after wishing out HU. ●——● : per cent
viable Con A-stimulated cells remaining in HU-treated cultures
at 48 hours, compared with HU-untreated controls.

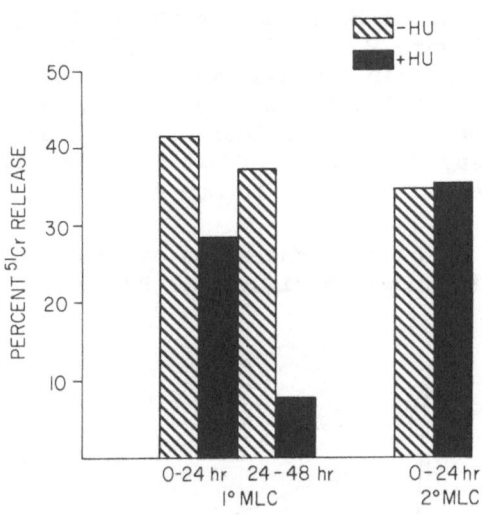

Figure 3. The effect of HU on generation of cytotoxicity in the primary and secondary MLC. Primary MLC: cultures were initiated using C57BL/6 lymph node cells and irradiated DBA/2 lymphocytes. 0.5 mM HU was added at the times indicated; cytotoxicity was assayed at 48 hours in a 10-12 hour assay at an effector's target ratio of 40:1. Secondary MLC: cultures were initiated using C57BL/6 anti-DBA/2 memory cells from primary MLC and irradiated DBA/2 lymphocytes. 0.5 mM HU was present from 0-24 hours of culture; cytotoxicity was assayed at 24 hours for 3 hours at a ratio of 100:1.

cytotoxic effects caused by prolonged exposure to HU, the effect of HU was tested for the time periods 0-24 and 24-48 hours in primary MLC. As can be seen from the data, HU has a slightly suppressive effect on generation of cytotoxicity when present from 0-24 hours, and a marked suppressive effect when present from 24-48 hours. This probably correlates with the period of active DNA synthesis. In Con-A transformed lymphocytes, there is very little DNA synthesis occurring in the first 24 hours of culture, but fairly vigorous synthesis in the second 24 hours of culture. A similar pattern of DNA synthesis has been inferred for lymphocytes reacting to allo-antigen in MLC (3,10), and the data presented here are consistent with this notion. As shown in Figure 2, exposure to HU for periods of 24 hours has only a slight effect on cell viability. In experiments not shown here, we have also found that cells exposed to HU for 24-48 hours recover their ability to become cytotoxic after removal of HU. Thus the suppressive effect on cytotoxicity is not likely due to selective elimination of antigen-reactive cells.

In contrast to the effect of HU seen in primary MLC, HU had no effect on the regeneration of cytotoxicity after restimulation in secondary MLC.

The effect of BUdR on DNA synthesis and generation of cytotoxicity in lymphocytes is shown in Figure 4. The effect of BUdR on DNA synthesis was examined in Con-A stimulated lymphocytes and in immune lymphocytes restimulated to proliferate in a secondary MLC. In a number of such experiments, the average concentration of BUdR required to reduce DNA synthesis and cell viability by 50% was approximately 200 μg/ml. In the primary MLC, BUdR caused a 50% inhibition of cytotoxicity at an average dose of 2.5 μg/ml. This differential sensitivity is consistent with patterns of selective "luxury gene" suppression in differentiating eukaryote cell systems (7). In the secondary MLC, on the other hand, BUdR had essentially no effect on the regeneration of cytotoxicity at doses less than those affecting general cell viability.

We propose the following model for terminal differentiation of cytotoxic T cells. Resting T cells, prior to encounter with the alloantigen for which they are precommitted, are not cytotoxic. Encounter with alloantigen leads to blastogenesis, DNA synthesis, and mitosis. Blastogenesis per se must be insufficient for expression of cytotoxicity, since 0.5 mM HU has no effect on the initial production of blast cells, but strongly suppresses generation of cytotoxicity. The mature, immunocompetent T cell prior to encounter with alloantigen must undergo one final differentiative event after antigenic contact before developing cytotoxic function. A round of cell division is required, during which a new genetic program is expressed (combined HU and BUdR data). This event is like the "quantal mitosis" event described by Holtzer for a variety of eukaryote cell systems (11). Once this program is established, it

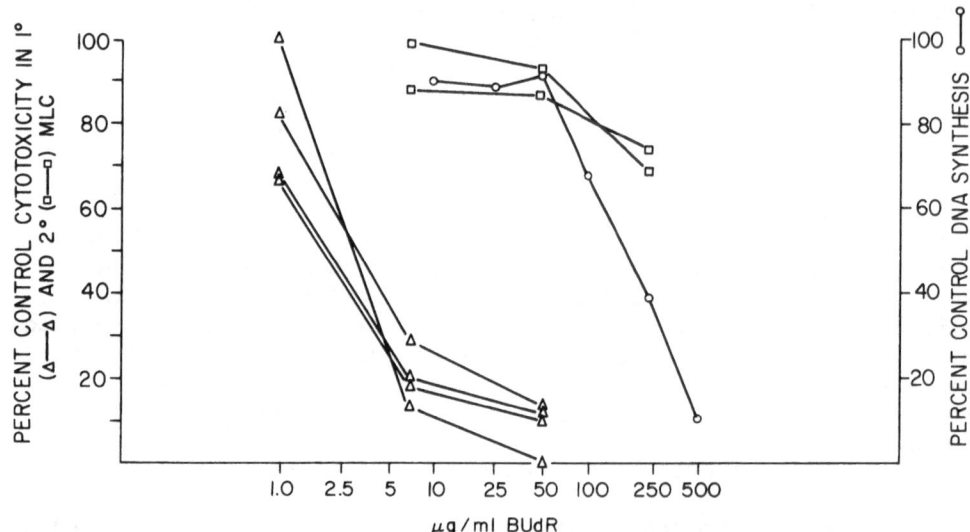

Figure 4. The effect of BUdR on generation of cytotoxicity in
primary and secondary MLC. Primary and secondary MLCs were
initiated as described in Figure 3. For primary MLC, BUdR was
present from 0-96 hours of culture, followed by a 3-hour cytotoxicity assay. For secondary MLC, BUdR was present from 0-72
hours of culture, followed by a 3-hour assay for either cytotoxicity or DNA synthesis.

is stable through the formation of cytotoxically inactive memory
cells, and into reactivation of the memory cells by exposure to
original stimulating antigen.

        The authors wish to thank Diane Heininger for technical
assistance. This study supported by NIH research grant HD-06071
and American Cancer Society research grant IM-48. WRC is the
recipient of NIH Career Development Award, AI-00009.

REFERENCES
1. Hirschberg, H. and E. Thorsby. Transplantation 16:451 (1973).
2. Zoschke, D. and F. Bach. Science 170:1404 (1973).
3. Cantor, H. and J. Jandinski. Eur. J. Immunol. 4:533 (1974).
4. Howe, M. et al. J. Immunol. 111:1234 (1973).
5. Eijsvoogel, V.P. et al. Transpl. Proc. 5:415 (1973).
6. Plant, M. et al. J. Immunol. 110:771 (1973).
7. Rutter, W.J. et al. Ann. Rev. Biochem. 42:601 (1973).
8. Cerrotini, J.C. et al. J. Exp. Med. 140:703 (1974).
9. Andersson, L. and P. Hayry. Eur. J. Immunol. 3:595 (1973).
10. Wilson, D. J. Exp. Med. 122:143 (1965).
11. Holtzer, H. Int'l Soc. Cell Biology, monograph 9, p.69 (1970).

A STUDY ON THE IMMUNOLOGICAL FUNCTION OF Fc RECEPTOR-BEARING CELLS AMONG ACTIVATED THYMOCYTES

B. Rubin, B. Hertel-Wulff and M. Høier-Madsen

Immunobiology Laboratory, Statens Seruminstitut

D-2300 Copenhagen S, Denmark

Injection of thymocytes into lethally irradiated mice generates in the spleen of the hosts a lymphoid cell population which consists mainly of T lymphocytes (1-5). This procedure has been used frequently in studies on the induction of T lymphocyte effector functions. Thus, the injection of parental thymocytes into 800 R irradiated Fl hybrid mice produces a cytotoxic T lymphocyte population specific for the H-2 antigens possessed by the other parent. The induction and expression of this particular T lymphocyte effector function have been shown not to depend on Fc receptor, C_3' receptor or membrane immunoglobulin (Ig) positive cells (2, 4). A majority of spleen cells from irradiated Fl hybrid mice injected with parental thymocytes acquire Fc receptors (3). Since, as stated above, cytotoxic T lymphocytes did not carry Fc receptors, we looked for Fc receptors (as measured by the EA-RFC assay; E = sheep erythrocytes, A = CBAxBalb/c anti-SRBC 7S antibodies, RFC = rosette forming cells (4)) on helper T lymphocytes induced by injecting syngeneic thymocytes into 800 R irradiated Fl hybrid mice together with the protein antigens: human serum albumin (HSA) or ovalbumin (OA), emulsified in complete Freund's adjuvant (CFA). In addition we investigated the development of Fc receptor bearing cells in the spleens of 800 R irradiated Fl hybrid mice injected with 1) saline, 2) syngeneic thymocytes, 3) syngeneic thymocytes and protein antigen in CFA, or 4) parental thymocytes. This was done in order to determine whether the Fc receptor bearing cells were of host origin or derived from the thymocyte inoculum and whether the Fc receptor bearing cells developed as a consequence of immunization.

As published elsewhere (4), we found that Fc receptor bearing cells may be generated by a process triggered by the physiological

Table 1.   HELPER EFFECT OF THYMOCYTES IMMUNIZED AGAINST HSA OR
            H-2 ANTIGENS IN 800 R IRRADIATED F1 HYBRID MICE

	Cells transferred			
Gr. No.	"B cells"[a]	"T cells"[b]	Antigen[c]	DNP-PFC ± SE[d]
1	DNP-KLH	-	DNP-HSA	193 ± 39
2	"	-	DNP-OA	175 ± 35
3	"	ATC-(2)	DNP-HSA	201 ± 81
4	"	ATC-(3) C	DNP-HSA	1,078 ± 105
5	"	ATC-(3) C	DNP-OA	149 ± 96
6	"	ATC-(3) P	DNP-HSA	1,288 ± 175
7	"	ATC-(3) P	DNP-OA	205 ± 55
8	"	ATC-(4)	DNP-HSA	113 ± 85

[a] Anti-Θ antiserum and complement treated spleen cells from DNP-
KLH immune mice. 20 x 10^6 cells injected per recipient mouse.

[b] 5 x 10^5 ATC was given per mouse. ATC:s harvested 7 days after
irradiation and thymocyte injection (P = passed on Ig:anti-Ig
column).

[c] 10 μg DNP-HSA or 2 μg DNP-OA was given together with immune
cells.

[d] DNP-specific plaque forming cells ± standard error of the mean
in the spleens of 500 R irradiated mice injected with the immune
cells and antigen (day 8). There were five mice per group.

Table 2.   MITOGENIC RESPONSES OF ACTIVATED THYMOCYTES AND NORMAL
            SPLEEN CELLS

	H^3-thymidine incorporation (cpm)[a]				
Mitogen/ml	N:Spl	Gr.(1)	Gr.(2)	Gr.(3)	Gr.(4)
-	1,076	856	1,258	636	1,521
1 μg PHA	42,494	3,819	28,337	27,749	4,183
1 μg Con A	60,625	1,359	31,223	27,955	2,547
10 μg LPS	37,100	723	881	507	959

[a] 5 x 10^5 spleen cells/ml cultured for 3 days, the last 18 hours
in the presence of 1 μCi H^3-thymidine (7). N:Spl = normal
spleen. Group designation, see text. ATC:s harvested 7 days
after transfer.

conditions in irradiated mice, since the percentage of Fc receptor
bearing cells in the four different groups ((1)-(4)) of mice was
very similar. However, probably due to the more pronounced proliferation of thymocytes upon immunization, the actual number of Fc
receptor bearing cells was higher (2-3 times) in groups (3) and (4)
compared with group (2) which was again 2-5 times higher than group
(1). In none of the four groups did the number of C_3'-receptor or
membrane-Ig positive cells exceed 5% (2, 4, 5). Thus, the Fc receptor bearing cells may be relatively radio-resistant, and therefore are enriched in group (1) mice, or other relatively radio-resistant cells (some T cells and macrophages (see also Table 2))
may acquire Fc receptors passively, due to the physiological conditions in irradiated mice.

Thymocytes immunized against HSA/CFA in 800 R irradiated mice
(group (3)) acquire a specific helper function, as shown in Table 1.
These helper cells were sensitive to anti-θ antiserum and complement and they passed through Ig:anti-Ig coated columns (6), indicating that they were θ positive, Fc receptor and membrane-Ig
negative cells in their effector state. Activated thymocytes
(ATC:s) from groups (1), (2) and (4) showed no helper capacity;
the same applied to group (2) and (4) cells even after Ig:anti-Ig
column passage. We have further shown that specific helper T
cells are generated from Ig:anti-Ig column passed thymocytes in
800 R irradiated mice and that the Fc receptor bearing cells among
ATC:s did not originate from the few Fc receptor bearing cells in
the thymus (0.7-3.2% EA-RFC in normal thymus, 0.01-0.05% EA-RFC in
Ig:anti-Ig column passed thymocytes (4). Thus, as was the case
with cytotoxic T cells, helper T cells were generated autonomously
and they did not express Fc receptors in their effector state.

By means of the anti-θ antiserum cytotoxicity test (6) and
the EA-RFC assay (4) we found that activated thymocyte populations
grom groups (2)-(4) contain more than 80% θ positive cells and between 20-90% EA-RFC:s (4). Thus, many EA-RFC:s must be T lymphocytes. Therefore, since the EA-RFC:s were neither cytotoxic nor
helper T cells, we tested whether the Fc receptor bearing cells
among ATC:s responded in vitro against the T cell mitogens (7):
phytohemagglutinin (PHA) and concanavalin A (Con A). The results
in Table 2 show that group (1) cells respond purely to the T cell
mitogens and not at all to a B cell mitogen, lipopolysaccharide
(LPS). In contrast, cells from groups (2) and (3) showed almost
normal responses to PHA and Con A, but did not respond to LPS.
Surprisingly, cells from group (4) only showed a very weak response to the T cell mitogens. The latter results may indicate
that T cells upon differentiation in a semiallogeneic milieu lose
their ability to respond to PHA and Con A, as was demonstrated
after in vitro mixed lymphocyte culture reactions (8). Then, are
the PHA or Con A responding cells among ATC:s Fc receptor bearing
cells? As can be seen in Table 3, PHA responding cells among

Table 3.   MITOGENIC RESPONSES OF Ig:ANTI-Ig COLUMN PASSED ATC:s
IN VITRO

| Mitogen/ml | H^3-thymidine incorporation (cpm)[a] | | | | | |
| | Gr.(2)[b] | | Gr.(3) | | Gr.(4) | |
	C[c]	P	C	P	C	P
*1 µg PHA	17,170	31,301	22,534	22,179	5,099	12,402
**1 µg "	3,227	-	4,677	-	1,390	-
*1 µg Con A	19,815	18,546	23,275	14,636	1,070	1,413
**1 µg "	4,450	-	3,165	-	114	-
*10 µg LPS	141	17	611	99	63	151
% EA-RFC	72.3	6.67	55.2	10.5	46.3	1.70
% reduction	-	90.8	-	80.9	-	96.3

a H^3-thymidine uptake in non-stimulated cultures subtracted (7).

b Group designation, see text.

c C = non-passed cells, P = Ig:anti-Ig column passed cells.

* 10 x 10^5 spleen cells/ml, ** 2 x 10^5 spleen cells/ml.

ATC:s did not express Fc receptors, whereas variable results were
obtained when testing the Con A response. However, similar results were obtained when we determined the PHA and Con A response
of normal spleen cells after fractionation on different kinds of
immunoadsorbent columns (7), i.e. the PHA response was performed
autonomously by T lymphocytes, whereas complicated effector mech-
aniams seemed to operate in the Con A response of θ positive cells.

Thus, the present results would indicate that Fc receptor
bearing cells among ATC:s did not function as T lymphocytes. However, they did not belong to the B lymphocyte population which re-
sponds to LPS (Tables 2-3). Finally, we tested whether the Fc receptor bearing cells would kill antibody coated chicken erythrocytes (CRBC) in vitro (i.e. could be defined as K lymphocytes?).
As demonstrated in Table 4, ATC:s from groups (2)-(4), but not
from group (1) did function as cytotoxic cells against antibody
coated CRBC (9). These data, together with the EA-RFC data (4),
strongly suggest that most of the Fc receptor bearing cells among
ATC:s (group (2)-(4) cells) derive from the thymocyte inoculum.
However, whether these cells (T cells?) synthesize their Fc receptors by themselves or the Fc receptors are passively adsorbed
(indicated from the EA-RFC data (4)) remains to be established.
It has been shown (10) that ATC:s can produce Fc receptor-like
substances in vitro, but it is not known whether these Fc receptor producing cells derive from the host or from the injected

Table 4. CYTOTOXIC ACTIVITY OF ATC:s AGAINST ANTIBODY COATED CHICKEN ERYTHROCYTES[a]

Effector cells	E/T ratio[b]	% ^{51}Cr release ± SD	% specific ^{51}Cr release[c]
25 x 10^5 N:Spl	50/1	61.6 ± 6.06	55.2
5 x " "	10/1	42.2 ± 2.66	35.8
1 x " "	2/1	22.6 ± 3.59	16.2
25 x 10^5 Gr.(1)	50/1	4.23 ± 2.57	2.73
25 x 10^5 Gr.(2)	50/1	29.8 ± 3.97	27.8
5 x " "	10/1	19.6 ± 2.47	17.6
1 x " "	2/1	10.0 ± 1.30	8.00
25 x 10^5 Gr.(3)	50/1	30.6 ± 2.20	28.5
5 x " "	10/1	20.7 ± 1.83	18.6
1 x " "	2/1	9.23 ± 0.40	7.16
25 x 10^5 Gr.(4)	50/1	35.0 ± 3.07	33.3
5 x " "	10/1	20.9 ± 3.38	19.2
1 x " "	2/1	12.3 ± 1.10	10.6
25 x 10^5 N:Thy	50/1	3.87 ± 0.59	1.45

[a] Spontaneous release of 5 x 10^4 CRBC/culture = 2.27 ± 0.76; N:Spl = normal spleen cells. N:Thy = normal thymocytes. SD = one standard deviation.

[b] E/T = effector cell/target cell ratio.

[c] % ^{51}Cr released by cells in presence of 10^{-3} diluted rabbit-7S-anti-CRBC antibodies minus % ^{51}Cr released by the cells without antibody.

thymocytes. Preliminary results have shown that the K lymphocytes among ATC:s were a) retained on Ig:anti-Ig columns, b) resistant to anti-θ antiserum and complement, and c) resistant to anti-H-2 antiserum and complement directed specifically against the F1 hybrid cells. Thus, even though the present data have shown that some of the Fc receptor bearing cells among ATC:s were θ negative K lymphocytes derived from the thymocyte inoculum, the biological significance of Fc receptor positive and θ positive cells is still unknown. However, the method of activation of thymocytes in 800 R irradiated mice has been shown in the present study to be of great importance in studies of both the nature of K lymphocytes and the cellular basis for autoimmunity (Fc receptors on ATC:s being rheumatoid-like factors?).

This study was supported partly by the Danish Medical Research Council.

The technical assistance of B. Rumler, L. Trier and J. Lieber-kind, and the expert secretarial assistance of A. Thorborg are gratefully acknowledged.

REFERENCES

1. Sprent, J. and Miller, J.F.A.P.: Nature New Biol. 234: 195, 1971.

2. Golstein, P., Wigzell, H., Blomgren, H. and Svedmyr, E.A.J.: Europ. J. Immunol. 2: 498, 1972.

3. Yoshida, T.O. and Anderson, B.: Scand. J. Immunol. 1: 402, 1972.

4. Rubin, B. and Hertel-Wulff, B.: Scand. J. Immunol. 4: 1975 (in press).

5. Hudson, L., Sprent, J., Miller, J.F.A.P. and Playfair, J.H.L.: Nature 251: 60, 1974.

6. Rubin, B. and Wigzell, H.: J. exp. Med. 137: 911, 1973.

7. Høier-Madsen, M. and Rubin, B.: Acta path. microbiol. scand. Section C, 1975 (in press).

8. Häyry, P. and Andersson, L.C.: Scand. J. Immunol. 3: 823, 1974.

9. Golstein, P., Schirrmacher, V., Rubin, B. and Wigzell, H.: Cell. Immunol. 9: 211, 1973.

10. Fridmann, W.H. and Golstein, P.: Cell. Immunol. 11: 442, 1974.

These references are given mostly for methodology.

RELATION OF ANTIGEN-BINDING CELLS TO IMMUNOLOGICAL MEMORY

R. Tanenbaum and D. Sulitzeanu

Lautenberg Center for General and Tumor Immunology

Hebrew University, Hadassah Medical School, Jerusalem
Israel

INTRODUCTION

It is generally accepted that a small proportion of lymphocytes
of normal animals can bind a given antigen by means of receptors
specific for that antigen (1, 2). It is assumed that a population
of lymphocytes carrying memory would contain a larger proportion of
antigen binding cells (ABC). This practically self evident point
has been extremely difficult to prove conclusively, however (3).
It is true that the number of ABC increases following immunization
(1-3), but since antibody forming cells (AFC) can also bind antigen
(1, 2, 4), the proportion of ABC which are actually memory cells
is not known. Basten et al (5) have attempted to define the
relation between ABC and the capacity to transfer memory adoptively,
but with inconclusive results.

We have approached the question as to whether memory involves
an increase in ABC by using a "pure priming" system (6). Mice were
primed to Human Serum Albumin (HSA) under conditions in which a
high level of memory was established, with minimal concomitant antibody production. ABC found in the spleens of these mice could be
consequently expected to contain very few AFC. ABC were determined
by means of a rosette technique (7), thus avoiding the difficulties
encountered by Basten et al (5) in their autoradiographic study.
An increased number of rosette forming cells (RFC) was found in the
spleen cells of primed mice. The RFC were separated by density
gradient centrifugation and used to transfer adoptively memory to
HSA. All the adoptive transfer capacity was found in the rosetted
fraction, indicating that the RFC included all the memory cells.

MATERIALS AND METHODS

HSA was coupled to sheep (SRC) or donkey (DRC) red cells by
means of conjugates of HSA with the respective anti red cell antibodies (7). Mice were primed to HSA by injecting 150 x 10[6] SRC
conjugated with HSA(SRC-HSA). The small dose of HSA contained in
the conjugate (1.8 μg) induced a high degree of sensitization (as
ascertained by response to secondary challenge with 500 x 10[6] SRC-
HSA) with very little antibody formation (pure priming). Adoptive
transfer experiments were performed by injecting spleen cells (10 x
10[6]) of normal or HSA primed donors, mixed with DRC-HSA (200 x 10[6])
where appropriate, to groups of mice irradiated with 600r. Antibody
response was measured using a hemaglutination technique. HSA specific
rosettes were prepared by centrifuging spleen cells mixed with DRC-
HSA. Suspensions enriched in rosettes were obtained by fractionating
rosette suspensions on BSA density gradients (8). Most of the spleen
cells remained on the top of the gradient, while the rosettes became
concentrated in a sharp band in the dense portion of the gradient.
Suspensions containing 12-16% RFC were routinely obtained from spleen
cells contain initially 0.4 - 0.6% RFC, i.e. up to 40 fold enrichment.
When used in adoptive transfer experiments, fractionated cells were
made up to 10 x 10[6] cells by mixing with normal spleen cells.

RESULTS

All memory cells are included in the RFC

RFC isolated by centrifugation on BSA density gradients were
tested in adoptive transfer experiments for capacity to confer
memory to irradiated recipients. As seen in Table 1, the fraction
containing rosettes contained all the memory cells, while the
rosette poor fraction was almost totally depleted of such cells.
To determine the minimal number of rosettes required for detectable
transfer of memory, graded doses of rosettes were transferred
adoptively. Memory was transferred to 5 out of 7 mice (Fig. 1) with
3000 rosettes (19.000 enriched primed cells).

The specificity of RFC for HSA was ascertained by inhibition
experiments. Treatment of spleen cells with various concentrations
of HSA before mixing with DRC-HSA resulted in a greatly diminished
number of rosettes. Similar doses of ovalbumin had no effect on
rosette formation.

A small number of HSA specific RFC was also found in the spleens
of normal mice (about 0.08%). Much smaller concentrations of HSA
were needed to inhibit rosette formation by primed cells, as compared
to normal cells, suggesting that primed RFC have a much higher
affinity for the antigen.

Table 1.   Adoptive transfer of memory by enriched rosettes

Cells transferred	Reciprocals of hemagglutinating titers
Non fractionated rosettes	920 ± 60
Rosette rich fraction	1000 ± 200
Rosette poor fraction	0
Reconstituted spleen cells	1000 ± 100

The rosette rich fraction contained 14% rosettes. Each mouse was given 10^7 cells. Antibody titers were assayed at 14 days after cell transfer.

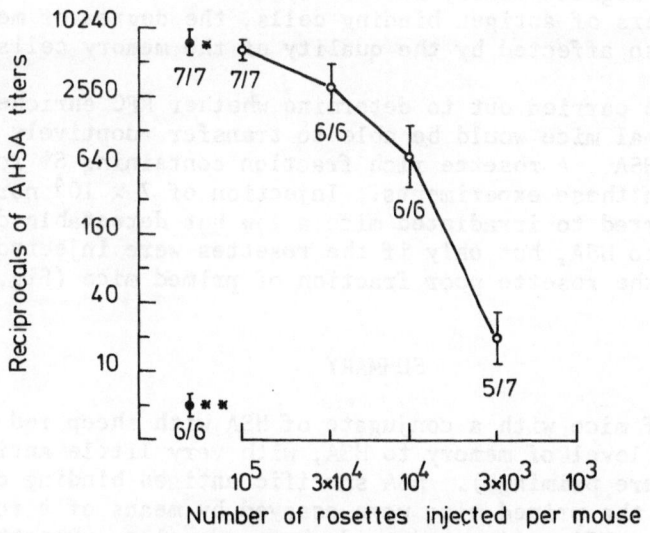

Fig. 1. Adoptive transfer of memory with graded doses of enriched rosettes. Figures indicate numbers of responding mice out of the total number injected. X: Non fractionated (4×10^4) rosettes. XX: Rosette poor fraction.

Immunological memory is associated with increased numbers of
antigen binding cells.

Having established that the antigen binding cells included the
cells carrying memory for HSA, it was possible to inquire whether
the level of RFC was or was not related to the level of immunological
memory. Primed mice were tested at various time intervals as follows
(Fig. 2): per cent RFC in the spleen and specificity of RFC for HSA;
level of anti HSA antibody in the serum before and at 14 days after
secondary challenge; capacity of the spleen cells to transfer
adoptively secondary responsiveness to HSA. Primed but non
challenged mice had negligible amounts of antibody throughout the
duration of the experiment. Progressively higher titers were
obtained following challenge, as the time intervals between priming
and challenge became greater. The number of RFC rose roughly in
parallel with the intensity of the secondary response and with the
adoptive transfer capacity of the spleen cells, up to 63 days after
priming. At all time intervals tested the rosettes preserved their
specificity to HSA. Mice examined at longer intervals after priming
(105, 230 and 390 days) had lower numbers of RFC in the spleen, yet
they possessed a high level of memory to HSA, as tested both by
direct challenge and by adoptive transfer. It was concluded that,
although immunological memory in this system is associated with
increased numbers of antigen binding cells, the degree of memory
is probably also affected by the quality of the memory cells.

Tests were carried out to determine whether RFC enriched from
spleens of normal mice would be able to transfer adoptively
reactivity to HSA. A rosette rich fraction containing 5% rosettes
was employed in these experiments. Injection of 7×10^4 normal
rosettes conferred to irradiated mice a low but detectable degree
of reactivity to HSA, but only if the rosettes were injected
together with the rosette poor fraction of primed mice (Fig. 3).

SUMMARY

Priming of mice with a conjugate of HSA with sheep red cells
induced a high level of memory to HSA, with very little antibody
production ("pure priming"). HSA specific antigen binding cells in
the spleens of the primed mice were assayed by means of a rosette
technique, using HSA conjugated to donkey red cells. Rosette
formation was almost completely inhibited by soluble HSA, thus
confirming that the RFC were specific for this antigen. Spleens
of primed mice contained up to 0.6% RFC, as compared to 0.08% HSA
specific RFC in the spleens of non immunized animals. Suspensions
enriched in rosettes (containing up to 16% RFC) were prepared by
centrifugation on BSA density gradients. Adoptive transfer
experiments showed that the rosette rich fraction contained all the
memory cells. A marginal level of memory could be transferred to

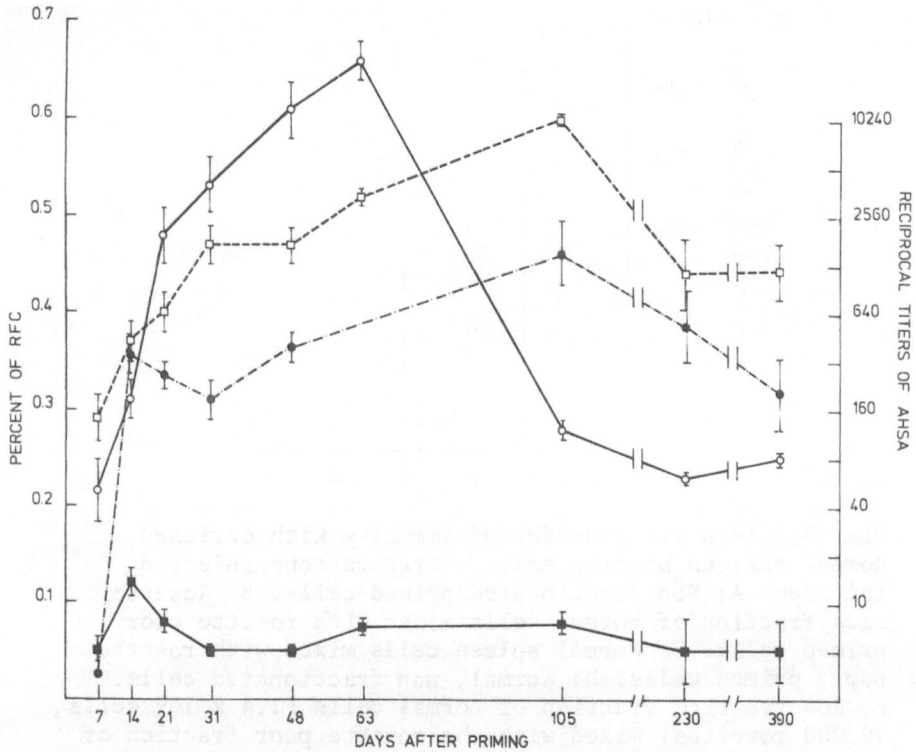

Fig. 2. Correlation of level of RFC with level of immunological memory. Primed mice were tested for: percent
RFC (o —— o), antibody titers following challenge (□---□),
antibody titers before challenge (■——■) and adoptive
transfer of memory (● --- ●). Right hand ordinate shows
haemagglutination titers.

irradiated recipients with 3000 rosettes. A comparable degree of
responsiveness to HSA could also be transferred with 70.000 RFC
enriched from spleens of non immunized mice, but only when injected
together with primed, RFC depleted spleen cells. Kinetic studies
showed that the level of memory correlated well with the number
of RFC up to two months after priming. The number of RFC decreased
at later time intervals (though remaining higher than in controls
at all times), without a corresponding decrease in the level of
memory. A change in the quality of the memory cell with time is
postulated.

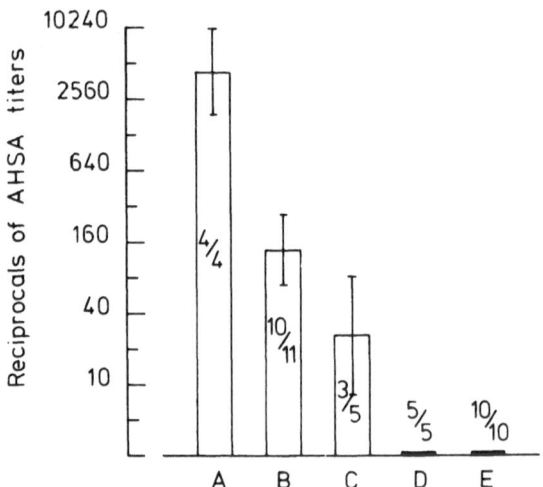

Fig. 3.   Adoptive transfer of immunity with enriched,
normal antigen binding cells.   Preparations injected
included: A: Non fractionated primed cells. B: Rosette
rich fraction of normal cells mixed with rosette poor
primed cells. C: Normal spleen cells mixed with rosette
poor, primed cells. D: Normal, non fractionated cells.
E: Rosette rich fraction of normal cells (1.4 x 10^6 cells,
70.000 rosettes) mixed with the rosette poor fraction of
normal cells.   Figures indicate number of responding mice,
out of the total injected.

REFERENCES

1.   Ada, G.L.   Transplant. Rev. 5: 105, 1970.
2.   Sulitzeanu, D.   Curr. Top. Microbiol. Immunol. 54: 1, 1971.
3.   Miller, J.F.A.P.   Immunological memory, In: Contemporary topics
     in Immunobiology, Vol. 2. Davies, A.J.S., and Carter, R.C.
     eds., p. 151, 1973.
4.   Naor, D., and Sulitzeanu, D.   Israel J. Med. Sci. 5: 217, 1969.
5.   Basten, A., Miller, J.F.A.P., Sprent, J., and Pye, J.   J. Exp.
     Med. 135: 610, 1972.
6.   Sulitzeanu, D., and Axelrad, M., Immunology, 24: 803, 1973.
7.   Sulitzeanu, D., and Haskill, J.S.   J. Immunol. Methods. 2: 11,
     1972.
8.   Tanenbaum, R., and Sulitzeanu, D.   Immunology, In press, 1975.

THE DETECTION OF IgD AND IgM ON MURINE B-LYMPHOCYTES IN CONDITIONS WHERE NO Ig CAN BE FOUND ON T-LYMPHOCYTES

Erika R.Abney and R.M.E.Parkhouse

National Institute for Medical Research

Mill Hill, London NW7 1AA, England

The crucial event in immune responses is recognition of antigen by lymphocytes. A massive body of evidence has established that the molecule responsible for antigen binding by B-lymphocytes is immunoglobulin. Curiously, there is little, if any, IgG on the surface of B lymphocytes. Instead, the major classes of Ig found are IgM and an Ig thought to be IgD (1,2,3). The presence of Ig on T-lymphocytes is not conclusively proved. Using the lactoperoxidase catalysed procedure for radiolabelling cell surfaces, some workers have prepared similar (4) or even greater (5), amounts of radioactive Ig from thymocytes as B-lymphocytes. Others (6,7,8) as well as ourselves (9), have failed to repeat this work. We can, however, demonstrate a component of thymocyte membranes which behaves like μ-chain on electrophoresis, but which is not immunoglobulin in nature.

METHODS

Spleen and thymus cell suspensions were labelled internally in the presence of ^{3}H-leucine (10), or externally with ^{125}I using lactoperoxidase (11). From the leucine-labelled cells, a plasma membrane fraction was isolated (12), which was solubilised in 1% (w/v) sodium deoxycholate. Cells labelled with ^{125}I were solubilised by a variety of procedures. In all cases Ig was purified from the soluble extract by precipitation with rabbit anti-(mouse Ig) and goat anti-(rabbit IgG) (10), and then characterised by electrophoresis in SDS-gels (13) with the addition of an internal ^{131}I-labelled marker consisting of Ig and Ig subunits (1).

Rabbits were immunised with purified MOPC 104E IgM (λ_1) or the Fab portion of Adj PC5 (γ_{2a}K) (14). After passage through

normal mouse Ig coupled to Sepharose 4B (15), the anti-IgM precipitated $\mu\lambda_1$ (MOPC 104E) and μK (TEPC 183), but was negative towards γ_1K (MOPC 21), γ_{2a}K (Adj PC5), γ_{2b}K (MOPC 195), γ_3K (FLOPC 21)
and $\alpha\lambda_2$ (MOPC 315)in a sensitive radio-immuno-assay (^{125}I-myeloma
proteins (5-10 ng) mixed with test serum (10 μl) and then precipitation of the rabbit Ig with goat anti-(rabbit Ig). The anti-Fab
reagent precipitated all classes of immunoglobulin but no other
serum protein. The IgG fractions of both antisera were prepared,
coupled to fluorescein isothiocyanate, and conjugates with fluores-
cein-protein ratios of 2-3:1 were selected by chromatography on
Whatman DE 52 (16). A goat antiserum specific for rabbit IgG was
similarly treated to yield a rhodamine conjugate. Rabbit antisera
specific for other mouse heavy chain classes were also prepared as
indicated above.

RESULTS

    B-lymphocytes. Spleen cells labelled with ^{125}I were lysed in
1% (w/v) Nonidet P40-0.1M iodoacetamide-1mM KI-1mM phenylmethylsulphonyl fluoride-PBS, centrifuged and the supernatant, containing
at least 95% of the acid-precipitable material, was passed over
Sephadex G:25 equilibrated with the solution used for cell lysis.
All operations, including precipitation of Ig, were carried out in
the cold in order to minimise proteolysis. When radioactive surface
Ig precipitated with polyspecific anti-(mouse Ig) was analysed on
SDS gels, the predominant component observed was a disulphide-link-
ed H_2L_2 structure, similar in size to monomeric IgM. Some H1 subunits were also present but neither IgG nor 19S IgM were observed.
Furthermore, on using antisera specific for mouse heavy chain
classes, we were unable to detect IgG or IgA. With anti-μ chain,
however, some, but not all, of the surface Ig was precipitated,
and on reduction yielded a heavy chain the same size as authentic
(secreted) μ chain. The Ig remaining after precipitation with anti-
μ chain was isolated by addition of anti-K chain, but in this case
reduction revealed a heavy chain of size intermediate between μ and
γ. Thus in addition to monomeric IgM, there exists on the surface
of mouse B-lymphocytes an Ig class which does not react with anti-μ,
anti-α or anti-γ chain sera. Because of similarities in heavy chain
size, susceptibility to proteolysis, and location (i.e. found on
lymphocyte surfaces), we have concluded that this Ig class is the
murine homologue of IgD. The size of the heavy chain excludes the
possibility of it being IgE.

    This candidate for IgD is a major cell surface component, com-
prising 40% of surface Ig from splenic lymphocytes and 70% of surface Ig from lymph node cells. Remaining Ig is entirely accounted
for as IgM. The difference between spleen and lymph nodes may reflect
the presence of a more mature population of B-lymphocytes in the
latter location. Interestingly, the ratio of IgM:IgD was the same

in spleen cells from normal, 6 week old, CBA mice and nude mice. Expression of IgD on the cell surface is therefore independent of T-lymphocytes. Furthermore, using the same methodology we never recovered either IgM or IgD from thymocytes or peripheral T-lymphocytes. In foetal liver or neonatal spleen and liver, however, only IgM was found. Thus IgM precedes IgD in embryological development in the mouse, as would be expected if, as seems the case, IgD appears subsequent to IgM in evolution (17). Earlier assumptions that IgD precedes IgM in the human were based on comparisons between cord and adult blood (18,19), and appear to be incorrect (20).

The distribution of IgM and IgD on individual cells was studied by staining live cells with fluorescent antibodies in an experimental design based on the radiolabelling experiments described above. The crucial assumption, which is supported by the labelling data (1,2) is that IgM and IgD are the major Ig classes present of lymphocyte surfaces. The possibility of very low numbers of IgG-bearing cells or the presence of very small amounts of surface IgG will not influence the experimental approach. Since IgM and IgD cap independently on human lymphocytes (18,19), our protocol consisted of first capping IgM using rabbit anti-(mouse μ chain) and rhodamine-labelled goat anti-(rabbit IgG). The cells were then reacted with a polyspecific fluorescein-coupled rabbit anti-(mouse γ_{2a} K Fab) under non-capping conditions (0.03M sodium azide, 0°). For reasons given above, the green rings visualised by the second reagent must represent IgD. Using this double staining procedure, splenic lymphocytes from 6 week old, SPF, female CBA mice could be classified into three groups. A large number (31-41% of total Ig-bearing cells) which were capped with anti-μ subsequently stained peripherally with anti-Fab (i.e. surface IgM and IgD simultaneously present). The remaining stained cells were divided between those showing only caps (i.e. surface IgM only) (17-29% of Ig-bearing cells) and those showing only green rings (i.e. surface IgD only)(37-45% of total Ig-bearing cells). In the doubly stained cell population there was considerable variation in the relative intensities of the two fluoorochromes, suggesting a variation in the IgM to IgD ratio from cell to cell. Complete capping of IgM occurred in the first stage, since fluorescein-labelled anti-μ failed to reveal ring staining of cells previously capped in the first staining step.

The biological significance of these subpopulations of B-lymphocytes remains to be established. However, the fact that IgM precedes IgD in ontogeny does suggest a developmental sequence. Thus the B-lymphocytes, originally expressing only IgM, matures to a cell expressing only IgD via an intermediate cell type with both classes of Ig on its surface.

The simultaneous expression of two Ig classes on the cell surface has implications for "switch" and V - C gene integration mech-

anisms. While it is quite possible that an explanation be sought
in the half-life of mRNA for μ and δ chains, it is intriguing to
consider that there is simultaneous transcription of the genes for
the two heavy chains. Were this to be so, then the possibility of
simultaneous integration of all C_H genes with V_H genes is raised.
Based on the probability that a given lymphocyte expresses only one
V_H gene (21), then simultaneous integration of all C_H genes would
require a copy-choice mechanism (22) for V - C gene integration.
The advantage of simultaneous integration of all C_H genes early in
the ontogeny of a B-lymphocyte is that questions relating to Ig
class expression would then revolve entirely around differential
gene activation and repression; the requirement to account for a
V - C gene integration event at this stage of differentiation
would no longer exist.

T-lymphocytes. We have been unable to demonstrate Ig on the
surface of thymocytes or peripheral T-lymphocytes (23) when the cells
were labelled externally with ^{125}I. The cells were extracted with
1% (w/v) Nonidet P40, 1% (w/v) sodium deoxycholate or 9M urea -
1.5M acetic acid. In all cases, essentially all of the radioactivity
incorporated into the cells was recovered in soluble form after
adding the extractant. Removal of low molecular weight material
by dialysis resulted in excellent recovery of TCA-precipitable material in detergent lysates; but aggregation caused highly variable
yields (10-80%)when acid-urea lysates were dialysed. Addition of a
variety of anti-(mouse Ig) reagents (with specificities to all
known classes of heavy and light chains) to dialysed lysates failed
to precipitate detectable amounts of mouse Ig. Ig was also absent
when inhibitors of proteolysis (Trasylol, phenylmethylsulphonyl
fluoride, iodoacetamide and ϵ -aminocaproic acid) were added at the
moment of cell lysis and during the isolation procedures. These
results contrast with those we obtained with splenic lymphocytes,
where Ig was readily detectable; Nonidet P40 gave best results,
sodium deoxycholate was satisfactory and acid-urea was erratic.
Because Marchalonis and Cone have emphasised that thymocyte Ig is
not solubilised by Nonidet P40, the pellet obtained after centrifuging Nonidet P40 extracts of labelled thymocytes was extracted
with acid-urea, but results were again negative.

If Ig was present on thymocytes, but inaccessible to iodination, then this should be revealed by internal labelling. Accordingly, thymocytes were labelled in vitro with ^{3}H-leucine for 4-24 hr
and their plasma membranes were prepared. However, we were unable
to detect Ig in these plasma membrane samples (detection limit:
0.1% of total radioactivity), although similarly prepared plasma
membranes from spleen cells contained easily demonstrable Ig (3%
of total radioactivity). When internally labelled spleen cells
were added either to a gross excess of unlabelled spleen cells or
thymocytes, the plasma membranes prepared in both cases contained

similar amounts of Ig. We are therefore confident that our negative
data for thymocytes is not due to proteolysis.

The experiments above argue against the presence of Ig on the
surface of thymocytes. In order to complete our study, we turned
to the system of "metabolic release" (24).

Here, ^{125}I-labelled thymocytes are incubated in vitro for 2-4
hours and the medium is used as a source of cell surface proteins.
Using this system it has been claimed (24) that Ig is released from
thymocytes and is cytophilic for macrophages. The Ig was characterised as a polypeptide with the mobility of a μ-chain on SDS-gels.
In our experiments, surface labelled thymocytes were cultured in
vitro for 4 hr. The culture medium was dialysed against cold PBS
and divided into three portions: (a) Control, no treatment, (b)
Nonspecific precipitation, normal rabbit IgG plus goat anti-rabbit
IgG (c) Anti-Ig precipitation, rabbit anti-(mouse IgM (λ_1), IgA
(λ_2), IgG$_1$ (K), IgG$_{2a}$ (K), and free K chains) plus goat anti-
(rabbit IgG). The precipitates were removed and the supernatants
were incubated with macrophages (peritoneal exudate cells from mice

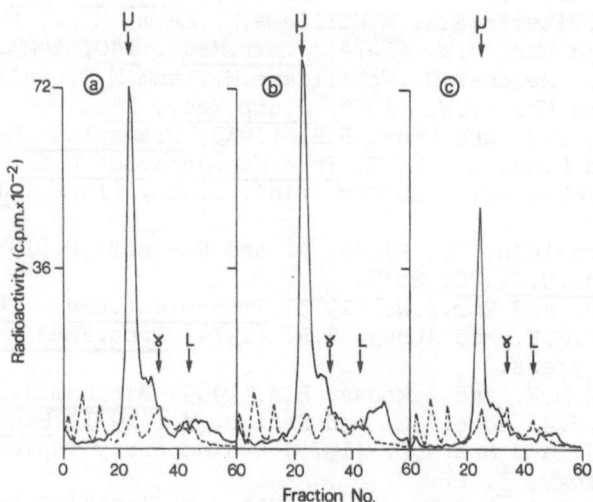

Fig.1. Absorption of material released from labelled thymocytes
in vitro to macrophages. Analysis on 4.2% (w/v) SDS gels of reduced samples. Macrophages incubated in (a) Control medium (b)
Medium after removal of non-specific Ag-Ag precipitate (c) Medium
after removal of anti-(mouse Ig) precipitate. ^{125}I-surface labelled material is represented by the solid line and ^{131}I-labelled
internal markers by the dotted line.

given 1 ml 2% protease peptone intraperitoneally 4 days previous to
sacrifice) for 90 min at 0°. The incubation conditions were such
that 2.5 x 10⁵ macrophages were mixed with released material from
2 x 10⁶ thymocytes. The cells were pelleted, washed in PBS and
applied to SDS gels with or without reduction in dithiothreitol.

Comparable amounts of radioactivity (about 4% total input) was
absorbed to macrophages when all three samples were tested. On gel
analysis of reduced samples, most of the absorbed material was found
to migrate in the same position as μ-chain (Fig.1). However this
component was found when the cells were incubated with all three
sources of cell surface material. Since one of the samples was
absorbed with polyspecific anti-(mouse Ig) (Fig.1c), the radioactive
material in the μ chain position cannot be immunoglobulin. Furthermore, when the samples were not reduced prior to gel analysis, the
major peak in the μ-chain position persisted in the absence of a
radioactive component in the position of monomeric IgM. It is
possible, but not conclusively proved, that this molecule has previously been mistaken for immunoglobulin.

References

1. Abney, E.R. and Parkhouse, R.M.E. (1974) Nature, 252,600.
2. Melcher, U.,Vitetta,E.S.,McWilliams,M.,Lamm, M.E., Phillips-Quagliata,
       J.M. and Uhr, J.W. (1974) J.exp.Med., 140, 1427.
3. Vitetta,E.S., Melcher,U.,McWilliams,M.,Lamm,M.E.,Phillips-Qaugliata,
       J.M. and Uhr, J.W. (1975) J.exp.Med., 141, 206.
4. Marchalonis, J.J. and Cone, R.E. (1973) Transplant.Rev., 14, 3.
5. Moroz,C. and Hahn, Y. (1973) Proc.Nat.Acad.Sci.U.S., 70, 3716.
6. Grey, H.M.,Kubo, R.T. and Cerottini, J.-C., (1972) J.exp.Med.,136,
       1323.
7. Lisowska-Bernstein, B., Rinuy, A. and Vassalli,P.(1973) Proc.Nat.
       Acad.Sci.U.S.,70, 2879.
8. Vitetta, E.S. and Uhr,J.W. (1973) Transplant.Rev., 14, 50.
9. Parkhouse, R.M.E. and Abney, E.R. (1974) Proc.FEBS meeting, 1974,
       in the press.
10.Parkhouse, R.M.E. and Askonas, B.A.(1969) Biochem.J., 115, 163.
11.Marchalonis,J.J.,Cone,R.E. and Santer, V. (1971) Biochem.J.,124,921.
12.Crumpton,M.J. and Snary,D. (1974) Contemporary Topics in Molecular
       Immunology, 3, 27.
13.Summers,D.F.,Maizel,J.V. and Darnell,J.E. (1965) Proc.Nat.Acad.Sci.
       U.S., 54, 505.
14.Knopf,P.M.,Parkhouse, R.M.E. and Lennox,E.S.(1967)Proc.Nat.Acad.Sci.
       U.S., 58, 2288.
15.Axen,R.,Porath,J.and Ernback,S.(1967) Nature, 214, 1302.
16.Cebra,J.J. and Goldstein,G. (1965) J.Immunol. 95, 230.
17.Spiegelberg,H.L. (1975) Nature, 254, 723.
18.Knapp,W.,Bolhuis,R.L.H.Radl,J. and Hijmans,W.(1973) J.Immunol.111,
       1295.
19.Rowe,D.S.Hug,K.,Forni,L. and Pernis, B. (1973) J.exp.Med.,138,965.

20. Vossen, J.M. and Hijmans,W. (1975) Ann.N.Y.Acad.Sci.,254, In the
        press.
21. Salsano, P., Froland,S.S.,Natvig, J.B. and Michaelsen, T.E.(1974)
        Scand.J.Immunol., 3, 841.
22. Williamson, A.R. (1971) Nature, 231, 359.
23. Julius, M.H., Simpson, E. and Herzenberg, L.A. (1973) Eur.J.Immunol.
        3, 645.
24. Cone, R.E.,Feldmann, M., Marchalonis, J.J. and Nossal, G.J.V. (1974)
        Immunology, 26, 49.

Acknowledgements

E.R.Abney thanks the Consejo Nacional de Ciencia y Tecnologia de
Mexico for financial support. We thank Iain Hunter and Gill Priestley
for their assistance in the experimental work.

THE INFLUENCE OF "I" REGION ANTIBODIES ON TRANSPLANTS

D.A.L. DAVIES AND N.A. STAINES

Searle Research Laboratories, Lane End Road

High Wycombe, Bucks, HP12 4HL ENGLAND

INTRODUCTION

The role of antibody in graft rejection is a vexed question. There are many reports of graft rejection apparently mediated by antibody but equally antibody clearly has protective effects under some circumstances. One has not been able to predict with total assurance the outcome of exposing a transplant to an antiserum directed against it. Clearly this multiparametric situation is amenable to analysis and it is desirable to do so because passive enhancement, by which we mean the prolongation of graft survival by passively administered anti-graft antiserum, is the one tangible hope at the present for generating donor-specific immunosuppression in transplantation. The inadequacies of drug and ALS therapy and the total failure to achieve transplant tolerance in adults makes this analysis all the more pressing.

The original definition of passive enhancement in tumour systems has created a (psychological) barrier to understanding its relevance to the transplantation of normal tissues. This is unjustified as passive enhancement has been unequivocally demonstrated in many animal species and with transplants of heart, kidney and skin.

A considerable effort has been invested in identifying the class of antibody involved in prolonging survival and this has been motivated partly by a lack of correlation between serological titre and enhancing activity and partly by the assumption that complement-fixing antibody must <u>a priori</u> be damaging to a graft. As far as we are concerned this argu-

ment must rest with the recent observations that several different
classes of antibody can enhance and that not any one in particular
possesses this property (1).

We have concerned ourselves with defining the specificity
of antibody responsible for mediating passive enhancement.
This was initially stimulated by the realization that there were
antigens, other than those easily detected serologically (i.e.
H-2, HL-A, Ag-B), of the major histocompatibility complex (MHC)
that were of crucial importance in determining the fate of a
transplant (2,3).

EXPERIMENTS IN RODENTS

Enhancement of Rat Heart Allografts

Antisera were raised between Ag-B (=H-1) different strains
of rats in the combination (Wag x A/gus) → A/gus. These sera,
used in 6 doses of 1ml each over the 9 days post transplantation
prolonged indefinitely the survival of hemizygous auxiliary heart
transplants.   The removal of conventional Ag-B antibody from the
sera by exhaustive absorption with donor strain red blood cells
(RBC) (4) or blood platelets (5) in no way diminished the
enhancing capacity of the antisera.   The enhancing activity of
the RBC absorbed antisera was shown not to be due to antigen-
antibody complexes as reabsorption with recipient strain spleen
cells (possessing F_c receptors for complexes) did not remove
activity whereas donor strain spleen absorption did (4).
Moreover one would not expect RBC to be a suitable source of
antigen for this anyway because RBC do not sensitize for graft
rejection (6).

The absorbed sera retained a small degree of lymphocytotoxic activity which was absorbable by donor strain lymphoid
cells but not liver, RBC or platelets (4).   These properties
clearly distinguished it from conventional Ag-B antibody and
showed its similarity to antibodies raised in mice to products
of the I region of the MHC (7). This indicated that these
enhancing sera had specificity for antigens of the I region of
the rat MHC (4).

Enhancement of Mouse Skin Allografts

These studies were extended to the mouse where there is
the advantage of more extensive genetic knowledge.   Although
mouse skin, unlike rat hearts, can never be enhanced indefinitely,
clear enhancing effects of RBC-absorbed H-2 sera were found,
confirming the rat experiments (8,9).   The absorbed antisera

had serological properties described above and further analysis showed they had specificity for Ia antigens (10) which are products of the I regions of the mouse MHC (11,12).

Not only was graft survival prolonged by sera that were unreactive with conventional H-2 antigens (K,D) but it was also prolonged by Ia antisera that gave only partial coverage of the Ia antigen incompatibility of the graft (12,13), demonstrated either in third party grafting combinations or by using sera fractionated into their constituent Ia specificities.   These results are of course relevant to the clinical situation where in active or passive enhancement a total coverage of the relevant antigens might not be achieved easily (see following sections).

The role of conventional K,D antibody in enhancement must be trivial.   Its removal from enhancing sera does not affect their potency and moreover the activity of K,D antibody recovered by acid elution from the absorbing RBC was either weak or immeasurable (12).   These results are reminiscent of earlier findings that D-end incompatible skin grafts were less easily enhanced than K-end incompatible grafts (14).   In most cases the K-end incompatibilities involved I region differences although that was not appreciated at the time the experiments were conducted.

The prolongation of graft survival by Ia sera is specific and in preliminary experiments we can find no evidence of any immunosuppressive effects of host directed Ia sera (unpublished).

The mechanism whereby anti-graft Ia sera exert their immunosuppressive effect is only partly defined.   In common with other observations on skin graft enhancement the sera are best administered at or near the time of grafting and there is no advantage in prolonged administration.   Grafts are still rejected within three weeks.   The recognition phase of the immune response against a graft is in some way inhibited (or diverted):   this is reflected by the fact that enhancing Ia sera will inhibit mixed lymphocyte culture (MLC) reactions when directed against the stimulating cell type (15,16).   Again, in this system pretreatment of stimulator cells is sufficient to suppress the MLC reaction even if no additional serum is added through the culture period (16).

The result of interfering with the effector phase in this way is, according to published data, to suppress in some rather ill-defined way the immune reactivity of host lymphocytes to graft antigens.   The nature of this suppression is not understood. nor is it clear why an enhanced skin graft, but not a kidney graft, is ultimately rejected, unless this can be attributed to the Ia positive character of skin itself while kidney may be Ia positive only by virtue of its passenger cells.

CLINICAL DATA

As far as one can tell, active enhancement has never been intentionally employed for kidney transplantation but it was reported some years ago to be effective for human skin transplants (17).   Passive enhancement of kidney transplants has been attempted, with rather little success, using F(ab')$_2$ fragments of HL-A antibodies (18).   We would attribute the failure of this trial to the use of the wrong antibody.

There is considerable evidence in a number of clinical studies that supports our theory that "I" region antibodies (or LD antibodies as they may be more conveniently called in man) are responsible for prolonging graft survival.   We would dismiss conventional SD HL-A antibody as an enhancing agent because it clearly can have profound graft damaging effects frequently leading to hyperacute rejection.   The evidence that LD antibodies prolong graft survival in man rests on the observations that transplant patients retain kidneys longer if they have preformed antibodies as a result of haemodialysis (19,20,21) and that transplanted hearts survive longer in patients that have previously undergone open-heart surgery and have been therefore polytransfused (22).   The in vitro detection of LD antibody has not been extensively pursued but in two cases (19,22) MLC blocking factors were present in recipient sera.   It has been shown very recently that platelet absorbed HL-A sera (i.e. LD reagents) will block MLC (23) in a way similar to Ia sera in the mouse (15,16).   Thus in these clinical studies, the exclusion of SD cross-match positive individuals leaves behind a number of recipients who have preformed blocking antibody which we believe mediates its effect by enhancement.   It is not directly damaging to the graft.   We therefore believe that LD sera (=Ia sera by homology) prepared by absorbing SD antibody from HL-A sera with donor-type platelets are the appropriate agents to generate donor-specific immunosuppression for clinical transplantation.

REFERENCES

1.   Rubinstein, P.,   Decary, F. and Streun, E.W., J. Exp. Med., 140:591, 1974.

2.   Amos, D.B. and Yunis, E.J., Cell Immunol., 2:517, 1971.

3.   Yunis, E.J. and Amos, D.B., Proc. Nat. Acad. Sci. U.S.A., 68:3031, 1971.

4. Davies, D.A.L. and Alkins, B.J., Nature, 247:294, 1974.

5. Davies, D.A.L., Transplant. Proc., 7:443, 1975.

6. Medawar, P.B., in Albert and Medawar (Eds.), "Biological Problems of grafting", Blackwell, Oxford, p.6, 1959.

7. Hauptfeld, V., Klein, D. and Klein, J., Science, 181:167,1973.

8. Staines, N.A., Guy, K. and Davies, D.A.L., Transplantation, 18:192, 1974.

9. Archer, J.R., Smith, D.A., Davies, D.A.L. and Staines, N.A., J. Immunogenetics, 1:337, 1974.

10. Shreffler, D.C. and David, C.S., Advs. Immunol., 20: in press.

11. Staines, N.A., Ashton, L.J., Cuthbertson, J.L. and Davies, D.A.L., Tissue Antigens, submitted.

12. Staines, N.A., Guy, K. and Davies, D.A.L., Eur.J.Immunol., submitted.

13. Staines, N.A., Behring Inst. Mitteilung., 57: in press, 1975.

14. McKenzie, I.F.C. and Snell, G.D., J. Exp. Med., 138:259, 1973.

15. Meo, T., David, C.S., Rijnbeek, A.M., Nabholz, M., Miggiano, V.C. and Shreffler, D.C., Transplant. Proc., 7:127, 1975.

16. Fish, F., Cuthbertson, J.L. and Staines, N.A., in preparation.

17. Rapaport, F.T., Dausset, J., Lawrence, H.W. and Converse, J.M., Surgery, 64:25, 1968.

18. Batchelor, J.R., Ellis, F., French, M.E., Bewick, M., Cameron, J.S. and Ogg, C.S., Lancet, 2:1007, 1970.

19. Sengar, D.P.S., Opelz, G. and Terasaki, P.I., Transplant. Proc., 5:641, 1973.

20. Opelz, G., Sengar, D.P.S., Mickey, M.R. and Terasaki, P.I., Transplant. Proc., 5:253, 1973.

21. Murray, S., Dewar, P.J., Uldall, P.R., Wilkinson, R., Kerr, D.N.S., Taylor, R.M.R. and Swinney, J., Tissue Antigens, 4:548, 1974.

22. Caves, P.K., Stinson, E.B., Griepp, R.B., Rider, A.K.,
    Dong, E. and Shumway, N.E., Surgery, 74:307, 1973.

23. vanRood, J.J., vanLeeuwen, A., Keuning, J.J. and
    Termijtelen, A., Transplant. Proc., 7:31, 1975.

VIRUS-IMMUNE CYTOTOXIC T CELLS ARE SENTIZED TO BY VIRUS SPECIFICALLY ALTERED STRUCTURES CODED FOR IN H-2K OR H-2D: A BIOLOGICAL ROLE FOR MAJOR HISTOCOMPATIBILITY ANTIGENS

ROLF M. ZINKERNAGEL and PETER C. DOHERTY

Department of Microbiology, The John Curtin School of

Medical Research, A.N.U. Canberra, Australia

We discovered quite fortuitously that specific T cell-mediated lysis (^{51}Cr release) of target cells (macrophages, tumor cells or fibroblasts) infected with lymphocytic choriomeningitis (LCM) virus occurs only if lymphocyte and target are compatible at the H-2 gene complex[1,2]. Experiments with ectromelia (mousepox)[3] and paramyxovirus (Sendai)[2] infection indicate that this may be a general phenomenon, as these three viruses differ considerably in their effects at the molecular level. This view is further reinforced by the demonstration, from other laboratories, that the same constraint applies in the cytotoxic T cell response to trinitrophenyl (TNP)-modified mouse lymphocytes[4], and in Rous sarcoma virus infection of chickens[5].

Genetic mapping studies[2,6] have shown conclusively that compatibility at either the K or the D region of one H-2 haplotype is sufficient for this lytic interaction to occur. Providing that this requirement is satisfied presence of unshared H-antigen specificities seems to have no inhibitory effect. Furthermore the Ir-Ss regions are not obviously involved, either in a primary or in a regulatory role. The phenomenon appears to be associated with identity at the serologically-defined H-2 private specificities, the strong transplantation antigens. Less detailed animal experiments indicate that the same constraint applies to T cell-mediated immunity _in vivo_, in LCM (immunopathology)[2], ectromelia[7] and _Listeria monocytogenes_[8] infection (protection).

This requirement for H-2K or H-2D compatibility may be explained in one of two ways[1,2,9,10]: 1. Genes mapping at, or near to, H-2K or H-2D code for physiological recognition structures, mutuality of which is mandatory for lymphocyte-target interaction. This is additional to recognition of virus-specified cell-surface antigens by an immunologically specific T cell receptor. 2. A single T cell receptor recognises 'altered self' antigens, the self components involved being coded for with the H-2K or H-2D regions. Altered self may be thought to reflect some complex of viral and H antigens, or more long range virus-induced changes of the H antigens themselves.

Two experimental protocols have been used to differentiate between these possibilities[1]: Further proliferation of antigen-stimulated lymphocytes in vivo, and 'cold-target' competitive inhibition of cytotoxicity in vitro. The results of both approaches indicate that different clones of virus-immune T cells are associated with each parental haplotype, in F_1 mice, and with H-2K or H-2D. The first possibility can only be true if the postulated physiological recognition structure exhibits allelic exclusion, and if only one of the gene products coded for at H-2K or H-2D is expressed in each clone of immune T cells[1,2]. The much more likely possibility would seem to be that T cells are sensitized to 'altered self' - structure coded for at H-2K or H-2D must form at least part of the sensitizing antigen. Recognition of virally or chemically modified cells[4], of allo-antigens[11] and of xenoantigens[12] may thus be accommodated within the same model.

An essential implication of these findings is that the surveillance (cytotoxic?) T cell is programmed to monitor H antigen structural integrity. A central function of the H antigens themselves may thus be to signal changes in self to the immune system. Furthermore, as a greater number of T cell specificities are induced in F_1 mice (4 instead of 2 in homozygotes), operation of such a mechanism provides a biological basis for overall selective advantage for heterozygotes[1,2]. Maintenance of the high level balanced polymorphism observed in the major H antigen systems is best explained by their being evolutionary advantage for heterozygosity, in the absence of positive selection for any particular H antigen type[13].

Also, in all of the virus models examined, some H-2K or H-2D types (which differ for each virus) are associated with low responsiveness[1,2,6]. Presence of a great variety of H antigen types thus decreases the chance of unresponsiveness being general throughout the population, whereas operation of many different selective forces would minimize evolutionary advantage for any particular H-2 type.

REFERENCES

1. Zinkernagel, R.M., Doherty, P.C.   Nature, 1974, 248, 701;
    251, 547. J.exp.Med. 1975, 141, 1427.

2. Doherty, P.C., Zinkernagel, R.M.   Transplant.Rev. 1974, 19,
    89. J.exp.Med. 1975, 141, 502. J.Immunol. 1975, 114, 30.
    Nature (in the press), Lancet (in the press). Unpublished
    data.

3. Gardner, I., Bowern, N.A., Blanden, R.V.   Eur.J.Immunol.
    1975, 5, 122.

4. Shearer, G.M.   Eur.J.Immunol. 1974, 4, 527.

5. Wainberg, M.A., Markson, Y., Weiss, D.W., Doljanski, F.
    F.Proc.Natl.Acad.Sci. U.S.A. 1974, 71, 3565.

6. Blanden, R.V., Doherty, P.C., Dunlop, M.B.C., Gardner, I.D.,
    Zinkernagel, R.M., David, C.S.   Nature, 1975, 254, 269.

7. Blanden, R.V., Bowern, N.A., Pang, T.E., Gardner, I.D.,
    Parish, C.R. Aust.J.exp.Biol.med.Sci. (in the press).

8. Zinkernagel, R.M.   Nature, 1974, 251, 230;   Ph.D Thesis,
    Australian National University, 1975.

9. Katz, D.H., Hamaoka, T., Dorf, M.E., Benacerraf, B.   Proc.
    Natl.Acad.Sci. U.S.A. 1974, 70, 2624.

10. Shevach, E.M., Rosenthal, A.S.   J.exp.Med. 1973, 138, 1213.

11. Bevan, M.J.   J. Immunol. 1975, 114, 317.

12. Lindahl, F.F., Bach, F.H.   Nature, 1975, 254, 607.

13. Burnet, F.M.   Nature, 1973, 245, 359.

RESTRICTION BY H-2 GENE COMPLEX OF THE TRANSFER OF DELAYED TYPE HYPERSENSITIVITY IN MICE

J.F.A.P. Miller and M.A. Vadas

Walter and Eliza Hall Institute of Medical Research

Royal Melbourne Hospital, Melbourne 3050, Australia

Specific lysis of virus infected cells in mice occurs when immune T cells and their targets share at least one H-2 haplotype. Homology is essential in the K or D region, not in the I region (1). On the other hand, optimal induction of helper T cells by macrophage associated antigen requires identity at the I-A region of major histocompatibility complex (2). In this paper, we present the results of preliminary investigations designed to determine whether the ability of sensitized lymphoid cells to transfer delayed type hypersensitivity (DTH) to normal mice is restricted by the H-2 complex.

MATERIALS AND METHODS

Mice

Highly inbred strains used were CBA, C57BL, B10.A(2R), B.10A(4R) and A.TL.

Sensitization

This was performed using fowl gamma globulin (FGG) or dinitro-fluorobenzine (DNFB) as described elsewhere (3).

Transfer of Sensitized State

Lymph node cells from sensitized donors were taken at the peak
period of sensitivity and injected intravenously into normal mice.
These were immediately challenged with the appropriate antigen to
test for transfer of the sensitive state as described in detail
elsewhere (4).

Test for DTH

This was performed by our radioisotopic method (3). In brief,
10 μl of the appropriate concentration of the test antigen was
injected intradermally (in the case of FGG) or painted (in the
case of DNFB) in or on the left pinna. A control solution was used
for the right pinna. 10 hours later 2 μCi of iododeoxyuridine-
^{125}I (^{125}I-UdR) (specific activity 4-6 μCi/μg) was given intravenously and the pinnae cut off at the hairline after a further 16
hours. The radioactivity of the pinnae was counted in gamma
spectrometer and the results expressed as the ratio of the radioactivity in counts per minute of the left pinna over that of the
right pinna (^{L}/R ^{125}I-UdR uptake). A ratio of around 1.0 implies no
sensitivity whereas a ratio of 1.5 or more indicates a state of
sensitivity. It has been demonstrated that this in fact reflects a
DTH response (3, 4), since (a) the ear reaction is not apparent
at 6 hours but is so at 26 or 48 hours; (b) it is associated with
a mononuclear cell infiltration (predominantly monocytic) in which
the cells are labelled in autoradiographs; and (c) it is T-cell
dependent since it fails to occur in athymic nu/nu mice or in normal
mice immunized with antigens known not to activate T cells, and it
can be transferred by purified T cells but not by lymphoid cells
depleted of T cells by pretreatment with anti-θ serum and complement.

RESULTS

Three types of experiments were performed to determine whether
the capacity of sensitized lymphoid cells to transfer sensitivity to
normal recipients might be restricted by the host's H-2 gene complex.

Experiment I

Lymphoid cells from mice sensitized to FGG were injected in
recipient mice which were then challenged intradermally in the ear
with FGG and tested for DTH by the radioisotopic assay method. The
results are shown in Table I. It is clear that maximal responses
occurred in syngeneic recipients and minimal or no responses in
allogeneic recipients. The response in semi-allogeneic recipients

was usually of an intermediate degree. Three explanations may be
given to account for the poor response in allogeneic recipients.
(1) It may be due to rejection of the injected cells. This is most
unlikely first because there is not sufficient time during the DTH
assay period to allow host sensitization to the allogeneic cells
and second because sensitized F_1 cells gave good responses in
parental recipients (group 2). (2) Alternatively, allogeneic cells
may be recruited into the spleen or liver, so that insufficient
numbers of cells are left in the circulation and hence available to
migrate to the site of challenge. This possibility deserves serious
consideration (and is the reason why expt. II was done). If,
however, recruitment accounts for the results, F_1 recipients of
sensitized parental cells should not develop such a marked ear
response (see e.g. response in F_1 recipients of CBA cells - group 1).
(3) A third possibility is that the capacity of sensitized cells
to be triggered into activity by antigen is restricted by gene
products of the H-2 complex, and will be examined in expt. III.

Table I. Effect of H-2 incompatibility on the adoptive transfer of DTH

Group	Source of lymphoid[1] cells transferred	DTH response in following recipients[2]		
		CBA	(CBAxC57BL)F_1	C57BL
1	CBA	100%[3] (2.58+0.14)	70% (2.17+0.15)	0% (1.12+0.11)
2	(CBAxC57BL)F_1	54% (1.56+0.25)	100% (2.40+0.20)	75% (1.78+0.22)
3	C57BL	6% (1.33+0.08)	30% (1.75+0.11)	100% (3.35+0.31)

[1] Donors sensitized to FGG.

[2] Recipients ear challenged with FGG and ear response measured by
radioisotopic method following IVI of ^{125}I-UdR. Approximately 5
mice per group.

[3] 100% is used for response in syngeneic system. Other percentages
derived from L/R [125] I-UdR data shown in brackets.

The above experiment has been repeated 5 times with similar results.
It has also given similar results, using DNFB.

Experiment II

A second experiment was performed to test the possibility that recruitment of sensitized cells into the spleen or liver plays a major role in dictating the magnitude of the ear response in hosts of different H-2 genotypes. Normal CBA mice were grafted on the left flank with 2 pieces of ear skin of approximately equal size, one from CBA, the other from C57BL. 4 days after grafting, when vascularization had just been established, the mice were given 2×10^7 cells from DNFB sensitized CBA or C57BL mice. The results are shown in Table II. It appears that sensitized cells produced a response of magnitude significantly greater in syngeneic than in allogeneic grafts, irrespective of the H-2 genotype of the recipient mouse. This tends to exclude recruitment of allogeneic cells to the spleen as the sole mechanism to account for the data in Table I. In the experiments in Table II, only 4 and 5 recipients, respectively, were used. These experiments are, however, being repeated using at least 10 mice per group in both CBA, C57BL and various congenic recipients.

Table II. Effect of H-2 genotype on reactivity of DNFB sensitized cells[1]

Source of sensitized lymph node cells	$\dfrac{\text{CBA ear graft}}{\text{C57BL ear graft}}$ ^{125}I-UdR uptake
	following DNFB painting of each graft 4 days after transplantation to CBA mice[2]
CBA	1.45 ± 0.09
C57BL	0.85 ± 0.17

[1] 2×10^7 lymph node cells from CBA or C57BL mice sensitized 5 days before to DNFB were given intravenously into CBA mice transplanted 4 days before with CBA and C57BL ear grafts.

[2] Each graft was painted with DNFB and the radioactivity incorporated following IVI ^{125}I-UdR measured.

Experiment III

Lymphoid cells from CBA or C57BL mice sensitized to FGG were transferred to normal recipients of strains of known H-2 genotypes and the state of sensitivity to FGG determined. The results shown in Table III indicate that identity at the I-A region, but not at the K or D regions, is required for successful transfer.

Table III. Effect of H-2 genotype on adoptive transfer of DTH
           (5 mice per group)

Strain of donor of FGG-sensitized lymphoid cells	Strain of recipients	Major histocompatibiltiy complex						$^L/_R$^{125}I-UdR uptake
		K	I-A	I-B	I-C	S	D	
CBA	CBA	k	k	k	k	k	k	2.81+0.12
	B10.A(2R)	k	k	k	d	d	b	2.45+0.31
	B10.A(4R)	k	k	b	b	b	b	2.52+0.35
	C57BL	b	b	b	b	b	b	1.11+0.08
	A.TL	s	k	k	k	k	d	2.54+0.22
C57BL	C57BL	b	b	b	b	b	b	1.63+0.14
	B10-A(2R)	k	k	k	d	d	b	1.11+0.03
	B10-A(4R)	k	k	b	b	b	b	1.05+0.03
No cells	CBA	k	k	k	k	k	k	1.10+0.04
No cells	C57BL	b	b	b	b	b	b	1.12+0.06

DISCUSSION

The preliminary results given here suggest that sensitized lymphoid cells can transfer a state of specific DTH to normal mice only if recipients share the I-A gene product of the major histocompatibility complex. Identity at K or D ends is apparently not essential. This is similar to the requirements for the induction of T helper cells by macrophage associated antigen (2), but not to specific lysis of virus infected target cells by killer T cells when homology at D or K is essential (1). We must stress that our conclusions may be premature as more experiments have to be performed to exclude other possibilities. Among these are the following. The sensitized cells may have been rejected in the allogeneic hosts or may have been diverted to organs such as liver or spleen. Alternatively, suppressor mechanisms may have prevented their ability to respond to the sensitizing antigen. Further experiments are in progress to evaluate such possibilities.

SUMMARY

Preliminary results suggest that the I-A region of the major
histocompatibility complex restricts the ability of sensitized
lymphoid cells to transfer a state of DTH to the specific antigen
in normal mouse recipients.

REFERENCES

1. Blanden, R.V., Doherty, P.C., Dunlop, M.B.C., Gardner, I.D.,
    Zinkernagel, R.M. and David, C.S. Nature 254, 269, 1975.
2. Erb, P. and Feldmann, M. in press, 1975.
3. Vadas, M., Miller, J.F.A.P., Gamble, J. and Whitelaw, A.
    Intern Arch. Allergy Appl. Immunol. in press, 1975.
4. Miller, J.F.A.P., Vadas, M.A., Whitelaw, A. and Gamble, J.
    Intern. Arch. Allergy Appl. Immunol. in press, 1975.

CHARACTERIZATION AND SPECIFICITY OF A T-CELL COOPERATIVE FACTOR

E. Mozes, R. Isac, D. Givol, R. Zakut and D. Beitsch

Department of Chemical Immunology

The Weizmann Institute of Science, Rehovot, Israel

One of the central problems in analyzing immune response phenomena, is the mechanism of thymus (T)-bone marrow (B) derived cell interactions. Investigations performed in the past few years resulted in the identification and characterization of various biologically active mediators produced by T cells which are capable of stimulating B cells. Some of these T cell factors have been shown to be antigen-specific (1-3) whereas others are non-specific (4,5), and their functional effects are either-enhancing (1-5) or suppressing (3) antibody production by B cells.

We have studied the properties of a cooperative T cell factor which is antigen specific (2). This antigen specific T cell factor is capable of replacing T cells in thymus dependent antibody responses. It is produced by antigen-educated thymocytes which are subsequently cultured for a short period in vitro in the presence of the inducing immunogen. These T cell factors have been successfully utilized in studying the cellular basis of genetic controls of immune responses to multichain synthetic polypeptide antigens since they can be used for measuring directly T and B cell functions (6-8).

The T cell factor specific to the synthetic polypeptide poly ($\underline{L}$Tyr,$\underline{L}$Glu)-poly($\underline{DL}$Ala)--poly($\underline{L}$Lys), designated (T,G)-A--L, has been the one most extensively studied. Its activity was found to be removed by passing on an antigen-immunoadsorbent, but not by anti-immunoglobulin Sepharose columns (9). The (T,G)-A--L specific T cell factor can also be adsorbed to columns coated with alloantisera specific for the major histocompatibility (H-2) haplotype of the strain in which the factor was produced and furthermore, it was removed with antisera against the I region of the same H-2 complex

(10) suggesting that the factor is a product of I region genes.

It is very likely that the specific T cell factor represents part of the recognition system of T cells for antigens. Hence it is important to establish the degree of specificity of such a factor and to find out how far the binding site of this factor resembles that of humoral antibody, as far as its specificity is concerned. Specific T cell factors to (T,G)-A--L or poly(LPhe,LGlu)-poly(DLAla)--poly(LLys), (Phe,G)-A--L were prepared as described (6). Briefly, irradiated C3H.SW mice were injected with 10^8 thymocytes and 10 µg antigen. Seven days later the spleens of these mice, which contain educated T cells, were cultured for 6 hours in serum free medium containing 2 µg/ml of antigen. The cells cultures were centrifuged and the supernatants were used as the T cell factors, and were analyzed for their cooperative activity with B cells in adoptive transfer experiments in irradiated mice. The mice were injected with either (T,G)-A--L, (Phe,G)-A--L, poly(LHis,LGlu)-poly (DLAla)--poly(LLys), (H,G)-A--L or poly(LTyr,LGlu)-poly(LPro)--poly (LLys), (T,G)-Pro--L and the immune responses were analyzed 12 days later. B cells of either C3H.SW or C3H/He mice were used according to their response to the above antigens. The specificity of the factors as measured by their helping effect is shown in Table 1. It is shown that there is a complete "cross-cooperative" effect between factors to (T,G)-A--L and (Phe,G)-A--L, i.e. when a factor to (T,G)-A--L was injected together with B cells and either (Phe,G)-A--L or (T,G)-A--L a significant immune response was obtained for both antigens. Similarly the factor to (Phe,G)-A--L was as active in eliciting immune response to either (Phe,G)-A--L or (T,G)-A--L. In addition the factor to (T,G)-A--L cross-reacted for helping the immune response to (H,G)-A--L, but failed to cooperate with B cells in eliciting antibody response to (T,G)-Pro--L. It is noteworthy that antibodies to (T,G)-A--L cross react with (Phe,G)-A--L, (H,G)-A--L and with (T,G)-Pro--L. However antibodies to (T,G)-Pro--L do not cross react with (T,G)-A--L or (Phe,G)-A--L since they are directed exclusively against the Pro--L moiety.

The specificity of the T cell factor produced with (T,G)-A--L was further analyzed using immunoadsorbent of antigens coupled to Sepharose. The (T,G)-A--L factor lost its cooperative activity in eliciting an immune response to either (T,G)-A--L or (Phe,G)-A--L after passage on immunoadsorbent of either antigen. However, no reduction in the helper activity of the (T,G)-A--L factor was detected after chromatography on an immunoadsorbent of multichain poly-DL-alanine (A--L), indicating that the cross-reactivity in the specificity of the factor between (T,G)-A--L, (Phe,G)-A--L and (H,G)-A--L is not due to the A--L moiety alone. An immunoadsorbent of (T,G)-Pro--L-Sepharose also failed to reduce the activity of the factor to (T,G)-A--L.

TABLE 1

Specificity of T cell factors

Cells and factors transferred into irradiated recipients	Antigen	Antibody titer Average $\log_2$ of hemagglutination
BM C3H.SW+Factor$_{(T,G)-A--L}$	(T,G)-A--L	6.5
BM C3H.SW+Factor$_{(T,G)-A--L}$	(Phe,G)-A--L	6.2
BM C3H/He+Factor$_{(T,G)-A--L}$	(H,G)-A--L	5.1
BM C3H.SW+Factor$_{(T,G)-A--L}$	(T,G)-Pro--L	1.1
BM C3H.SW+Factor$_{(Phe,G)-A--L}$	(Phe,G)-A--L	6.1
BM C3H.SW+Factor$_{(Phe,G)-A--L}$	(T,G)-A--L	6.0

In these experiments effort was also made to recover the factor from the immunoadsorbents and to analyze its activity in helping B cells to mount an immune response. 25 ml of (T,G)-A--L-educated T cells supernatant, derived from 50 spleens (6) were passed through a 2 ml column of (T,G)-A--L-Sepharose. The column was washed with PBS and eluted with 0·1M NH$_4$OH. The eluate, containing about 50 µg of protein was neutralized with NH$_4$HCO$_3$ and acetic acid and dialyzed against PBS. Portions of this eluate equivalent to a volume of 0.5 ml of the original T cell supernatant were injected to irradiated recipients together with B cells and antigen. As is shown in Table 2 this eluate was as active as the T cell supernatant in helping B cells to mount an immune response to (T,G)-A--L. It is also shown that the antigen immunoadsorbent eliminated the helping activity from the effluent which passed through the column.

The eluate possessing the activity of this (T,G)-A--L specific T cell factor was injected into rabbits. The activity of the rabbit antiserum was checked by mixing the T cell factor with 0.75 ml of the antiserum before the addition of B cells and antigen, and the transfer into irradiated recipients. The results given in Table 3 demonstrate that over 90% of the cooperative activity of the T cell factor is inhibited by the antiserum, whereas the normal rabbit serum used as a control did not interfere with the specific activity of the factor.

Preliminary characterization of the T cell factor purified by affinity chromatography on (T,G)-A--L-Sepharose was performed on SDS polyacrylamide gels. The major peptide chains revealed on the gel were of molecular weights of 45,000 and 70,000.

TABLE 2

Activity of a purified T cell factor specific for (T,G)-A--L

Cells and factors transferred into irradiated recipients[a]	Mean PFC/spleen	Average log$_2$ of hemagglutination titer
10^7 C3H.SW BM cells	1096 (1.10)[c]	0.8
10^7 C3H.SW BM cells + 10^8 C3H.SW thymocytes	28457 (1.11)	4.4
10^7 C3H.SW BM cells + C3H.SW T cell factor[b]	32558 (1.16)	5.7
10^7 C3H.SW BM cells + T cell factor eluted from a (T,G)-A--L Sepharose column	32774 (1.22)	5.4
10^7 C3H.SW BM cells + Effluent from a (T,G)-A--L Sepharose column	1345 (1.15)	1.6

a) Cells and factors from C3H.SW mice were transferred together with (T,G)-A--L (10 µg/mouse) into syngeneic irradiated recipients.

b) Produced by 1 spleen equivalent of "educated" T cells.

c) Geometric means of hemolytic direct PFC. Standard errors are given in parenthesis.

TABLE 3

Inhibition of the activity of a specific T cell factor by antiserum

Cells and factors transferred into irradiated recipients[a]	Mean PFC/spleen	Average $\log_2$ of hemagglutination titer
10^7 C3H.SW BM cells	1020 (1.04)[b]	1
10^7 C3H.SW BM cells + 10^8 C3H.SW thymocytes	31666 (1.12)	4.8
10^7 C3H.SW BM cells + C3H.SW T cell factor	32713 (1.14)	6.3
10^7 C3H.SW BM cells + C3H.SW T cell factor + antiserum	1794 (1.19)	0.5
10^7 C3H.SW BM cells + C3H.SW T cell factor + normal rabbit serum	32863 (1.09)	6.2

a) Cells and factors from C3H.SW mice as well as the sera were transferred together with (T,G)-A--L (10 µg/mouse) into syngeneic irradiated recipients.

b) Geometric means of hemolytic PFC. Standard errors are given in parenthesis.

Further purification and characterization of T cell specific factors to synthetic polypeptides as well as for other antigens will shed light on the nature of T cell receptors and their function in triggering B cells for antibody production or in cell mediated immunity

REFERENCES

1. Feldmann,M. (1972) J. Exp. Med. 136: 737.
2. Taussig, M.J. (1974) Nature 248: 234.
3. Tada, T. (1975) In Immune Recognition. Proceedings of the Ninth Leukocyte Culture Conference. A.S. Rosenthal, ed., Academic Press, New York, in press.
4. Schimpl, A. and Wecker, E. (1972) Nature New Biol. 237: 15.
5. Armerding, D. and Katz, D.H. (1974) J. Exp. Med. 140: 19.
6. Taussig, M.J., Mozes, E. and Isac, R. (1974) J. Exp. Med. 140: 301.
7. Mozes, E., Isac, R. and Taussig, M.J. (1975) J. Exp. Med. 141: 703.
8. Mozes, E. (1974) Progr. Immunol. II Vol. 2, L. Brent and J. Holborow, eds., North-Holland Publishing Co., p. 191.
9. Taussig, M.J. and Munro, A.J. (1974) Nature 251: 63.
10. Taussig, M.J. and Munro, A.J. (1975) In Immune Recognition. Proceeding of the Ninth Leukocyte Culture Conference. A.S. Rosenthal, ed., Academic Press, New York, in press.

Supported in part by a grant 1R01 A I 11405-03 from the National Institutes of Health, U.S. Public Health Service.

RAT ANTI-LYMPHOCYTE ALLOANTIBODIES BLOCK CON A-STIMULATION OF T

LYMPHOCYTES: INHIBITION OF A POLYCLONALLY SPECIFIC T CELL REACTION

Hartmut Wekerle

Max-Planck-Institut für Immunbiologie

D-78 Freiburg, Western Germany

Alloantisera induced in rats by immunization against allogeneic lymphocytes contain antibodies that prevent non-sensitized, immuno-logically competent T lymphocytes from recognizing foreign cellular antigen. Absorption of such blocking antisera on various tissues combined with immunogenetic analyses revealed that these blocking antibodies act by binding to a constant part of the T cell receptor, which is a non-SD product of the major histocompatibility gene locus (1).

These results were obtained in a test system that measures specific antigen binding by T lymphocytes capable of differemtia-ting to effector cells in transplant reactions. Graft rejection, however, is only <u>one</u> of the functions exerted by T lymphocytes. Other T cells, that act as regulators in humoral or in cellular immune responses (2) might differ in their receptor properties. In order to learn, how far our previous findings on the graft reactive cells are valid for the entire T cell pool, one could screen the effect of the test antisera on all the functionally different T subpopulations, or, on the other hand, check their influence on a reaction that (a) involves the vast majority of all T lymphocytes, and which (b) is triggered via the receptor structures acting in antigen mediated lymphocyte triggering.

In this communication, evidence is presented that stimulation of T lymphocytes with the lectin ConA reflects polyclonally specific activation of the majority of all T lymphocytes. Since the early stages of the ConA reaction can be effectively blocked by T cell receptor blocking antisera, we conclude that (a) ConA acts via the T cell receptor, and (b) that a large proportion, if not all popula-tions of the T cell pool share identical antigen receptor properties.

MATERIALS AND METHODS

We used Lewis,BN and congenic L.BN and L.BDV inbred rat strains. The elicitation and absorption of the antisera was carried out as previously described (1).

Blocking of ConA stimulation was tested in microtiter culture plates (Fa. Greiner, Nürtingen, Germany). Each experimental group consisted of 6 parallel culture wells. 100 µl lymphocyte suspension ($10x10^6$ cells/ml Eagle's medium, supplemented with 5% horse serum and 0.05 mMol 2-mercaptoethanol) were pipetted into each well, and, sequentially, 50 µl of antisera (diluted 1:5 in phosphate buffered saline) or BN normal control sera, respectively, and 50 µl ConA solution (20 µg/ml) were added. Thus, the final dilution of the antisera was 1:20, and the ConA concentration was 5 µg/ml. After 30 hr. we labelled the cultures with 20 µCi ^{3}H-thymidine and harvested them with a multiple harvester after a total culture period of 48 hr.

Primary mixed lymphocyte cultures were established by incubating $10x10^6$ Lewis responder lymph node lymphocytes with the same number of L.BN stimulator lymphocytes (2 000 R irradiated) in 60 mm plastic Petri dishes (Fa. Greiner) in 6 ml culture medium. After 5 days incubation, the lymphoblasts were isolated in discontinuous Ficoll density gradients (density range: 1.05 - 1.10 g/ml; centrifugation: 10 000 g, 60 min., 4°C). The purified blast cells were reincubated for 5 days without antigen ($1x10^6$ blast cells in 6 ml medium) to let them revert to medium sized memory cells. For secondary stimulation, fresh cultures of 6 ml volumes were set up that contained $1x10^6$ secondary memory cells, and, as stimulants, either $10x10^6$ irradiated lymphocytes or 300 µg ConA (final concentration: 50 µg/ml). After another 48 hr., the boosted lymphocytes were assayed for specific cytotoxicity in a ^{51}Cr release assay against L.BN and L.BDV target fibroblast cultures (3).

RESULTS AND DISCUSSION

In a first attempt to monitor the effect of blocking anti-lymphocyte alloantisera on ConA stimulation of rat lymphocytes, we cultured Lewis lymph node cells with 5 µg/ml ConA in the presence of BN-anti-Lewis anti-lymphocyte alloantisera, either unabsorbed (L), or absorbed on Lewis liver homogenate (A) to remove anti-Lewis SD alloantibodies (1). As shown in Tab.I, Exp.1, the blocking sera, applied at a dilution of 1:20, reduced ConA stimulation up to 90%. This blocking effect was strain specific, for the same antisera scarcely affected the ConA reactivity of BN (Exp.2) or congenic

Tab.II: Blocking of ConA stimulation of rat lymphocytes by BN-anti-Lewis anti-lymphocyte alloantibodies, unabsorbed (L), orabsorbed on Lewis liver homogenate (A):

responding lymphocytes	addition of sera (hr)	pretreatment	sera	^{3}H thymidine incorporation (CPM)	inhibition (%)
Exp.1					
Lewis	0		BN	11 075 ± 1 713	--
"	0		L	7 612 ± 1 210	36
"	0		A	561 ± 69	95
Exp.2					
BN	0		BN	13 232 ± 2 416	--
"	0		L	15 586 ± 1 222	-18
"	0		A	11 445 ± 3 331	14
Exp.3					
Lewis		pretreat-ment	BN	33 701 ± 3 703	--
"		"	L	24 708 ± 2 294	27
"		"	A	16 308 ± 4 454	52
Exp.3					
Lewis	0		BN	55 348 ± 3 129	--
"	0		L	18 227 ± 2 819	64
"	4		L	25 238 ± 4 238	54
"	20		L	56 407 ± 5 548	-1

L.BN lymphocytes. Furthermore, the antisera were found to act in the
early phase of the reaction, since the mitogenic activity could be
significantly reduced by pretreatment of the reactive Lewis lymphocytes with the antisera before confrontation with the mitogen ConA.
When, on the other hand, the blocking sera were added after a delay
longer than 4 hr. to ConA cultures, the blocking effect was lost
(Exp.4). These data are compatible with the ones reported by
Schlesinger et al., who found that ConA reactivity of murine thymus
and spleen cells could be effectively depressed by anti-H2 alloantibodies (4). Our findings suggest, moreover, that ConA activation is
blocked by competition for a non-SD structure of the major histocompatibility gene locus, and that this competition must take place
at the initial stage of the reaction.

     Further interpretation of these data was limited by the lack
of information concerning the functional character of T lymphocyte
stimulation by ConA. It is true that this reaction closely resembles
lymphocyte activation by specific antigen in morphologic as well as
in certain functional aspects. Both reactions, however, clearly
differed from each other in one crucial point: no _specific_ activity
could yet be ascribed to ConA activated blast cells. It was thus
open, whether ConA stimulation of T lymphocytes represents an
activation process fundamentally different from antigen stimulation.
Alternatively, ConA could be a polyclonal lymphocyte activator,
possibly functioning via lymphocyte surface structures involved in
the chain of events leading to antigen stimulation.

     This question is technically difficult to approach as long as
multiclonal lymphocyte populations have to be investigated. We
therefore tried to overcome this problem by analysing the effect of
ConA on functionally restricted memory cell populations which can
be readily generated _in vitro_ (5-7). In a first step, we stimulated
Lewis lymph node cells against irradiated L.BN lymphocytes. The
resulting blast cells were isolated by discontinuous Ficoll density
gradient centrifugation, and transferred to antigen free "resting
cultures". Within 5 days, the blast cells reverted back to medium
sized secondary lymphocytes with reduced metabolism. These cells
were antigenically committed memory cells, since they vigorously
responded, when reexposed to the relevant primary antigen, viz.
L.BN stimulator cells. Their reactivity against unrelated third
party stimulator cells was ,however, low.

     In order to learn, whether memory cells can be reactivated by
ConA, Lewis secondary lymphocytes primed against L.BN were incubated with varying ConA doses. We found that ConA at a concentration
of 50 µg/ml restimulated these cells as effectively as relevant
antigen. Lower doses proved to be ineffective, which explains the
obvious contrast to the data of Andersson and Häyry (7), who were
unable to stimulate similar memory cells by 10 µg/ml ConA.

To determine the specific cytotoxic activities by both types of restimulated memory cells, equal samples of each $3x10^6$ viable cells of each restimulated cell population were transferred to relevant L.BN, and, as a specificity control, to third party L.BDV fibroblast target cultures. Thier lytic capacities were compared in addition to the one of dormant memory cells. As shown in Tab.II, Lewis-anti-L.BN memory cells reactivated either by L.BN stimulator cells or by ConA displayed cytotoxic values similar in their amplitude as well as in the degree of their specificity.

Tab.II: Specific ^{51}Cr release from fibroblast target cultures after 20 hr. incubation with Lewis-anti-L.BN memory cells reactivated either by L.BN lymphocytes or ConA.

Target fibroblasts	2° Stimulans		
	none	L.BN	ConA
L.BN	2 $\pm$ 0.1	63.5 $\pm$ 0.5	45.6 $\pm$ 0.6
L.BDV	4 $\pm$ 0.2	29.7 $\pm$ 1.7	24.0 $\pm$ 1.5
% Blast Cells	2	80	69

ConA thus appears to activate specific immune capacities programmed for in given lymphocyte clones. In non-selected lymphocyte populations it therefore probably activates all accessible clones on a random base, and thus acts as a polyclonally specific lymphocyte activator. The activation process in that case could take place by 2 different mechanisms: (a) by complexing of the mitogen to a lymphocyte structure critically necessary for lymphocyte activation, albeit distinct from the receptor for antigen, a mechanism analogous to polyclonal B cell activation by LPS (8), or (b) by binding to a constant part of the T cell antigen receptor, thus directly mimicking antigen triggering.

We showed that ConA stimulation of rat T cells can be prevented by anti-lymphocyte alloantisera.These sera contain antibodies

that are presumably directed against the constant part of the T cell
receptor for cellular antigen, since they directly interfere with
antigen binding to the complementary receptors. Provided that in
both cases the same antibodies are responsible for the prevention
of lymphocyte activation, it seems reasonable to conclude that ConA
activates T lymphocytes via constant determinants present on T cell
antigen receptors, probably carbohydrate moieties. The fact that
most of the T cell pool seems to be activated by ConA suggests that
a very high proportion, if not all of the T lymphocytes share a
similarly structured antigen receptor, which contains a component
coded for in the major histocompatibility gene locus.

Acknowledgements: The excellent technical assistence by Ms.
Marlot Prester is gratefully acknowledged. This work was supported
by the Deutsche Forschungsgemeinschaft.

LITERATURE

1) H. Wekerle, Z. Eshhar, P. Lonai, and M. Feldman: Proc. Nat. Acad.
   Sci. (US): 72: 1147 (1975).
2) Transpl. Rev.: 23: (1975).
3) G. Berke, W. Ax, H. Ginsburg, and M. Feldman: Immunol.: 16: 643
   (1969).
4) M. Schlesinger, M. Chaouat, and I. Gery: Proc. 8th Leucocyte
   Confer. (K. Lindahl-Kiessling, and D. Osoba, Ed.), p.645 (1974).
5) N. Hollander, H. Ginsburg, and M. Feldman: J. Exp. Med.: 140:
   1057 (1974).
6) H.R. Macdonald, H.D. Engers, J.-C. Cerottini, and K.H. Brunner:
   J. Exp. Med.: 140: 718 (1974).
7) L. C. Andersson, and P. Häyry: Eur. J. Immunol.: 3: 595 (1973).
8) A. Coutinho, and G. Möller: Scand. J. Immunol.: 3: 133 (1974).

RECOGNITION OF ANTIGEN BY B AND T LYMPHOCYTES

G.E. Roelants

Basel Institute for Immunology

487 Grenzacherstrasse   CH-4058 Basel,   Switzerland

At the end of the session on "Lymphoid cell receptors and antigen recognition", I would like to make a few brief remarks about a subject which paradoxically has barely been touched: that of the recognition structure of B and T lymphocytes. I wish to do this in the form of three questions:

1) Do B and T cells have receptors of refined specificity? The numerous studies demonstrating the refined specificity of the Ig combining site are by now classics and it is generally admitted that the B cell receptor is a sample of the Ig that it would make upon activation. Thus the receptor of B cells has all the refined antigen specificity of Ig. This has been amply confirmed by antigen binding studies and functional analysis.

Soluble T cell receptors are not available to date and precise studies on specificity of recognition are scarce. Indeed, while numerous studies on activation or inactivation of T cell functions clearly show that they are not wholly unspecific, immunochemical studies on the discriminatory power of T cells are not as abundant as for B cells. However, Schlossman et al. (1) demonstrated that T cells could discriminate between a series of DNP-nonalysines differing in the position of the DNP group and of one D-lysine residue. Goodman and his coworkers (2) showed that there was no cross reaction between small compounds of the general structure L-tyrosine-p-azobenzene-R which induce pure T responses in guinea pigs when the radical R was arsonate, carboxylate, sulfonate, acetamide, sulfonamide, nitro- or trimethyl ammonium chloride. Becker et al. (3) found that T cells could discriminate between p-azobenzene arsonate (ABA)-L-Tyr, ABA-Tyr (L-Tyr)$_3$

ABA-L-Tyr (L-Ala)$_3$ and (L-Tyr)$_3$-ABA-L-Tyr. These studies show
that T receptors have a highly refined degree of discrimination
comparable to that of B receptors. Another question is whether
they recognize the same determinants.

2) Do B and T cell receptors have the same repertoire?
Here two main approaches were used: The study of cross-activation
or cross-tolerance compared at the level of B and T cells and the
direct visualization of T and B antigen binding cells.

Rajewsky and Mohr (4) using a system of cross induction and
cross tolerance to various albumins in primed and unprimed mice
concluded that B and T cells not only have the same highly refined
specificity but also recognize the same determinants and have the
same system of antigen binding receptors. However, in other
systems it appeared that the T cell specificity was not as refined
as the B cell. This included lysozyme and carboxymethyllysozyme (5),
flagellin and acetoacetylated derivatives (6), flagellins of various
serological specificities (7) and native and methylated BSA (8).
This discrepancy may be due to the fact that B cross-reactions are
studied at the level of soluble antibody while T cross reactions
are studied at the level of the T cell itself where multiple points
attachment to the receptors lattice may amplify weak cross reactions.
Thus the broader specificity of T cells may be more apparent than
real.

Studies with better chemically defined antigens clearly show
that the dichotomy between epitopes recognized by T cells or B
cells is only apparent.

Glucagon, a polypeptide of 29 amino acids induces both T and B
cell responses in guinea pigs (9). The B response is directed towards the amino terminal part, the T response towards the carboxy-
terminal part (9). However, when glucagon is conjugated to a
carrier, good antibody is produced against both moieties and delayed
hypersensitivity is not elicited (10).

Small bifunctional molecules of the general type dinitrophenyl-6-
amino caproyl-tyrosine-azobenzene arsonate (DNP-SAC-RAT) induce B
responses against the DNP moiety and T cell responses against RAT
(2). Again there is a dichotomy of recognition, again this dichotomy is only apparent: thus T cell responses can be induced to
DNP and other small conventional haptens (11-14), B cells can
respond to RAT (15).

Thus it appears that B and T receptors have the same dictionary,
i.e., recognize the same determinants. However, the mode of presentation of the epitope will determine whether one or the other will be
preferentially triggered. This phenomenon has a close parallel in

activation of lymphocytes by lectins *(16)*.

If this is so we should find antigen binding cells largely for any epitope in both the T and B series. This was indeed the case for all antigens we have studied so far (17) which included proteins: MSH, KLH, HGG; synthetic polypeptides: (T, G)-A--L native or heavily iodinated, GT; haptens: NNP, NAP, DNP, TNP.

3) Do T and B receptors share the same set of V genes? The answer to this question is not definitely clear at present. Indeed the parallel and similar recognition of epitopes by B and T receptors may not be due to shared V genes but to a convergent evolution of both recognition structures. However, recent studies appear to show that both B and T receptors in addition to sharing the same specificity also share the same idiotype (18-20). These studies if confirmed would definitely show that the variable, i.e. the antigen specific, part of the recognition structure of B and T cells is identical.

REFERENCES

1. Schlossman, S.F., Herman, J. and Yaron, A. 1969. J. Exp. Med. 130:1031.
2. Alkan, S.S., Williams, E.B., Nitecki, D.E. and Goodman, J.W. 1972. J. Exp. Med. 135:1228.
3. Becker, M.J., Levin, H. and Sela, M. 1973. Eur. J. of Immunol. 3:131.
4. Rajewsky, K. and Mohr, R. 1974. Eur. J. Immunol. 4:112.
5. Thompson, K., Harris, M., Benjamini, E. Mitchell, G. and Noble, M. 1972. Nature, New Biol. 238:20.
6. Parish, C.R., 1971. J. Exp. Med. 134:21.
7. Cooper, M.G., and Ada, G.L. 1972. Scand. J. Immunol. 1:247.
8. Schirrmacher, V. and Wigzell, H. 1972. J. Exp. Med. 136:1616.
9. Senyk, G., Williams, R., Nitecki, D.E. and Goodman, J.W. 1971. J. Exp. Med. 133:1294.
10. Senyk, G., Nitecki, D.E., Spitler, L. and Goodman, J.W. 1972. Immunochemistry 9:97.
11. Taylor, R.B., and Iverson, G.M. 1971. Proc. Roy. Soc. B 176:393.
12. Benacerraf, B. and Gell, P.G.H. 1959. Immunology 2:219.
13. Henry, C. and Trefts, P.E. 1974. Eur. J. Immunol. 4:824.
14. Janewey, C.A., Cohen, B.E., Ben-Sasson, S.Z. and Paul, W.E. 1975. J. Exp. Med. 141:42.
15. Bush, M.E.,Allan, S.S., Nitecki, D.E. and Goodman, J.W. 1972. J. Exp. Med. 136:1478.
16. Loor, F. 1974. Eur. J. of Immunol. 4:210.
17. Roelants, G.E. In "Membrane receptors of lymphocytes" M. Seligmann, J.L. Preud'homme and F.M. Kourilsky, eds. North

Holland Publishing Co., Amsterdam. In press.

18. Binz, H. and Wigzell, H. In "Membrane receptors of lymphocytes"
     M. Seligmann, J.L. Preud'homme and F.M. Kourilsky, eds. North
     Holland Publishing Co., Amsterdam. In press.

19. Eichmann, K., Black, B., Hammerling, G. and Rajewsky, K. In
     "Membrane receptors of lymphocytes", M. Seligmann, J.L. Preud'-
     homme and F.M. Kourilsky, eds. North Holland Publishing Co.,
     Amsterdam. In press.

20. Cosenza, H., Augustin, A., Loor, F. and Roelants, G.E.
     Unpublished.

Tumor Immunology:
Interactions between Lymphocytes,
Antibodies and Neoplastic Cells

HOST PROTECTION BY THE ANTIBODY-FORMING SYSTEM IN MALIGNANCY

T. Juhani Linna, Cheng-po Hu and Kenneth M. Lam

Department of Microbiology and Immunology

Temple University School of Medicine

Philadelphia, PA 19140, USA

We have previously reported, that not only impairment of cell-mediated immunity, but also impairment of bursa-dependent, antibody-producing capacity decreases host defense to tumors induced by the avian reticuloendotheliosis (RE) virus, strain T, indicating that both parts of the immune system have a host-protective function in this malignancy(1, 2). In order to study whether the antibody-forming system may have a host-protective function in oncogenesis in general, unrelated tumors were studied with regard to tumor development in bursectomized and control animals. The tumors chosen for this purpose were tumors induced by XC cells, a Rous sarcoma-derived tumor line, and a chemical carcinogen-induced transplantable fibrosarcoma. The three malignancies chosen for study are of widely different genesis, and convergent results could therefore illustrate a common principle in host defense in oncogenesis.

We will report here that crippling of the antibody-forming capacity by surgical bursectomy results in an increased tumor growth rate for the Rous sarcoma-derived malignancy and for the chemical carcinogen-induced transplantable tumor, thus adding support to the concept of a host-protective function for the antibody-forming system. We will also report successful tumor therapy experiments, using immune serum or immune gammaglobulin in the cure of RE virus-induced malignancy, thus further emphasizing the host-protective capacity of antibodies.

MATERIALS AND METHODS

Induction of immunodeficiency: Hy-Line line WC chickens were used in all these studies. Surgical bursectomies or thymectomies

were performed on the day of hatching using the standard technique
(3). Selective destruction of the bursa and of antibody-forming
capacity was obtained by treatment with 4mg of cyclophosphamide
each day during the first three days of life.

Tumor induction: RE virus, strain T, (originally obtained
from Dr. R. Fischer, Univ. of North Dakota), was injected into the
wing web. Surgically bursectomized and normal birds were given the
virus on the third day. Cyclophosphamide bursectomized birds and
their controls were inoculated when one month old. The dose of RE
virus varied with the design and purpose of the different experiments,
but experimental and control groups in each study were given the
same dose of RE virus. XC cells were obtained from the Wistar
Institute (Dr. A.J. Girardi), and maintained in vitro. Five
million viable (0.1% trypan blue-excluding) cells were injected into
the wing web of three-day-old surgically bursectomized, thymectomized or control chickens. The transplantable fibrosarcoma
was derived from a neonatally thymectomized WC chicken,
which received an injection of 1.0 ml 1% (w/v) benzo(a)pyrene
in trioctanoin intramuscularly when five weeks old. The
tumor was harvested five months later and was serially transplantable.
One thousand live cells were used as the inoculum to one-day-old
bursectomized and control chickens in this study.

Immune serum, RE virus-absorbed immune serum, and gammaglobulin: Three-day-old WC chickens were given 0.1 LD_{50} of RE
virus. At 1 month of age, they were challenged with 5 LD_{50}'s of RE
virus. The survivors were exsanguinated from the heart 6
weeks later. Serum was obtained in the usual manner, and heated
at 56°C for 30 minutes. Normal control serum was purchased from
GIBCO, Grand Island, N.Y. To remove antiviral antibodies, the
immune serum was absorbed extensively with RE virus obtained from
tissue culture supernatants of RE virus-infected chick embryo
fibroblasts. Absorption was continued until the band obtained on
counterimmunoelectrophoresis between the immune serum and RE virus
had disappeared. A gammaglobulin fraction was obtained from
immune and control sera by precipitating 3 times with $(NH_4)2 SO_4$
at the 35% saturation.

Evaluation of tumor development: The local tumors were
measured with a caliper. The animals were checked for tumor
mortailty daily. A few animals dying from causes other than
tumor were excluded from the evaluations. Presence of tumors
was determined macroscopically, and microscopically when necessary.
Inoculation of sufficient doses of RE virus and of XC cells results
in the death of the recipient. The chemical carcinogen-induced
tumor line grows in the recipients without causing death. Differences
in tumor mortality and progression were evaluated with Fisher-Yates
exact test using fourfold tables, and differences in tumor size with
analysis of variance and student's t-test.

Tumor immunotherapy studies: Three-day-old chickens were given one LD_{50} of RE virus into the wing web. Six days later, about 60% of the animals were tumor bearing, and a few days later, virtually all animals had measurable tumors. Tumor treatment was initiated six days after RE virus inoculation. A total of 9 intravenous injections were given every other day, 0.5 ml each time. The group of animals were treated either with immune serum, normal serum, or were untreated. To exclude the influence of the antibody-forming system of the host on tumor development, the same studies were done in cyclophosphamide-treated month-old animals, which were tumor-bearing after administration of one LD_{50} of RE virus into the wing web six days previously. To eliminate the effect of anti-viral antibodies on tumor cure, tumor-bearing animals were treated with immune serum which had been extensively absorbed with RE virus, and with appropriate control sera. To exclude that the host-protective effect was afforded by a mechanism not related to antibodies, tumor-bearing animals were treated with the gammaglobulin fraction of immune or normal serum. The curative effect of these preparations was compared with that of immune and normal serum.

RESULTS

Bursectomy experiments.

XC cells. Tumors induced by XC cells were significantly (P < 0.01) larger in the animals which had been surgically bursectomized in the newly hatched period than in the control birds. Surgical bursectomy in the newly hatched period had no clear effect on tumor frequency or mortality. In animals which were thymectomized in the newly hatched period, larger tumors were also observed (Fig. 1). In addition, tumor frequency and mortality was also significantly higher in thymectomized than in control animals.

Benzo(a)pyrene-induced transplantable tumor line. Also in this tumor model, a standard inoculum of cells grew significantly (P = 0.01) faster in bursectomized than in control animals (Figure 2). However, there was no difference in tumor frequency between bursectomized and control birds.

RE tumor therapy studies: Immune serum treatment of RE virus-induced tumors in normal tumor-bearing animals resulted in significant regression of normally progressing tumors and lowered tumor mortality when compared with normal serum-treated or untreated birds (4). Similar data were obtained in cyclophosphamide bursectomized, RE-tumor bearing birds treated with immune serum (4). Immune serum which was extensively absorbed with RE virus was at least as effective as non-absorbed immune serum in accomplishing tumor regression and host survival. 80% of the RE virus-absorbed immune serum-treated animals regressed their tumors, and 73% survived the tumor challenge, while 65% of the non-absorbed serum-

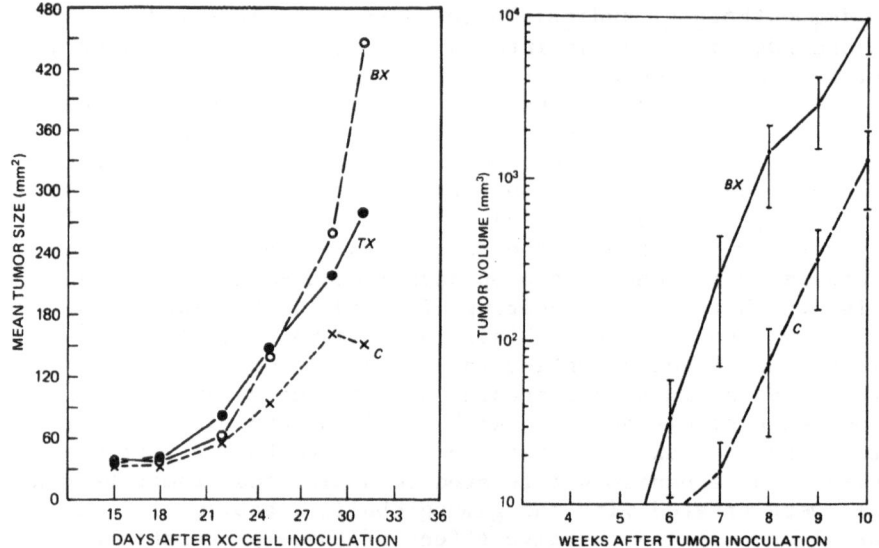

Figure 1. Growth of XC cell induced tumors in bursectomized, in thymectomized and in control animals.

Figure 2. Growth of benzo(a)pyrene-induced tumor in bursectomized and control animals.

TABLE I

Effect of serum γ-globulin on the development of RE tumors

Treatment	Regression of local tumors	Survivors
Immune serum γ-globulin	17/20 (85%) p<0.05	17/20 (85%) p<0.02
Normal serum γ-globulin	10/20 (50%)	9/20 (45%)
Immune serum	15/20 (75%) p<0.002	15/20 (75%) p<0.002
Normal serum	3/18 (17%)	2/18 (11%)
None	8/20 (40%)	8/20 (40%)

treated animals regressed their tumors and 59% survived. In the non-treated control group, 23% were able to regress their tumors, and 15% survived. Thus, both absorbed and non-absorbed immune serum had significant curative effect in terms of regression, and survival. Thus, the curative effect may be mediated by antibodies directed against transplantation-type antigens on tumor cells. To further substantiate that the effect was mediated by the gamma-

globulin fraction of immune serum, this fraction of immune serum and appropriate controls were used to treat tumor-bearing animals, with a dose schedule corresponding to that used in immune serum therapy studies. Treatment with immune gammaglobulin and with immune serum resulted in significant (P < 0.05 and P < 0.002, respectively) tumor cure, as compared with the other treatments, both in terms of survival and tumor regression (Table 1).

DISCUSSION

We have demonstrated that surgical as well as chemical (cyclophosphamide) bursectomy in the newly hatched period significantly impairs host resistance to tumors caused by the avian reticuloendotheliosis virus, strain T. A similar effect can be demonstrated after thymectomy in the newly hatched period. The data have been obtained both after systemic (1, 5) and after wing web (2, 5) administration of the RE virus, and can be demonstrated both in terms of tumor mortality and local tumor development. The work presented here is an extension of these findings. We have studied the development of unrelated tumors in bursectomized and control animals, as well as performed immune serum therapy experiments with RE tumor-bearing animals.

We have now extended the studies to include a classical member of the avian tumor virus complex, Rous sarcoma. Since the Bryan strain (6) and the Carr-Zilber strain (7) have been studied earlier with regard to tumor development in bursectomized birds, with essentially negative results, we have used a different approach. XC cells, a cell line carried in vitro for more than a decade, were originally derived from the tumor of a rat inoculated with the Prague strain of Rous sarcoma virus (RSV) (8). When XC cells are inoculated into chickens, tumors are formed (9, 10). We studied the influence of surgical bursectomy in the newly hatched period on the development of these tumors and found that when bursectomized animals were inoculated with a standard dose of XC cells, they developed significantly larger tumors than the non-bursectomized controls. In these studies, there was no significant effect of bursectomy on tumor frequency or mortality. Thymectomy in the newly hatched period, on the other hand, was associated with a clear increase not only in tumor size but also in tumor frequency and mortality. Whether this reflects true differences in the influence of thymus-dependent, cell-mediated immunity, and of bursa-dependent, humoral immunity on tumor development can not be stated at present, since neither thymectomy nor surgical bursectomy in the newly hatched period, without adjunct treatment, completely abolishes cell-mediated or humoral immunity, respectively. Suffice it to state that these studies demonstrate that not only cell-mediated immunity, but also the antibody-forming system has a host-protective effect also on this Rous sarcoma-derived tumor.

When growth of a standard inoculum of a chemical carcinogen-induced transplantable tumor was compared between bursectomized and control birds, a similar finding was made as in the previous study: the tumors were significantly larger through the observation period in bursectomized than in control birds, but tumor "take" frequency was not significantly different between the bursectomized and the control group. We do not know if this latter parameter would also be affected if a method such as treatment with high doses of cyclophosphamide in the newly hatched period (11), which would more completely destroy antibody-producing capacity, were to be used.

Thus, we now have data in three widely different tumor systems, demonstrating that the antibody-forming system performs a host-protective function - "surveillance" if you will. Because of the convergent findings in the three widely different tumor models, we propose that these data reflect a general mechanism in host influence on tumor development, well realizing that the mechanism may oftentimes not be sufficiently effective, and may well work in concert with other host-protective mechanisms such as cell-mediated immunity (12) and the mononuclear phagocyte system (13).

The demonstration of the impairment of host defense mechanisms by crippling of the bursa-dependent, antibody-forming system raises the question whether immune serum has a sufficient host-protective effect to be useful in tumor therapy. Such experiments have been reported in the literature in other tumor models (14, 15). We have demonstrated here that immune serum, obtained from birds which survived sublethal challenges of RE virus, can be used to treat this malignancy. This treatment results in regression of normally progressing tumors, and in survival of animals after inoculation of a virus dose which results in death of most non-immune serum treated animals. The host's own antibody-forming system does not significantly contribute to this curative effect, since similar results are obtained in tumor-bearing recipients, profoundly deficient in antibody-forming capacity. The curative effect is not due to the presence of antiviral antibodies, since extensive absorption with RE virus does not decrease the efficacy of immune serum. The treatment has immunologic specificity, since it has no effect on the development of a laboratory strain of Marek's disease (Hu and Linna, unpublished). The effect is in the gammaglobulin fraction of immune serum, since this fraction is effective in tumor cure. Thus, our studies on RE virus-induced tumors demonstrate that impairment of antibody-forming capacity results in decreased ability to combat tumor development, while immune serum and immune gammaglobulin is effective in accomplishing tumor cure, probably due to antibodies directed against determinants other than those present on the virus. These data further support the host-protective function of the antibody-forming system.

ACKNOWLEDGEMENTS

The work presented here was supported by USPHS, NIH grant CA-13347 from the National Cancer Institute, an NIH General Research Support grant to Temple University, and grant IN-88F from the American Cancer Society.

REFERENCES

1. Thompson, K. D. and T. J. Linna. Nature, New Biol. 245:10-12, 1973.
2. Linna, T. J., C. Hu and K. D. Thompson. J. Natl. Cancer Inst. 53:847-854, 1974.
3. Peterson, R. D. A., B. R. Burmester, T. N. Frederickson, H. G. Purchase and R. A. Good. J. Natl. Cancer Inst. 32:1343-1354, 1964.
4. Linna, T. J. and C. Hu. Rad. Res. (in press), 1975.
5. Linna, T. J., C. Hu and K. D. Thompson. In Virus Tumorigenesis and Immunogenesis, pp. 141-165. Academic Press, New York-London, 1973.
6. McArthur, W. P., E. A. Carswell, and G. J. Thorbecke, J. Natl. Cancer Inst., 49:907-909, 1972.
7. Radzichovskaja, R. Nature, 213:1259-1260, 1967.
8. Svoboda, J. Folia Biol. (Praha), 7:46-70, 1961.
9. Svoboda, J., P. Chyle, D. Simkovic, and I. Hilgert. Fol. Biol. (Praha), 9:77-81, 1963.
10. Lam, K. M., and T. J. Linna. Fed. Proc., 34:963, 1975.
11. Linna, T. J., D. Frommel and R. A. Good. Int. Arch. Allergy 42:20-39, 1972.
12. Smith, R. T. and M. Landy (eds.): Immune Surveillance. New York, Academic Press Inc., 1970.
13. Evans, R., H. Cox and P. Alexander. Proc. Soc. Exp. Biol. Med. 143:256-259, 1973.
14. Gorer, P.A. Ann. N. Y. Acad. Sci. 73:707-721, 1958.
15. Hersey, P. Br. J. Cancer 28 (Suppl. I):11-18, 1973.

TUMOUR RESISTANCE OF TETRAPARENTAL

AKR↔CBA CHIMAERAS

R. D. Barnes

Clinical Research Centre

Harrow

Mouse chimaeras derived by early embryo aggregation (EEA) have been used for a variety of purposes including a study of tumour development which is discussed here.

On comparison with the lymphoma susceptible AKR the incidence of tumours were both delayed (1) and markedly reduced (2) in a group of EEA derived susceptible (S) ↔ (R) resistant AKR↔CBA chimaeras. Since this observation various factors have become apparent suggesting how tumour resistance has been achieved in this situation.

Although embryo transplantation derived CBA born from AKR retain their innate lymphoma resistant (3) one of the six lymphomas seen in eighteen AKR↔CBA/H-T6 chimaeras was found to be CBA/H-T6 in origin when examined cytogenetically (4). This clearly points to a (S)→(R) activity. However the overal lymphoma resistance of the chimaeras suggesting (R)→(S) activity appears more important. Although reduction in lymphoma incidence from 100% to 30% might be considered only relative the fact that the majority of chimaeras (12/18) lived and were found to be free of lymphomas at an age up to three times the average life span of the parental AKR (5), is evidence of (R)→(S) activity. It remained to determine the mechanism involved and in this respect the following findings appear important.

I)   In respect of mixed coat colour composition and in the distribution of the gametes, the chimaeras were roughly 'balanced' (neither one or the other strain component was always dominant) (4).

II)   In spite of this there was an overwhelming preponderance of AKR cells in:-
   a)   PHA stimulated blood cultures (>99%) (4).
   b)   in 'direct' cytogenetic analysis of the lymphomyeloid complex (>90%) (6).

and c) somatic tissues (>80%) (6).

Therefore it cannot be argued that the relative tumour
resistance of the chimaeras was due to the lack of lymphoma-prone
AKR cells.

III) AKR predominance was also matched at a cell product
level since analysis of the:-

a) red cell isoenzyme - glucose phosphate isomerase (7)
b) serum allotype (7).

and c) serum complement (C'5 - MuB1) (unpublished data) also showed
an overwhelming preponderance of the corresponding AKR cell
product, in the case of C'5 this was shown by the relative
lack of the associated antigen MuB1 (CBA).

IV) Lymphoma resistance of the chimaeras also could not be
attributed to absence of the oncogenic virus since:-

a) numerous type-C murine leukaemia virus-like particles were
found to be present upon electron microscopy (8)

and b) Gross antigen specificity was subsequently confirmed (9).

V) In spite of levels of murine leukaemic group specific antigen
titres comparable and on occasion in excess of the parental AKR there
was very little evidence of renal antibody-antigen complexes visible
on fluorescent microscopy (9). Investigation on both light and
electron microscopy also failed to demonstrate renal lesions that are
generally associated with soluble antibody - antigen complex
deposition (9). These findings were in marked contrast to the AKR
where antibody - antigen complex associated renal lesions are a
prominent feature (10). The findings in the chimaeras were
particularly remarkable since as mentioned above the chimaeras were
predominantly AKR in respect of both cellular and cell product
composition - the latter including the allotype defined antibody
status (7).

VI) Although the relative lack of renal antibody - antigen
complexes could have been explained in several ways renal elution
(11) and immunoabsorption (12) studies have since suggested that
this was due to absence of anti-Gross antibody activity which is a
'normal' characteristic of the parental AKR (10).

VII) This led us in turn to suggest that in absence of masking
antibody - viral antigen complexes 'normal' tumour immunity may have
been effected and that this was responsible for the relative tumour
resistance of the chimaeras (13). Although this has yet to be proven
this concept remains our working hypothesis concerning the situation
in the AKR↔CBA/H-T6 chimaeras.

A recent report by Kassel and his colleagues (14) suggested the
possibility of an alternative explanation. The AKR like many other
strains of mice are deficient in C'5 and on noting in-vivo regression
of their lymphomas following infusion of 'normal' serum possessing
the full spectrum of complement components, Kassel suggested that
C'5 was an anti-leukaemic component in serum (14). In the case of
the AKR↔CBA chimaeras we have a C'5 deficient ↔ C'5 normal situation
and it was therefore conceivable that the C'5 component derived from
the CBA may have corrected the 'deficiency' of the AKR and this turn

may have played a part in the overal lymphoma resistance of the chimaeras. This view however appears unlikely. Although C'5 or rather its associated antigen MuBl were on occasions demonstrated in the sera of the chimaeras levels obtained in a modified Ouchterlony technique (15) showed that MuBl (CBA) levels were minimal and generally less than 10% in the chimaeras serum (unpublished data). Similarly although MuBl was detected by means of immunofluorescence in the renal lesions of the chimaeras staining was minimal and in marked contrast to staining seen in another group of C'5 deficient ↔ C'5 normal NZB↔CFW chimaeras (15). There is other evidence that makes the role of C'5 in the tumour resistance of the AKR↔CBA chimaeras appear even less likely. Unlike the AKR x CBA Fl which are relatively tumour resistant lymphomas are seen in some of the (AKR x CBA) x AKR backcross - however this is not confined to mice which are MuBl (C'5) negative (unpublished data).

Returning to the concept of tolerance to the oncogenic Gross virus playing a major role in ensuring the relative tumour resistance of the AKR↔CBA/H-T6 chimaeras the question remains how this was achieved. There originally appeared to be a vital clue since in spite of an overwhelming excess of AKR T cells in PHA stimulated peripheral blood cultures (4) analysis upon the basis of θ surface antigen determinants showed roughly equal numbers of AKR and CBA T cells (16). These two findings appeared to be paradoxical. More recently the paradox appears to have been resolved. Cytogenetic analysis following treatment of chimaera thymus cell suspensions with anti-θ^{AKR} (in the presence of C') and subsequent selective T cell mitogenic stimulation (CON. A) showed a significant number of AKR cells (unpublished data). This suggested the possibility of AKR T cells having been processed with θ^{CBA}. Thus it would appear that θ processing had occurred independent of the cellular genome. This phenomenon, if confirmed, has certain biological precedence since certain red blood group antigens in man, sheep and goats are acquired from a source other than the red cell or its precursor (17).

Theta processing independent of the cellular genome - interesting in its own right - led us to consider whether this may have played any part in the tumour resistance of the chimaeras. In this context we were led to question whether CBA^θ processing of AKR cells was in any way responsible for the tumour resistance of the chimaeras. There initially seemed to be some evidence in favour of this view since Acton and his colleagues had noted that AKR/FuA and AKR/Cum were not only atypical in possessing θ^{C3H} rather than θ^{AKR} but also were lymphoma resistant (18). This seemed to support the view that the tumour resistance of the chimaeras might involve θ status. However, this now seems unlikely since we have noted that the incidence of lymphomas in the θ^{C3H} AKR/Cum is comparable with the highly susceptible θ^{AKR} AKR/J (unpublished data). This in turn has thrown doubt upon the association of θ processing of AKR cells and tumour resistance in the chimaeras.

Although C-type murine leukaemia virus like particles were
identified in all the chimaeras their numbers varied (8).
Similarly although the presence of the murine leukaemia group
specific (gs) antigen was confirmed in each case, the titre varied
(9). Curiously enough in each case viral replication appeared
related to coat colour composition. (Viral replication is used
here in context of numbers of C-type particles and levels of gs
antigen). Although it was not surprising to note that viral
replication was maximum in the chimaeras that were predominantly
albino (AKR) what is remarkable is the fact that viral replication
was notably less in the more agouti (CBA) chimaeras - mice that
were still predominantly AKR at a cellular level (4,6,7). In other
words, oncogenic viral replication in cytogenetically defined AKR
cells varied in relation to coat colour composition of the chimaeras.
Re-examination of our earlier findings (16) has since showed that
the proportion of the two θ defined cell populations also paralleled
coat colour composition.

Like skin the stroma of the thymus is also derived from
ectoderm. In chimaeras derived by aggregation of very early
undifferentiated embryos, it might therefore be anticipated that
the composition of ectodermally derived thymic stroma might parallel
that of the coat. Although this has yet to be proven this assumption
does not appear unreasonable. One is therefore left to consider how
the coat/thymic stromal composition can influence oncogenic viral
replication and furthermore in what now appears to be genotypically
essentially an AKR chimaera. It must be presumed that the influence
is manifest through some soluble factor. In this context we were
interested to note a recent report by Tennant and his colleagues
(19) in defining the influence of a soluble factor that diminished
in-vitro infectivity of the N-associated Gross virus. The question
remains, are we seeing the effect of the same or similar factor in
the chimaeras in-vivo. Although there are obvious differences
between the in-vitro and in-vivo conditions -if the phenomenon was
the same then the in-vivo situation offers the distinct advantages
in further investigation. Isolation, definition and determination
of the source of the factor appear tremendously important in
respect of influencing oncogenic viral replication and therefore
tumour development in general. The possibility that the source of
this factor being stromal elements of the thymus has to be
considered. Its role in tumour resistance of the chimaeras still
has to be determined.

Since our experiments were originally commenced, the field of
murine tumour genetics has emerged. The Fv-1 locus is known to
determine permissiveness of cells to infection with endogenous
murine leukaemia virus (20) and it is also known that mice that are
$H-2^k$ are especially susceptible to virus associated tumours (21).
It is therefore not surprising to note that the AKR are $Fv-1^n$ and
$H-2^k$ and consequently both permissive to n-tropic virus (Gross)
infection and susceptible to associated lymphoma development. What

is surprising, is that this is also the situation in the lymphoma resistant CBA (3). This has argued the existence of another and furthermore dominant factor in the CBA that leads to its lymphoma resistance (3) and it is presumed that this factor is responsible for (R)→(S) activity in the AKR↔CBA/H-T6 chimaeras. Upon the basis of the above mentioned findings it is unlikely that C'5 or θ is this dominant (R) resistance factor.

In terms of genetics we can assume that there is a factor in the CBA associated with its lymphoma resistance. We tentatively have designated this the (R) (resistance) factor. It's dominance is not only argued by the lymphoma resistance of the CBA (3) the chimaeras (1,2) but also by findings in the naturally derived AKR x CBA hybrid which as mentioned earlier is also relatively lymphoma resistant. Whilst currently attempting to map the (R) area by means of various isozymal and antigenic markers we are also trying to determine whether the (R) locus may be dominant over Fv-1, H-2 and also the Fv-2 locus - the latter which determines permissiveness to the Friend group of exogenous murine leukaemia viruses (22).

There is a possible clue as to the location and mode of activity of the (R) factor. The fact that unlike the AKR tolerance to the Gross virus appears to have been maintained in the AKR↔CBA chimaeras points to clear differences in the immune response of the two parental strains, at least in respect to the Gross virus. There is possibly other, although circumstantial evidence to suggest that the overal immune response of the two strains differ. Unlike the AKR↔CBA/H-T6 chimaeras the incidence of lymphomas in AKR↔C3H/He chimaeras appeared remarkably similar to the parental AKR (23). Whereas originally considering differences between the AKR and CBA we are now examining possible differences between the CBA and the C3H/He. In this context we were intrigued to note one major difference especially since it concerns the immune response of the two strains. Unlike the C3H/He, thymus cells from the CBA appear atypical in showing auto-reactivity against syngeneic spleen cells in mixed lymphocyte culture (24). This atypical self thymus → spleen CBA auto-reactivity apparently is short lived and is lost within the first few days of life (25). Studying the interaction between the two strains in culture showed that unlike the transient reactivity of CBA thymocytes against syngeneic spleen cells the reaction of C3H/He thymocytes against CBA spleen cells is maintained. However, it is the 'switching off' of CBA thymocyte activity that appears important. This finding suggests clear differences between the immune response of the CBA and C3H/He and moreover since this difference concerns tolerance this might explain the difference in the tumour susceptibility of the AKR↔C3H/He chimaeras and the tumour resistance of the AKR↔CBA/H-T6 mice. In this respect it should be remembered that in spite of early acquisition upon the germ line, tolerance to the oncogenic Gross virus is not maintained in the AKR. One possible explanation is that this is due to the late exposure of the associated viral antigens. There is some evidence to support this since in spite of extensive

examination viral antigens have rarely been detected until after
birth (26). The question is - is this too late for tolerance to
be maintained in the AKR and furthermore is this the CBA with its
remarkable ability to recognise and 'switch off' self reactivity
stopped any AKR anti-Gross activity in the AKR↔CBA/H-T6 chimaeras.
In contrast the C3H without such ability is unable to 'switch off'
anti-Gross activity and in the presence of masking anti-viral
antigen complexes tumours are not eliminated. This would
therefore explain why lymphomas were invariable in the AKR↔C3H
situation and why the AKR↔CBA/H-T6 chimaeras remained relatively
tumour resistant - a possibility that continues to be examined
in a comparative study of further chimaeras and also the naturally
derived hybrids.

REFERENCES

1. Barnes, R.D., Tuffrey, M., and Kingman,   Clin exp. Immunol.,
        1972, 12, 541.
2. Barnes, R.D., Tuffrey, M., and Ford, C.E., Nature New Biol.,
        1973, 244, 282.
3. Barnes, R.D., and Tuffrey, M., Europ. J. Cancer, 1974, 10, 575.
4. Tuffrey, M., Barnes, R.D., Evans, E.O., and Ford, C.E.,
        Nature New Biol., 1973, 243, 207.
5. Barnes, R.D., and Tuffrey, M., Brit. J. Cancer, 1974, 29, 400.
6. Ford, C.E., Evans, E.P., Burtenshaw, M.D., Clegg, H., Barnes,
        R.D., and Tuffrey, M., Differentiation, 1974, 2, 321.
7. Barnes, R.D., Tuffrey, M., Drury, L., and Catty, D.,
        Differentiation, 1974, 2, 257.
8. Barnes, R.D., Tuffrey, M., Holliday, J., Hilgers, J., and
        Souissi, A., Europ. J. Cancer, 1975, (in press).
9. Wills, E.J., Tuffrey, M., and Barnes, R.D., Clin. exp. Immunol.,
        1975, 20, 563.
10. Oldstone, M.B.A. Aoki, T., and Dixon, F.J., Proc. Nat. Acad.
        Sci., 1972, 69, 134.
11. Barnes, R.D., Tuffrey, M., and Holliday, J., Brit. J. Cancer,
        1974, 31, 1.
12. Barnes, R.D., Tuffrey, M.A., and Bourne, R.C., Cancer Res.
        1975, (in press).
13. Barnes, R.D., Europ. J. Cancer, 1975, (in press).
14. Kassel, R.L., Old, L.J., and Carswell E.A. J. exp. Med.,
        1973, 138, 925.
15. Barnes, R.D., Tuffrey, M., Kingman, J., Thornton, C., Turner,
        M.W., Clin. exp. Immunol., 1972, 11, 605.
16. Bona, C., Tuffrey, M., and Barnes, R.D., Tissue Antigens,
        1974, 4, 31.
17. Race, R.R., and Sanger, R., Blood Groups in Man, 1958.
18. Acton, R.T., Blankenhorn, E.P., Douglas, T.C., Owen, R.D.,
        Hilgers, J., Hoggman, H.A., and Boyse, E.A., Nature New
        Biol., 1973, 245, 8.

19.   Tennant, R.W., Schluter, B., Wen Kuang Yang and Brown, A.,
         Proc. Nat. Acad. Sci. U.S.A.,1974,11, 4241.
20.   Lilly, F., and Pincus, T., Adv. Cancer Res.,1973,17, 231.
21.   Lilly, F., Bibl. Haematol.,1970,36, 213
22.   Lilly, F., J. Nat. Cancer Inst.,1970,45, 163.
23.   Mintz, B., Fund. Cancer. Res. M.D. Anderson Hospital and
         Tumour Inst.,1970,477.
24   Howe, M.L., Goldstein, A.L., and Battisto, J.R.,
         Proc. Nat. Acad. Sci. U.S.A.,1970,67, 613.
25.   Carter, J., and Wegmann, T., Cellular Immunol.,1973,7, 402
26.   Hilgers, J., Decleve, A., Galesloot, J., and Kaplan, H.S.
         Cancer Res.,1974,34, 2553.

LOW NUMBERS OF TUMOR CELLS SUPPRESS THE HOST IMMUNE SYSTEM

Eckehart Kölsch and Rudolf Mengersen

Heinrich-Pette-Institut für experimentelle Virologie und
Immunologie an der Universität Hamburg
2 Hamburg 20, Martinistrasse 52, Fed. Rep. Germany

Most spontaneous tumors are of clonal origin, evidence coming
from the analysis of myeloma proteins and from other biochemical
data (1,2). Therefore, in experimental tumor immunology emphasis
must be put on the analysis of effects caused by small numbers of
tumor cells. An immunological approach to tumor elimination might
have a greater chance to be successful in early states of tumorigenesis than in late states of tumor growth. Many experiments
with transplantable syngeneic and allogeneic tumors demonstrate
that injection of a small dose of cells leads to an unexpected
high take of tumors. The terms "sneaking through" (3) and "dilution escape" (4) have been coined to describe this phenomenon
which could be either immunological or non-immunological. Recently, experiments have been put forward suggesting that dilution
escape might be the result of non-specific inhibition of anti-
allograft reactions by tumor cell populations too small to be immunogenic (5). In contrast, we have suggested, on the basis of
our experiments, that sneaking through might be an immunological
process by which a growing tumor specifically paralyzes the immune
system at a cell concentration too low to be immunogenic (6,7).

The tumor used is a BALB/c mastocytoma BM3 with a long transplantation history which shares some antigenic determinants with
DBA/2 P 815 mastocytoma cells and which, apart from growing best
in BALB/c mice, can kill animals from other inbred strains when
cells are inoculated in sufficiently large numbers. For the purpose of our experiments it was necessary to have a tumor which because of its cell size remains in the peritoneal cavity, allowing
permanent exposure to immunocompetent cells.

Tumor incidences after injection of graded numbers of living

431

Table 1. Incidence of tumors in BALB/c mice injected
with a single dose of living BM3 cells

Number of living cells injected	Percentage of tumors
2×10^1	16
1×10^2	32
5×10^2	58
1×10^3	17
1×10^4	20
3×10^4	45
1×10^5	75
5×10^5	95
6×10^6	100

tumor cells are given in Table 1. The frequency decreases from
100% upon injection of 10^6 cells to a plateau of 20% when 10^3 - 10^4
tumor cells are transferred. If, however, 5×10^2 cells are injected, the tumor frequency rises again to 58% (sneaking through).
For further analysis mice were injected with graded numbers of X-
irradiated tumor cells and subsequently challenged with living BM3
cells. It can be seen (Table 2) that animals pretreated with 10^2
- 10^3 irradiated tumor cells develop more tumors when challenged
with living tumor cells than those pretreated with 10^0 - 10^1 cells.
Animals pretreated with 10^4 - 10^6 irradiated tumor cells develop
immunity. Thus, sneaking through conditions can be induced by

Table 2. Tumor incidences in BALB/c mice pretreated
with irradiated and challenged with living BM3 cells

Pretreatment (irradiated cells)	Tumor incidence after challenge with living cells
10^0 - 10^1	11/20
10^2 - 10^3	18/20
10^4 - 10^6	0/40

Table 3. Tumor incidence in animals pretreated before challenge

Challenged with	Pretreated with	
	saline	5×10^1 irradiated BM3 cells
Living BM3 cells	8/20	17/20
Living EL4 cells	0/20	0/20

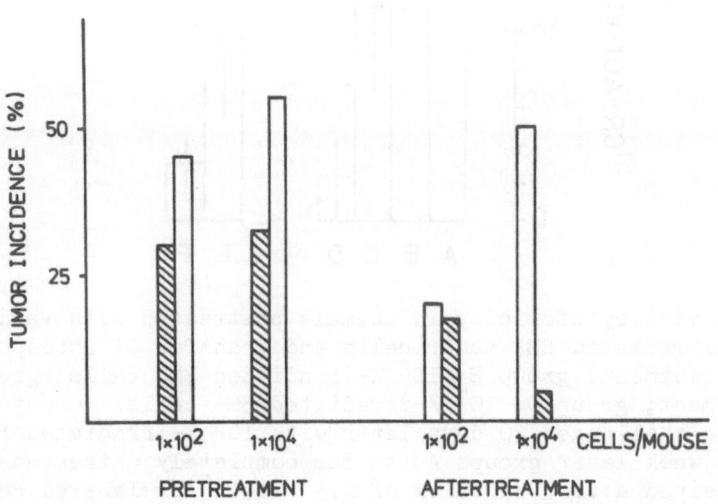

Fig. 1. Effect of pre- and aftertreatment with 10^4 glutaraldehyde-fixed BM3 cells on the tumor incidence in animals injected with 10^2 (sneaking through dose) or 10^4 living tumor cells. Dashed bars represent treatment with glutaraldehyde, open bars are controls. Pretreatment: 10^4 glutaraldehyde-fixed cells 14 days before injection of living cells. Aftertreatment: 10^4 glutaraldehyde-fixed cells 21 days after injection of living cells. Forty animals per group. No tumors arose in animals receiving only glutaraldehyde-fixed cells. Analysis by χ^2-test: pretreatment, 10^2: $p < 0.15$; pretreatment, 10^4: $p < 0.05$; aftertreatment, 10^2: $p = 1$; aftertreatment, 10^4: $p < 0.001$.

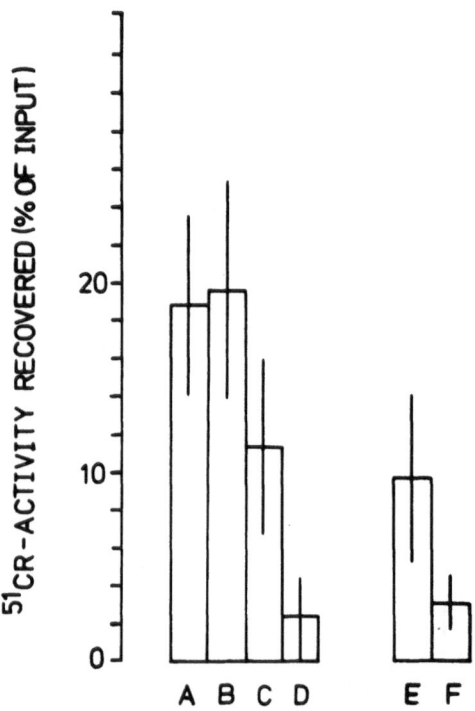

<u>Fig. 2</u>. In vivo cytotoxicity in animals pretreated with various
doses of X-irradiated BM3 tumor cells and transfer of unresponsiveness. Pretreatment: group B: 10^2 X-irradiated BM3 cells; group C:
no pretreatment; group D: 10^7 X-irradiated BM3 cells. Groups B,
C and D were challenged 30 days later with 10^5 X-irradiated BM3
cells. One week later groups A (so far completely untreated), B,
C and D received a test inoculum of 2.5 x 10^5 ^{51}Cr-labeled BM3
cells (9 x 10^4 cpm). ^{51}Cr retention was measured 20 h later by
collecting peritoneal cells and counting the radioactivity retained. Groups E and F were assayed in a similar way. Animals
were immunized with 10^5 X-irradiated BM3 cells. Twelve days later
they received 3 x 10^7 spleen cells/mouse i.p. from animals pretreated as group B (group E) or normal spleen cells (group F).
Four days after transfer of spleen cells mice were challenged with
10^5 BM3 cells. Another 12 days later the in vivo cytotoxicity was
measured.

subimmunogenic numbers of irradiated tumor cells. A full documentation of several experiments can be found elsewhere (6,7).

The next experiments show that sneaking through is not due to general immune suppression since the allogeneic lymphoma EL4 does not grow in animals showing sneaking through for BM3 cells (Table 3), nor is the T cell-mediated cytotoxicity against EL4 suppressed in these mice (7).

In a further attempt to demonstrate immunological specificity of sneaking through we used glutaraldehyde-fixed BM3 cells to test the immunological reactivity of animals confronted with subimmunogenic doses of antigen. Preliminary experiments had shown that injection of glutaraldehyde-fixed BM3 cells given after the injection of 10^4 living BM3 cells reduced tumor incidences. Thus, glutaraldehyde-fixed BM3 cells can induce immunity as already demonstrated for other systems (8). We suspected, however, that subimmunogenic doses of 10^2 living tumor cells in contrast to 10^4 cells could induce specific unresponsiveness; therefore, in this case a subsequent injection of 10^4 glutaraldehyde-fixed cells should not reduce tumor incidences. That is exactly what has been found. The induction of a primary as well as an anamnestic response to glutaraldehyde-fixed BM3 cells is suppressed in animals injected with 10^2 living tumor cells followed by 10^4 glutaraldehyde-fixed BM3 cells (Fig. 1). The third approach to test for specificity in the sneaking through experiment was made by an in vivo ^{51}Cr release assay (6). Pretreatment of mice with 10^2 X-irradiated tumor cells induces unresponsiveness as measured by ^{51}Cr retention (Fig. 2). Furthermore, spleen cells from these unresponsive animals are able to suppress immune reactivity upon transfer into primed animals (Fig. 2).

In conclusion, sneaking through of BM3 mastocytoma cells carries features of low zone tolerance (9) since it is induced with very small subimmunogenic doses of antigen. It differs from classical enhancement (10), from which it is separated by a dose range inducing immunity. The mechanism by which sneaking through is achieved is still unknown. It is possible that antibodies other than those cytotoxic in C'-dependent lysis or K cell activity are involved. In addition to such stimulating antibodies (11), suppressor T cells need to be considered. So far, our data demonstrate the following important finding. Specific unresponsiveness is induced by tumor cells too low in number to elicit effective immunity, suggesting that a growing tumor successfully undermines and paralyzes the host immune system, counteracting immune surveillance in an early state of tumorigenesis.

ACKNOWLEDGMENT

This work was supported by the Deutsche Forschungsgemein-schaft.

REFERENCES

1. Murray, R.F., Jr., Hobbs, R.F., and Payne, B. (1971): Nature 232, 51.
2. Fialkow, P.J., Klein, E., Klein, G., Clifford, P., and Singh, S. (1973): J. exp. Med. 138, 89.
3. Old, L.J., Boyse, E.A., Clarke, D.A., and Carswell, E.A. (1962): Ann. N.Y. Acad. Sci. 101, 80.
4. Bonmassar, E., Goldin, A., and Cudkowicz, G. (1971): Trans-plantation 12, 314.
5. Bonmassar, E., Menconi, E., Goldin, A., and Cudkowicz, G. (1974): J. Natl. Cancer Inst. 53, 475.
6. Kölsch, E., Mengersen, R., and Diller, E. (1973): Europ. J. Cancer 9, 879.
7. Mengersen, R., Schick, R., and Kölsch, E. (1975): Europ. J. Immunol. 5, in press.
8. Sanderson, C.J., and Frost, P. (1974): Nature 248, 691.
9. Kölsch, E., Stumpf, R., and Weber, G. (1975): Transplant. Rev. 26, in press.
10. Voisin, G.A. (1971): Progr. Allergy 15, 328.
11. Fink, M.P., Parker, C.W., Shearer, W.T. (1975): Nature 255, 404.

STUDIES ON EFFECTOR CELL - TARGET CELL INTERACTIONS IN VITRO BY MEANS OF THE QUANTITATIVE IMMUNOADHERENCE TECHNIQUE

F. DOLJANSKI, Y. MARKSON, S. KATZAV, AND D.W. WEISS

LAUTENBERG CENTER FOR GENERAL AND TUMOR IMMUNOLOGY, AND
DEPARTMENT OF EXPERIMENTAL MEDICINE AND CANCER RESEARCH
HEBREW UNIVERSITY - HADASSAH MEDICAL SCHOOL, JERUSALEM,
ISRAEL

We have previously reported the development of a quantitative immunoadherence (IA) test for the in vitro detection of effector cells specifically reactive with allogeneic and autochthonous tumor target cells (1, 2). The test is performed by labeling lymphoid tissue cells with ^{51}Cr and placing them in contact with target cells in stationary cultures for 2h. The nonadhering lymphoid cells are then removed by washing, and the extent of adherence of effector cells from tumor-bearing and normal animals determined by measuring the radioactivity remaining in the target cultures and that present in the non-adherent lymphoid cells. The degree of adherence capacity is calculated by the formula:

$$\% \text{ adherence} = \frac{\text{cpm of adherent lymphoid cells}}{\text{cpm of adherent} + \text{cpm of nonadherent lymphoid cells}} \times 100$$

The IA test was developed in the model system of Rous sarcomas (RS) of chickens (1), and it was found that lymphoid tissue cells of tumor-bearing hosts ("sensitized lymphoid cells") consistently show greater adherence for RS cells than do lymphoid cells from normal donors ("normal lymphoid cells"). Moreover, the adherence of lymphoid cells to the autochthonous tumor was invariably greater than that to allogeneic RS target cells. In contrast, lymphoid cells from tumor-bearing and normal donors reacted to a similar extent with a variety of normal target cells. The preferential adherence capacity of sensitized lymphoid cells correlated well with their cytotoxic competence. Preliminary observations with syngeneic mouse tumors suggested that specific IA is even more pronounced (2) in these models.

The advantages of the quantitative IA test for estimating the levels of specific reactivity in effector cell populations lie with its rapidity, reproducibility, the opportunity to detect reactivity against individual-specific tumor-associated antigens even against a background of strongly expressed group-specific immunogenicities, and the consideration that the assay focuses on the earliest stages of effector - target cell interactions.

The present communication reports the results of further studies conducted with the IA method in three directions: Analysis of the specificity of effector cell reactivity, by comparing the adherence capacity of lymphoid cells from mice bearing different tumors against the corresponding and against other syngeneic neoplasms; attempts to correlate the degree of IA in vitro with the progress of tumor development in vivo; and, initiation of steps towards the identification of the tumor cell surface antigens responsible for effector cell IA.

SPECIFICITY OF IMMUNOADHERENCE OF EFFECTOR CELLS FROM TUMOR BEARING MICE

Pooled lymph node (LN) cells of mice bearing syngeneic tumor isografts or spontaneously developing mammary adenocarcinomas were tested for adherence capacity in syngeneic interactions with the corresponding and with other tumor target cells. (Mouse LN cells appear more reactive in IA than mouse splenocytes (2).) The results of several representative experiments are presented in Figure 1, which also shows, for purposes of comparison, the adherence of normal chicken splenocytes and of splenocytes from birds with tumors induced by the Schmidt-Ruppin (SR) strain of Rous Sarcoma Virus (RSV) with target cells of the same RS. The sensitized chicken lymphoid cells again exhibited greater adherence to the RS targets than did normal lymphoid cells, with preferential autochthonous interaction. LN cells from tumor bearing mice displayed much greater adherence in interaction with the corresponding tumor target cells than did LN cells from a normal donor with any of the targets, but did not react more pronouncedly in contact with other syngeneic neoplasms. These findings, confirmed in a number of additional experiments, point to the high specificity of the IA reaction.

IMMUNOADHERENCE CAPACITY OF SPLENOCYTES FROM CHICKENS BEARING RS OF DIFFERENT SIZE FOR ALLOGENEIC RS CELLS.

The growth kinetics of Rous sarcomas in the primary chicken host vary from bird to bird; this is shown for 4 tumors in Figure 2. It is noted that the tumors appearing early after virus inoculation tend to grow more rapidly than those making their appearance later; this has been a consistent observation. An experiment was now

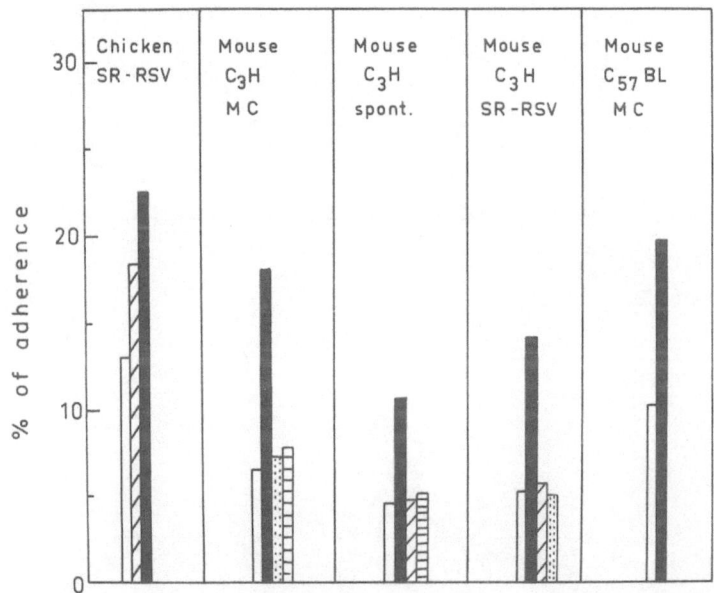

Figure 1: Adherence of chicken (White Leghorn) spleen and mouse LN
cells to the tumor target cells indicated in each compartment.
Chicken system: Splenocytes from normal bird (open bar), bird bearing RS allogeneic to RS target cells (striated bar), and bird with
tumor autochthonous to same target cells (filled bar). Mouse
systems: LN cells from normal mice and from mice bearing a primary
spontaneous mammary carcinoma ("spont") or isografts of a
methylcholanthrene induced sarcoma ("MC") or a RS induced by the
SR-RSV ("SR-RSV"), interacting with target cells of the syngeneic
neoplasms indicated in each rubric. Effector cells from a normal
mouse, open bars; from a mouse bearing the corresponding tumor,
filled bars; and, from a mouse bearing one of the other tumors,
dotted and striated bars.

conducted in which 9 chickens were inoculated with RSV on the same
day, and sacrificed 25 days later, when the tumors had reached
various sizes in different birds. The adherence ability of
splenocytes from each host was assessed simultaneously for the target
cells of a RS allogeneic to all the spleen donors. It is seen
(Figure 3) that splenocytes from hosts with small tumors had similar
adherence capacity as those from birds with medium-sized growths
(ca. 100 cu.mm.), and that adherence was less when effector cells

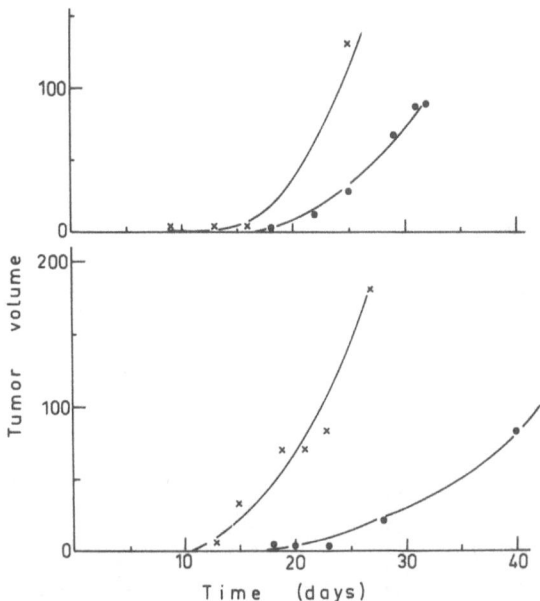

Figure 2: Growth kinetics of 4 RS in the primary chicken hosts
inoculated with SR-RSV. Tumor volumes (in cu.mm.) approximated by
calculation V=ab x h, where a and b are largest and smallest
diameters evenly bisecting tumor at right angles to each other, and
h height of the tumor. Time in days after virus inoculation.

were from chickens with large sarcomas (ca. 200 cu.mm.). Decline
of splenocyte adherence capacity was confirmed in 20 additional
experiments comparing the reactivity of effector cells from birds
infected with RSV simultaneously and having either medium or large
tumors at given times of testing.

It is not possible, however, to infer that tumor size as such
is the sole determinant of host effector cell adherence ability.
Patterns of tumor development undoubtedly reflect ongoing interactions between inherent growth capacity of neoplasms, differential
host immunological responsiveness, and other factors defining the
tissue microenvironment (3). The vigorous adherence capacity of
splenocytes from chickens with even small tumors could be interpreted
as indicating either that once a minimal tumor has formed, host
splenocyte recognition is generally already pronounced, or that the
small size of the tumors 25 days after RSV infection manifests
potent host surveillance. The reduced splenocyte adherence of birds
with large tumors could be ascribed to weak immunogenicity of rapidly

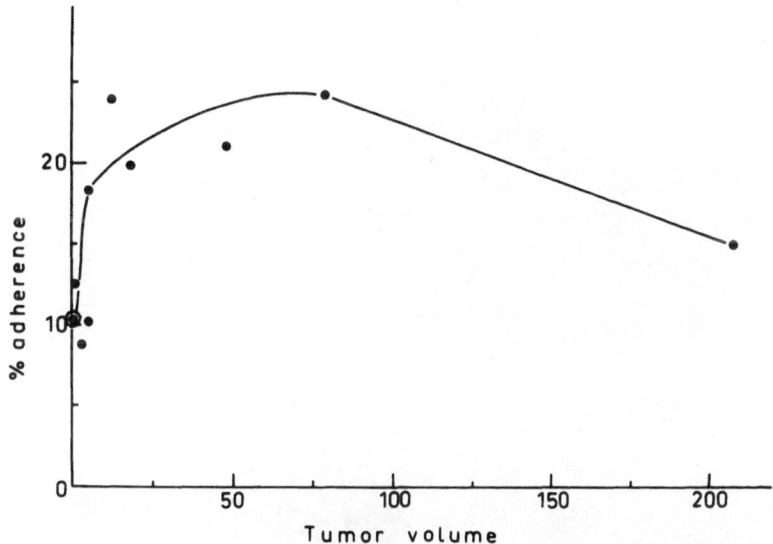

Figure 3:   Adherence of splenocytes from chickens with RS of
different size 25 days after inoculation of SR-RSV. Each point
represents results with effector cells from one host, interacting
with the same allogeneic RS targets. Circled point represents
result of interaction of normal chicken splenocytes with same RS
targets.

growing tumors, generalized immunological dyscrasia, or specific
blocking of effector cell receptors by surface antigens shed from
the tumor cells (4). To discriminate between these and other
possibilities, it will be necessary to ascertain the adherence
capacity of effector cells from the same hosts at progressive
stages of tumor development.

APPROACH TOWARDS THE IDENTIFICATION OF TUMOR-ASSOCIATED
CELL SURFACE ANTIGENS

Specific IA in tumor systems is based on the recognition by
sensitized effector cells of tumor-associated antigenic determinants
on the surface of the target cells. Since such specific determinants
probably represent only a small portion of the total surface
antigenic entities, their identification poses considerable
difficulty. The task would be made easier if it were possible to
compare the surface composition of populations of tumor cells with
that of similar neoplastic clones but which fail to express the

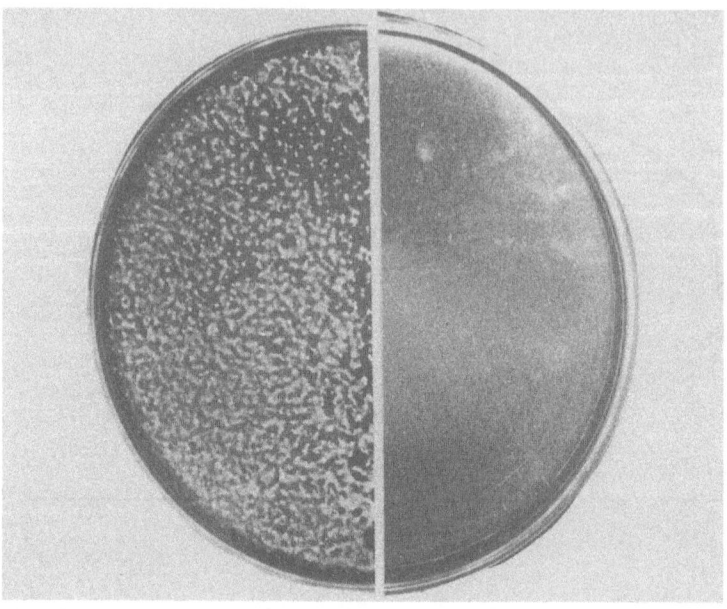

Figure 4: Growth of untreated (left) and BUDR treated (right) chicken RS cells in plates, with standard culture medium (1); appearance after 14 days incubation. Magnification x 1.

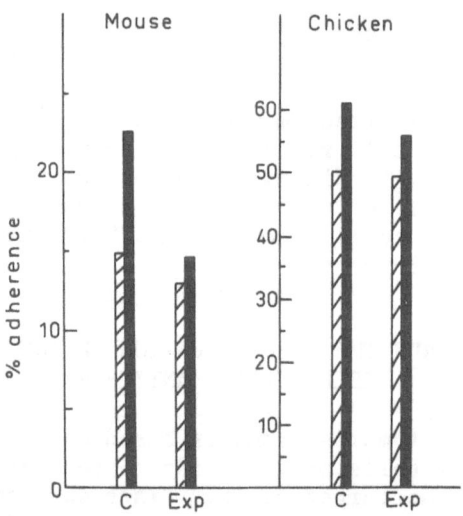

Figure 5: Adherence of mouse LN and chicken spleen cells from normal hosts (striated bars) or hosts bearing RS tumors (filled bars) with syngeneic (mouse) or allogeneic (chicken) RS target cells. C = RS target cells not treated with BUDR; Exp = RS target cells treated with BUDR.

antigenic markers with which sensitized effector cells interact. 5-bromo-2'-deoxyuridine (BUDR) selectively inhibits the expression of differentiated cell characteristics without impinging on more basic cell properties, such as cell division (5-7). BUDR also inhibits the phenotypic expression of neoplastic properties, at least for some tumors (8-10). Accordingly,we tested the IA ability of sensitized effector cells for BUDR treated and untreated RS targets.

BUDR treatment of chicken RS cells resulted in striking morphological changes. Whereas untreated cells are round and highly refractile, growing in plates as clusters discernible with the naked eye, BUDR treated cells adhere closely to the plate surface, forming a flat, transparent, non-refractile monolayer of cells having some resemblance to normal fibroblasts (Figure 4). Similar, although less striking, morphological changes were observed for mouse RS cells. The adherence of sensitized lymphoid cells to BUDR treated RS targets was less than that for untreated RS cells. This reduction was small in the chicken system, and marked in case of the mouse model. Figure 5 presents the results of one of 3 experiments, each yielding very similar findings. This observation paves the way for experiments to identify bio-chemically the RS cell surface constituents diminished after exposure to BUDR and responsible for IA.

REFERENCES

1. Wainberg, M., Markson, Y., Weiss, D.W., and Doljanski, F. P.N.A.S. 71: 3565, 1974.
2. Doljanski, F., Markson, Y., Wainberg, M.A., and Weiss, D.W. Transp. Proc. Vol. VII. No. 1. Supp. 1. M. Schlesinger and R.E. Billingham, eds., Grune and Stratton, N.Y., p. 519, 1975.
3. Weiss, D.W. In: International Symposium on the Spontaneous Regression of Cancer. The Johns Hopkins Hospital, N.C.I. Monograph. In press, 1975.
4. Ben-Sasson, Z., Weiss, D.W., and Doljanski, F. J. Natl. Cancer Inst., 52: 405, 1974.
5. Abbott, J., and Holtzer, H. P.N.A.S. 59: 1144, 1968.
6. Turkington, R.W., Majumder, G.C., and Riddle, M. J. Biol. Chem. 246: 1814, 1971.
7. Levitt, D., and Dorfman, A. P.N.A.S. 70: 2201, 1973.
8. Silagi, S., and Bruce, S.A. P.N.A.S. 66: 72, 1970.
9. Kreider, J.W., Del Villano, B., Shoff, W.H., and Davidson, E.A. Cancer Research, 32: 2148, 1972.
10. Rothschild, H., and Black, P.H. J. Cell. Physiol. 81: 217, 1973.

IMMUNOLOGIC RESPONSES OF THE AUTOCHTHONOUS HOST AGAINST TUMORS INDUCED BY ULTRAVIOLET LIGHT

Margaret L. Kripke and Michael S. Fisher

Basic Research Program, Frederick Cancer Research
Center, Frederick, Maryland, and Department of
Pathology, University of Utah College of Medicine,
Salt Lake City, Utah

Skin cancer can be induced in mice by exposing them repeatedly to ultraviolet (UV) light over a long period of time. Recently, we reported that tumors with spindle cell morphology, induced in inbred mice by chronic UV irradiation, are highly antigenic and have individual or non-crossreacting, tumor specific transplantation antigens (1). Most tumors of this type are immunologically rejected after transplantation to normal syngeneic recipients and grow only in immunologically deficient hosts. In spite of their strong antigenicity, these tumors grow progressively in the primary host and rarely undergo regression in situ. Thus, the animal in which the tumor has arisen is incapable of mounting an effective immunologic attack against the developing tumor, even though a normal syngeneic recipient will reject the tumor after primary transplantation. This suggests that mechanisms exist that enable these tumors to escape immunologic destruction in situ, and/or that the immune response of the primary host is altered in a way that favors, rather than hinders, tumor growth. Here, we address the following question: Why does the primary host fail to reject its own highly antigenic tumor?

Our first step was to determine whether the inability of the host to reject its tumor is a local phenomenon, restricted to the site of the tumor, or whether it is expressed systemically. Skin tumors were induced on the backs of C3Hf/Sm mice by chronic UV irradiation. The backs of the animals were shaved weekly and exposed to UV light for 60 seconds, 3 times per week, until tumors developed (an average of 45 weeks). The light source was an intermediate pressure 100-W quartz-mercury arc lamp (Hanovia) which delivered a dose rate of approximately

3×10^5 ergs/cm^2/sec. over a wavelength range of 280-320 nm.
Primary spindle cell tumors of approximately 10mm in diameter
were surgically excised, cut into 1mm^3 fragments and retransplanted
subcutaneously on the ventral (non-irradiated) side of the
tumor donor. At the same time, tumor fragments were transplanted
into groups of 3-5 syngeneic age-matched normal animals and
groups of recipients immunosuppressed by adult thymectomy and
450r whole body X-irradiation (ATX recipients). The tumor
recipients were palpated once a week for at least 10 weeks and
the tumor sizes recorded.

    Only 2 tumors grew progressively in 1 or more normal recipients,
while 11 out of 12 grew in at least 1 immunosuppressed recipient
(table 1). All 12 grew progressively when retransplanted to the
primary host, indicating that at the time when tumors are
detectable grossly, the primary host is systemically altered in
a way that favors tumor growth.

    We then asked whether this inability to reject tumors in vivo
is restricted to an animal's own tumor (tumor-specific), or whether
it extends to tumors induced by UV light in other syngeneic mice.
If it is tumor-specific, then the ability to reject other UV-induced
tumors should remain intact, since these tumors do not cross-react
antigenically in vivo (1,2). Six of the tumors tested in their
autochthonous hosts were also transplanted, at the same time, into
7 different primary tumor hosts. In every case, the tumors grew
progressively (table 1: syngeneic host). This suggests that the
major mechanism underlying the inability of the primary host to
reject its own tumor may not involve such tumor-specific phenomena
as immunological tolerance or serum blocking factors.

Table 1--Growth of transplanted syngeneic UV-induced spindle
cell tumors

Recipients	No. of transplantable tumors	No. of progressively growing implants
	No. tested	No. mice implanted
Normal	2/12	4/58
ATX	11/12	27/56
Autochthonous host	12/12	12/12
Syngeneic host	6/6	7/7

This systemic alteration of the primary host could be generated by either the presence of the tumor itself, or by the chronic exposures to UV light. To distinguish between these possibilities, we implanted fragments of UV-induced spindle cell tumors into groups of mice that had been UV irradiated (60 sec., 3x/wk) for various lengths of time. Age-matched normal controls and ATX positive controls were included in each testing. Under our conditions of UV irradiation, the first tumors are detectable macroscopically after 25-30 weeks of treatment, with a mean time of appearance of about 45 weeks. The results are summarized in table 2. Most of the tumor implants grew progressively in UV irradiated mice, while none grew in normal age-matched controls. Even with only 2 weeks of UV treatment, some of the mice were unable to prevent the progressive outgrowth of the transplanted tumors. This suggests that exposure to the carcinogen itself induces a systemic alteration that promotes tumor growth and/or prevents immunologic destruction of the tumor.

One possible explanation for our observation is that UV treatment might lead to a state of general immune depression, thereby rendering the animals susceptible to the growth of a highly antigenic tumor. To explore this possibility, we tested the reactivity of UV irradiated mice against an allogenic UV-induced tumor. Groups of mice treated with UV for 8 or 17 weeks were implanted with a C3Hf (syngeneic) or an A/J (allogeneic)

Table 2--Growth of a syngeneic UV-tumor in UV
irradiated C3Hf mice

Weeks of UV treatment	UV irradiated	Normal	ATX	Transplant generation of challenge tumor #2:3
30	5/5	0/5[*]	5/5	5
26	5/5	0/5	4/5	4
15	6/9	0/10	3/5	4
8	12/15	0/15	16/20	4
4	5/5	0/5	3/7	3
2	3/5	0/5	2/10	3

[*]Number of progressively growing implants/number of mice challenged

Table 3--Tumor allograft rejection in UV irradiated mice

Weeks of UV treatment	Challenge tumor	UV treated C3Hf	Normal C3Hf	Syngeneic ATX
8	C3Hf	3/5*	0/5	7/10
	A/J	0/5	0/5	5/5
17	C3Hf	10/10	1/10	5/5
	A/J	0/10	0/10	5/5

*Number of progressively growing implants/number of mice challenged

UV-induced tumor. The strain A tumor is only weakly immunogenic and grows progressively in normal syngeneic mice. As is shown in table 3, all of the UV-treated mice rejected their tumor allografts, while the syngeneic tumor implants grew progressively in most of these recipients.

We then tested the effect of UV irradiation on the reactivity of mice that were pre-immunized against a syngeneic UV-induced tumor. Animals were implanted with fragments of tumor #2:3 subcutaneously. Following regression of the implants, these mice and a group of nonimmunized controls were UV irradiated for 15 weeks. The mice were then challenged with either the immunizing tumor (#2:3) or a non-crossreacting UV-induced tumor (#861). The results, summarized in table 4, show that UV irradiation does not abrogate the ability of immunized mice to resist challenge with the immunizing tumor, and only affects the first-set rejection reaction.

From these experiments, we conclude that UV irradiation does not lead to a state of complete immune depression. Even though they fail to reject primary implants of a syngeneic UV-induced tumor, UV irradiated mice still exhibit a second-set response to these tumors, and can reject a primary challenge with a UV-induced tumor allograft. It is possible that UV treatment induces a very moderate degree of immunosuppression, detectable upon primary exposure to weak cellular antigens, but insufficient to affect either the amplified second-set rejection of weakly antigenic cells, or the primary rejection of grafts across the major histocompatibility barrier.

Table 4--Effect of UV treatment on tumor immune mice

Challenge tumor	2:3 Immune + 15 wks UV	15 wks UV	Normal	ATX
2:3	0/10	6/9	0/10	3/5
861	6/10	8/10	1/10	5/5

*Number of progressively growing implants/number of mice challenged

Alternatively, UV irradiation might adversely affect a population of effector cells that functions to a greater degree upon first challenge to a syngeneic tumor than on second challenge. Consistent with this possibility is the finding that trypan blue treatment, which inhibits the cytotoxic activity of macrophages (3,4), greatly delays the primary rejection of syngeneic UV-induced tumors, but has no effect on the rejection response of pre-immunized mice (5). Thus, it is possible that direct inactivation of macrophages by UV treatment, or inhibition of macrophage function by a humoral factor induced by UV treatment, could account for our findings.

A third possibility is that tumor growth promoting substances are produced or released in response to UV irradiation, and that these factors enable the tumor to overcome immunologic defense mechanisms. Further experimentation is required to determine whether any or all of these possibilities actually contribute to the survival of these tumors in the autochthonous host.

ACKNOWLEDGMENTS

Research supported by the U.S. Public Health Service Contract NOI-CP-45600 from the National Cancer Institute

REFERENCES

(1) Kripke M.L., J Natl Cancer Inst 53:1333, 1974.
(2) Pasternak, G., Graffi, A., and K. Horn. Acta Biol Med Ger 13:276, 1964.
(3) Hibbs, J.B., Jr. Science 184:468, 1974
(4) Hibbs, J.B., Jr. Transplantation 19:77, 1975.
(5) Kripke, M.L., Gruys, M.E., and J.B. Hibbs, Jr. Submitted for publication.

THE IN VIVO COATING OF TUMOR CELLS BY POTENTIALLY CYTOTOXIC ANTI-TUMOR ANTIBODIES[1]

Maya Ran[*], Isaac P. Witz[*] and George Klein[†]

[*]Department of Microbiology, The George S. Wise Center for Life Sciences, Tel Aviv University, Tel Aviv, Israel
[†]Department of Tumor Biology, Karolinska Institutet, Stockholm, Sweden

INTRODUCTION

Masking of cell surface antigens was first suggested as one of the mechanisms by which enhancing antibodies operate in a tumor bearing host (1). Such a masking, inferred also from studies showing that in vivo growing tumor cells are coated with immuno-globulin (Ig), is lately considered a key event in many alternative pathways by which the tumor escapes the immune reactivity of the host (2). This consideration is supported by the following indirect evidence: 1. Enhancement of tumor growth by immunoglobulin (Ig)-containing tumor eluates (3-4). 2. Blocking of in vitro cell mediated antitumor activity by tumor eluates, of human and animal origin (4-6). 3. Demonstration of an increased ability of human tumor cells to stimulate DNA synthesis in autochthonous lymphocytes following "unmasking" of tumor antigens (7). The association between tumor cell surface and Ig has been demonstrated directly (8). Yet it is not clear whether the coating of tumor cells by Ig and the masking of cell surface antigens is the very same phenomenon. This study was aimed to determine whether part of the Ig coating of Polyoma virus induced mouse tumor cells (SEYF-a, 9) consists of specific antibodies.

[1]This study was supported by NCI Contract No.NOI-CB-43858

EXPERIMENTAL

Detection of Circulating Antibodies Mediating Complement-dependent Lysis of SEYF-a Cells in Tumor Bearing Mice

Sera collected from SEYF-a bearing mice on different days after tumor inoculation were assayed for their capacity to mediate complement-dependent lysis (CdL) towards ^{51}Cr labelled SEYF-a cells propagated in vivo for 7 days. The source of the complement in these experiments was normal rabbit serum (NRS). The range of the cytotoxicity index (CI) for 1:16 serum dilution as well as the range of the cytotoxicity titers is presented in Table I. No demonstratable level of cytotoxicity was mediated by serum drawn during the first week after tumor inoculation. Circulating cytotoxic antibodies appeared during the second week after inoculation and markedly increased during the second half of that week. Cytotoxicity titers remained high throughout the entire survival time.

Table I

Antibodies mediating complement dependent cytotoxicity towards SEYF-a cells, in the circulation of SEYF-a bearing mice

Days after inoculation[1]	No. of assayed mice	CI given by a 1:16 serum dilution	Titer[2]
5	1	0	<2
7	5	0–0.15	<2
8	4	0–0.15	<2
9	3	0.05–0.30	<2; <2; <4
11	3	0.05–0.45	<2; 32; 128
12	4	0.60–0.70	16; 32; 128; 128
13	3	0.50–0.80	16; 32; 256
14	3	0.50–0.90	16; 128; 128–256
17	2	0.60–0.90	16–32; 32
19	4	0.40–0.90	16–32; 32–64; 32–64; 64–128
24	2	0.85–0.90	64–128; 128
30	2	0.70–0.75	128; 128–256

1) 2×10^6 cells were injected i.p. to each mouse. Mice were bled from the retro-orbital sinus on the day recorded.

2) Titer of cytotoxic antibodies = reciprocal of serum dilution causing a CI of 0.50. Individual results are presented.

Demonstration of Cell-bound Cytotoxic Antibodies on the Surface of in vivo Propagated SEYF-a Cells

The appearance of circulating cytotoxic antibodies during
in vivo propagation of SEYF-a cells was associated with the presence
of such antibodies on the surface of cells propagated in vivo for
two or three weeks. This was demonstrated by adding NRS, as a source
of complement (C'), to the cells. The results are summarized in
Table II. Two weeks old cells were much more sensitive to the cytotoxic effect of normal rabbit serum than 7 days old cells. The
cytotoxic effect of NRS towards older cells was not eliminated by
absorption of natural rabbit anti mouse antibodies. Thus, a higher
amount of cell bound cytotoxic antibodies was detected on two weeks
old cells than on one week old cells, by NRS absorbed either with
mouse liver powder or with SEYF-a cells.

Table II

Cell-bound cytotoxic antibodies on in vivo propagated SEYF-a cells[1]

Treatment of complement	CI of cells propagated in vivo for the indicated post inoculation period [2]		
	1 week	2 weeks	3 weeks
None	0.30 ± 0.30[3]	0.85 ± 0.15[3]	0.90 ± 0.15
Absorption with mouse liver powder	0.10 ± 0[4]	0.80 ± 0.30[4]	0.95 ± 0.05
Absorption with 1,2 or 3 weeks old SEYF-a cells	0.45 ± 0.10[5]	0.80 ± 0[5]	

1) Cell lysis caused by adding C' alone at a final dilution of 1:15
   to ^{51}Cr labelled cells was measured. The NRS which served as
   source of C' was complementary in all the dilutions recorded.
   A mean calculated from 2-6 experiments is given.

2) Cells harvested one, two or three weeks after injection were
   used as targets.

3) 4) 5)
   Values marked with the same number are significally different
   (P < 0.01 as measured by t test) from each other.

The Antigenic Expression of in vivo Propagated SEYF-a Cells

The question whether antigenic determinants on SEYF-a cells were in fact masked during in vivo propagation was investigated. SEYF-a cells propagated in vivo for 7 days were compared to three weeks old cells in their capacity to compete against ^{51}Cr labelled 7 days old cells for hyperimmune syngeneic anti SEYF-a antibodies. The results shown in Table III demonstrate that the competition capacity of 7 day old cells was higher than that of cells propagated in vivo for 20 days. In addition the competition capacity of 7 day old cells, but not of 20 days old ones, was proportional to the amount of cells present in the cytotoxicity mixture.

The availability of antigenic determinants on in vivo propagated SEYF-a cells was also measured by their capacity to absorb hyperimmune syngeneic anti SEYF-a antibodies. As demonstrated in Table IV, 7 days old cells absorbed the cytotoxicity of anti SEYF-a antiserum while cells propagated for 20 days did not (experiment No.I., serum dilution 1:16). Transferring the cells propagated in vivo for 20 days into short term culture (a treatment causing a

Table III
The Availability of Antigenic Determinants on in vivo Propagated SEYF-a Cells, as Measured by Competition Assays

Propagation time in vivo of unlabelled competitor cells[1]	Exp	Inhibition of cytotoxicity (%)[2] unlabelled/labelled cells ratio				
		0.6	1.25	2.5	5.0	10.0
First week	I	28	35	45	60	
	II		25	45	55	100
Third week	I	30	25	20	25	
	II		5	25	0	20

1) Unlabelled competitor cells were allowed to porpagate in vivo for either one or three weeks.

2) Inhibition of cytotoxicity was calculated as % of controls performed in the absence of competitor cells. (CI levels of controls was around 0.50).

Table IV

The Availability of Antigenic Determinants on in vivo Propagated SEYF-a Cells Measured by Absorption Experiments

Treatment of absorbing cells after explantation	Propagation time in vivo	Inhibition of Cytotoxicity (%)[1] serum dilutions					
		1:16	1:32	1:64	1:16	1:32	1:64
		Exp.I			Exp.II		
None	7 days	80[3]	30	30			
	20 days	40[3]	0	0	15[3]	16[3]	30
Incubation[2]	7 days	75[3]	30	30			
	20 days	50[3]	40	20	25[3]	25[3]	40

1. Inhibition of cytotoxicity (%) was calculated from CI values given by the same dilutions of non-absorbed antiserum.

2. Cells were cultured for 3 hours at 37°C and the culture medium changed every hour. The cells were then adjusted to the desired concentration and mixed with antiserum for absorption.

3. Seven days old cells had a significantly higher absorption capacity than 20 days old ones (P < 0.01). The absorption capacity of 20 days old cells incubated for 3 hours at 37°C was significantly higher than the absorption capacity of non-incubated 20 days old cells (P < 0.05 in experiment I and P < 0.01 in experiment II).

spontaneous release of absorbed Ig into the supernatnant (10)) significantly increased the absorption capacity of these cells (experiments I & II).

The antigenic expression of in vivo propagated SEYF-a cells was also evaluated directly by measuring their sensitivity to CdL mediated by syngeneic hyperimmune anti SEYF-a antisera. The net sensitivity of 7-11 days old cells to antibody mediated CdL (i.e. cytotoxicity caused by antibody + C' minus cytotoxicity caused by C' alone - see above) was high. The net sensitivity to antibody mediated CdL decreased thereafter.

All these results indicate that antigenic determinants on the cells were progressively being covered by antibodies capable of complement fixation.

CONCLUSIONS AND DISCUSSION

Evidence for the masking of surface antigenic determinants of in vivo propagated SEYF-a tumor cells, has been presented. This evidence is based on the following results: 1. The appearance of cytotoxic anti SEYF-a antibodies in the sera of tumor bearing hosts is followed by the presence of a cell bound cytotoxic anti-body on the cell surface. 2. Concomittantly with the increase in the amount of cell bound cytotoxic antibody on in vivo propagated cells there is a decrease in the amount of free antigenic deter-minants capable of binding anti tumor antibodies. An increase in the antigenic expression has been demonstrated by unmasking of the antigenic determinants.

The presence of cytotoxic anti tumor antibodies on the surface of in vivo propagated tumor cells raises two basic questions: 1. What role do cytotoxic anti tumor antibodies play in the anti tumor activity of the host in this particular host tumor combination? 2. What escape mechanism is responsible for the fact that SEYF-a bearing hosts do in fact die in spite of the presence of high levels of cytotoxic antibodies in their sera and on the tumor cells ? Is it an inefficiency of the host complement system in reacting with cytotoxic antibodies coating the cells ?

The presence of cell-bound antibody on the cell surface may prevent a specific cellular anti tumor reactivity. Experiments designed to answer these questions are presently under way.

REFERENCES

1. Moller, G. Nature, 204: 846, 1964.
2. Witz, I.P., Levy, H.S., Keisari, Y. and Izsak, F. Ch. In: "The Role of Immunoligical Factors in Viral and Oncogenic Processes" (Bears, R.S. Jr., Tilghman, R.C., Bassett, E.G. eds.) Baltimore, Maryland, John Hopkins University Press. 289, 1974.
3. Bansal, S.C., Hargreaves, R. and Sjogren, H.O. Int. J. Cancer, 9: 97, 1972.
4. Ran, M. and Witz, I.P. Int. J. Cancer, 9: 242, 1972.
5. Sjogren, H.O., Hellstrom, I., Bansal, S.E. Warner, G.A. and Hellstrom, E.K. Int. J. Cancer 9: 274, 1972.
6. Sjogren, H.O. and Bansal, S.C. Prog. Immunol., 1: 921, 1971.
7. Stjernsward, J. and Vanky, F. Natl. Cancer Inst. Monogr. 35: 237, 1972.
8. Witz, I.P. Current Topics in Microbiol. & Immunol. 61: 151, 1973.
9. Sjogren, H.O. J. Nat. Cancer Inst. 32: 361, 1964.
10. Ran, M., Fish, F., Witz, I.P. and Klein, G. Clin. Exp. Immunol. 16: 335, 1974.

MODULATION OF THE IMMUNE RESPONSE IN VITRO AND IN VIVO BY SPLENOCYTES FROM TUMOR-BEARING MICE

Steven C. Specter, Isao Kamo and Herman Friedman

Department of Microbiology and Immunology, Albert Einstein

Medical Center, Philadelphia, Pa. USA

Individuals with neoplasia often show markedly suppressed immune responses (1-3). However, the nature and mechanism of immune dysfunction in individuals with malignancy is still far from clear. In this regard, it is now generally accepted that oncogenic viruses, as well as some carcinogenic agents are immunosuppressive (4,5). Furthermore, immunologic impairment is often observed in experimental animals transplanted with tumor cells which appear free of oncogenic viruses. In addition, soluble factors capable of inhibiting immune responses have been found in serum and ascitic fluids in tumor bearing individuals (6-8). Much attention has been focused in recent years on purification and characterization of such immunosuppressive factors, including those associated with neoplasia as well as other "natural" immunosuppressive substances, presumably alpha globulins, in serum from patients with a variety of diseases. However, the target cell(s) involved in tumor associated immunosuppression induced by such substances is unknown. Indeed, several studies have revealed that lymphoid cells from tumor-bearing mice with suppressed immune competence are immunocompetent when used to repopulate heavily irradiated recipient mice (9,10). Thus immunosuppression is not always accompanied by irreversible depletion of immunocompetent cells.

In the present study several distinct model systems were used in regards to tumor-associated immunosuppressive factors, i.e. immunosuppression induced by a murine leukemogenic virus and by a plasmacytoma or a mastocytoma. Mice infected with either the leu-

kemia virus or given transplants of the two tumor cell lines were
studied in terms of immune responsiveness of their splenocytes
in vivo and in vitro to sheep erythrocytes. Subcellular factors
related to tumor growth were also studied in regards to effects on
antibody formation in vitro.

GENERAL METHODS AND MATERIALS

For these studies inbred Balb/c or DBA/2 mice obtained from
Cumberland View Farms, Clinton, Tennessee or Flow Laboratories,
Dublin, Va., were used as the experimental animals. The tumor
model consisted of either Friend leukemic cells induced by Friend
virus (FLV) or a plasmacytoma cell line (MOPC 173) or a mastocytoma (P815X). FLV has been passaged in this laboratory through
adult Balb/c mice for at least 10 years and consisted of both the
lymphatic leukemia and spleen focus forming virus components.
The virus preparation was free of contaminating lactic dehydrogenase or lymphocytic choriomeningitis viruses. Aliquots of clarified infected Balb/c spleen homogenates frozen at -70°C were
used as the stock virus preparation and contained approximately
1000 ID_{50} virus doses per 0.1 ml. The plasmacytoma was obtained
originally from Dr. M. Bosma, Institute for Cancer Research,
Philadelphia, Pa. and has been passaged through Balb/c mice by intraperitoneal (i.p.) injection of 10^5 or 10^6 cells. The tumor
grows progressively in the peritoneum of the animals, resulting
in death within 3 to 4 weeks. The mastocytoma cells were obtained
originally from the American Type Culture Collection and is passaged by (i.p.) injection in susceptible DBA/2 mice.

Mice given either the Friend virus or graded numbers of the
transplantable tumor cells were challenged by intravenous injection with 0.5 ml of a 2% suspension of sheep erythrocytes. The
number of antibody plaque forming cells (PFC) appearing in the
spleen of these animals on the 4th day after immunization was determined by the localized hemolytic plaque assay in agar gel specific for 19S IgM hemolysins (11). For in vitro studies spleen
cells from control or tumor bearing mice were obtained at autopsy,
dispersed cell suspensions prepared and 5×10^6 viable nucleated
cells cultured on a dialysis membrane in the inner chamber of Marbrook culture vessels using Minimal Essential Medium (MEM) and
10% fetal calf serum (12,13). The outer reservoir chamber contained 11 ml of the same medium. The splenocytes were immunized
with 2×10^6 RBCs added at the time of culture initiation. Subcellular extracts were prepared from either the spleen or tumor
per se and clarified by centrifugation. Graded amounts of the extracts were added to the inner chamber of the Marbrook vessels at
the time of immunization. In addition, plasma or ascites fluid
from tumor-bearing mice were also added to other cultures to test
their affect on PFC responsiveness.

Table 1. Effect of length of time of tumor growth on PFC response of mice to SRBC.

Tumor system[a]	Percent PFC response to SRBC (time of challenge in days)[b]		
	5-7	14-20	30-40
Friend leukemia	15	5	5
Plasmacytoma (MOPC 173)	120	66	13
Mastocytoma (P815)	115	78	35

[a]Groups of 6-10 mice each immunized i.p. with 4×10^8 SRBC at indicated time after either injection i.p. with FLV (0.1 ml of 10^{-1} virus dose) or 10^6 plasmacytoma or mastocytoma tumor cells.

[b]Average response of mice 4 days after immunization at indicated time after tumor induction as percent of responses of control mice.

EXPERIMENTAL RESULTS

Immunosuppression was evident in all mouse groups given either Friend virus or transplantable plasmacytoma or mastocytoma cells. However, whereas FLV induced a rapid depression of the immune response so that mice infected for as short a time as 5-7 days showed a 70 to 90% or greater suppression of the PFC response, mice inoculated with either of the transplantable cell lines showed significant immunosuppression only after 2-3 weeks or longer (Table 1). Immunosuppression was evident throughout the time of expected PFC formation after immunization with SRBC.

Spleen cells from FLV-infected animals as well as from mice given plasmacytoma or mastocytoma cells 2 to 4 weeks earlier evinced marked inhibition of immunocompetence when cultured in vitro with SRBC. Spleen cells from these Friend virus infected or mastocytoma bearing mice showed a 90% or greater suppression of the expected PFC response as compared to spleen cells from normal control animals (Table 2). Spleen cells from the plasmacytoma bearing mice showed a greater than 50% suppression.

In all three situations addition of 10^5 splenocytes from suppressed animals to other Marbrook chambers containing 50 times more splenocytes from normal mice resulted in a significant level of immunologic impairment, indicating that small numbers of spleen cells from tumor-bearing animals are capable of influencing adversely the immunocompetence of normal splenocytes (Table 3).

Table 2.   Antibody responsiveness of splenocytes from tumor bearing
mice immunized in vitro with SRBC.

Mouse Spleen Source [a]	Antibody response per culture[b]	
	PFC/10^6 spleen cells	Percent of control response
Normal controls	968 ± 128	–
FLV infected	32 ± 5	4.2
Plasmacytoma-bearing	445 ± 87	46.0
Mastocytoma-bearing	45 ± 12	5.9

[a]Indicated spleen cells (5x10^6) cultured in vitro in Marbrook culture vessels and immunized with 2 x 10^6 SRBCs; spleen cells obtained 7-10 days after i.p. injection of Balb/c mice with 10^{-1}
dose of virus or 20-30 days after i.p. inoculation of 10^6 plasmacytoma cells.   DBA/2 mice used 20-30 days after inoculation of 10^5
mastocytoma cells i.p.

[b]Average PFC response for 6-8 cultures in each group 5 days after
in vitro immunization with SRBC; viability of all cell cultures
approximately 25-30%.

Table 3.   Effect of spleen cells from tumor-bearing mice on hemolytic PFC responsiveness of normal spleen cell cultures.

Source of Spleen cells added to cultures[a]	Antibody response per culture[b]	
	PFC/10^6 spleen cells	Percent of control response
Normal	653 ± 120	–
FLV-infected	246 ± 106	38
Plasmacytoma-bearing	310 ± 95	47
Mastocytoma-bearing	205 ± 72	31

[a]10^5 spleen cells from tumor bearing mice per culture of 5x10^6 normal
splenocytes.

[b]Average PFC responses of 6-8 Marbrook cultures 5 days after in vitro
immunization.

In all three cases it appeared that a soluble factor(s) present in the splenocytes was responsible for immunologic impairment since clarified homogenates of spleens of either FLV-infected mice or mice bearing a plasmacytoma or mastocytoma significantly depressed the PFC response of splenocytes in vitro. In addition, ascitic fluid or plasma from tumor-bearing animals, when added in 0.1 ml volumes to the normal spleen cell cultures, also resulted in a significant immunosuppression (30-60% inhibition).

DISCUSSION AND CONCLUSIONS

The results of these experiments indicate that immunosuppression observed in mice infected with either a leukemogenic virus or bearing a tumor induced by small numbers of transplantable plasmacytoma or mastocytoma cells continued in vitro as shown by the depressed immune response of spleen cells from these animals after challenge immunization in vitro with SRBC. It is noteworthy that the leukemia induced by FLV is characterized by the continued replication of the virus, which continues to transform normal lymphoid cells during the progression of the disease. On the otherhand, the plasmacytoma, although showing evidence of the presence of intracellular virus particles (14), nevertheless, is considered a non-virus tumor; tumor progression occurs due to direct multiplication of neoplastic cells per se. Similarly, the mastocytoma cells, although also probably infected or contaminated with viruses, increase in number and cause disease by rapid division of the tumor cells. However, in all three cases splenocytes from animals bearing these tumors showed marked immunologic impairment, and furthermore could induce immunologic impairment of much larger numbers of normal splenocytes in vitro.

The suppressive activity associated with these tumor cells appears to be mediated by a subcellular factor(s) present in the spleen of the tumor bearing animals. Cell free extracts from spleen cells of FLV-infected or plasmacytoma or mastocytoma-bearing animals were capable of suppressing the immune response of normal splenocytes in vitro. In the case of FLV the suppressive factor most likely was either the virus itself or a virus associated product, since other experiments had shown that anti-FLV serum could neutralize the suppressive activity of the extracts from FLV-infected mice. Furthermore, the suppressive factor(s) was able to pass through a 0.4 u Nucleopore membrane but not a 300,000 molecular weight filter, suggesting a role for a virus per se (13). Giacomoni et al have also reported that a virus present in plasmacytoma cells or an RNA rich material derived from the pelleted virus material could suppress the immune response of mice when injected together with sheep RBCs (15).

In the present study clarified extracts of spleens from plasmacytoma-bearing mice were suppressive. It seemed unlikely that a

virus per se would be responsible since other experiments indicate that even supernatants after high speed centrifugation are
still suppressive. Similarly, Zolla and colleagues have shown
that normal splenocytes cultured in cell impermeable Millipore
chambers in the peritoneal cavity of Balb/c mice bearing a plasmacytoma show marked immunosuppression (16). Those results have
been interpreted to indicate that a "chalone"-like substance secreted by the plasmacytoma cells might be the mediator of the immunosuppression. Although no such chalone has been actually identified or characterized, it does seem likely from the results
obtained in the present study that a soluble factor(s) related
to the tumor process, possibly derived from the tumor cells per
se, can affect normal immunocompetence of uninfected splenocytes.

The studies with the mastocytoma cells, which are often used
in cellular immunology as indicators for cell mediated immune assays, provided further evidence that a generalized immunosuppressive soluble factor(s) is associated with rapid tumor growth. Extracts from the mastocytoma cells, as well as from ascitic fluid
of mastocytoma-bearing mice, were immunosuppressive in vitro (17).
The factor(s) was heat labile (56°C) and probably had a macro-mol-
ecular size since activity was not sedimented by ultracentrifugat-
ion at 100,000 x g for 90 minutes. Furthermore, the suppressive
activity was resistant to irradiation, suggesting that a virus per
se was not involved.

Recent studies concerning the target cell affected by the mastocytoma supernatant indicated that "educated" T-cells from irradiated recipient mice infused with thymocytes from normal syngeneic
donor animals and sheep RBCs were capable of restoring the immune
responsiveness of mastocytoma treated normal splenocytes (17).
This suggested that a specific "target cell" was involved in immunosuppression. Similar studies are in progress with the suppressive factor(s) associated with the plasmacytoma and Friend virus
infection. Physicochemical and immunochemical studies are in
progress in attempts to characterize the soluble factors associated
with these three tumor systems in order to determine whether they
are similar or distinctive. In addition, further studies concerning the mechanism of action of these factors on immunocytes and
their precursors are in progress. It seems likely that the results
of such studies should provide valuable information as to the complex interaction between the malignant process, at least in terms
of a rapidly growing transplantable or virus induced tumor, and the
equally complex immune response mechanism of the host.

SUMMARY

Immunosuppression in mice infected with either a leukemia virus
(Friend virus) or bearing a rapidly growing transplantable tumor
(either a plasmacytoma or mastocytoma) was studied at the level of
individual immunocytes to sheep erythrocytes both in vivo and in
vitro. Immunization of mice with progressing tumors showed

markedly depressed hemolytic antibody plaque responses in the spleen. Furthermore, spleen cell cultures derived from immuno-depressed mice with the tumors revealed the continued impairment of antibody formation in vitro. Relatively small numbers of splen-ocytes from the tumor-bearing mice suppressed larger numbers of nor-mal spleen cells from control mice. Immunosuppression in all three tumor systems could be related to subcellular factors in that cell-free extracts of the spleens and tumor bearing mice or even ascites fluid or plasma could suppress the normal antibody respon-siveness of normal spleen cell cultures. The virus per se or a virus associated factor seemed important in the leukemia virus model but non-virus tumor associated or related substances seemed to be involved in the immunosuppression induced by the plasmacy-toma or mastocytoma. Such results support the view that tumor re-lated subcellular factors may be important mediators of immunologic impairment of a host's immune defense mechanism to a neoplasm.

ACKNOWLEDGEMENT
The capable technical assistance of Mr. Navin Patel and Mr. Chandu Patel during various portions of this study is gratefully acknowledged.

REFERENCES

1. Burnet, H.M., Brit. Med. Bull. 20:159, 1967.
2. Miller, D.E., Cancer Res. 28:1441, 1968.
3. Aisenberg, A.C. in Proc. Internat'l. Conf. Leukemia Lymphoma, Zarofonetis, C.J.D. (ed) p. 873 Lea and Febiger, Phila., 1968.
4. Dent, P., Prog. Med. Virol. 14:1, 1972.
5. Ceglowski, W.S. and Friedman, H., (eds) Virus Tumorigenesis and Immunogenesis. Academic Press, New York, 1973.
6. Mocarelli, P., Villa, L.V., Garotta, G., Porta, C., Bigi, G. and Clerici, E., J. Immunol. 111:873, 1973.
7. Chan, P.L. and Sinclair, N.R.S.C., J. Nat. Cancer Inst. 48: 1629, 1972.
8. Hrsak, I. and Marotti, T., Eur. J. Cancer 9:717, 1973.
9. Loring, M. and Schlesinger, M., Cancer Res., 30:2204, 1970.
10. Laux, D. and Laush, R.N., J. Immunol. 112:1900, 1974.
11. Jerne, N.K., Nordin, A.A. and Henry, C., in Cell Bound Antibodies Amos B. and Koprowski, H. (eds) p. 109: Wistar Inst. Press, Phila, 1963.
12. Marbrook, J., Lancet 2:1279, 1967.
13. Kateley, J.R., Kamo, I., Kaplan, G. and Friedman, H., J. Nat'l Cancer Inst. 53:1371, 1974.
14. Potter, M., in The Molecular Biology of Cancer, Busch, H. (ed) p. 536, Academic Press, New York, 1974.
15. Giacomoni, D., Katzmann, J., Chandra, S. and Heller, P. in "Tumor Virus Infection and Immunity", ASM Symposium, Friedman, H., Crowell, R. and Prier, J. (eds), University Park Press, in press, 1975.
16. Tanapatchaiyapong, P. and Zolla, S., Science 186:748, 1974.
17. Kamo, I., Patel, C., Kateley, J. and Friedman, H., J. Immunol. 114:1749, 1975.

DIVALENT CATION REQUIREMENTS AS A TOOL FOR THE STUDY OF CELL-MEDIATED CYTOTOXICITY SYSTEMS

Pierre GOLSTEIN

Tumour Immunology Unit
Department of Zoology
University College London, London, WC1E 6BT

Cells mediating cytolysis of other cells in vitro can be classified into two broad classes, namely T cells (sensitised thymus derived cells lysing the relevant target cells, which they recognise through specific cell surface receptors) and non-T cells (unsensitised cells, not thymus-derived, lysing antibody-coated target cells which they recognise through cell surface Fc receptors). Cytolytic non-T cell populations are ill-defined as to their exact identity, and moreover, are very probably heterogeneous. The mechanism of lysis can be divided into at least three stages: recognition, post-recognition hit, and target cell disintegration which can occur in the absence of effector cells. The physiology of the post-recognition hit stage is unknown, and moreover, may be different from one type of cytolysis to the other.

We have studied the cation requirements of a variety of mouse and human cell-mediated cytolytic systems. We found that different systems had different cation requirements, either for Ca^{++} or for Mg^{++}, or for both, or for neither, which can be used for the functional fractionation of the corresponding cytolytic subpopulations. Also, we studied in more detail two systems with mouse cells, and found that the differences in cation requirements were essentially at the post-recognition hit stage. Finally, we characterised a 'cation pulse' method for the analysis of this stage.

1. MATERIALS AND METHODS

The materials and methods used were described elsewhere (1-3). Briefly, effector cells were mouse spleen cells or Ficoll-Isopaque fractionated human peripheral blood cells, either unsensitised or

sensitised in vitro against allogeneic cells. Target cells were
either the mouse mastocytoma cell line P815, phytohaemagglutinin-
stimulated human blast cells, antibody-coated sheep red blood cells
(SRBC-Ab), or human Chang cells uncoated (Chang) or antibody-coated
(Chang-Ab). Target cells were prelabelled with ^{51}Cr and mixed with
effector cells in V-shaped wells of plastic microplates. The latter
were centrifuged, incubated for 4 h at 37°C and centrifuged again.
Sequential addition of 50 μl volumes of cations and/or EDTA at
times indicated below did not macroscopically affect the cell
pellet at the bottom of each well. Cytolysis was assessed by
measuring the radioactivity of samples of supernatants at the end
of the 4 h incubation period.

2. DIFFERENT CYTOLYTIC SYSTEMS HAVE DIFFERENT CATION REQUIREMENTS

We investigated the cation requirements of various types of
cell-mediated cytolytic systems, using relatively cation-free conditions and adding, at the beginning of the cytotoxicity test,
graded amounts of either Ca^{++} or Mg^{++}, or both. A summary of the
results is given in Table 1.

The T cell-mediated systems were essentially Ca^{++} dependent
with both human (2) and mouse cells (3). The mouse data confirmed
previous results by others showing that the inhibitory effect of
EDTA could be reverted by Ca^{++} more efficiently than by Mg^{++} (4,5).
Non-T cell-mediated lysis of Chang-Ab was also essentially Ca^{++}
dependent (2). In sharp contrast, lysis of SRBC-Ab by mouse spleen
cells was Mg^{++} dependent (1,3), whereas their lysis by mouse

Table 1: Cation requirements of various types of cell mediated
          cytolytic systems

Effector cells*	T	Non-T against		
		SRBC-Ab	Chang-Ab	Chang
Mouse spleen cells	Ca^{++}	Mg^{++}		
Human peripheral blood cells	Ca^{++}	$Mg^{++}/-$	Ca^{++}	Mg^{++} & Ca^{++}

* Mouse spleen cells or Ficoll-Isopaque fractionated human peripheral blood cells were used either without sensitisation (non-T
systems) or after in vitro sensitisation against allogeneic cells
(T systems).

peritoneal cells did not require the presence of extracellular cations (6). Also, lysis of SRBC-Ab by human cells probably involves two subpopulations, one which requires Mg^{++} and another one which does not require extracellular cations (2). Finally, the 'background' lysis of uncoated Chang cells by normal peripheral human blood cells was specially marked in the presence of both Ca^{++} and Mg^{++} (2). Thus, the overall cation requirements are widely different for different systems of cell-mediated cytolysis.

3. TWO MOUSE CELL-MEDIATED CYTOLYTIC SYSTEMS HAVE DIFFERENT CATION REQUIREMENTS AT THE POST-RECOGNITION HIT STAGE

We looked more closely at two mouse systems, namely T cell mediated cytolysis and non-T cell-mediated cytolysis of SRBC-Ab, and asked at which stage of the lytic process one could locate the differences in cation requirements. A summary of the results is given in Table 2.

For T cell-mediated cytolysis, the recognition stage was investigated using specific adsorption of effector cells on fibroblast monolayers, in the presence of various concentrations of divalent cations. We found that specific adsorption could occur in the presence of Mg^{++} as well as in the presence of Ca^{++} (3), which confirmed earlier results by others (7). The target cell disintegration stage does not require any divalent cations, since it can occur in the presence of EDTA (4,8,9). Since neither of these stages

Table 2: Cation requirements, at various stages, of two types of mouse cell-mediated cytolysis

	T	Non-T anti-SRBC-Ab
Overall	Ca^{++} necessary	Mg^{++} necessary
1. Recognition	Mg^{++} sufficient	Cations not necessary
2. Post-recognition hit	Ca^{++} necessary	Mg^{++} necessary
3. Target cell disintegration	Cations not necessary	Cations not necessary

requires Ca^{++}, and since Ca^{++} is necessary for this type of lysis, it follows that Ca^{++} is necessary at the post-recognition hit stage of T cell mediated cytolysis.

For non-T cell mediated cytolysis of antibody-coated sheep red blood cells, the recognition stage was investigated using preblocking of effector cells with aggregated IgG. We found that incubation of effector cells in the presence of aggregated IgG blocked any subsequent cytotoxicity, and that this was not affected by a concentration of EDTA which would block the cytolytic process (3). The target cell disintegration stage did not require any cations either (3). Since neither of these stages requires Mg^{++}, and since Mg^{++} is necessary for this type of lysis, it follows that Mg^{++} is necessary at the post-recognition hit stage of non-T cell mediated cytolysis.

Thus, for two different systems of cell-mediated cytolysis, the cation requirements are different at the post-recognition hit stage, which suggests differences in the actual mechanism of lysis.

4.   CHARACTERISATION OF A 'CATION PULSE' METHOD
FOR THE STUDY OF CELL-MEDIATED CYTOLYTIC SYSTEMS

From the results described in the previous section and from Table 2, it can be concluded, not only that cation requirements are different from one system to another, but also that within each system they are different from one stage to the other. This provided the basis for an analytical 'cation pulse' method (3), schematised in Table 3.

For T cell mediated cytolysis, effector and target cells were mixed in the presence of Mg^{++} and the plates were centrifuged. A Ca^{++} pulse was made at 40 min, for 20 min as a rule. Without Ca^{++} pulse, minimal lysis was obtained. A significant increase in lysis was observed with a Ca^{++} pulse as short as 5 min. Substitution of Mg^{++} for the Ca^{++} pulse resulted in a far lower level of cytolysis. Also, we checked that under these timing conditions most of the recognition events occurred before the Ca^{++} pulse, and most of the target cell disintegration events occurred after the Ca^{++} pulse. Similar results were obtained with an Mg^{++} pulse in non-T cell mediated cytolysis of antibody-coated erythrocytes.

Thus, a cation pulse method timed as described in Table 3 enables us to experimentally isolate the post-recognition hit stage of two systems of cell-mediated cytolysis.

Table 3: An analytical 'cation pulse' method

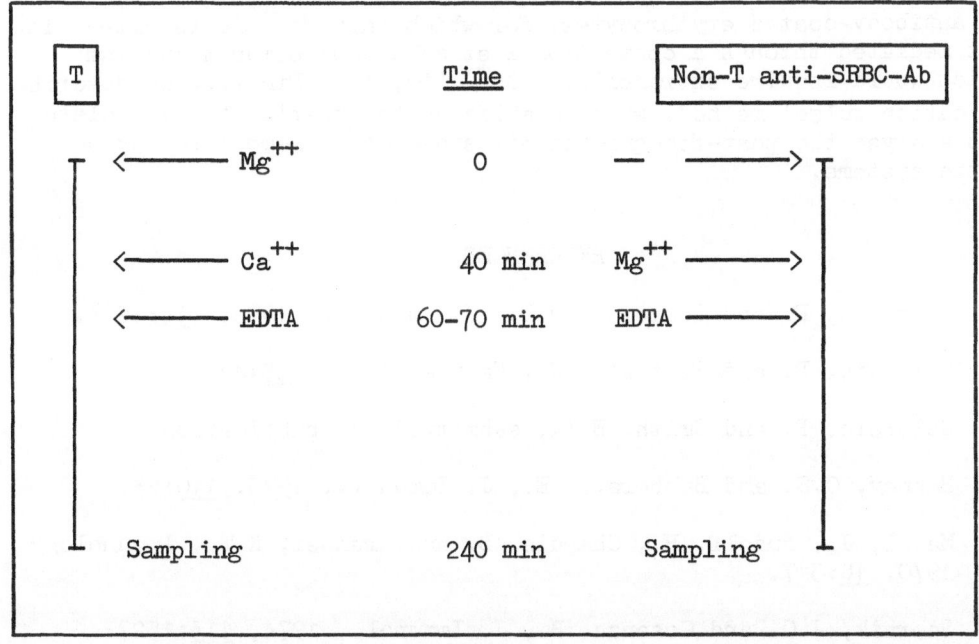

5. CONCLUSIONS

These results have some implications in two directions. First, the fact that several types of cell-mediated cytolysis, implying different effector cells, have different cation requirements can be used to distinguish the corresponding effector cell subpopulations. For instance, subpopulations fractionated through physical means can be better characterised through their cation requirements, which would then be used as a marker. Also, cation requirements can be used as a functional fractionation device, since the type of cyto- toxicity that is obtained varies as a function of the presence of Ca^{++} and/or Mg^{++}. Two components of lysis by human cells against SRBC-Ab could thus be detected, presumably corresponding to different subpopulations. Also, in anti-tumour research in man, one may hope that Mg^{++} free conditions would depress the 'variable background' cytotoxicity by control blood cells more than specific anti-tumour cytotoxicity by blood cells from tumour-bearing patients.

Second, a detailed study of cation requirements can contribute to our knowledge of the mechanism of cell-mediated cytolysis. Thus, two systems have been shown to have different cation requirements at the post-recognition hit stage, which suggests the possibility of the existence of different mechanisms of cell-mediated lysis. Also, lysis of antibody-coated erythrocytes, for which only Mg^{++} is required, is not mediated through a conventional stimulus-secretion mechanism which would require extracellular Ca^{++} (10,11). Finally, we described a 'cation pulse' method, which enables us to experimentally isolate and analyse the post-recognition hit stage of cell-mediated cytolytic systems.

REFERENCES

1. Golstein, P. and Gomperts, B.D., J. Immunol., 1975, 114:1264.

2. Golstein, P. and Fewtrell, C., Nature, 1975, 255:491.

3. Golstein, P. and Smith, E.T., submitted for publication.

4. Henney, C.S. and Bubbers, J.E., J. Immunol., 1973, 110:63.

5. Mauel, J., Rudolf, H., Chapuis, B. and Brunner, K.T., Immunology, 1970, 18:517.

6. Scornik, J.C. and Cosenza, H., J. Immunol., 1974, 113:1527.

7. Stulting, R.D. and Berke, G., J. Exp. Med., 1973, 137:932.

8. MacDonald, H.R., Eur. J. Immunol., 1975, in press.

9. Martz, E., J. Immunol., 1975, in press.

10. Rubin, R.P., Pharmacol. Rev., 1970, 22:389.

11. Becker, E.L. and Henson, P.M., Adv. Immunol., 1973, 17:93.

MACROPHAGE KILLING CAPACITY.   ASPECTS OF MECHANISM

Ruth Gallily, Hannah Eliahu and Zina Ben-Ishay*

Departments of Immunology and Anatomy*

Hebrew University - Hadassah Medical School
Jerusalem, Israel

The heterogeneity of effector cells and killing mechanisms against normal and tumor allografts has been frequently emphasized. It is generally believed that rejection of foreign graft tissue is mediated mostly by cellular immune mechanisms where the T derived lymphocytes are the most important cells which recognize and lyse foreign target cells. However, during the last few years, evidence has been accumulating demonstrating the participation of macrophages in graft rejection and tumor destruction (Reviewed by Nelson (1)). In vitro studies have shown that isolated immune macrophages were cytotoxic to tumor cells bearing alloantigens used for immunization (2,3). However, the mechanism by which macrophages gain their cytotoxic capacity as well as their killing mechansim is still far from clear.

In the present investigation the capacity of immune macrophages to kill other macrophages in a mixed macrophage culture (MMC) system was studied. Attempts were also made to elucidate the mechanism of macrophage killing.

MATERIALS AND METHODS

Essentially the same methods for immunization and cultivation of cells were used as previously described (4). Thioglycollate stimulated macrophages were withdrawn from the peritoneum of non-immunized and immunized mice (nonimmune and immune macrophages). The immune macrophages were obtained 10 days after the last of 3 successive weekly intraperitoneal injections of 3-5 x 10^7 suspended allogeneic spleen cells. In mixed macrophage cultures (MMC) immune macrophages (1.5 x 10^6) were cultured together in the same petri dish (3.5 cm, Falcon) with allogeneic nonimmune or immune macrophages (1.5×10^6) of the strain used for immunization. Control cultures consisted of 3×10^6 peritoneal cells from one donor only. The cells were allowed to adhere to the plates and rinsed vigoursly twice (every 3 hours) with a jet of PBS. After the rinsing only 1-2% lymphocytes could be detected in the cultures. Cytotoxicity in MMC was usually tested 4 days after cultivation, by ^{86}Rb uptake assay (4,5) which serves as an index of viable cell number. The percentage of killing was calculated as follows:

$$\% \text{ killing} = [1 - \frac{^{86}\text{Rb cpm in allogeneic mixed culture}}{1/2 \ (^{86}\text{Rb cpm in parental syngeneic}}] \times 100$$
cultures.

"Arming" of normal macrophages by alloimmune lymphocytes was obtained by adding $2-3 \times 10^7$ unfractionated or fractionated sensitized spleen cells to monolayers of 1.5×10^6 syngeneic nonimmune macrophages. After 24 hours of incubation the lymphocytes were removed and 1.5×10^6 nonimmune macrophages from the allogeneic strain used for immunization were added. After rinsing, the MMC were further incubated for 4 days before assaying for cytotoxicity. Fractionation of immune spleen cells to T enriched cell population was obtained by passing the cells through Degalan beads coated with anti-mouse immunoglobulins (6). Enriched B cell population was obtained by incubating immune spleen cells with heterologous anti-θ serum (7) and complement. The values given in the tables are the mean of 3-5 experiments done in triplicate. Cytotoxicity of less than 25% was not considered significant.

EXPERIMENTAL RESULTS AND DISCUSSION

Macrophage Cytotoxicity

While no killing was observed when nonimmune C57B1/6 macrophages were grown together with nonimmune BALB/c macrophages, a pronounced cytotoxicity of 55-68% was detected when immune C57B1/6 or BALB/c macrophages derived from alloimmunized donors were cultivated with macrophages bearing the alloantigens used for immunization. In MMC in which both populations of macrophages were immune, i.e. cross immunization, 83% killing was observed (Table 1). No killing was detected when immune macrophages were cultivated on separated glass slides placed in the same dish (Table 1). It seems therefore that physical contact between the cells in MMC is required for the elicitation of cytotoxicity. The killing observed was found to be specific as killing by immune macrophages was expressed only against macrophages bearing the alloantigens used for immunization (4). To determine whether cytophilic antibodies are responsible for the capacity of macrophages to recognize and kill allogeneic cells, the

Table 1: Killing in immune allogeneic separated
and mixed macrophage cultures (MMC's).

Type of Culture	Macrophages	% killing
MMC	BALB/c + C57Bl/6	0
MMC	BALB/c im* + C57Bl/6	68
MMC	BALB/c + C57Bl/6 im	55
MMC	BALB/c im + C57Bl/6 im	83
Separated slides	BALB/c im + C57Bl/6	-4
Separated slides	BALB/c im + C57Bl/6 im	-6

* im immunized against the culture partner's alloantigens.

immune macrophages were treated with trypsin (0.05 - 0.10 mg/ml
for 5-15 min); no decrease of cytotoxicity was detected. In another
set of experiments 1 mg rabbit anti-mouse γ globulin was added
daily to the medium of MMC's; here too no decrease in immune
macrophage cytotoxicity was observed following this treatment.
On the other hand, daily addition of 10% anti-macrophage serum
pronouncedly decreased (30-50%) the cytotoxicity of immune
macrophages. Thus, no indication could be obtained suggesting
that cytophilic antibodies are taking an active part in cytotoxicity
expressed by immune macrophages in our system.

The Killing Mechanism

Suspended spleen cells derived from immunized mice were
incubated for 24 hr with nonimmune syngeneic macrophages. After
removing the lymphocytes, normal allogeneic macrophages from the
strain used for immunization were added to the cultures.
Cytotoxicity of about 50% was expressed by normal macrophages
armed by sensitized lymphocytes (Table 2). T enriched cell
population isolated from sensitized spleen cells demonstrated a
similar capacity to "arm" normal macrophages for cytotoxicity.
On the other hand, B enriched population had a negligable capacity
to "arm" macrophages. One may assume therefore that T lymphocytes,
rather than B cells, secrete or release mediator(s) and/or membranal
factors which attach to the macrophages and render them cytotoxic.

To asses the possible participation of T lymphocytes in the

Table 2:   Arming of non immune macrophages in vitro by
           unfractionated and fractionated immune spleen
           lymphocytes.

Nonimmune macrophages	Immune lymphocytes	Target macrophages	% killing*
	'unfractionated'		
BALB/c	BALB/c im	C57B1/6	37
C57B1/6	C57B1/6 im	BALB/c	42
	'T enriched'		
BALB/c	BALB/c im	C57B1/6	49
C57B1/6	C57B1/6 im	BALB/c	47
	'B enriched'		
BALB/c	BALB/c im	C57B1/6	15
C57B1/6	C57B1/6 im	BALB/c	9

$$* = 1 - \left[\frac{{}^{86}Rb \text{ cpm in MMC armed by immune spleen lymphocytes}}{{}^{86}Rb \text{ cpm in MMC armed by nonimmune unfractionated}} \right] \times 100$$
spleen lymphocytes.

killing process observed in immune MMC, the peritoneal cells were
treated before cultivation, with either heterologous anti-θ antiserum (7) or allogeneic anti-θ antiserum [AKR anti-C3H(8)] and
complement. It was found that cytotoxicity expressed by immune
macrophages was totally abolished. One may argue that the few T
lymphocytes detected in the MMC (about 1%) are the cells that
actually kill target macrophages. However this is quite unlikely
as the addition of 5% allogeneic immune peritoneal lymphocytes to
target macrophages were unable to kill the target macrophages
during 4 days of cultivation. We suggest that the presence of T
lymphocytes or their secretion of mediator(s) is a prerequisit for
the expression of cytotoxicity by effector macrophages or that
membranal components, recognized by anti-θ serum, are being released
from T cells and bind to macrophages thus enabling the later to
recognize and kill foreign cells. In order to elucidate further
the mechanism of macrophage killing, an electron microscopic
(E.M.) study was undertaken. No phagocytosis of cells could be
detected during cultivation of MMC. After 48 hrs of cultivation
the monolayers of MMC consisted of pairs or small clusters of normal
and necrotic macrophages in close contact (Fig. 1). By using
cationized ferritin which binds to negative surface charges (9) we
could not detect fusion of membranes between effector and target
cells (Fig. 2). Thus, killing by immune macrophages apparently
occurs via a lytic process.

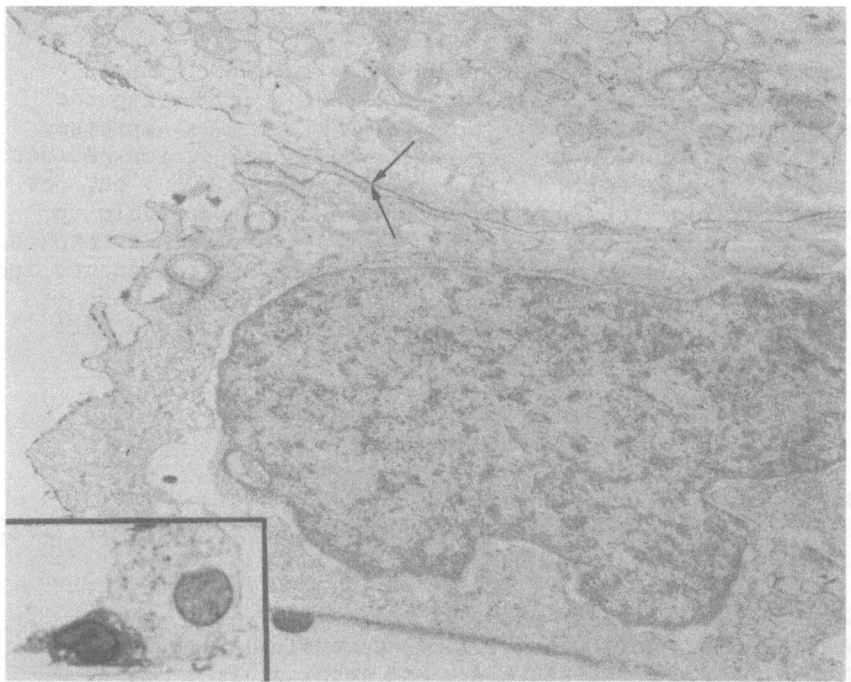

Fig. 1: Killer and target macrophages in ᴹMC. The macrophage at
lower part of electronmicrograph (effector cell) is of normal
appearance while part of the macrophage seen at upper side displays
signs of lysis (Target cell). Note ferritin (black dotes) at outer
surface of cells and in intercellular space (specimen unstained).
Insert: the normal macrophage is seen darkly stained and the lysed
macrophage appears swollen with a rarified cytoplasm. (light
micrograph of a 1 mµ thick section of epon embedded material.
Toluidine blue staining.
16,500 x, (insert) 1,200 x.

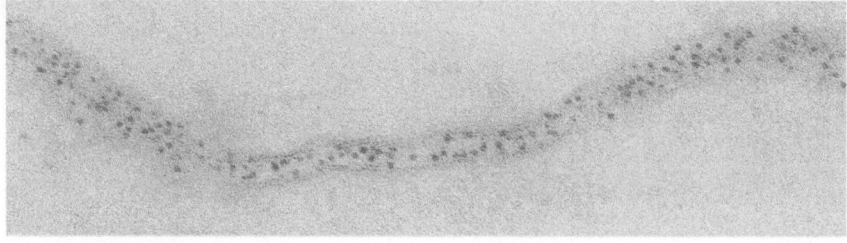

Fig. 2: Intercellular space between the cells in Fig. 1. demarcated
by cationized ferritin particles.
153,000 x.

CONCLUSION

Immune macrophages have the capacity to kill in mixed macrophage cultures (MMC) allogeneic macrophages bearing the alloantigens used for immunization. The killing is expressed by a lytic mechanism as neither phagocytosis nor fusion between effector and target cells could be detected by E.M. T but not B lymphocytes isolated from immune spleen cells, are able to "arm" syngeneic nonimmune macrophages and render them cytotoxic. It is suggested that mediator(s) and/or membranal components are released from T cells and attach to macrophages. Such an "arming" factor enables the macrophage to recognize and kill target cells.

REFERENCES

1. Nelson, D.S., Trans. Rev. 19: 226, 1974.
2. Evans, R., and Alexander, P. Immunology, 23: 615, 627, 1972.
3. Lohmann-Matthes, M.L., Schipper, H., and Fischer, H. Eur. J. Immunol. 2: 45, 1972.
4. Gallily, R. Cell. Immunol. 15: 419, 1975.
5. Walker, S.M., and Lucas, Z.T. J. Immunol. 109: 1223, 1973.
6. Wigzell, H., Sundqvist, K.G., and Yoshida, T.O. Scand. J. Immunol. 1: 75, 1972.
7. Golub, E.S. Cell. Immunol. 2: 353, 1971.
8. Schlesinger, M., and Hurvitz, D. Transplantation. 7: 132, 1969.
9. Dannon, D., Goldstein, Y., Marikovsky, Y., and Skutelsky, E. J. Ultrastruct. Res. 38: 500, 1972.

ACKNOWLEDGEMENTS

This work was supported by research grant from the Leukemia Research Foundation, Inc.

A NEW T CELL NEOPLASM EXPRESSING SURFACE ANTI-DNP ACTIVITY, DE-

VELOPED FROM THE THYMUS OF MICE BEARING MOPC-315 PLASMA CELL TUMORS

Nitza Lahat and Chaya Moroz

Rogoff-Wellcome Med. Res. Inst. and Tel-Aviv University

Med. School, Beilinson Medical Center, Petah Tikva, Israel

The plasmacytoma of BALB/c mouse has become an important model for the study of some clinical and immunochemical aspects of human multiple myeloma. The characteristics of multiple myeloma is the high level of monoclonal immunoglobulin (Ig) accompanied by diminished production of all classes of Ig and by immunological deficiency consisting mainly of the primary response to antigen (1,2,3). Yakulis et al have demonstrated that upon implantation of plasmacytoma into normal BALB/c mice a large percentage of circulating lymphocytes aquired on their surface the idiotypic specificity of the Ig produced by the plasmacytoma (4). This phenomenon could be reproduced in-vitro by incubating normal lymphocytes with an RNA preparation from the plasmacytoma (5).

The current study was designed to investigate the possible effect of a developing plasmacytoma on T cells in the host's thymus, both as to oncogenic transformation and the expression of myeloma protein on the T cell surface. The MOPC-315 plasmacytoma was chosen since the monoclonal γA globulin produced by the plasma cells has anti-DNP activity (6) and enables therefore the use of erythrocytes coated with the antigen to demonstrate lymphocytes bearing anti-DNP surface receptors. Indeed, a tumor was developed from the thymus of mice bearing MOPC-315 plasmacytoma, the cells of the new Mouse T Cell Tumor-315 (MTCT-315) carry θ antigen, synthesize γA globulin and form rossettes with DNP-SRBC.

Development of T Cell Tumor (MTCT-315)

BALB/c MOPC-315 plasmacytoma was transplanted subcutaneously

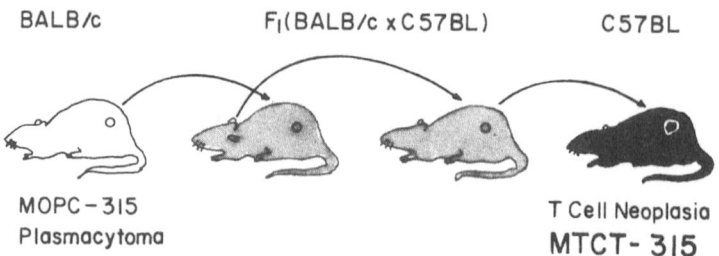

BALB/c   F₁(BALB/c x C57BL)   C57BL

MOPC-315   T Cell Neoplasia
Plasmacytoma   MTCT- 315

Fig. 1.   Development of T cell tumor MTCT-315

into 6 weeks old (BALB/c x C57BL) F_1 hybrid mice (BALB/BL). Large
tumors developed in all mice 14 days following inoculation. The
thymuses of the plasmacytoma bearing F_1(BALB/BL) mice were removed
and transplanted subcutaneously into a second group of F_1(BALB/BL)
mice (Fig. 1).   Following 45 days all (20/20) inoculated mice developed subcutaneous tumors.   This finding suggested that oncogenic
transformation of thymocytes had occurred in F_1(BALB/BL) mice
bearing plasmacytoma.

H-2 differences are known to represent a strong barrier against
the grafting of neoplastic tissues. However, it has been demonstrated that F_1 heterozygous tumors throw off variants selectively
compatible with one parental strain (7,8,9). Based on these observations, we transplanted subcutaneously the thymus derived F_1
(BALB/BL) tumor cells into C57BL mice.   Following 7 days, 70% (19/28)
of the inoculated C57BL mice gave rise to tumors half of which
regressed secondary at day 10 following inoculation. 35% (9/28) of
the inoculated C57BL mice gave rise to fairly large tumors which
were not rejected until sacrificed at day 17. The thymus derived
tumors raised in C57BL mice were designated MTCT-315 (Fig. 1).

Serologic Analysis of MTCT-315 Tumor Cells

In order to demonstrate that a new tumor originated from
transformed F_1 (BALB/BL) thymocytes of mice bearing MOPC-315 plasmacytoma, the thymus derived tumors raised in F_1 (BALB/BL) and in
C57BL mice were tested in a cytotoxic assay for their sensitivity
to anti-BALB/c, anti-C57BL H-2 isoantibodies as well as to anti-

Table 1. Serologic Analysis of Tumors Developed from Transformed
Thymocytes of Mice Bearing MOPC-315 Plasmacytoma[a]

Tumor	Host of Origin	Cytotoxic Index[b]		
		Anti-BALB/c[c]	Anti-C57BL[d]	Anti-θ[e]
MOPC-315	BALB/c	0.976	0.02	0
MTCT-315	F_1(BALB/cxC57BL)	0.96	0.9	0.83
MTCT-315	C57BL	0.08	1.0	0.95

[a] for serologic analysis cell suspensions (2×10^5 cells/0.05 ml PBS)
were mixed with antiserum (0.05 ml) for 1 h at 4°C, washed 1 x
with cold PBS and incubated with guinea-pig complement (0.05 ml)
for 30 min. at 37°C. The percentage of cells excluding trypan
blue was determined before and after incubation.

[b] Cytotoxic index $=$ $\dfrac{\text{\% unstained cells in control-\% unstained cells in test}}{\text{\% unstained cells in control}}$

[c] C57BL anti-BALB/c dil. 1:4

[d] BALB/c anti C57BL dil. 1:4

[e] AKR anti-θ-C3H dil. 1:8

θ-C3H serum and complement. The serologic analysis of the new tumor
was compared to that of BALB/c MOPC-315 plasmacytoma. As seen in
Table 1 the cytotoxic index for MOPC-315 plasmacytoma indicates
that the tumor cells are of BALB/c origin and do not carry θ antigen on the surface. In contrast the thymus derived MTCT-315 tumor
cells raised in heterozygous F_1 (BALB/BL) mice were affected to a
similar extent by isoantibodies directed against either of the two
parental strains. 83% of the cells in this tumor were killed by
anti-θ-serum and complement (θ^+). It is likely that the anti-θ
resistant cells (θ^-) in the tumor represent BALB/c plasma cells
which infiltrated the thymus of BALB/BL mice bearing the plasmacytoma and were carried over with the transplanted thymus. In contrast the variant tumor capable of growing in the homozygous C57BL
parental strain lost the sensitivity toward antibodies directed
against the opposite parental strain (BALB/c), all cells in this
tumor were sensitive to anti-C57BL isoantibodies and almost all
(95%) carried θ antigen. We conclude that oncogenic transformation
of T cells occurred in the thymus of F_1 hybrid mice bearing MOPC-315
plasmacytoma. Subcutaneous grafting of the transformed F_1 (BALB/BL)
T cells into C57BL mice resulted in a tumor variant which is a
C57BL T cell neoplasia.

Table 2. ^{14}C Amino Acids Incorporated into Intracellular Proteins
and Isolated IgA of MOPC-315 and MTCT-315 Tumor Cells in
Culture[a]

| Tumor | Host of Origin | Radioactivity cpm x 10^{-4}[b] | |
		Intracellular Proteins[c]	IgA[d]
MOPC-315	BALB/c	3.5	1[e]
MTCT-315	C57BL	11.75	1.7[f]

[a] 3×10^6 tumor cells suspended in 0.2 ml Spinner medium containing
   1/100 the amino acid concentration were incubated with a mixture
   of ^{14}C amino-acids (1 μCi) for 180 min. at 37°C.
[b] Figures in columns have been multiplied by 10^{-4}.
[c] Precipitated with 5% cold TCA.
[d] Isolated by immunoprecipitation with goat anti-mouse α chains
   serum, and corrected for non-specific counts in immunoprecipitate.
[e] Corrected for 1×10^3 non-specific cpm.
[f] Corrected for 4×10^3 non-specific cpm.

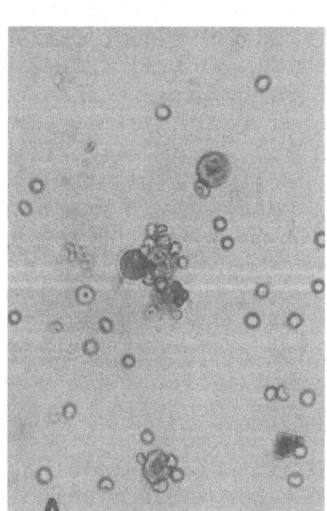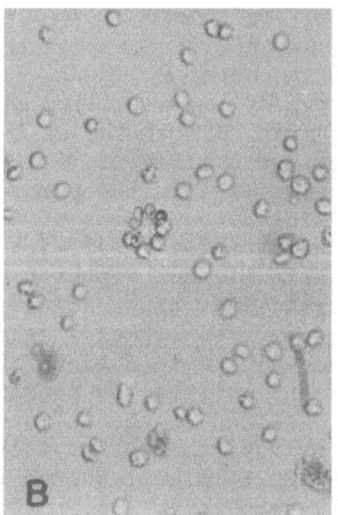

Fig. 2.   Tumor cells forming rossettes with DNP-SRBC x 250
         A. BALB/c plasmacytoma MOPC-315. B. C57BL T cell
         tumor MTCT-315

Some Functional Characteristics of MTCT-315 Tumor Cells

The biosynthesis of proteins and Ig in C57BL MTCT-315 tumor cells was compared to that of BALB/c MOPC-315 plasmacytoma and determined by incubating the tumor cells in short term tissue culture in the presence of ^{14}C amino acids for 180 min. as described before (10). ^{14}C amino acids incorporated into intracellular protein was determined by acid precipitation, whereas nascent intracellular Ig was precipitated with anti-mouse α chain serum (10). As seen in Table 2, the T cell tumor MTCT-315 incorporated 3 times more radio-active amino acids into intracellular protein than MOPC-315 plasma cells. Both types of tumor cells synthesize IgA, in plasmacytoma MOPC-315 28% of the nascent protein was isolated as Ig whereas in the T cell tumor MTCT-315 it amounted to 15% only. The ability of the tumor cells to form rossettes with DNP-SRBC was determined according to the method of Hannestad et al (11). As seen in Fig 2, the T cell tumor C57BL MTCT-315 was able to form rossettes with DNP-SRBC.

The results of this study demonstrate that oncogenic transformation of T cells occures in mice bearing plasmacytoma, the transformed T cells synthesize Ig of the class identical to that synthesized by the plasmacytoma, and express similar surface receptors. These observations may suggest that the agent causing the oncogenic transformation as well as the message for the synthesis of the myeloma Ig are transferred from the plasma cell tumor to normal T cells of the host.
Further experiments are carried out to study this suggestion.

REFERENCES

1. Cwynarski, M.T. and Cohen, S. Clin. Exp. Immun., 8,237;1971
2. Fahey, J.L., Scoggins, R., Utz, J.P. and Szwed, C.F. Am. J. Med., 35,698;1963
3. Cone, L. and Uhr, J.W. J. Clin. Invest., 43,2241;1964
4. Yakulis, V., Bhoopalam, N., Schade, S. and Heller, P. Blood, 39, 453;1972
5. Giacomoni, D., Yakulis, V., Ruey Wang, S., Cooke, A., Dray, Sh. and Heller, P. Cellular Immunol., 11,389;1974
6. Eizen, H.N., Simms, E.S. and Potter, M. Biochemistry, 7,4126; 1968
7. Klein, E., Klein, G. and Reverz, L. J. Nat. Cancer Inst., 19,95;1957
8. Hellstrom, K.E. J. of Nat. Cancer Inst., 25,237;1960
9. Klein, E., Klein, G. and Hellstrom, K.E. J. Nat. Cancer Inst. 25, 271;1960.
10. Moroz, C. and Lahat, N. Cellular Immunol., 13,397;1974
11. Hannestad, K., Kao, M.S. and Eizen, H.N. Proc. Nat. Acad. Sci. 69,2295;1972

LYMPHOCYTE-TARGET CELL CONJUGATION: MEMBRANE RECEPTORS FOR ALLOANTIGENS

Gideon Berke

Department of Cell Biology, The Weizmann Institute of Science, Rehovot, Israel

It is generally accepted that interactions between cytotoxic T-lymphocytes (CTL) and target cells (TC) are involved in allograft rejection. This interaction is a complex process initially involving a distinct and specific CTL-TC binding step which then leads to TC lysis (1-3). Several indirect methods are available for the study of the binding of CTL and TC (4-7). In this paper a new approach to the direct analysis of the binding of CTL and TC is presented.

MATERIALS AND METHODS

BALB/c and C57BL/6 mice, 2-4 months old, were used. Leukemia EL4 of C57BL/6 mice was carried in the ascites form in C57BL/6 mice. BALB/c mice were immunized against leukemia EL4 by a single intra-peritoneal injection of 25×10^6 tumor cells in 0.5 ml phosphate-buffered saline (PBS). BALB/c anti-EL4 peritoneal exudate cytotoxic lymphocytes (PEL) were obtained 11 days after immunization as described before (8). Binding of PEL and EL4 was achieved by centrifuging a suspension of 1×10^6 PEL and 1×10^6 EL4 in 1 ml PBS supplemented with 10% fetal calf serum (PBS-FCS) at 250 x g, 10 min at room temperature. The cell pellet was resuspended vigorously with a Pasteur pipette and the resulting cell suspension was examined microscopically for lymphocyte target cell conjugates.

RESULTS

The centrifugation of suspensions containing PEL and EL4 cells resulted in the formation of PEL–EL4 conjugates. Various types of PEL–EL4 conjugates were observed. For example, simple conjugates of one PEL and one EL4 (PEL_1–$EL4_1$) as well as more complex conjugates ($PEL_{n>1}$–$EL4_{n>1}$) were found. In Fig. 1 PEL_1–$EL4_1$ and PEL_2–$EL4_1$ conjugates are shown. Different types of conjugates were obtained at different PEL–EL4 ratios during centrifugation, but a conjugate of one PEL and one EL4 (PEL_1–$EL4_1$) was usually the predominant type. The specificity and the quantitative aspects of PEL–EL4 conjugation will be presented elsewhere (9).

Conjugate formation between lymphocytes and EL4 cells was used to directly determine the frequency of lymphoid cells capable of binding. BALB/c mice were immunized against EL4 leukemia and spleen, lymph node and thymus cells were prepared 11 days later. The lymphoid cells were mixed with EL4 cells, conjugates were formed by centrifugation of the mixtures and the number of conjugates was determined. Evaluation of the frequency of lymphoid cells capable of specific binding to target cells revealed that 35% of the PEL, 10% of the spleen cells, 8% of the lymph node cells and 2% of the thymus cells formed conjugated with EL4 cells (9).

It was then of interest to examine whether each individual EL4 cell was capable of conjugating with EL4. Mixtures containing a

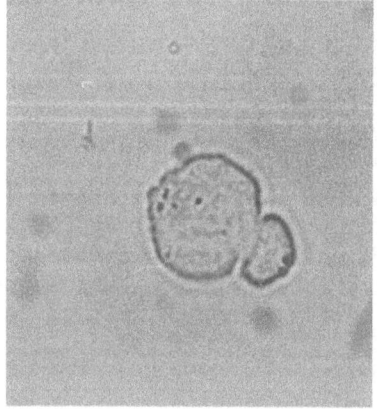 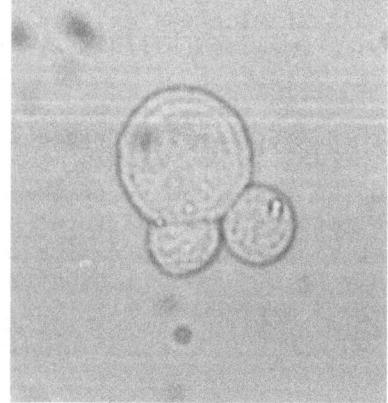

Fig. 1. PEL–EL4 conjugates. The small cells are PEL, the large are EL4.

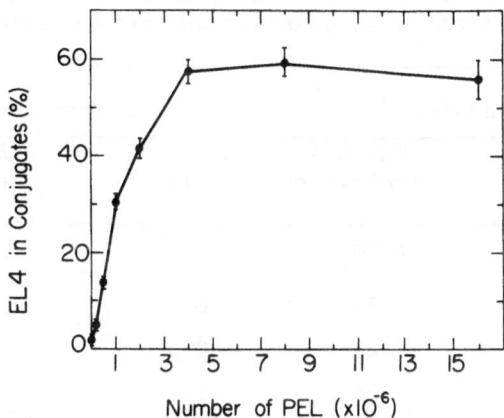

Fig. 2. Percent EL4 capable of conjugation with PEL.

fixed number (1×10^6) of EL4 cells and increasing numbers of PEL were centrifuged and the percentage of EL4 in conjugates was determined following centrifugation. The results of this (Fig. 2) and other experiments were that 60-75% of the target cells were capable of conjugation. Similar experiments were performed with other target cells of C57BL/6 origin. For example, thymocytes and radiation leukemia cells were as efficient as EL4 cells in binding to PEL. Lymph node cells and tissue cultured fibroblasts were less efficient. Red blood cells did not bind at all.

An insight into the nature of the PEL receptors which play a role in the binding of EL4 was obtained by examining the effects of trypsin on PEL. It was found (Table 1) that trypsin had a marked suppressive effect on the binding capacity of PEL. Additional experiments have shown that full regeneration occured 2-3 hrs after removal of the enzyme.

DISCUSSION AND CONCLUSIONS

Excellent methods are available for evaluating the number of antibody producing cells, but as yet there has been no satisfactory

Table 1. Effect of trypsin of PEL-EL4
conjugation: suppression and regeneration

Suppression [a)		Regeneration [b)	
Trypsin concentration	PEL-EL4 conjugates	Time	PEL-EL4 conjugates
(μg/ml)	($\times 10^{-4}$)	(hrs)	(%)
0	30	0	26
0.1	28	0.5	51
1	24	1	59
10	17	2	84
100	10	3	104
1000	6	4	100

[a) PEL, (1×10^6/ml PBS-FCS) were treated with trypsin (Worthington TR-TPCK) at the indicated concentrations for 30 min at 37^0C. Treatment in PBS-FCS was necessary to avoid clumping of PEL.

[b) PEL were treated with trypsin (1mg/ml); cells were allowed to regenerate at 37^0C in MEM + 10% FCS. Results are expressed as percent of the number of conjugates obtained with untreated PEL.

method available for directly determining the actual number of effector T cells in a given lymphoid population. In this paper, a method for enumerating the number of effector cells in lymphoid populations containing CTL is presented. It is based on the specific binding of CTL and TC and the formation of CTL-TC conjugates. Because the PEL and EL4 cells differ in size, the PEL being small-to-medium sized lymphoid cells and the EL4 lymphoblastic, analysis of conjugates is done by microscopy of unstained material. PEL-EL4 binding is optimal at room temperature (9), therefore binding experiments have been carried out at this temperature. Further, at room temperature virtually no lysis of target cells could be detected (1,10), thus enabling a clear separation of the binding stage from the ultimate lytic process.

Following alloimmunization, cells obtained from different
lymphoid organs possess different cytolytic activity against a
particular target cell (11). These differences may be due to quantitative differences in the content of effector cells in various
lymphoid sites or to qualitative differences or to both. We have
shown (9) that the majority of lymphocytes which bind to TC are
also cytotoxic cells. The evidence presented here and elsewhere (9)
suggests that the differences between lymphoid cells from various
sources are likely to be quantitative. This is because a positive
correlation exists between the number of lymphoid cells from a
given lymphoid site which are capable of binding to EL4 and their
lytic activity (see also Ref. 8).

The reason why only 60-75% of the target cells are competent
of conjugating with effector lymphocytes is not clear. It may
indicate that target cells are unable to bind at a particular phase
of their cycle. It is interesting to note that evidence which shows
differential expression of cell surface antigens at various stages
of the cell cycle has been reported (12).

The binding of PEL and EL4 is undoubtedly mediated by specific
PEL cell-surface receptors. The chemical nature of these receptors
is unknown. Their susceptibility to the proteolytic action of
trypsin (13, Table 1), suggests that the PEL receptor involved in
binding is a protein. Trypsin treated PEL regains full binding
capacity in 2-3 hrs, indicating de novo production of the binding
capacity and excluding the possibility that the receptor is an
adsorbed molecule. The results on the regeneration of the binding
capacity of PEL are in contrast to those obtained by Wekerle et al.
(14) in another system, the binding of unsensitized antigen-reactive
lymphocytes to mouse fibroblasts, where no regeneration of binding
activity could be demonstrated following trypsin treatment. The lack
of regeneration of the binding activity of unsensitized lymphocytes
(14) may indicate that the receptors for alloantigens on these cells,
in contrast to sensitized lymphocytes (PEL) are adsorbed molecules.

REFERENCES

1. G. Berke, and D.B. Amos, Transplant. Rev. 17:71, 1971.
2. J.-C. Cerottini, and K.T. Brunner, Adv. Immunol. 18:67, 1974.
3. C.S. Henney, Transplant. Rev. 17:67, 1973.
4. B.D. Brondz, and A.E. Snegirova, Immunol. 20:457, 1971.
5. R.D. Stulting, and G. Berke, J. Exp. Med. 137:932, 1973.
6. G. Berke, and R.H. Levey, J. Exp. Med. 135:972, 1972.
7. P. Golstein, E.A.J. Svedmyr, and H. Wigzell, J. Exp. Med. 134:
   1385, 1971.

8. G. Berke, K.A. Sullivan, and D.B. Amos, <u>J. Exp. Med.</u> <u>135</u>:1334, 1972.

9. G. Berke, D. Gabison, and M. Feldman, Submitted for publication.

10. G. Berke, K.A. Sullivan, and D.B. Amos, <u>J. Exp. Med.</u> <u>136</u>:1594, 1972.

11. T.G. Canty, and J.R. Wunderlich, <u>Transplant.</u> <u>11</u>:111, 1971.

12. M. Cikes, and S. Friberg,Jr., <u>Proc. Nat. Acad. Sci.</u> <u>68</u>:566, 1971.

13. B.D. Brondz, A.E. Snegirova, Yu.A. Rassulin, and O.G. Shamborant <u>in</u>: Prog. in Immunology, ed. D.B. Amos, Academic Press, N.Y. 1971, p.447.

14. H. Wekerle, P. Lonai, and M. Feldman, <u>Proc. Nat. Acad. Sci.</u> <u>69</u>: 1620, 1972.

OBSERVATIONS IN VITRO REGARDING THE MECHANISM OF THE CELL DESTRUCTION BY STIMULATED LYMPHOCYTES

H.Oerkermann,N.Paweletz and D.Gerecke

Medizinische Universitätsklinik,Cologne

and Krebsforschungszentrum,Heidelberg,W.-Germany

Many studies have focussed the interest on the cell destructive properties of lymphocytes (1,2).However,little is still known about the mechanism of this cell destruction.The behaviour of the lymphocytes has been observed in vitro,and it was found that they always entered into a close contact with the other cells they destroyed (3). This contact seemed to be necessary,since no cell destruction occurred when the lymphocytes were separated from the target cells by a millipore membrane (4).Furthermore,the lymphocytes developed a remarkable motility moving about upon the target cells (5,6).

In our studies we used purified human lymphocytes from the peripheral blood which were stimulated with phytohaemagglutinin (PHA).The cell destructive reaction of such stimulated lymphocytes was not considerably different from that of immune lymphocytes (lymphocytes from donors immunized with the special target cells) or lymphocytes in a mixed leukocyte culture (MLC) .Monolayers of HeLa cells or mouse fibroblasts served as target cells.The lymphocytes were added to the target cell cultures together with PHA in a culture medium consisting of 20% human AB serum and 80% TC 199.The observations were done by use of time lapse microcinematography.Besides electron microscopy and radioautography were performed.

The lymphocytes started to kill the target cells very early in the experiments,already a few hours after their addition to the target cell cultures.The death of the target cells happened as a sudden break-down of the whole

cell and a rapid change into debris.No previous necro-
biotic changes announced the sudden death of the single
cell.

We observed that the lymphocytes always touched the
surface of the target cells with fine processes,and we
assumed that they might cause lesions of the target
cell membrane which seemed to explain the typical disintegration of the cells best.Numerous electron microscopic preparations of those cultures,however,did not
reveal such lesions(Fig.1).

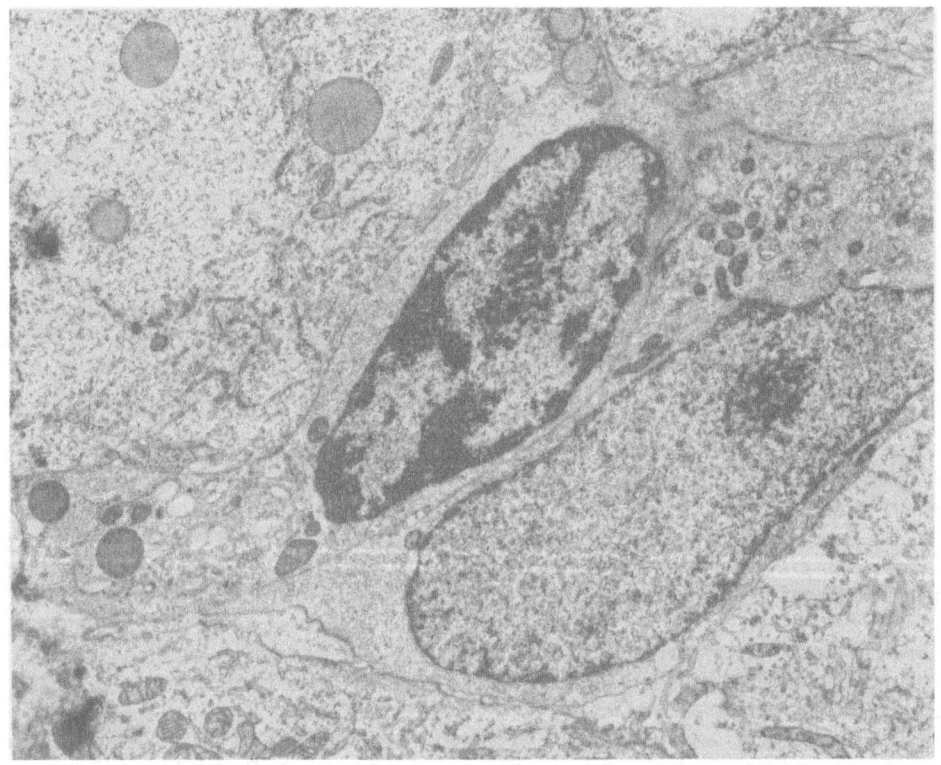

Fig.1: Electron microscopic picture demonstrating the
close contact between a stimulated human lymphocyte and
the target cells.No membrane lesions or cell bridging
is observable.

Wondering whether the lymphocytes released cytotoxic
substances or took material away essential for the
target cells,we performed radioautographic studies.
Either the stimulated lymphocytes or the taget cells
were protein-labeled with 3H-Leucine.It was found
that the lymphocytes released labeled material (Fig.2),
whereas the target cells did not,nor took the lymphocytes labeled material away from them.Electron microscopic radioautographic pictures of the target cells
showed that the labeled material derived from the
lymphocytes had been incorporated by the target cells.
Since the radioactivity was distributed irregularly in
all parts of the target cells no conclusions could be
drawn about the manner of a possible cytotoxic action
of these substances.

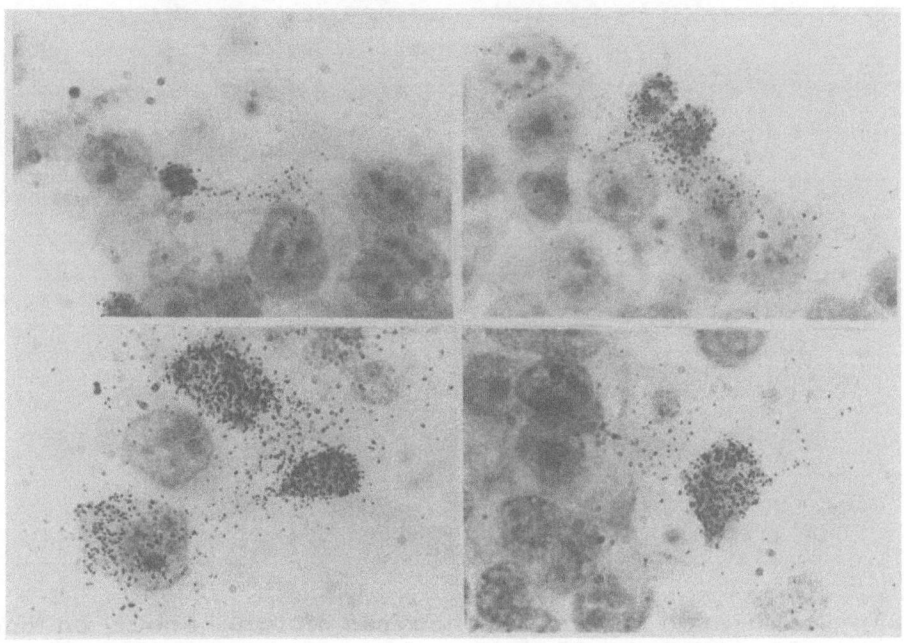

Fig.2: Radioautographs showing the release of radioactivity by stimulated human lymphocytes labeled with 3H-Leu-
cine,in a monolayer culture of HeLa cells.The lymphocytes
are surrounded by an area of radioactivity.

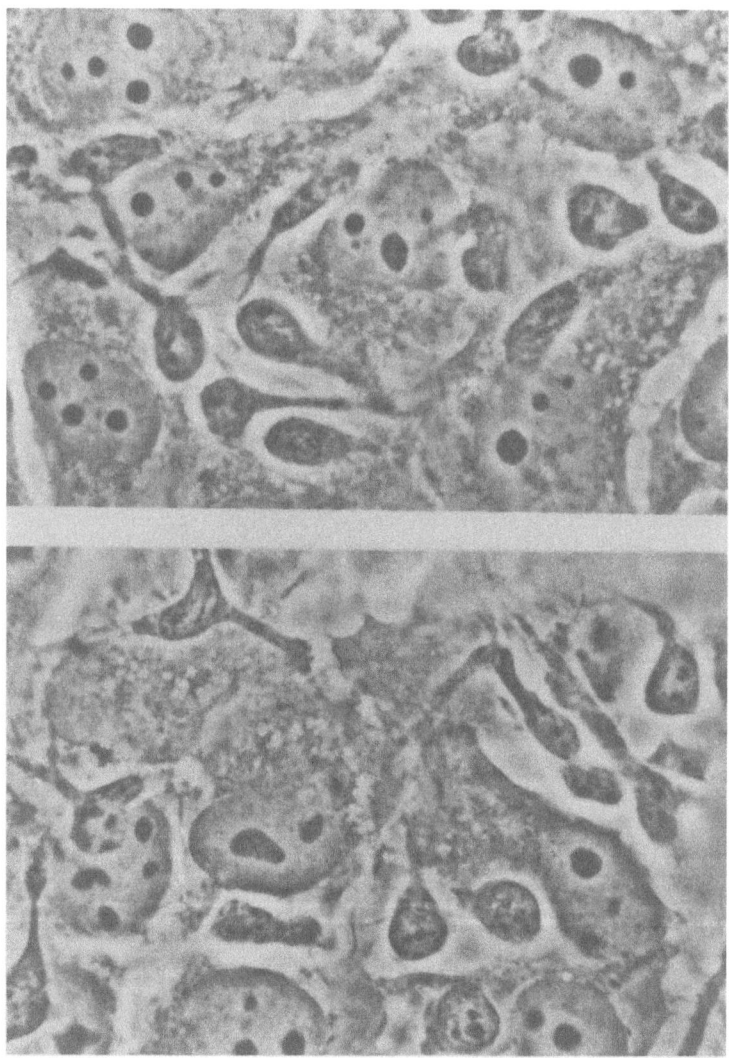

Fig.3: Stimulated human lymphocytes moving about on the target cells (HeLa cells).They have developed the uro-pod from where fine processes are extended on to the target cells.

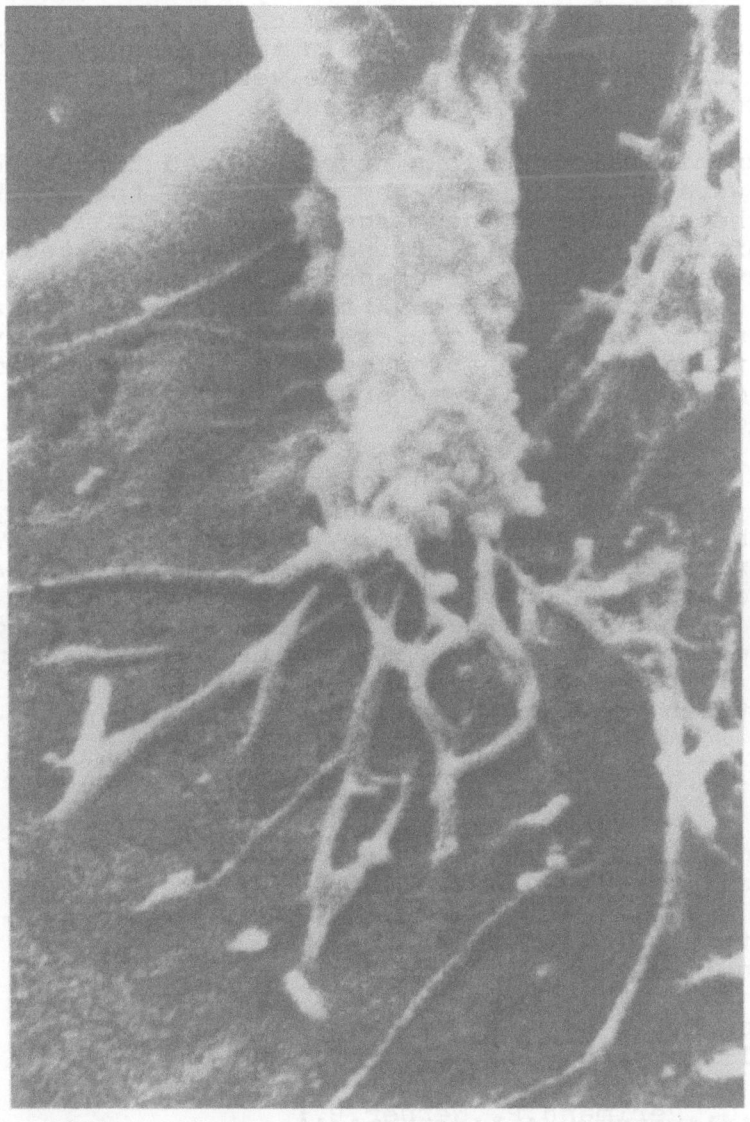

Fig.4: Scanning electron microscopic picture of the uropod end of a stimulated lymphocyte touching the surface of a target cell.Fine processes are torn off and by and by incorporated by the target cell.

Small vesicles were often observed sticking at the uro-
pod region of the lymphocytes.This seemed to explain
how the lymphocytes released the cytotoxic substances.
However,in all of our electron microscopic studies no
secretion was really observed in the lymphocytes.This
made it rather unlikely that the vesicles at the uropods
were produced by the lymphocytes.

The microcinematographic pictures showed that fine processes were extended from the uropods of the lymphocytes
on to the surface of the target cells (Fig.3),and that
parts of them were torn off when the lymphocytes moved
about.By and by these fragments were incorporated by the
target cells.Similar observations were made in scanning
electron microscopic pictures (Fig.4).These observations
gave a possible explanation by which means the lymphocytes released cellular material and passed it to the
target cells.

SUMMARY AND CONCLUSION: In contrast to other cells stimulated lymphocytes release substances probably cytotoxic which are incorporated by the target cells.The
cellular material is released by tearing off parts of
fine processes which the lymphocytes extend on to the
surface of the target cells.This explains the before
mentioned observations that the cell destruction mediated by lymphocytes depends absolutely on a close contact between the lymphocytes and the target cells.

REFERENCES

1) Perlmann,P.,Holm,G.:
   Advan.Immunol. 11:117   (1969)

2) Cerottini,J.C.,Brunner,K.T.:
   Advan.Immunol. 18:67   (1974)

3) Wilson,D.B.:
   J.Cell Comp.Physiol. 62:273   (1963)

4) Holm,G.,Perlmann,P.,Werner,B.:
   Nature 203:841 (1964)

5) Ax,W.,Malchow,H.,Zeiss,I.,Fischer,H.:
   Exper.Cell Res. 53:108 (1968)

6) Oerkermann,H.,Hirschmann,W.D.Schumacher,K.,Alzer,G.,
   Uhlenbruck,G.,Gross,R.:
   Klin.Wschr. 48:1368 (1970)

THE PRESENCE OF CELLS EXPRESSING IMMUNE-COMPLEX RECEPTORS IN NON-LYMPHOID MURINE TUMORS*

Gary R. Braslawsky, Margalith Yaakubowicz, Asher Frensdorff and Isaac P. Witz

Department of Microbiology, The George S. Wise Center for Life Sciences, Tel Aviv University, Tel Aviv, Israel

INTRODUCTION

Tumor cells, whether of lymphoid or non-lymphoid origin, are coated in vivo with a surface layer of immunoglobulin (Ig) (1). At least some of this surface Ig may represent anti tumor antibody (1,2) that is most likely attached to the surface through the Fab portion of the molecule. However, there have been reports that some non-lymphoid tumors contain cells which bear an Fc or Fc-like receptor (3-5,11). The Ig-coat of these Fc-reactive cells could contain anti tumor antibodies, as well as non-tumor antibodies, attached to the surface through the Fc part of the molecule (most likely as immune complex). In this paper we present evidence that non-lymphoid tumor populations can fix both in vivo and in vitro tumor unrelated antibodies or immune complexes.

EXPERIMENTAL

The Demonstration of Non-tumor Antibodies on the Surface of TA3/St Cell Populations

Table I shows the capacity of TA3/St (a transplantable ascitic mammary carcinoma) cells propagated in either OA or BSA preimmunized mice to react in vitro with both ^{125}I-OA and ^{131}I-BSA. Results clearly show that those tumor populations propagated in OA-immunized mice bound more OA than either the BSA-immunized or control (unimmunized) animal groups. Conversely, tumor populations originating from BSA-immunized mice bound more BSA than that bound to cells from either the OA-immunized or control animal groups.

*This study was supported by NCI Contract No. NOI-CB-43858

Table I

The Fixation of Radioiodinated Albumins to TA3/St Cells
Propagated in Albumin Immunized Animals

Animal group	Mice pre-immunized with	Exp[1]	Amount antigen fixed (ηg)			
			Tumor cells[2]		Spent-media[3]	
			OA	BSA	OA	BSA
1	ovalbumin (OA)	I	18.5	8.0	6.6	0.1
		II	19.2	7.8	N.T.	N.T.
2	unimmunized controls	I	6.5	5.5	0.1	0.1
		II	6.1	5.5	0.1	0.1
3	bovine serum albumin (BSA)	I	6.6	10.5	0.1	6.8
		II	6.6	12.7	0.1	5.4

1) Results of each experiment are averages of 4-6 animals
   tested individually.
2) TA3 populations were collected after 7 days growth in the
   pre-immunized animals, washed and incubated with ^{125}I-OA
   and ^{131}I-BSA (0.5 μg each) at 4°C for 30 min. Cells were
   again washed before counting.
3) The amount of labelled antigen bound by the cell-free
   supernatant after 4 hours incubation at 37°C.

It had been previously shown that if in vivo coated cells
were placed at 37°C in vitro, the Ig coat disappeared from the
surface and Ig was subsequently detected in the supernatant (6).
The capacity of culture supernatants of tumor cells propagated
in OA or BSA pre-immunized mice to bind the corresponding antigen
was measured by the 50% NH_4SO_4 precipitation test of Farr (7)
(Table I). Anti-OA antibody was detected only in supernatants from
tumor populations that were propagated in OA pre-immunized mice.
Anti-BSA antibody was detected only in supernatants from tumor cell
populations originating from BSA pre-immunized animals. Tumor
eluates from the control animal group did not show either OA or BSA
antibody activity. Thus, in these experiments we demonstrated that
tumor cell populations propagated in animals hyperimmunized to non-
tumor antigens could bear the corresponding antibodies on their
surface.

In Vitro Fixation of Immune Complexes by Various Cell Populations

The adherence of antibodies to Fc-receptors is stabilized by
prior complexing of the antibody with antigen (8). The ability of
various tumor or normal cell populations to bind purified anti-OA
antibody (PAOA) or its soluble immune complex (cPAOA) is given in

Table II
The Fixation of Radioiodinated C3H anti-OA antibody (purified by
affinity chromatography) or its Soluble Immune Complex to Various
Tumor or Normal Cells

Mouse strain	Cell[1] type	Tumor cell origin	Cell concentration[2] per reaction	ng-Antibody protein fixed per reaction[3]	
				PAOA	cPAOA
A/Sn	TA3	mammary carcinoma	1.0×10^7	20	54
C57B1	EL4	T-cell-lymphoma	1.4×10^7	22	54
A/Sn	YAC	T-cell-lymphoma	1.4×10^7	25	52
BALB/c	S-19	plasmacytoma	1.1×10^7	22	52
A.BY	SEYF-a	fibrosarcoma	0.7×10^7	21	63
C57B1	Spleen	-	4.0×10^7	11	24
BALB/c	PEC	-	1.0×10^7	8	30
C57B1	Thymocytes	-	1.0×10^7	2	4

1) Cells originating from unimmunized animals were incubated
   with ^{125}I-PAOA or its soluble complex with unlabelled OA.
   Cells were washed 4 times before counting.
2) Cell concentrations adjusted to give surface area approximately
   equal to 1×10^7 TA3 cell populations.
3) Average of 2-8 experiments consisting of 6-24 replicates.

Table II. Cell populations were adjusted in each case to give a
roughly similar surface area per reaction. Enhanced binding of
cPAOA over free PAOA was observed with each tumor cell population
tested, regardless of the tumor type. Three populations of normal
cells were also tested for their ability to bind cPAOA (Table II).
Two of the populations (spleen and induced peritoneal exudate cells-
PEC), containing known Fc-reactive cells showed enhanced binding of
the cPAOA, while thymocytes which do not bear such a receptor, did
not bind appreciable amounts of PAOA or cPAOA.

Some Characteristics of the Receptors for Immune Complexes on TA3/St Tumor Cell Populations

Table III shows that unlabelled homologous or heterologous
immune complexes or heat aggregated antibody but not free antibody
had the capacity to inhibit fixation of radioiodinated cPAOA. The
inhibition experiments were performed by preincubating TA3/St cell

population with unlabelled inhibitor at various concentrations followed by addition of ^{125}I cPAOA to the washed cells.

Binding of the cPAOA to the tumor cell population was not effected by pretreatment of the cell population with trypsin pronase or pepsin.

Steps Towards Identification of the Immune Complex Binding Cells

The identification of the complex binding cell within the tumor cell population is under active investigation. Removal of macrophage-like cells by adherance or by phagocytic ability will remove only about 50% of the enhanced cPAOA binding (Table IV). Depletion of Fc-receptor bearing cells (by rossette formation with 7S antibody coated sheep erythrocytes) removed all cPAOA binding cells (Table IV). However, the identity of the depleted cells must still be considered. Visual observation of rossette formers within a certain tumor cell population (SEYF-a) indicated that, morphologically, some of these cells may be tumor cells.

Binding to the Fc receptor of lymphocytes could be inhibited by preincubation of the cells with alloantisera (9). Using a similar approach we were able to obtain inhibition of cPAOA binding to TA3 cells with C3H antisera directed against TA3 (H-2^k anti H-2^a)

Table III
Inhibition of cPAOA Fixation to TA3/St Cells by Complexed
or Aggregated PAOA

Antibody source	Unlabelled antibody inhibitor	Treatment	% Inhibition of cPAOA binding at various inhibitor concentrations (µg) [4]		
			10	5	1
C3H	PAOA[1]	immune complex[2]	52.4	33.5	29.0
C3H	PAOA	heat aggregated[3]	36.0	50.4	16.4
C3H	PAOA	none	1	1	0
Rabbit	PABSA[1]	none	0	1	1
Rabbit	PABSA	immune complex[2]	63.5	41.1	15.6

1) C3H anti OA was purified on OA-conjugated Sepharose beads (PAOA) and rabbit anti BSA purified on BSA-conjugated Sepharose beads (PABSA).
2) Soluble immune complex prepared at antigen excess.
3) Antibody was heat aggregated at 63°C (10).
4) Inhibition of enhanced complex binding over free PAOA binding.

Table IV
Inhibition of cPAOA Fixation to Tumor Cell Populations

Cell source	Antiserum added[1]	Cell type removed	Inhibition of enhanced cPAOA binding[2]
TA3	–	adherent	49%
"	–	phagocytic	54%
"	–	Fc-receptor	100%
"	C3H anti TA3	–	91%
"	Normal C3H	–	0%
"	A anti C57Bl	–	0%
SEYF-a	A.BY anti SEYF-a	–	41%
"	Normal A.BY serum	–	0%
"	A.BY anti SEYF-a	phagocytic	77%

1) Tumor cells were incubated with antisera (diluted 1:10),
   washed and incubated with either PAOA or cPAOA.
2) See Table III footnote 4.

(Table IV). There was no inhibition of cPAOA binding by prior
incubation of the cells with normal mouse sera or with A anti C57Bl
antiserum (H-2^a anti H-2^b). Similar inhibitions were obtained with
SEYF-a cells (a polyoma virus induced tumor) treated with syngeneic
anti-SEYF-a antisera that were not cytotoxic to normal syngeneic
A.BY lymphocytes. Thus, at least a portion of the complex binding
cells in the SEYF-a population are tumor cells. Moreover, enriching
the relative percentage of tumor cells by removal of host phagocytic
cells increased the inhibition of cPAOA by the anti-SEYF-a antiserum (Table IV).

DISCUSSION

Evidence has recently been accumulating showing that cells
present in various murine tumors have Fc-like surface receptors.
The expression of such receptors has been evaluated by the in vitro
capacity of certain cells in the tumor to fix antibody-coated
erythrocytes (3-6,11) or by the ability of such cells to act as
effectors in antibody dependent cellular cytotoxicity (11,12). The
present paper adds a previously uninvestigated finding by showing
that fixation of unrelated antibody (or soluble immune complex) by
murine ascitic tumors cells was not a laboratory artifact, but
occured in vivo as well.

One of the main questions raised by this and other findings is
the exact nature of the immune-complex binding cells. Although
removal of macrophage-like cells from ascites tumors lowered complex
binding, it was not eliminated. Our results with SEYF-a cell
populations showed that both tumor and host cells may be involved.

Complex binding to SEYF-a tumor cells could be inhibited by
pretreatment with syngeneic antisera directed against tumor cells.
These antisera had no demonstrable activity towards the syngeneic
normal lymphoid cells. Furthermore, enrichment of tumor cells in
the ascitic suspension by removal of phagocytes, increased inhibition
by anti tumor antibodies. These results provide strong evidence
that receptors for immune-complexes can also be present on some
types of non-lymphoid tumor cells. Ralph et al (11) using a murine
reticulum-cell sarcoma reached the same conclusion.

SUMMARY

     In this study we demonstrated that cells lodging in tumors
have the capacity to fix antibody or immune complexes in vivo and
in vitro. Although some of the fixation is probably by host, at
least in one system studied, tumor cells, per se, were found to
exhibit immune complex fixation.

REFERENCES

1. Witz, I.P. Current Topics in Microbiol. Immunol. 61: 151, 1973.
2. Ran, M. and Witz, I.P. Int. J. Cancer 9: 242, 1972.
3. Humphrey, L.J., Milgrom, F., Tønder, O. Yasuda, J. and
   Witebsky, E. Int. Arch. Allergy, 30: 474, 1966.
4. Cohen, D., Gurner, B.W. and Coombs, R.R.A. Brit. J. Exp.
   Path. 52: 447, 1971.
5. Tønder, O. and Thunold, S. Scand. J. Immunol. 2: 207, 1973.
6. Ran, M., Fish, F., Witz, I.P. and Klein, G. Clin. Exp.
   Immunol. 16: 335, 1974.
7. Farr, R.S. J. Infect. Dis. 103: 239, 1958.
8. Basten, A., Warner, N.L. and Mandel, T. J. Exp. Med. 135:
   627, 1972.
9. Dickler, H.B. and Sachs, D.H. J. Exp. Med. 140: 779, 1974.
10. Dickler, H.B. and Kunkel, H.G. J. Exp. Med. 135: 627, 1972.
11. Ralph, P., Prichard, J. and Cohn, M. J. Immunol. 114: 898, 1975.
12. Tracey, D.E., Pross, H.F., Jondal, M. and Witz, I.P. (Submitted)

T AND B IMMUNODEPRESSION DURING 7,12-DIMETHYLBENZ(α) ANTHRACENE (DMBA) CARCINOGENESIS IN MICE*

C. D. Baroni, R. Scelsi, M. Scelsi, G. Soravito, L. Ruco and S. Uccini

Institute of Pathological Anatomy II, Experimental Pathology Unit, University of Rome, Viale Regina Elena 324, 00161 Rome, Italy

Certain chemical carcinogens administered to animals either at birth or later in life induce a marked and long-lasting reduction of both humoral and cellular T-dependent immune responses (1—7). Both responses are thymus-dependent, requiring either cooperation (8) or direction action of T lymphocytes (9). Recent reports indicate the existence of antigens inducing humoral antibody formation independent of thymus cell action (10). The present experiment was undertaken to study a B lymphocyte immune response in DMBA-treated mice. For comparison, a T-dependent humoral response was also studied using the same model. Moreover, in view of the fact that changes in normal rate of cellular proliferation in lymphoid tissues could be an important phenomenon during the early phases of carcinogenesis (11), we concomitantly studied the rate of cellular proliferation in central and peripheral lymphoid tissues of mice treated with DMBA at birth.

MATERIALS AND METHODS

Newborn Charles-River mice were injected s.c. with 100 μg of DMBA (Eastman Organic Chemicals) in 0.05 ml of olive oil. Controls were untreated. The animals were separated at 5 weeks of age.

*Investigation supported by a contract from the Consiglio Nazionale delle ricerche (C.N.R.), Rome, Italy.

Polyvinylpyrrolidone (PVP) (K90) m. w. 360,000 (Fluka AG, Switzerland), and sheep red blood cells (SRBC) were used respectively as B and T dependent antigens. Groups of 25, 70, 95, 145 and 195 day old DMBA treated and untreated mice were given an intravenous injection of PVP (10^{-12} μg in 0.1 ml of PBS) or of SRBC (4 x 10^8 in 0.1 ml of PBS).

Anti-PVP antibody activity was determined 5 days after immunization by passive immune hemolysis of PVP K15 (m. w. 10,000) coated SRBC (12). Anti-SRBC antibody activity was assayed 5 days after immunization, using uncoated SRBC.

Lymphoid proliferation was measured in lymphoid tissues of DMBA treated and control mice, by incorporation of ^{3}H-thymidine. Mice were given an i. p. injection of 0.8 μc of ^{3}H-thymidine (^{3}H-TdR; Radiochemical Center at Amersham, England; specific activity 3,000 mCi:mM) per gram of body weight, and sacrificed 24 h after. From each animal, thymus and spleen were removed and weighed; bone marrow cells were obtained from the femur that was previously weighed. Bone marrow cells were adjusted to a final concentration in absolute ethanol of 1 x 10^6 cells per milliliter.

A Tricarb-Packard liquid scintillation spectrometer was used. After correction for quenching the results were expressed as ^{3}H-TdR uptake in d. p. m. /10^6 bone marrow cells or /10 mg of thymus and spleen. The mice in each experimental group were 2, 4, 8, 16, 24, and 32 days of age.

RESULTS

The incidence of the tumors observed in the various experimental groups is reported in Table 1. The antibody response against SRBC in all five DMBA treated groups of various ages was significantly less compared to untreated animals. The reduction of the anti-SRBC response was sustained but did not diminish with increased intervals of time between administration of DMBA and SRBC immunization.

The response against PVP was constantly impaired in DMBA treated mice (Table 1). Although the anti-PVP response was less depressed than the anti-SRBC response, the degree of inhibition was sustained for the duration of the experiment, regardless of the presence of tumors and of the age of the animals at time of sacrifice.

Bone marrow cellularity was markedly affected in DMBA treated mice (Text-fig. 1). In all cases, the numbers of bone marrow cells were

TABLE 1. Humoral antibody response of untreated and DMBA-treated
Swiss mice to SRBC and PVP, and tumor incidence

Age at killing (days)	Carcinogen	Antigen	Log_{10} hemol. titer ± S.E.	Total No. of tumor-bearing mice with:		
				M.L.	L.T.	S.T.
30	—	SRBC (5)	10.3 ± 0.30^a	—	—	—
30	DMBA	SRBC (7)	7.1 ± 0.27	—	—	—
30	—	PVP (10)	13.2 ± 0.37^a	—	—	—
30	DMBA	PVP (13)	10.7 ± 0.18	—	—	—
75	—	SRBC (5)	12.6 ± 0.28^a	—	—	—
75	DMBA	SRBC (8)	8.0 ± 0.26	—	—	—
75	—	PVP (10)	14.8 ± 0.47^a	—	—	—
75	DMBA	PVP (10)	11.8 ± 0.34	1	5	—
100	—	SRBC (5)	12.3 ± 0.34^a	—	—	—
100	DMBA	SRBC (10)	8.3 ± 0.24	2	7	3
100	—	PVP (10)	15.3 ± 0.29^a	—	—	—
100	DMBA	PVP (10)	11.7 ± 0.22	3	4	1
150	—	SRBC (5)	12.4 ± 0.30^a	—	—	—
150	DMBA	SRBC (6)	8.9 ± 0.26	5	6	3
150	—	PVP (10)	13.7 ± 0.30^a	—	—	—
150	DMBA	PVP (10)	11.1 ± 0.51	3	6	3
200	—	SRBC (5)	12.1 ± 0.38^b	—	—	—
200	DMBA	SRBC (5)	8.8 ± 0.40	1	3	—
200	—	PVP (9)	13.0 ± 0.22^b	—	—	—
200	DMBA	PVP (8)	10.9 ± 0.46	1	6	1

No. of mice sacrificed at each time shown in parentheses. M. L. = malignant lymphoma; L. T. = lung tumors; S. T. = subcutaneous tumors.
[a]Significantly greater (P < 0.01).   [b]Significantly greater (P < 0.05).

decreased except for the mice tested at 2 days of age, where an equal number of cells in control as well as in DMBA treated mice was noted. Similarly, the uptake of ^{3}H-TdR in bone marrow of normal mice was greater
than in DMBA injected groups from days 4 to 32, thus suggesting decreased
cellular proliferation in bone marrow of carcinogen treated mice. The uptake of ^{3}H-TdR by the thymus of DMBA injected mice was depressed in the
4- and 8-day age groups of mice compared to controls (Text-fig. 1). In the
16, 24 and 32 day age groups there was an increased ^{3}H-TdR uptake by the
thymus of the DMBA treated mice.

There was no significant difference in ^{3}H-TdR uptake of the spleen between the groups injected with DMBA and the untreated mice (Text-fig. 1).

DISCUSSION

Our data indicate that the humoral response to a T-dependent antigen
is constantly and markedly depressed in mice treated at birth with DMBA.
These findings support previously reported observations (5, 6) that T-cell
function is impaired during DMBA carcinogenesis, regardless of the presence of tumors. This is well illustrated by the fact that DMBA-treated
mice sacrificed at 30 and 75 days of age had an impaired anti-SRBC response although they had no tumors (Table 1). Thus, DMBA-treatment at
birth may lead to a depression of a T cell function during the early stages
of carcinogenesis.

A depression of B cell dependent humoral antibody response was observed regardless of the age and presence of tumors at time of sacrifice
(Table 1). It follows, therefore, that there is impairment of immunologic
reactivity against both T- and B-dependent antigens in mice given DMBA at
birth. This conclusion is strengthened by the fact that neonatal injection of
DMBA induces a permanent and selective impairment of bone marrow cellularity. It was found that while cellular proliferation was constantly depressed in bone marrow and unchanged in the spleen, it was initially depressed and subsequently increased in the thymus (Text-fig. 1), perhaps
as a result of an early tumor initiation in this tissue (13).

Taking together all our data, we believe that DMBA injected at birth in
mice acts by a double mechanism, i.e., as a suppressor mainly of bone
marrow T- and B-cellular precursors before they have migrated to the
thymus and periphery, and as carcinogen primarily on thymus cells.

In conclusion, an overall consideration of the reduction of both T and
B immunity observed in the present and other experiments (1, 2, 5, 7)

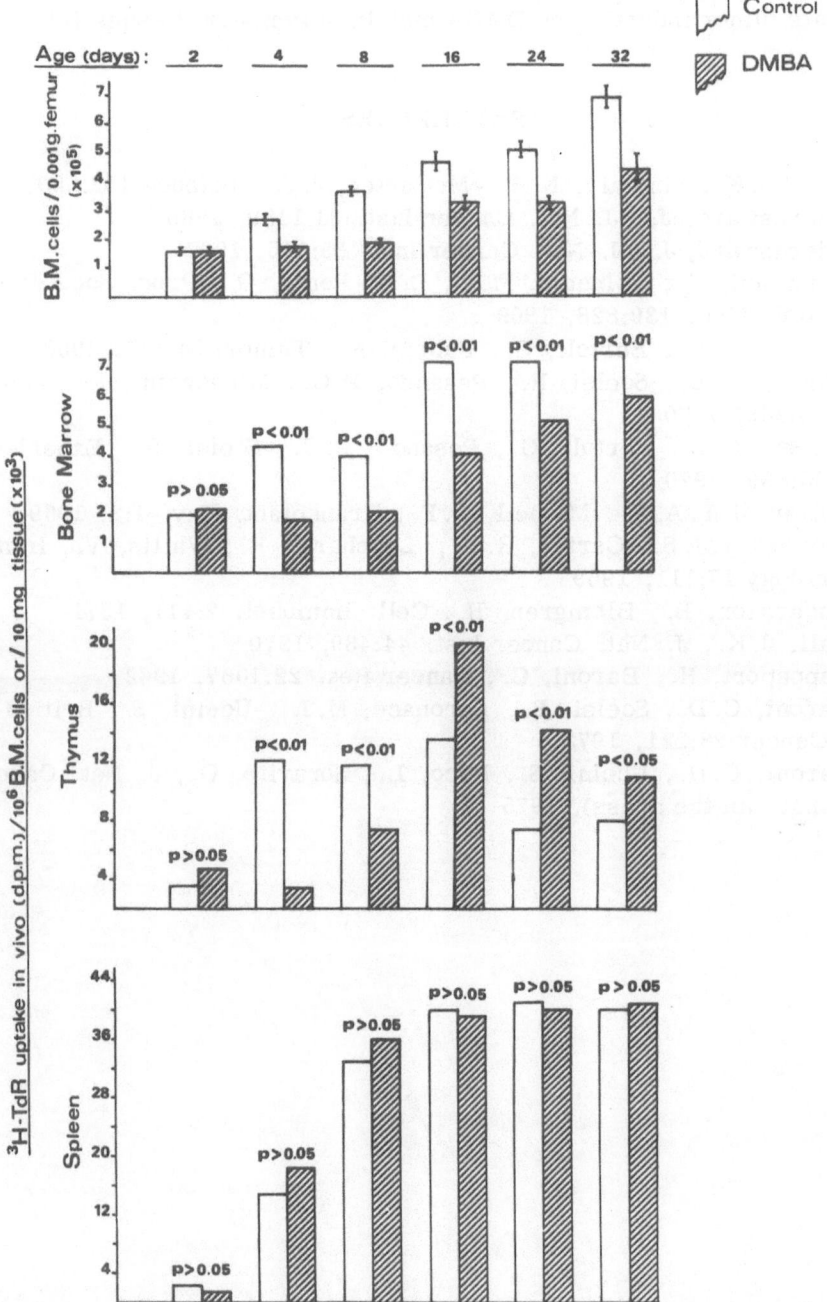

Text-fig. 1.   Bone marrow cellularity and ^{3}H-thymidine uptake in central and peripheral lymphoid tissues of control and DMBA-treated mice.

could be compatible with the indication that immunodepression may facilitate tumor induction by DMBA mainly in lymphoid tissues (14, 15).

REFERENCES

(1) Ball, J.K., Sinclair, N.R., McCarter, J.A., Science 152:650, 1966

(2) Stjernsward, J., J. Nat. Cancer Inst. 36:1189, 1966

(3) Stjernsward, J., J. Nat. Cancer Inst. 38:515, 1967

(4) Parmiani, G., Volnaghi, M.I., Della Porta, G., Proc. Soc. Exp. Biol. Med. 130:828, 1969

(5) Baroni, C.D., Bertoli, G., Fabris, N., Tumori 54:117, 1968

(6) Baroni, C.D., Scelsi, R., Pesando, P.C., Mingazzini, P., Tumori 56:269, 1970

(7) Baroni, C.D, Bertoli, G., Pesando, P.C., Scelsi, R., Experientia 26:899, 1970

(8) Miller, J.F.A.P., Michell, G.F., Transplant. Rev. 1:3, 1969

(9) Davies, A.J.S., Carter, R.L., Leuchars, E., Wallis, V., Immunology 17:111, 1969

(10) Andersson, B., Blomgren, H., Cell. Immunol. 2:411, 1971

(11) Ball, J.K., J. Nat. Cancer Inst. 44:439, 1970

(13) Rappaport, H., Baroni, C., Cancer Res. 22:1067, 1962

(14) Baroni, C.D., Scelsi, R., Peronace, M.L., Uccini, S., Brit. J. Cancer 28:221, 1973

(15) Baroni, C.D., Uccini, S., Ruco, L., Soravito, G., J. Nat. Cancer Inst. (in the press), 1975

REVERSAL OF A LEUKEMIA VIRUS-INDUCED IMMUNODEPRESSION BY MACROPHAGES IN VITRO AND IN VIVO

M. Bendinelli, A. Toniolo and H. Friedman

Departments of Microbiology,University of Pisa (Italy)and

Albert Einstein Medical Center, Philadelphia (U.S.A.)

The immunodepressive properties of many oncogenic viruses are well documented but the mechanisms involved and the significance of immunodepression to oncogenesis remain obscure (9).

Previous studies (2-4, 6-8) have characterized the immunological deficit produced in mice by Rowson-Parr virus (RPV), one of the lymphatic leukemia viruses isolated from the Friend leukemia complex (14). More recently it has been shown that the splenocytes of RPV-infected mice mount reduced antibody responses when cultured in vitro in the presence of sheep red cells (SRC), as antigen (5). Among other analogies, in culture the relationship between extent of hyporesponsiveness and time of infection is similar to that observed in the intact animal: an early phase of profound and constant suppression is followed by a long-lasting period of variable, though generally reduced responsiveness. In this paper we report that the in vitro antibody response of RPV-infected splenocytes during the phase of more intense immunodepression can be restored by cocultivation with small numbers of peritoneal macrophages but not by addition of other cell types and that a similar reversal of immunodepression can be obtained in vivo by administering small numbers of peritoneal exudate cell (PEC) together with the antigen.

MATERIALS AND METHODS

Mice. Inbred male BALB/c mice weighing 20-25 grams were used.
Viral infection. Mice were infected by i.v. or i.p. inoculation of 0.1-0.2 ml of various RPV preparations consisting of plasma or 10% spleen extract obtained from 8-day infected mice. The history of the virus is given elsewhere (2). The preparations used were free of lactic dehydrogenase and choriomeningitis viruses.
Cell suspensions. PEC were harvested by washing the cavity with

5 ml medium containing 5 U.I. heparin/ml five days after i.p. inoculation with 1-2 ml of 2% proteose peptone in saline. In some experiments PEC were depleted of T cells by treatment with absorbed anti-
C3H-theta AKR serum and complement (5). Spleens, thymuses and bone
marrows were brought into single cell suspension in culture medium.
Adherent spleen cells were obtained according to Mosier (13) and
detached from culture vessels with the help of a rubber policeman.
T cells educated to SRC were prepared according to Hartmann (10).
All cells were washed once, viability tested by the trypan blue
exclusion method and resuspended in culture medium at the concentration required.

Antibody response in vitro. 5×10^6 spleen cells, either alone
or with varying numbers of cells to be tested for restorative activity,
were cultured in Marbrook chambers (12) with or without 2×10^6 SRC.
The medium was Eagle's MEM with Hanks' base supplemented with nones-
sential aminoacids, sodium pyruvate, glutamin and 10% fetal calf
serum, and buffered with bicarbonate. Mycostatin, streptomycin and
penicillin were added to the medium. After 5 days incubation in 10%
CO_2, 7% O_2 and 83% N_2 the cultured cells were tested for viability
and for direct plaque-forming cells (PFC). Duplicate cultures were
done for each assay. The results are expressed as mean number of PFC/
10^6 viable cells recovered at the end of the experiment.

Antibody response in vivo. Groups of 7 mice were i.v. inoculated
with 10^8 SRC in 0.8 ml of medium either alone or mixed with varying
numbers of PEC. Four days later the spleens were weighed and assayed
for PFC. For each group the geometric mean of PFC per spleen was
calculated, together with its 95% confidence limits; the statistical
significance between groups was assessed by the Student's t test.

RESULTS

Spleen cells from mice infected with RPV five days earlier, when
cultured in the presence of SRC in Marbrook chambers, undergo consistently reduced PFC responses. As shown by Table 1, the PFC produced by infected splenocytes range between 3% and 25% of those formed by uninfecetd splenocytes although the survival of infected cells
in culture was normal. Table 2 gives the results of attempts to restore
the reactivity in vitro of RPV-infected splenocytes by adding graded
numbers of various cell types derived from normal syngeneic mice at
the beginning of cultivation. Spleen,thymus or bone marrow cells had
no effect on the response of infected splenocytes. Similarly T cells
educated to SRC were ineffective. A slight enhancement of the response
was produced by addition of adherent cells prepared from normal
spleens.

A more effective restoration of the PFC response in vitro of
infected splenocytes was achieved by adding PEC. In fact, the addition of these cells to the infected cultures brought the PFC response to normal levels. The effect of PEC was dose dependent:

TABLE 1. Results of eight representative experiments comparing the in vitro PFC response of splenocytes from normal and RPV-infected mice.

exp.	uninfected splenocytes		RPV-infected splenocytes		
	viability*	PFC	viability	PFC	% of normal
1	0.98	1610	0.67	120	7
2	1.10	1140	1.06	135	12
3	1.10	727	1.29	124	17
4	1.40	729	1.12	35	5
5	1.14	1070	1.24	73	7
6	1.69	598	1.72	20	3
7	1.60	1174	1.37	225	19
8	0.91	854	0.91	211	25

* Number of viable nucleated cells present in the cultures at the end of the experiment (x 10^6).

as shown by Table 3, as few as 3×10^4 PEC gave a marked enhancement and maximum restoration was produced in some experiments by 1×10^5 PEC and in others by 3×10^5 PEC. As the dose of PEC was further increased, inhibition of the PFC response ensued. No PFC were produced by 5×10^6 PEC cultured alone and the response of uninfected spleno-

TABLE 2. Effect of cocultivation with uninfected cells of various source on the PFC response in vitro of RPV-infected splenocytes.

exp.	cells added		PFC No. of cells added**						
	source	PFC*	0	1×10^3	3×10^3	3×10^4	1×10^5	3×10^5	1×10^6
1	thymus	0	76	141			141		182
	bone marrow	40		79			123		228
	spleen	950		172			135		276
2	T_{SRC}educat.	104	211	73			65		147
3	spleen adher.cells	65	88		94	162		236	312

* PFC produced by 5×10^6 cells cultured alone with SRC.
** The numbers of cells indicated were added to cultures containing 5×10^6 infected splenocytes.

TABLE 3. Effect of cocultivation with peritoneal exudate cells on the PFC response _in vitro_ of RPV-infected splenocytes.

exp.	cells added source	PFC	PFC — uninfected splenocytes, No. of cells added						PFC — RPV-infected splenocytes, No. of cells added					
			0	3×10^3	3×10^4	1×10^5	3×10^5	1×10^6	0	3×10^3	3×10^4	1×10^5	3×10^5	1×10^6
1	PEC	0[†]	1140	1260	1040	1810	1610		135	149	324	724	1020	
2	PEC	0	650	600	795	210		79		99	530	685	433	55
	RPV-inf.PEC[*]	0	1000		600			87				655		240
3	PEC	0	729	936	552	803			35		286	358	575	
	Tdep. PEC[**]	0		1303	641	842					217	282	627	

[†] PFC produced by 5×10^6 cells cultured alone with SRC.
[*] PEC collected from mice infected with RPV 5 days earlier.
[**] PEC pretreated with AKR anti-theta serum and complement. Control PEC were treated with normal AKR serum and complement.

TABLE 4. Effect of administering peritoneal exudate cells simultaneously with the antigen on the PFC response of RPV-infected mice.

| No.PEC | uninfected mice | | RPV-infected mice | |
	mean spleen weight (mg)	PFC/spleen[†]	mean spleen weight (mg)	PFC/spleen
0	177	53,460 (22,860-125,100)	270	3,945 (1,960-7,925)
2×10^5	242	141,000 (60,810-326,600)	299	23,390* (4,498-121,600)
2×10^6	253	55,210 (47,530-64,130)	296	22,600** (10,940-46,670)

† Geometric mean (in parenthesis the 95% confidence limits).
*,** The difference with the infected group not receiving PEC is significant at $P < 0.05$ (*) or $P < 0.01$ (**).

cytes was not substantially altered by PEC at the doses that reversed the immunodepression of infected splenocytes. With larger doses of PEC also the response of normal splenocytes was inhibited. PEC derived from 5-day infected mice proved as active as PEC collected from normal mice (Table 3, exp.2). After depletion of theta-positive cells by treatment with anti-theta serum, PEC maintained their restoring activity unmodified (Table 3, exp.3).

Similar attempts to reintegrate the immunoresponsiveness were done in intact animals. As shown by Table 4, 5-day infected mice given 2×10^5 or 2×10^6 PEC mixed with SRC developed numbers of PFC significantly higher than infected animals given SRC alone. Although the mean number of PFC was slightly lower than controls the difference was not significant. The PFC response of uninfected mice was not modified by 2×10^6 PEC and not significantly potentiated by 2×10^5 PEC.

DISCUSSION

Small numbers of PEC reverse the depression of antibody response to SRC in mice acutely infected with RPV. In these experiments as few as 3×10^4 PEC markedly increased the PFC response _in vitro_ of 5×10^6 splenocytes and as few as 2×10^5 PEC strongly potentiated the response of intact animals. There appears to be little doubt that the cells responsible are macrophages. The PEC used were more than 85% macrophages and the activity was present in the anti-theta serum resistant cells. The finding that adherent spleen cells, but not other cell types, are capable of some restorative activity also points to the macrophage as the active cell.

Macrophages may act with two mechanisms. The first possibility is that they substitute for macrophage functions impaired by RPV. The primary antibody response to multideterminant antigens in vitro requires macrophages (13) and a similar requirement is believed to take place in vivo (16). Moreover, macrophages have been implicated as the site of block in RNA-induced immunodepression (11) and in antigenic competition (15). Alternatively, macrophages might provide an extra stimulus to the precursors of antibody-forming cells that in RPV-infected spleens, though normal in number (5), might be less susceptible to be triggered to proliferate or to differentiate. Previous results showing that RPV-infected spleens have reduced numbers of cells with demonstrable Ig receptors and of cells exhibiting cap formation (4) permit to envisage an alteration that might justify the need for an extra stimulus. The observation that PEC restore the response even if collected from RPV-immunodepressed mice is in keeping with this interpretation, although it is possible that RPV differently affects peritoneal and splenic macrophages (1).

Whatever the mechanism of reversal, the demonstration that a leukemia virus-induced immunosuppression can be cured by grafting few macrophages offers a rational approach to evaluate whether the immunological impairment facilitates the tumorigenic process. Preliminary results showing that also the early phases of the immunodepression caused by Friend leukemia complex can be reversed in vitro by macrophages streghten the significance of the present findings(17).

REFERENCES

1. Bendinelli, M.(1968). Immunol. 14, 837.
2. Bendinelli, M.(1971). Infect.Immun. 4, 1.
3. Bendinelli, M., Campa, M. and Toniolo, A.(1975). Infect.Immun. 11, 1031.
4. Bendinelli, M. and Friedman, H. (1975). In press.
5. Bendinelli, M., Kaplan, G.S. and Friedman, H. (1975). In press.
6. Bendinelli, M. and Nardini, L. (1973). Infect.Immun. 7, 152.
7. Bendinelli, M. and Nardini, L. (1973). Infect.Immun. 7, 160.
8. Bendinelli, M., Toniolo, A. and Campa, M. (1975). Infect. Immun. 11, 1024.
9. Dent, P.B.(1972). Progr.med.Virol. 14, 1.
10. Hartmann, U÷K.(1970). J.exp.Med. 132, 1267.
11. Londoner, M.V., Morini, J.C., Amerio, M., Fout, M.T. and Rabasa, S.L. (1972). J.Immunol. 108, 552.
12. Marbrook, J.(1967). Lancet ii, 1279.
13. Mosier, D.E.(1967). Science (Wash. D.C.) 158, 1573.
14. Rowson, K.E.K. and Parr, I. (1970). Int.J.Cancer. 5, 96.
15. Schrader, J.W. and Feldman, M. (1973). Eur.J.Immunol. 3, 711.
16. Unanue, E.R.(1972). Adv.Immunol. 15, 95.
17. Supported by grants from the U.S.National Science Found., the U.S. National Inst.of Health and the Italian National Res. Council.

TUMOR IMMUNOLOGY--INTERACTION BETWEEN LYMPHOCYTES, ANTIBODIES AND NEOPLASTIC CELLS: A SUMMARY

M. G. Hanna, Jr.

Basic Research Program
Frederick Cancer Research Center
Frederick, Maryland 21701

There are great expectations for tumor immunology
in the belief that it will provide more alternatives to
clinicians in the management and control of neoplasia.
This is due to the fact that the immunologic approach to
the elimination of total tumor burden offers the aspect
of specificity that other therapeutic modalities lack at
the present time. Since cancer is a systemic disease and
since the intrinsic aggressiveness of tumor cells varies
not only among different classes of tumors but also
tumors of similar histologic type, the commonality
of the tumor cell surface is a major prospect for
immunotherapy. Currently, one of the major questions
concerning tumor immunologists is the ability of antigenic tumors to develop and the nature of the immune
status of the host against its own primary tumor.
Reasonable estimates are that not more than 10% of human
cancer is associated with viruses, and less than 5% is
associated with radiation. The increasing percentage of
spontaneous cancers in man, especially lung cancer, is
associated with combinations of environmental factors,
presumably in the form of chemical and physical carcinogens. Thus, information about the success of antigenic
tumors should continue to be developed from models based
on various modes of carcinogenesis.

Results from earlier studies have suggested that
induced tumors may express variability in antigenicity.
These experimental studies have revealed information
regarding the host's immunologic reactivity to its own
primary tumor, where the question of "immunescape" and

513

immune-selective pressures is to be evaluated. The
papers of Kölsch and Mengersen as well as Kripke and
Fisher are highly relevant to this effect. The latter
have demonstrated that ultraviolet (UV) induced sarcomas
in C3H/F mice, in spite of their strong antigenicity,
grow progressively in the primary host and rarely
undergo regression. These results clearly demonstrate
that the inability of the primary host to reject its
own tumor is systemic, not a local phenomenon. Furthermore the autochthonous tumors succeed in the primary
host in spite of the fact that these animals are immunologically competent at least by the criteria of allograft rejection. The primary defect in the host seems
to be induced by the UV irradiation rather than by the
development of the tumor.

Using a BALB/c transplantable mastocytoma model,
the Kölsch and Mengersen studies demonstrate the effect
of low, subimmunogenic numbers of tumor cells to para-
lyze the immune system before an immunogenic dose of
tumor antigen has accumulated. This paralysis is presumed to be accompanied by the activity of a suppressor
cell. Both of these papers are important for a more
complete understanding of the possible mechanisms of
escape from "immune surveillance". A most relevant
question related to both of these studies, however,
is whether the basis of the host response in either
tumor system is immunologic in nature or does it involve some nonspecific component of the host. For
further evaluation of this point, it would seem that
the most relevant model would be a UV induced tumor
system since it is an autochthonous tumor compared
with the allogeneic tumor system of Kölsch and Mengersen
and since it does not involve specific blocking factors.
With respect to blocking factors, suppressor cells, or
tolerance, it would have to be assumed that in the UV
system, during the course of carcinogenesis, the animal
becomes hypo-responsive to all possible tumor-specific
antigens. This speculation is highly improbable.

Virus-induced tumor models have played an important role in experimental basis for tumor immunology.
In reviewing the host response to virus-associated
cancers, it is important to consider the relevance of
experimental models and to distinguish between endogenous versus exogenous oncogenic virus infections.
With respect to the exogenous and horizontally transmitted oncogenic virus infections, two papers presented
suggest that virion-specific antibody has a role in
host protection of tumorigenesis. Linna, Lam, Hu and

Thompson show the cooperative effect of antibodies and
cytotoxic cells in reticuloendotheliosis virus infection
in chickens. Ran, Klein and Witz, using a polyoma-viral
system, demonstrate the presence of antibodies specific
to polyoma-induced cell surface antigens and suggest
that the humoral component of the immune system may be
effective in host control of this oncogenic virus-
induced lesion.

Possibly more important is the question of host
control of endogenous oncogenic viruses, such as the
murine leukemia viruses, which have been shown to be
endogenous and vertically transmitted. The role of the
host-immune system in control of endogenous oncogenic
viruses has undergone a drastic change in the last few
years. It is now known that there is an age-associated
development of autogenous humoral immunity to the
vertically transmitted endogenous murine leukemia virus
both of the xenotropic as well as ecotropic classes.
While definitive evidence is lacking that this autogenous immunity may be one of the major host regulatory
mechanisms which controls viral carcinogenesis, it is
clear that there is specific recognition of virion
type-specific envelope antigens and that this natural
antibody may be important in limiting virus expression
as well as virus-mediated neoplasia.

A most interesting and relevant paper related to
the genetic basis of host control to endogenous virus
was presented by Barnes. He demonstrated tumor resistance of tetraparental AKR-CBA chimaeras. The chimaeras
derived by early embryo aggregation show a tumor resistance which cannot be attributed to either the absence
of AKR cells or AKR-cell products. The presence of
numerous type-C leukemia virus with gross antigenic
specificity suggested that the tumor resistance of the
chimaeras could not be attributed to the absence of the
oncogenic gross virus. The basis in the host of the
resistance appears to be systemic since chimaeras, which
are only 5% CBA and 95% AKR, continue to retain the
tumor resistance. The possibility that this chimeric
condition establishes an animal which has a more functional autogenous immunity to endogenous leukemia virus,
than exists in the pure AKR, is a real possibility and
needs to be determined.

In the last few years, there has been a re-
evaluation of the effective arms of the immune response
with respect to tumors, and a major consideration has

been given to the role of cells of the histocyte-
macrophage compartment. While it is recognized that
antibodies as well as sensitized lymphocytes may play
an important role in in vitro cytotoxicity of tumors,
a large number of in vivo studies has emphasized the
role of the "macrophage". Questions also exist with
respect to the mechanism of macrophage involvement in
host control of neoplasia. The cytotoxic properties of
immune macrophages were studied by Gallily, Eliahu and
Ben-Ishay using a mixed macrophage culture system.
Their finding suggests that macrophage cytotoxicity may
be due at least in part to mediators released from
sensitized T lymphocytes and attached to the macrophage
surface. Their results indicate that cytophilic antibodies are not involved in the cytotoxicity expressed
in the mixed macrophage culture and that macrophage
target cell contact rather than phagocytosis is a
primary mechanism of cell killing. These studies,
while carried out in a non-tumor system, agree with
previous literature associated with the role of macrophages in transplantable and autochthonous tumor systems.

In general, this session has provided a variety of
experimental tumor systems. It appears that each study
exploited a major effector component of the immune
system and most dealt with host-tumor interaction. It
is apparent that the behavior of malignancies is determined in part by the host-immune response to them. In
addition, it is apparent from the papers presented that
variations exist in the balance between the behavior of
experimental tumors and the limiting factors in the host.
It is also expected that experimental models in tumor
immunology will attempt to minimize these individual
variations. While providing valuable insights, such
models are understandably limited when converting their
usefulness to cancer patients.

It appears, even at this time, that one of the
more important aspects of modern tumor immunology is
still to develop models which more closely associate
with the clinical reality. These models should provide
a variety of mechanisms which could be studied both
in vitro and in vivo utilizing a relevant histologic
type of tumor. With many of the experimental models
being studied, caution must be exercised in the translation of information from experimental to clinical
tumor immunology.

The potential methods of specific and nonspecific
tumor immunotherapy are limited at the present time.

Clinically these procedures have been problematic
especially when attempts have been made to increase
immunologic reactivity in either a specific or non-
specific manner. In individuals with established
tumors, the success of immunotherapy depends upon the
stage, type, and location of the tumor; the level of
antigenic specificity of the target cells; the status
of the host-immune response to the tumor; and the
particular mode of immunostimulation. Thus, investigations of relevant carcinogenesis and immunotherapy
models are urgently needed before any tangible progress
can be made in understanding progressive tumor growth
in the face of the various known immunologic factors of
the host.

Round-Table Discussion:
Definition and Functions of IR Genes

IR GENES, PHENOTYPIC EXPRESSIONS AND
THEIR INTERPRETATION

P. Lonai

Department of Chemical Immunology

Weizmann Institute of Science, Rehovot, Israel

The purpose of this introduction is to present the basic data and their various possible interpretations in a concise form for our discussion on the function of Ir genes.

From a genetical point of view the different immunological phenomena controlled by Ir genes, or by loci situated closely to it, can be regarded as phenotypic expressions of the H-2 gene complex. The strong point of this approach is that it allows the differentiation of various experimental phenomena into separate individual genetic traits separable as loci on the genetic map. The accuracy of such a separation is subject to the resolution of the genetic map. The advantage of this approach is in the strong heuristic value of genetic separation; namely, on the one hand it can be assumed that genetically separable phenomena are regulated by different genes involving different proteins, and on the other, that different experimental phenomena not separable by genetic means can be assumed to be controlled by the same gene or genes despite their different appearance in the experiments.

Five genetic traits observed as distinct immunological phenomena have been linked to the I region of the H-2 complex of the mouse. These are briefly described in Table 1. It is apparent from the table that all the five: H-2 linked Ir genes, cooperative interaction structures, lymphocyte stimulating determinants, Ia antigens, and the antigen specific T helper cell factor, however different they may be, are regulated by genes localized in the I-A and I-B subregions of the H-2 complex. Presently

Table 1

Term	Localization	Definition	Phenotypic Expression of the I-Region Experimental observation	Remark	Literature
Ir	I-A, I-B	Immune response gene	Dominant, determinant specific genes. Humoral immune reactions and delayed type hypersensitivity. Expressed on T and B lymphocytes.	Possibility raised for 2 closely linked Ir-s within the H-2 for one antigen.	1, 2, 3
C.I.	I-A, I-B (only?)	Cooperative interaction structures	Syngeneicity of C.I.-s required for T-B and T-macrophage cooperation.	Antigen specific? Required for all antigens?	4, 5
Lad	H-2 and M (Strongest I-A and I-B)	Lymphocyte (T) activating determinants	Main activators of MLR, GvH, and possibly graft rejection. Weak CML target. Expressed on T and B and other cells.	Physiological function besides allogeneic reactions?	6–11
Ia	Whole I region	Alloantigens, polymorphic	M.W. 3×10^4 present mainly on B and probably on some T lymphocytes, present on other cells also. Inhibits stimulation in MLR. At least 3 genes.	Ia = Lad (?)	3, 12
Specific T cell factor	I-A, I-B (only?)	Humoral factor of helper T cell activity. Some antigenic specificity. Under Ir control.	Its production and effect on antibody production under separate control. Anti-Ia column does, anti Ig column does not retain it.	T cell receptor? identical with Ia?	13, 14

neither the separation nor the identification of these traits with each other is possible. Therefore, we cannot tell for instance whether the Lad determinants are only alloantigens for lymphocyte stimulation, or Ir gene products recognized as alloantigens. Similarly, we do not know with any certainty whether the C.I. products influencing lymphocyte cooperation are merely regulators of lymphocyte cooperation or experimental representations of the Ir gene product or of the T cell factor-B cell acceptor complex. Despite our uncertainties but justified by the importance of the problem, several interpretations of the function of Ir genes have been proposed. Before briefly covering these, I would like to mention two groups of data not included in Table 1.

In H.O. McDevitt's laboratory I performed a series of experiments with the aim of identifying two of these five genetic traits. The question was whether Lad determinants are expressed on both B and T lymphocytes and whether these products could be identical with the Ia antigens. It was found that both T and B cells could stimulate the MLR in strain combinations differing in the I region only. This finding demonstrated that I region gene products are most likely expressed on both T and B lymphocytes (11). Further experiments have shown that the stimulator T or B cells, but not the responder cells, are sensitive to anti Ia serum, both upon pretreating the cells before culturing with immune serum and complement, and to direct anti Ia serum treatment (experiments of T. Meo), suggesting that the Ia antigens and Lad determinants may be identical (12). In these studies a very large number of congenic and congenic intra H-2 recombinant combinations were used, allowing a more accurate localization of the strongest Lad loci. In agreement with earlier studies (7-9) it was found that while the whole H-2 complex contains determinants capable of allogeneic lymphocyte stimulation, the strongest loci are those to be found in the I-A and I-B subregions of the I region (12 and unpublished). This observation is worth additional consideration. While humoral immune reactions can be induced against a vast number of dissimilar macromolecules, allogeneic reactions, MLR and GvH specially, are induced only by a small sample of all the possible allelic products, which are different between two individuals of the same species, suggesting that some T cells may have exclusive vocabulary for non self histocompatibility antigens.

Another group of observations important to consider deals with the immune recognition of antigen modified self H-2 products. Zinkernagel, Doherty and Blanden (15) using virus infected cells as well as Shearer using TNP modified lymphocytes (16) have found that the target antigens for killer lymphocytes are modified H-2K or H-2D. Since both these experiments are restricted to the study of cell mediated killing, and the main antigen of these reactions in allogeneic situations is H-2K and H-2D therefore, as was pointed out by R. M. Zinkernagel in these proceedings, it is not improbable that in other lymphocyte interactions, like, e.g., in reactions against soluble antigens, antigen modified self I region products should be involved. Such an observation has not yet been made, nevertheless, this possibility, if proven true, could resolve some of the uncertainties of our present interpretation of the function of Ir genes.

The punctum saliens of the interpretation of Ir genes is whether we regard them as structural or regulator genes. If Ir genes are regulator genes their role can be interpreted within the framework of any one of the unitarian - one receptor, one endproduct = immunoglobulin - hypothesis of immunity. However, if Ir genes are structural genes, their interpretation as antigen receptor cannot be avoided. The antigen specific and dominant nature of the Ir genes seems to favour this second alternative. Because the nature of the Ir gene product is not known, it cannot be ruled out whether Ir genes control immunoglobulin-like receptors. Since most of the experiments on the role of immunoglobulins in Ir gene controlled T cell reactions are negative, most of the hypotheses interpreting the function of Ir genes are of dualistic nature, predicting basic differences between the T and B cell receptors.

In the early stages of the research, on the basis of the antigen specific and dominant nature of Ir genes, and because of the lack of evidence for the control of immunoglobulins by the H-2 complex, and because of the lack or uncertainty of evidence for immunoglobulins on T cells, it was suggested that Ir genes code for T cell receptors. This hypothesis suggests that Ir genes should be expressed exclusively on T cells (2). As additional data became available, this view had to be modified. The new evidence suggested on one hand that Ir genes may be expressed on both B and T cells (limiting dilution experiments (17), the existence of receptor and acceptor molecules suggested by the T cell factor experiments (13,14), experiments suggesting two Ir genes, (Dorf personal com.)), and on the other hand, evidence was found for additional traits controlled by the I region expressed on both B and T lymphocytes (Ia, C.I., Lad, see Table 1). These data could be interpreted within the framework of the original Ir gene product-T cell receptor hypothesis by predicting separate roles for the different I region products. Thus, McDevitt et al. suggested that the Ia antigens should have different roles from the Ir gene products proper (18). More recently Katz and Benacerraf published a comprehensive hypothesis suggesting the interaction of four presumably I region coded units, T cell receptor, Ir-gene product, C.I., and T cell factor, in immune recognition (19).

A common feature of this series of hypotheses is that they do not interpret that the H-2 complex is a complex of histocompatibility genes. The observations of the Canberra group and those of G. M. Shearer suggest that the antigen for lymphocyte mediated target cell killing is altered self H-2K and H-2D. Would this finding be generalizable for helper cells and antigen modified Ia antigens, the role of Lad, C. I. and Ia products could be interpreted in one coherent framework together with the Ir genes. To end this introduction I will summarize the elements of such a generalization in a few points:

1. A class of T cells recognizes and reacts to non-self Ia-Lad products.

2. The Ia-Lad gene products can become specifically modified by antigen, either through directly binding the antigen (in analogy to the antigen specific T cell factor), or through their proximity to the antigen bound by immunoglobulin on the cell membrane.

3. This H-2 product-antigen complex represents a "T cell signal" recognized by T cells sensitive to non-self I region products.

4. The vocabularies represented by the T cell signal and the receptor recognizing it are genetically determined.

5. Any immunocyte carrying Ia antigens may play a role in the representation of the T cell signal.

6. The T cell recognizing the T cell signal cooperates with the presenting cell by stimulating it.

The justification of this interpretation as well as that of all hypotheses depends on whether they present questions for further experimentation.

Literature

1. McDevitt, H.O., Deak, B.D., Shreffler, D.C., Klein, J., Stimpfling, J.G. and Snell, G.D. J. Exp. Med. 135: 1259. 1972.
2. Benacerraf, B. and McDevitt, H.O. Science 175: 273. 1972.
3. Shreffler, D.C. and David, C.S. Adv. Immunol. 20: 125. 1975.
4. Katz, D.H., Hamaoka, T., Dorf, M.E. and Benacerraf, B. Proc. Nat. Acad. Sci. U.S.A. 70: 2624. 1973.
5. Katz, D.H., Graves, M., Dorf, M.E., DiMuzio, H. and Benacerraf, B. J. Exp. Med. 141: 263. 1975.
6. Bach, F.H., Widmer, M.I., Bach, M.L. and Klein, J. J. Exp. Med. 136: 1430. 1972.
7. Meo, T., David, C.S., Nabholz, M., Miggiano, V. and Shreffler, D.C. Transplant. Proc. 5: 377. 1973.
8. Klein, J. and Park, J.M. J. Exp. Med. 137: 1213. 1973.
9. Alter, B.J., Schendel, D.J., Bach, M.L., Bach, F.H., Klein, J. and Stimpfling, J.H. J. Exp. Med. 137: 1303. 1973.
10. Nabholz, M., Vives, J., Young, H.M., Meo, T., Miggiano, V., Rijnbeek, D. and Shreffler, D.C. Eur. J. Immunol. 4: 378. 1974.
11. Lonai, P. and McDevitt, H.O. J. Exp. Med. 140: 1317. 1974.
12. Lonai, P. in Immune Recognition (ed. A.S. Rosenthal), Acad. Press. 1975. pp. 683-704.
13. Taussig, M.J. and Munro,   in Immune Recognition (ed. A.S. Rosenthal), Acad. Press. 1975. pp. 791-804.
14. Taussig, M.J., Mozes, E. and Isac, R. J. Exp. Med. 140: 301.1974.
15. Doherty, P.C. and Zinkernagel, R.M. J. Exp. Med. 141: 502. 1975.
16. Shearer, G.M. Eur. J. Immunol. 4: 527. 1974.
17. Lichtenberg, L., Mozes, E., Shearer, G.M. and Sela, M. Eur. J. Immunol. 4: 450. 1974.
18. McDevitt, H.O., Bechtol, K.B., Hammerling, G.J., Lonai, P. and Delovitch, T. in The Immune System - Genes, Receptors and Signals, Acad. Press, 1974.
19. Katz, D.H. and Benacerraf, B. Transpl. Revs. 22: 175. 1975.

T HELPERS MAY BE SENSITIZED BY ANTIGEN-SPECIFICALLY ALTERED STRUCTURES, WHICH ARE CODED BY THE I REGION OF THE H-2 GENE COMPLEX

R. M. Zinkernagel

Department of Microbiology, John Curtin School of Medical Research, Canberra, Australia

We have shown that virus immune cytotoxic cells are specific for virus-altered structures (1—4). These structures are coded for in the H-2 $\underline{K}$ or the H-2 $\underline{D}$. Accordingly, virus immune cytotoxic CBA/H (H-2^k) T cells sensitized in vivo will react in vitro only with 'altered' H-2^k, not with 'altered' H-2^d. The alteration can be envisaged as biochemical modifications of the protein or carbohydrate part of the private specificity of major transplantation antigens or of structures coded very closely to them. Alternatively, it could be formation of a complex of these structures and viral antigens (1—4). Structures coded for in the I region of the H-2 complex could not be shown to be relevant at the effector level (2, 3). However, this H-2 region may be involved in the initial sensitization and/or proliferation step(s). The requirement for compatibility at H-2 $\underline{K}$ or H-2 $\underline{D}$ of in vitro T cell-mediated cytotoxicity against virus-infected target cells is apparently not due to an inherent incapacity of these T cells to interact with allogeneic infected target cells. This observed requirement may be purely manifestation of specificity (1, 4). It is expected that experiments with zygote fusion chimeras (tetraparental mice) now in progress should provide direct evidence for this argument (4).

Scripps Clinic and Research Foundation, La Jolla, California 92037, U. S. A .

527

We suggest that the apparent requirement for H-2 I region or subregion compatibility in T helper function (5—7) and possibly for DTH
effector T cells (8) could be explained in a similar way.   This concept
results from many discussions with associates in the Department of
Microbiology at this Institution, mainly with Drs. R. V Blanden, P. C.
Doherty, and also L. Pilarski, P. A. Bretscher and A. J. Cunningham.

T cells may have quite generally the function of surveillance of cell
surface structures coded for in the H-2 gene region.   These may be
reacting mainly against alterations of these structures.   On the basis of
this one simple model, one can explain a variety of observations, e. g ,
reactivity to modified self caused by virus (1—4), intracellular bacteria
(4), probably soluble antigens (2—4), or by chemical modification (9), as
well as reactivity to genetic differences (alloantigens).

According to this concept, there is no need for postulation of physiological cell interactions (6).   Thus, two functional groups of T cells
differing also with regard to serologically detectable surface markers
as described by Cantor and Boyse (10) could be distinguished.

Surveillance T cells

Cytotoxic T cells are representatives of this group, which are very
easily demonstrable in vitro.   They are sensitized to altered structures
coded in H-2 K or H-2 D.   In this respect, alloantigens can be regarded as
a special case of altered self.   Effector activity against altered self is
very potent;   it is 100 times more effective as compared with any other
cytotoxic activity to other antigens.   Several reasons which are by no
means mutually exclusive, may account for this.   H-2 K or H-2 D could
represent sites at the cell membrane where damage causing ^{51}Cr release
is most effectively performed.   On the other hand, as proposed by Drs.
P. A. Bretscher (11), K. J. Lafferty (12, 13) and A. J. Cunningham, these
structures may be more immunogenic than others when they are associated in a certain particular way with a mitogenic or a second signal, or
with a stimulatory capacity present only on cells with some level of immunocompetence (12, 13).   It is in fact interesting that the viruses (LCM,
ecteromelia, etc.) generating in vivo strong cytotoxic T cell responses
are known to infect lymphoid tissues (2—4).

Helper T cells

These cells do not seem to interact lytically with other cells as far as detectable. They can be sensitized to structures created by antigen-specific alterations, coded for in the I region (i. e. , altered Ia). Altered I structures could be envisaged as a complex of antigen and structures coded for by H-2 I. Phagocytic cells, like macrophages, may play an important role by phagocytizing soluble and/or corpuscular antigens, degrading or "processing" them, and subsequently exposing them partially on the cell surface, for example, as altered self (4).

The results of Bechtol et al. (14) using tetraparental mice could be interpreted to support this view (15, 4). The recent studies of von Boehmer et al. (16) may offer an extension of this scheme. They showed that irradiation chimeras, reconstituted with bone marrow of one or both parental type(s) generate T helper cells (tolerant to alloantigens of the other parental type) which can cooperate with B cells either syngeneic or parental allogeneic with respect to I region. This could suggest that the apparent requirement for H-2 I compatibility for T—B or T—macrophage—B cell interactions may also be in principle a question of specificity (4, 2).

References

1. Zinkernagel, R. M. , Doherty, P. C.   Nature 1974, 248:701;   251:547; J. exp Med. 1975, 141:1427.
2. Doherty, P. C. , Zinkernagel, R. M.   Transplant. Rev. 1974, 19:89; J. exp. Med. 1975, 141:502; Lancet (in press), and personal communication.
3. Blanden, R. V. , Doherty, P. C. , Dunlop, M. B. C. , Gardner, I. D. , Zinkernagel, R. M. and David, C. S.   Nature 1975, 254:269, and unpublished results; personal communication.
4. Zinkernagel, R. M.   Nature 1974, 251:230; Ph. D. Thesis, Australian National University 1975.
5. Katz, D. H. , Hamaoka, T. , Dorf, M. E. , Benacerraf, B.   Proc. Natl. Acad. Sci. U. S. A. 1973, 70:2624.
6. Katz, D. H. , Benacerraf, B.   Transplant. Rev. 1975, 22: 175.
7. Erb, P. , Feldmann, M.   J. exp. Med. 1975, in press.
8. Miller, J. F. A. P. , personal communication.
9. Shearer, G. M.   Eur. J. Immunol. 1974, 4:527.
10. Cantor, H. , Boyse, E. A.   J. exp. Med. 1975, 141:1376, 1390.
11. Bretscher, P. A. , personal communications.
12. Lafferty, K. J. , Cunningham, A. J. , Austr. J. exp. Biol. Med. Sci. 1975, 53:27.

13. Lafferty, K. J. , Misko, I. S. and Cooley, M. A.   Nature 1974, 249: 275.

14. Bechtol, K. B. , Wegmann, T. G. , Freed, J. H. , Brumet, F. C. , Chesebro, B. W. , Herzenberg, L. A. , McDevitt, H. O.   Cell. Immunol. 1974, 13:264.

15. Pilarski, L. , personal communications.

16. Von Boehmer, H. , personal communication.

MULTIGENIC I REGION CONTROL OF THE IMMUNE RESPONSES OF MICE TO THE GLØ AND GLT RANDOM TERPOLYMERS

Paul H. Maurer and Carmen F. Merryman

Department of Biochemistry, Jefferson Medical College

1020 Locust Street, Philadelphia, Pa.   19107

Studies in several species have shown that immune responsiveness to random polymers of amino acids is controlled by histocompatibility-linked immune response genes (Ir genes) (McDevitt and Landy 1972). In mice, we have characterized Ir genes controlling responsiveness to the terpolymers, poly(Glu^{58}Lys^{38}Phe^4) (GLØ) (Merryman et al. 1972), poly(Glu^{57}Lys^{38}Tyr^5) (GLT^5) and poly(Glu^{55}Lys^{34}Tyr^{15}) (GLT^{15}) (Merryman and Maurer 1975). The gene(s) controlling the responses to GLØ and GLT^5 were mapped to the IC subregion of H-2 (or to the right of the IB subregion) (Merryman and Maurer 1975). At the time we were aware of some "nonconcordant" negative responses obtained with some recombinant strains which had a responder allele in IC, i.e. IC^d. Here we present: a) the positive responses to GLT and GLØ obtained by F$_1$ (C57BL/6 x A/J) derived from two non-responder parental strains which help explain the "nonconcordant" data, and b) data with H-2 recombinant mice that indicate the presence of another gene to the left of IC, making the GLØ response under the control of at least two genes which map in two different subregions of the I region.

METHODS

Mice. Inbred and congenic strains were obtained from the Jackson Lab., Bar Harbor, Maine. Recombinant strains B10.A(1R), B10.A(3R), B10.A(4R), B10.A(5R), B10.M(11R), B10.M(17R), B10.P(10R), B10.G, B10.S(7R), B10.S(9R) and B10.T(6R) were bred in the laboratory of Dr. Jack H. Stimpfling. F$_1$ hybrids (C57BL/6J x A/J and B10.A(2R) x A/J) were bred in our lab.

Polymers. GLØ^5 (molecular weight 55,000), GLT^5 (molecular

TABLE 1

Immune Response Patterns of Inbred and Congenic Strains of Mice
Immunized with GLØ or GLT[15]

Strain	H-2 Haplotype	Percent Antigen Bound $\pm$ S.E.	
		GLØ	GLT[5]
A/J	a	3 ± 3	6 ± 6
B10.A/SgSn	a	7 ± 2	3 ± 3
C57BL/6J	b	1 ± 2	0 ± 0
C57BL/10Sn	b	5 ± 6	5 ± 4
BALB/cJ	d	82 ± 6	69 ± 4
B10.D2/nSn	d	97 ± 6	53 ± 15
NZB/B1NJ	d	96 ± 6	97 ± 6
A.CA/Sn	f	6 ± 6	0 ± 0
B10.M/Sn	f	4 ± 3	
Wb/ReJ-W	ja	70 ± 3	36 ± 3
B10.BR/SgSn	k	9 ± 7	8 ± 2
CBA/J	k	7 ± 10	0 ± 0
C3H/HeJ	k	9 ± 5	0 ± 0
AKR.M	m	11 ± 5	
B10.AKM	m	0 ± 0	
P/J	p	22 ± 9	12 ± 6
AU/SsJ	q		62 ± 16
BUB/BnJ	q		81 ± 2
B10.G	q	94 ± 9	
C3H.Q	q	94 ± 14	
DBA/1J	q	102 ± 2	33 ± 2
SWR/J	q	67 ± 8	71 ± 11
T138	q	108 ± 2	
SJL/J	s	7 ± 4	2 ± 3

weight 50,000) and GLT[15] (molecular weight 70,000) were polymerized
starting with the N carboxyanhydrides of the α-L amino acids
(Katchalski and Sela 1958). Before use, the polymers were dialyzed
free of salt, lyophilized and dissolved in saline. Concentrations
were determined by micro-Kjeldahl (Markham 1942). GLT[5] or GLT[15]
was radioiodinated by a modification of the chloramine-T procedure
(Hunter 1969) adapted for 1-5 mg quantities of polymer as we have
previously reported (Maurer and Merryman 1974). The specific
activities of the polymers were 1-2 Ci/g.

Immunization. Ten or 100 μg of the polymers were emulsified
in complete Freund's adjuvant and injected into the hind foot pads
of groups of 5-10 mice. Three weeks later, an aqueous injection of
the same polymer concentration was given intraperitoneally. Only
results of secondary responses (day 31) are presented.

Antigen-Binding Assay. Antibody activity against the polymers
was measured using an antigen-binding assay (Herzenberg et al. 1965).
Responses against GLØ were measured with iodinated GLT[5] or GLT[15]
which cross react with mouse anti-GLØ sera. 50 μl of ^{125}I polymer
(3 ng) and 25 μl of a 1:2 dilution of serum were incubated with
500 μl of goat anti-mouse gamma globulin antisera. Following a two-
hour period of incubation at 37° C, samples were centrifuged and
aliquots counted. Binding values of not more than 10% were observed
with the nonimmune normal mouse sera.

RESULTS

The strain distribution immune response pattern against GLØ
was previously characterized as well as the linkage to the H-2 locus
(Merryman et al. 1972). The responses of additional inbred and
congenic strains to GLØ and GLT[5] are presented in Table 1. Positive
responses are associated with the H-2[d,ja,p] and q haplotypes, and
negative responses with H-2[a,b,f,k,m] and s haplotypes.

The responses of the recombinant strains to GLØ and GLT[5] are
presented in Table 2. B10.A(3R) and B10.A(5R) mice are responders.
However, the B10.S(9R) mice repeatedly responded only to GLØ but
not to GLT[5]. B10.A, B10.A(1R), B10.A(2R), B10.A(4R) and B10.M(17R)
mice did not respond at all. F[1] hybrids of the two nonresponder
strains (B10.A(2R) x A) were nonresponders, whereas the F[1] hybrids
of two other nonresponder strains (C57BL/6 x A) were responders to
both polymers.

DISCUSSION AND CONCLUSION

We have postulated that a series of related GL polymers containing 4-15% of a third aromatic amino acid, i.e. GLT[5], GLT[15] and

TABLE 2

Immune Response Patterns of F₁ Hybrids and Recombinant Strains of Mice Immunized with GLØ or GLT⁵

Strain	H-2 Haplotype	Regions of the H-2 Complex						Percent Antigen Bound ± S.E.	
		K	Ir-IA	I Region Ir-IB	Ir-IC	S	D	GLØ	GLT⁵
B10.A/SgSn	a	k	k	k	d*	d	d	2 ± 3	1 ± 2
A.AL	al	k	k	k	k	k	d	0 ± 0	0 ± 0
HTG	g	d	d	d	d	d	b	91 ± 7	80 ± 6
B10.A(1R)	h1	k	k	k	d	d	b	14 ± 4	11 ± 2
B10.A(2R)	h2	k	k	b	d	d	b	2 ± 1	0 ± 0
B10.A(3R)	i3	b	b	b	b	b	d	60 ± 9	69 ± 5
B10.A(4R)	h4	k	k	b	d	d	b	5 ± 2	8 ± 3
B10.A(5R) SgSn	i5	b	b	b	d	d	d	42 ± 18	49 ± 10
AKR.M	m	k	k	k	k	k	q	11 ± 5	
B10.AKM	m	k	k	k	k	k	k	0 ± 0	
C3H.OL	o1	d	d	d	d	d	q	73 ± 17	70 ± 4
C3H.OH	o2	d	d	d	d	d	k	84 ± 17	80 ± 20
B10.S(9R)	t4	s	s	s	d	d	d	36 ± 7	17 ± 2
AQR	y1	q	k	k	q	q	d	5 ± 3	13 ± 2
B10.T(6R)	y2	q	q	q	q	q	d	94 ± 13	
B10.M(17R)	aq1	k	k	q	q	q	f	11 ± 2	13 ± 13
F1(A/J × C57BL/6)	a/b	k/b	k/b	k/b	d/b	d/b	d/b	47 ± 8	49 ± 9
F1(A/J × B10.A(2R))	a/h	k/k	k/k	k/k	d/d	d/d	d/d	10 ± 3	5 ± 3

*Indicates position of crossover event

GLØ may be under the same Ir gene(s) control (Merryman and Maurer 1974). Data in Table 1 show that the response patterns for these polymers, i.e. are generally indistinguishable. However, the level of antibody produced when GLØ is the immunogen may be greater than the levels against GLT[5].

We also mapped the Ir GLØ-GLT gene(s) to the right of IB, i.e. IC subregion (Merryman and Maurer 1975), whereas Dorf et al. (1974) initially mapped the gene to IB. Because of the uniqueness of our first finding of an Ir gene localized to the right of IB, additional recombinant and F1 mice were studied. B10.A(3R), B10.A(5R) and B10.S(9R) recombinant strains responded to GLØ. These results were unexpected since the B10.A(3R) and B10.A(5R) were derived from independent crossovers between two nonresponder haplotypes, H-2^a and H-2^b which had IA^{k}IB^{k}IC^d and IA^{b}IB^{b}IC^b haplotypes, respectively, and resulted in the indicated (Table 2) haplotypes of IA^{b}IB^{b}IC^d. These positive responses indicated the presence of a gene to the right of IB. However, the lack of responses of the recombinant strains B10.A, B10.A(1R), B10.A(2R) and B10.M(17R) with responder haplotypes in IC, i.e. IC^d, and the AQR strains with responder haplotypes in K and IC, was nonconcordant and indicated the possible presence of another gene in the IA or IB interacting with the gene located to the right of IB. That the second gene may not be to the right of IC, i.e. in S, is shown by the good response of C3H.OL mice having IC^d and S^k alleles, and that it is not in K is shown by nonresponsiveness of the AQR mice. We therefore mated several combinations of inbred strains which were nonresponders and had similar I region alleles as the parental strains of the 3R and 5R recombinant mice. The F1 (C57BL/6 x A/J) were responders to GLØ and GLT[5]. Another nonresponder, F1 (A x B10.A(2R)), did not respond.

The explanation offered for these apparent nonconcordant data invokes the concept of at least two gene control of the response as follows: One Ir gene is in IC where the d or q allele behaves as a dominant responder gene (Ir-GLØ$_A$); the other gene is present in IA-IB where the K allele behaves as a recessive nonresponder gene, and the d, g, b and s alleles behave as dominant responder gene(s) (Ir-GLØ$_B$). The interaction between these 2 gene loci results in an immune response, i.e. when the IC haplotype is d (or g) and the IA and/or IB subregions have a 'double dose' of the K allele, k-k, nonresponsiveness is present; however, if b-b, s-s, or k/b is present, responsiveness ensues. The positive results obtained with F1 (C57BL/6 x A/J) indicate gene complementation. Whether the above concept and the assignment of dominant and recessive traits to the indicated haplotypes in the I subregion is more general, is being studied with other F1 and backcross mice. Independently, Dorf et al. (1975) have concluded the need for two H-2 complex Ir genes for the response to GLØ.

One can only speculate about the roles for the two different genes for the response against GLT and GLØ polymers. Whether each gene(s) codes for a different set of determinants in the terpolymer, wherein one set is present on T cells and the other on B cells, as previously speculated for the responses of mice against the glutamic acid-lysine-alanine terpolymers (Maurer and Merryman 1974), is presently under study. However, the problem here is especially puzzling as in repeated experiments in our laboratory, neither GL nor GT copolymers, nor mixtures of both polymers over a wide range of concentrations are immunogenic in inbred strains of mice.

ACKNOWLEDGMENTS

    This study was supported by N.I.H. Research Grant AI07825 and Amer. Cancer Soc. Grant IM-5C. We thank Drs. A. Zeiger for the tyrosylated polymers, D. Ganfield for the iodination, and J. H. Stimpfling for the recombinant mice. The technical assistance of Mrs. J. Jones and Mrs. R. Rayachoti is gratefully acknowledged.

REFERENCES

Dorf, M.E., Lilly, F. and Benacerraf, B. (1974) J. Exp. Med. 140: 859.
Dorf, M.E., Stimpfling, J.H. and Benacerraf, B. (1975) J. Exp. Med. 141: 1459.
Herzenberg, L.A., Warner, N.L. and Herzenberg, L.A. (1965) J. Exp. Med. 121: 415.
Hunter, W.M. (1969) in Handbook of Experimental Immunology, 608, D.M. Weir (ed.), F.A. Davis and Co., Philadelphia, Pa.
Katchalski, E. and Sela, M. (1958) Adv. in Prot. Chem. 13: 243.
Markham, R. (1942) Biochem. J. 36: 790.
Maurer, P.H. and Merryman, C.F. (1974) Immunogenetics 1: 174.
McDevitt, H.O. and Landy, M. (eds.) (1972) Proc. of an Int'l. Conf., Brook Lodge, Augusta, Michigan, Academic Press, New York.
Merryman, C.F., Maurer, P.H. and Bailey, D.W. (1972) J. Immunol. 108: 937.
Merryman, C.F. and Maurer, P.H. (1975) Immunogenetics 1: 549.

OVERCOMING Ir GENE CONTROL OF THE RESPONSE TO THE LYSOZYMES

S.W. Hill[*], R.L. Yowell[*], D.E. Kipp[*], R.J. Scibienski[+],
A. Miller[*] and E.E. Sercarz[*]

[*]Department of Bacteriology, University of California,
 Los Angeles, California 90024 USA
[+]Department of Microbiology, University of California,
 Davis, California 95616 USA

INTRODUCTION

In studying the genetics of immune response capacity, it is
of importance to work in a molecular system in which it might be
possible to obtain knowledge of the exact antigenic determinant(s)
under the genetic influence. It was with this in mind that synthetic, random polypeptides were first used in genetic studies (1),
since it was assumed that these polymers had simpler structure than
the average multideterminant antigen. Recent evidence (e.g.2,3)
clearly suggests that there are multiple unknown specificities in
an antigen such as (T,G,)-A--L, making precise analysis difficult.

A structurally well-characterized, highly immunogenic molecule
such as hen lysozyme seemed to offer an immense advantage, in that
nature has prepared "derivatives", related lysozymes which are altered at a small number of amino acid residues. The observation
that different strains of mice showed disparate reactivity to various lysozymes has allowed detailed analysis of the epitopes
involved in regulation.

Fine Specificity of Genetic Control

In fact, we found during an extensive strain survey that several H-2[b] strains were unresponsive to immunization with HEL in
complete Freund's adjuvant, given intraperitoneally, but were highly
responsive to the structurally related, cross-reactive JEL.
(Table 1).

Table 1. Frequency of C57BL/6 responders to various lysozymes.
Known sequences are indicated by asterisks.

IMMUNOGENIC LYSOZYME		# a.a. Difs.	Ratio of Resp.
JEL*	Japanese quail	6	45/45
REL	Ringed-neck pheasant	~12	10/10
TEL*	Turkey	7	9/10

NON-IMMUNOGENIC LYSOZYME			
HEL*	Hen (chicken)	-	32/307
BEL*	Bob-white quail	4	1/10
NEL*	Guinea-hen	12	0/20
PEL	Peafowl	~4	2/25
HUL*	Human	51	3/11

$H-2^b$ strains such as C57BL/6 and its congenic resistant partner A.BY were highly responsive to JEL and REL and moderately responsive to TEL. However, 90% of the mice were completely unresponsive to a variety of related gallinaceous lysozymes which differed
by as many as 12 amino acid residues. Sera from these mice were
completely negative by the sensitive assay of isoelectric focusing,
and the parathymic lymph nodes, which have been found to contain a
many-fold greater concentration of PFC than the spleen (4), had no
detectable PFC.

What distinguishes the immunogenic lysozymes of known sequence
(JEL and TEL) from the non-immunogenic lysozymes (HEL, BEL and NEL)
are two amino acid changes in the region from residues 99 to 103.
(5). This region is located at the top of the substrate-binding
cleft in the molecule. Apparently, the decision to make a response
to any epitope of lysozyme is a resultant of an encounter between
a very limited area on the molecule and a regulatory receptor.

There are two interesting aspects of the fine specificity
distinctions made by Ir-GEL gene products. On the one hand, there
are the very closely related JEL and HEL which are perceived differently by the immune systems of $H-2^b$ mice. On the other hand,
there is the similar regulatory recognition of the very disparate
human and hen lysozymes. Despite differences in almost half their
amino acid residues, and an almost complete lack of cross-reactivity
at the B-cell level, their immunogenic ranking within our panel of
mouse strains is closely comparable, with the exception of the Balb/c
strain (Figure 1). This evidence speaks for a small area on both
HEL and HUL that is recognized by the same regulatory element on
the T cell. This area must also be different from that on JEL
which narrows the possibilities greatly, but still doesn't permit
a final assignment.

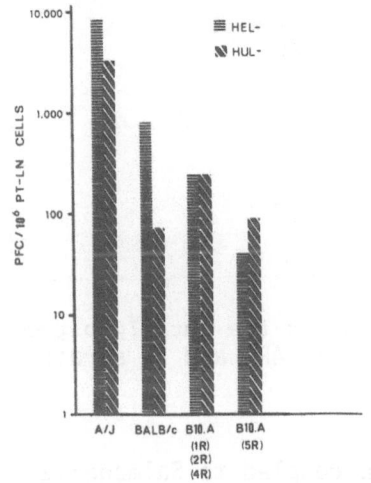

Fig. 1. Comparison of Responsiveness to HEL and HUL in several mouse strains. PT-LN = parathymic lymph nodes. The B10 strain is a nonresponder to both HUL and HEL (not plotted).

Overcoming Ir-GEL Control

By overcoming the I-A-linked genetically controlled unresponsiveness of the $H-2^b$ strains, it could be demonstrated that a full B-cell spectrum of v-regions was present in these animals.

Genetic modulation. The primary genetic control which is expressed as an all-or-none reactivity to a particular lysozyme, maps within I-A (or K) in the H-2 complex. The critical evidence for this comes from the B10.A (4R) recombinant strain (Fig.2). The "k" responder alleles at K and I-A suffice to make the B10.A. (4R) a responder, despite the fact that the "b" nonresponder alleles are present in the rest of the H-2 complex.

B10.A (3R) and B10.A (5R) possess the "b" allele of the nonresponder C57BL/10 haplotype in the I-A region while the H-2 regions from 1-C to D contain the "d" alleles of the responder B10.A haplotype. Yet, unlike the characteristic nonresponder phenotype of the $H-2^b$ C57BL/10 parent, most members of these 2 strains demonstrate a low anti-HEL response. Thus, there are additional H-2 linked loci which can modify the expression of the I-A-linked nonresponder "b" allele, allowing a low response. Supporting the notion that HEL and HUL are subject to the same control, this modulator gene also influences the anti-HUL response (Fig. 1).

Provision of T-cell help. In the responses to JEL, REL and TEL, the antibodies produced were highly cross-reactive with HEL, suggesting that HEL-recognizing B-cells were fully competent to respond, given an immunogen with effective T-cell induction properties. Furthermore, the attachment of HEL itself to immunogenic carriers such as sheep erythrocytes (SRC), allowed stimulation of HEL-specific B cells. This could be observed <u>in vitro</u> (S. Adler, unpublished) or in adoptive transfer studies.

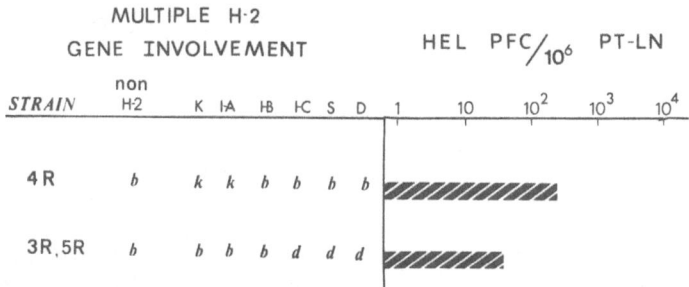

Fig. 2. *Multiple H-2 gene involvement in the anti-lysozyme response.* PT-LN= parathymic lymph node. 3R, 4R, and 5R strains are on a B10 background.

Mitogenic signal. Making use of HEL coupled to <u>Salmonella enteritidis</u> LPS (HEL-LPS) to directly stimulate B cells, both an IgM and an IgG response to HEL-LPS could be induced in C57BL/6 mice. LPS itself, or unconjugated LPS plus HEL could not trigger an anti-HEL response. The specificity of this response was similar to that triggered by HEL-LPS in the responder CBA/J strain mice, and included a significantly large component of anti-HEL plaques which produced antibody directed against epitopes present on the HEL molecule, but absent on the JEL molecule. This indicates that there is no defect in the population of HEL-specific B-cell v-regions in the H-2^b non-responder mice. (Data in Fig. 3)

Repeated exposure to HEL. 10% of any H-2^b strain will make a very weak anti-HEL secondary response following I.P. challenge. Most of the remaining C57BL/6 mice could be driven to produce antibody after repeated injection of soluble HEL. At each boost, a fairly constant percentage of the previously nonresponding mice

Fig. 3. *IgM and IgG response to HEL-LPS in C57BL/6 mice.* (10 µg HEL, 20 µg LPS). IgG plaques are total plaques minus direct plaques.

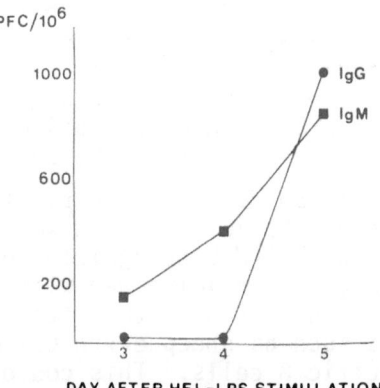

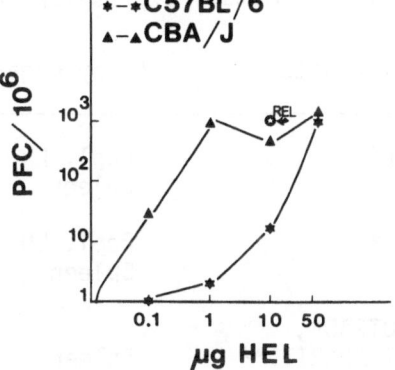

Fig. 4. Anti-HEL dose response.
Antigens given in complete
Freund's adjuvant in the
hind footpads. The response
to REL in C57BL/6 is shown
for 10 µg.

were converted to responsiveness, until after seven injections, only
5% of the initial mice remained persistently unresponsive. In many
cases, the characteristically restricted initial antibody patterns
became increasingly heterogeneous after repeated exposure to HEL,
until they were indistinguishable from serum patterns exhibited by
responder haplotypes. This suggests that the genetic "lesion" in
these animals is one of a regulatory balance rather than lack of
appropriate T-cell or B-cell recognition units. A second possibility is that recognition potential is being gradually acquired
through mutational or other genetic mechanisms.

   Peripheral priming. This second possibility seems unlikely
in the light of recent evidence that a response can be obtained
in H-2^b mice by injection of HEL in complete Freund's adjuvant in
the hind footpads. At a dose of 50 µg of HEL, the peak response
of popliteal lymph nodes from C57BL/6, CBA (Figure 4) and A/J
(data not shown) mice are equivalent. At suboptimal doses, however,
C57BL/6 mice still demonstrate their preference for the lysozymes
that are immunogenic when given I.P., e.g. at the intermediate dose
of 10 µg. The response to ring-necked pheasant lysozyme (REL) is
60 times the response to HEL, indicating no difficulty in antigen-
stimulated cell proliferation in the H-2^b strain.

   The spleens of footpad-injected C57BL/6 mice show no anti-HEL
PFC at any time during the primary popliteal lymph node response,
whereas, responder strains do develop some splenic PFCs following
primary footpad immunization. When footpad-primed C57BL/6 mice are
subsequently boosted I.P. with a dose of soluble HEL, a low level
of splenic anti-HEL PFCs can be demonstrated (Table 2). Apparently,
conditions favorable to successful cell cooperation in the HEL
system exist in the popliteal lymph nodes of H-2^b mice whereas
in the spleens of these animals, conditions for response are less
advantageous. Thus, stimulation of splenic responses occurs in a
majority of the H-2^b animals only after repeated I.P. injection, or

Table 2. Memory Expression in the Spleen in C57BL/6 Mice

Injection site	Assay organ	Time after injection	Anti-HEL PFC/10^6
FOOTPAD*	Popl. LN	2 weeks	966
	Spleen	2 weeks	<1
FOOTPAD*	Popl. LN	4 weeks	57
	Spleen	4 weeks	<1
1°--FOOTPAD*, 2°--INTRAPERIT.**	Spleen	11 weeks 7 days	25

*50 µg HEL in complete Freund's adjuvant; **100 µg soluble HEL.

after memory cells generated at more favorable sites (popliteal lymph nodes) have migrated into the spleen.

CONCLUSIONS

There can be little doubt that a broad potential for reactivity to HEL is present in the H-2^b mouse. Not only are there ample numbers of B-clonotypes present throughout the animal available for triggering, but they also can be induced to make IgM and IgG antibody in the popliteal node through local footpad immunization. Furthermore, memory cells which migrate to the spleen can be stimulated there by soluble antigen to antibody formation.

The balance between regulatory (suppressor) cells and cooperating, helper cells appears to be very different in the many lymphoid compartments of the mouse (6). It is possible that the very dramatic response to HEL in the parathymic lymph nodes compared to the spleen relates to this balance. We have studied carrier-primed T-cell suppression in another system (7) and found that the spleen is richest in cells exhibiting this effect, and it is most pronounced within the first week following immunization.

It is possible that in the spleen, the regulation in H-2^b strains is such as to not generally permit stimulation by HEL to advance beyond its initial suppressive phase. Because of a different mixture of cells in the popliteal lymph node and its access to antigen prior to the spleen, the response can progress to a helper, cooperative phase. In any event, the problem is now being subjected to detailed scrutiny in reconstitution and cell-mixing experiments.

It remains puzzling why evolution would have chosen to preserve this most complex control system in which a single epitope can prevent the entire response to a multideterminant antigen, and yet allow a response elsewhere in the animal. This may be one expression of a mechanism maintaining stern, central self-surveillance while also encouraging defensive surveillance at the outposts of the system, in the local lymph nodes.

REFERENCES

1. McDevitt, H.O. and Sela, M., J. Exp. Med. 122, 517, 1965.

2. Rüde, E., and Günther, E., In "Progress in Immunology, II" edited by L. Brent and J. Holborow, Elsevier, New York, p. 223, 1974.

3. Mozes, E., Schwartz, M., and Sela, M., J. Exp. Med. 140, 349, 1974.

4. Hill, S.W., Submitted for publication

5. Hill, S.W. and Sercarz, E.E., Europ. J. Immunol. 5, 317, 1975.

6. Gershon, R.K., In "Immunological Tolerance" edited by D.H.Katz and B. Benacerraf, Academic Press, New York, p. 413, 1974.

7. Eardley, D.D. and Sercarz, E.E., Submitted for publication.

ACKNOWLEDGMENTS

Supported in part by a grant from the National Institutes of Health (AI-08198), contract NCI-CB-43972, and support for R.L.Y. by a stipend from grant 5T01-AI-00431 in Clinical and Fundamental Immunology. We thank Joel Sercarz for photographic assistance.

GENETIC CONTROL OF THE IMMUNE RESPONSE TO ORDERED PEPTIDES OF TYROSINE AND GLUTAMIC ACID

Michal Schwartz, Edna Mozes and Michael Sela

Department of Chemical Immunology, The Weizmann Institute

of Science, Rehovot, Israel

One of the important problems in understanding the genetic regulation of the immune response potential to random synthetic polypeptides is to establish the major determinant(s) of all possible
amino acid combinations which is responsible for the phenotypic expression of the immune response to the whole immunogen. The random
synthetic immunogen poly(LTyr,LGlu)-poly(DLAla)--poly(LLys) abbreviated (T,G)-A--L is one of the antigens most extensively used in
studies of the genetic control of the immune responses. Therefore,
in order to elucidate the above-stated problem we have prepared
several ordered tetrapeptides composed of tyrosine and glutamic
acid which were attached to multichain poly-DL-alanine (A--L).
Only one of the antigenic determinants, namely Tyr-Tyr-Glu-Glu,
resembled the random peptide (T,G) in the pattern of immune responses elicited against it and in the cross-reactivity of the specific antibodies with (T,G)-A--L. The immune response pattern to
the other ordered tetrapeptides tested was different from that obtained with (T,G)-A--L, and no cross-reactivity was detected between the antibodies provoked with these peptides and (T,G)-A--L (1).
The gene(s) controlling the ability to respond to the random polypeptide (T,G)-A--L was found to be linked to the major histocompatibility (H-2) locus of the mouse (2). Genetic analysis experiments
demonstrated a close linkage between the ability to respond to (Tyr-
Tyr-Glu-Glu)-A--L and the H-2 complex. In contrast, no linkage was
observed between the immune response potential to another ordered
tetrapeptide (Tyr-Glu-Tyr-Glu)-A--L, to which the pattern of response
was different from that observed for (T,G)-A--L, and H-2 as indicated
by the pattern of response of different inbred and congenic mouse
strains and by genetic analysis (3). It is noteworthy that two congenic mouse strains C3H.SW and CWB which possess the H-2^b type and

differ only in their allotypes are high and low responders, respectively, to this immunogen. This observation suggests a possible linkage between the ability to respond to (Tyr-Glu-Tyr-Glu)-A--L and allotypes. Thus, the two ordered tetrapeptides Tyr-Tyr-Glu-Glu and Tyr-Glu-Tyr-Glu are composed of the same amino acids and differ only in their order. Nevertheless, they were found to be under qualitative different genetic controls, indicating the high degree of discrimination of the genes involved in the immune response.

The antibody levels of low responder mice to (T,G)-A--L was shown to be enhanced to that observed in high responders, following immunization with a complex of (T,G)-A--L with methylated bovine serum albumin (MBSA) (4). This could be due to enhancement in antibody levels to any of the possible determinants which exist in the random immunogen. Therefore, it was of interest to immunize low responder mice to (Tyr-Tyr-Glu-Glu)-A--L with the complex of this antigen with MBSA.

A significant enhancement in the antibody titers produced by low responder mice was observed following immunization with the complex. The antibody titers reached the levels of that obtained in high responder mice when immunized with the antigen alone. Since (Tyr-Tyr-Glu-Glu)-A--L possesses a single determinant, the results suggest that, following immunization with the antigen complexed with MBSA, low responder mice to the random (T,G)-A--L produce antibodies with the same specificity as that elicited by the high responders.

The possibility still existed that the antibodies produced by high and low responders to (Tyr-Tyr-Glu-Glu)-A--L differed in their affinity. Therefore, the relative association constants of antibodies elicited by high responders to (Tyr-Tyr-Glu-Glu)-A--L as well as by high and low responders upon immunization with a complex of (Tyr-Tyr-Glu-Glu)-A--L with MBSA were measured. No significant differences were observed between the association constants of the above antibody populations.

It thus appears that upon immunization with a complex of (Tyr-Tyr-Glu-Glu)-A--L and MBSA, low responder mice produce antibodies similar in their level, specificity and affinity to that elicited by high responders to the above immunogen.

REFERENCES

1. Mozes, E., Schwartz, M. and Sela, M. (1974) J. Exp. Med. 140: 349.
2. McDevitt, H.O. and Tayan, M.L. (1968) J. Exp. Med. 128: 1.
3. Schwartz, M., Mozes, E. and Sela, M. Eur. J. Immunol., in press.
4. McDevitt, H.O. (1968) J. Immunol. 100: 485.

Supported in part by a grant 1RO1 AI 11405-03 from the National Institutes of Health, U.S. Public Health Service.

ANTIGEN SPECIFIC T CELL FACTORS IN THE GENETIC CONTROL OF THE

IMMUNE RESPONSE TO POLY(TYR,GLU)-POLY(PRO)--POLY(LYS)

Edna Mozes and Ronit Isac

Department of Chemical Immunology

The Weizmann Institute of Science, Rehovot, Israel

The antibody response of mice to poly(LTyr,LGlu)-poly(LPro)--poly(LLys), abbreviated (T,G)-Pro--L, is specific for the Pro--L region of the immunogen and is genetically controlled. SJL mice are high responders to this immunogen, whereas DBA/1 and SWR mice are low responders. DBA/1 mice do not produce antibodies to Pro--L, but respond well to antigenic determinants attached to this moiety, while SWR mice do not respond to Pro--L or to any determinant attached to this carrier.

The gene(s) controlling antibody response to this immunogen has been designated Ir-3 (1). Genetic analysis of the immune response to (T,G)-Pro--L performed in SJL and DBA/1 mice, their F_1 hybrids as well as in the backcross progeny, showed no linkage between the immune response potential to (T,G)-Pro--L and the major histocompatibility (H-2) locus of the mice (2).

The cellular basis of the immune response to (T,G)-Pro--L has been studied using antigen specific T-cell factors. These factors are able to replace T cells, when transferred together with B cells and (T,G)-Pro--L into irradiated, syngeneic recipients. Cellular analysis of the genetic control of the immune response to another synthetic polypeptide, poly(LTyr,LGlu)-poly(DLAla)--poly(LLys), (T,G)-A--L has been performed also using the specific cooperative T-cell factors (3,4).

T cells of SJL (high responder mice to (T,G)-Pro--L) were compared with T cells of DBA/1 and SWR mice for their ability to produce cooperative factors. In parallel B cells of these strains were tested for their response to the T cell product. It was found that T cells of both SJL high and DBA/1 low responder strains produced active cooperative factors to (T,G)-Pro--L, whereas supernatants of cultures from educated T cells of SWR low responder mice

were not effective. The factors of SJL and DBA/1 origin cooperated efficiently in eliciting antibodies to (T,G)-Pro--L only with B
cells of SJL and SWR mice and hardly at all with marrow cells of
DBA/1 low responders. Thus, the cellular genetic defect is on the
level of the B cell population in DBA/1 mice and on the level of the
T cells in SWR mice. These observations confirmed previous findings
of limiting dilution experiments (5,6).

Studies on the molecular nature of the T-cell factor produced
to (T,G)-A--L to which the response is H-2 linked, suggested that it
is a product of a gene in the I region of the H-2 complex (7). It
was, therefore, of interest to establish the nature of the T cell
factor specific for (T,G)-Pro--L to which the immune response was
found not to be linked to H-2.

Preliminary data obtained with a T-cell factor produced with
(T,G)-Pro--L suggest that this factor is similar in its nature to
the (T,G)-A--L specific factor. Thus, the factor produced by SJL
(high responder to (T,G)-Pro--L) educated T cells was removed by an
antigen-coated column, whereas its activity was not reduced after
transfer through an anti-immunoglobulin immunoadsorbent. This
factor was absorbed by a column coated with an antiserum against
the H-2^S haplotype. These results suggested that the (T,G)-Pro--L
specific factor is a product of the H-2 complex. Further studies
using alloantisera raised against subregions of the H-2 complex
(kindly supplied by Drs. Dorf and Benacerraf, Harvard Medical
School, Boston, Mass.) were performed. It was shown that the
(T,G)-Pro--L specific factor was not removed by an immunoadsorbent
prepared with antisera to the D end of the H-2 complex. However,
it lost its activity when passed on columns coated with antisera to
the K+I subregions of H-2.

The contradiction between results showing that the (T,G)-Pro--L
specific T-cell factor is a product of the H-2 complex and results
of genetic analysis which show no linkage of the response to H-2,
could be explained if the existence of two genes regulating this
immune response is taken into consideration. In this case one of
the genes is linked to H-2 and is involved in the production of the
T-cell factor, and the second gene is not H-2 linked and is expressed in the B cell population.

REFERENCES

1. Mozes, E., McDevitt, H.O., Jaton, J.-C. and Sela, M. (1969) J.
   Exp. Med. 130: 493.
2. Mozes, E., McDevitt, H.O., Jaton, J.-C. and Sela, M. (1969) J.
   Exp. Med. 130: 1263.
3. Taussig, M.J., Mozes, E. and Isac, R. (1974) J. Exp. Med. 140:
   301.
4. Mozes, E., Isac, R. and Taussig, M.J. (1975) J. Exp. Med. 141:
   703.

5. Mozes, E. and Shearer, G.M. (1971) J. Exp. Med. 134: 141.
6. Mozes, E. and Sela, M. (1974) Proc. Nat. Acad. Sci. 71: 1574.
7. Taussig, M.J. and Munro, A.J. (1975) In Immune Recognition. Proceedings of the Ninth Leukocyte Culture Conference. A.S. Rosenthal, ed., Academic Press, New York, in press.

Supported in part by a grant 1RO1 AI 11405-03 from the National Institutes of Health, U.S. Public Health Service.

A MODEL FOR GENETIC CONTROL OF THE IMMUNE RESPONSE

M. J. Taussig

Department of Pathology, University of Cambridge

Cambridge CB2 1QP, ENGLAND

From our work, and that of Benacerraf and colleagues, it seems reasonable to expect that at least two genes linked to the major histocompatibility locus will be found to determine the response levels to each thymus-dependent antigen. Our experiments take these findings further by defining the mode of action of the genes and their products. Thus, one type of Ir gene codes for the antigen-specific T cell regulators of the immune response, and thus, by inference, the T cell antigen recognition system. The second type of gene, by coding for an acceptor for the T cell regulators on lymphocytes, determines the ultimate response of the cell to antigen (Fig. 1).

We must now consider how the two genes would incorporate the antigen-specificity which is the remarkable feature of the genetic control of the immune response. In the case of T cell defects in response an obvious possibility is that failure to respond to an antigen is due to the absence of the specific binding site for that antigen from the repertoire of T cell antigen receptors. The presence of Ir genes expressed in the B cell, however, requires a more complex explanation for the apparent antigen specificity of Ir gene control. A model to account for the findings is as follows:

1. We propose that there must be several "classes" of T cell factor, analogous in a sense to the classes of immunoglobulin and that for each factor class there exists a corresponding acceptor. The genes for a T cell factor class and the corresponding acceptor for that class comprise a "set." Note that the T factor is assumed to be clonally expressed,

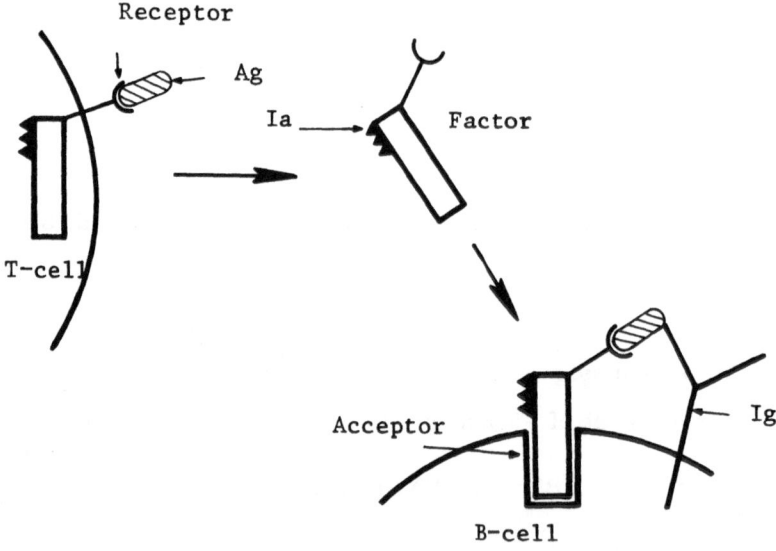

Fig. 1.   A model for T cell—B cell interaction

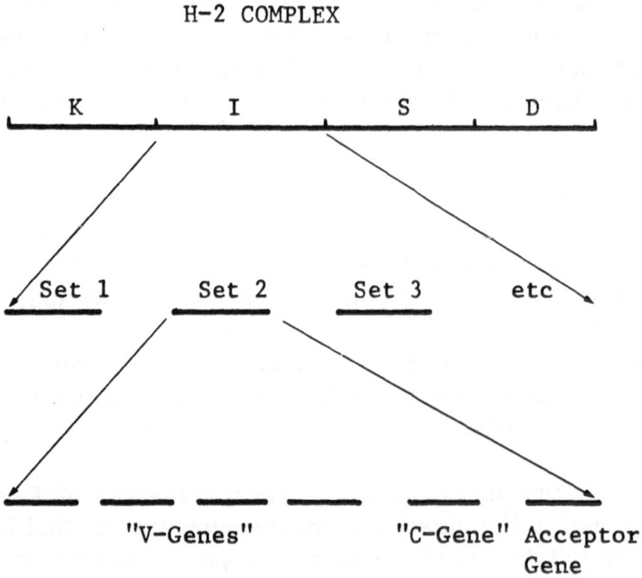

H-2 COMPLEX

Fig. 2   Immune response genes of the H-2 complex.   Schematic representation of the possible arrangement of genes in the I region of H-2

while each B cell would carry all classes of acceptor site.

2. Within each set there would be genes which contribute to the antigen-binding sites carried by that class of factor. Taking again the analogy with immunoglobulin genes, each set would contain a number of "variable" (V) genes which could become associated with the "constant" (C) gene for the T factor of that set (Fig. 2).

3. An important point is that the V genes of any one set will only code for part of the total binding site repertoire of T cell factors. In this way, there will be antigens which will only react with the binding sites of one set, although there will be other antigens for which several sets are available.

4. The loss of a B cell acceptor for one class of T factor will render the B cell incapable of response to factor of that class, and thus to any antigen which is dependent solely on that set for cell cooperation. This would predict that all antigens which are restricted to that defective set would fail to give responses.

5. Two types of T cell defect are possible, namely (a) a defect in a specific antigen-binding site, as already mentioned, and (b) a defect in the constant region of the T cell factor, leading to the effective inactivation of the entire set.

6. A consequence of the model is that "Ir-gene" control will only be noticeable for antigens which are restricted to the binding sites of one set. This explains the well-known observation that genetic control is in general only observed for antigens where a limited number of determinants are presented to the system, e. g., synthetic polypeptides, proteins in limiting dose, alloantigens, etc.

7. The different patterns of response which antigens show in different strains arise in part because of the different genetic causes of low responsiveness. Furthermore, there is the possibility of genetic rearrangements, so that the genes comprising each set can vary between strains.

Regulation of Immune Responses:
Suppressor Cells, their Nature and Function.
Enhancing Factors

THE ROLE OF SUPPRESSION IN IMMUNOREGULATION

Richard K. Gershon

Yale University, School of Medicine

310 Cedar Street, New Haven, Connecticut 06510

INTRODUCTION

The classical notion of tolerance as a deletion of antigen reactive clones has recently come under a two-pronged attack. It has been suggested that at least some forms of tolerance (if there is more than one form) are due to active suppression of potentially reactive clones by antigen antibody complexes and/or suppressor T cells. At this moment the latter mechanism of suppression seems to be in ascendency in immunological thought. This is mirrored in the papers being presented at this conference, as well as in its organizational hierarchy; a suppressor T cell maven is the chairman of the session on suppression while the originator of the antigen antibody complex notion has been relegated to co-chairman status. However, front runners have been known to fade and if one thing is clear about the subject, it is that the final answer is not yet in. Hopefully, at the conclusion of the conference we will be closer to it than we are at the moment of this writing.

What has caused immunologists to re-evaluate their thinking about the basis for the specific lack of immunological reactivity due to prior exposure to antigen (i.e.: tolerance) has been the multiple demonstrations in recent years of cells or serum factors which are present in operationally tolerant animals and which specifically suppress the immune response of normal cells (reviewed in 1-5). While not all seekers have found these suppressors, the large number of ones that have and the diversity of the situations in which they have been found, make it seem at least plausable that suppression is the main mechanism of tolerance maintenance, if not the actual causative agent.

PROBLEMS IN INTERPRETATION

In most cases in which the cellular basis for the suppression has been examined it has been found to be T dependent. T dependence has most commonly been shown indirectly by removal of suppression and T cells concomitantly. Direct suppression by isolated T cells has also been shown and several workers have actually demonstrated that T derived factors are suppressive. Although these results make it seem likely that the T cells can produce suppressive factors it is hard to categorically rule out the possibility that the T cells are turning on B cells to make a highly suppressive form of antibody. Thus, if the assay for an immune response is antibody production there is no way, within the limits of our present technology, to rule out a T to B to B mechanism of suppression.

However, since there are immune responses which do not require the presence of B cells there are ways of demonstrating a pure T to T form of suppression. At present this has not been achieved although some approaches have been made which indicate that it is likely to be successful. What is required is for isolated T cells to be put together with antigen, either in B deprived mice or tissue culture, and to then retrieve the T cells and show that they can suppress an immunological response of other T cells, again either in B deprived mice or tissue culture. We have approached this problem by mixing various T cell populations together in lethally irradiated mice, stimulating them with antigen and measuring their DNA synthetic response. Using this technique we have been able to demonstrate suppressive interactions between the T cells in several situations (6-9). Whereas these experiments demonstrate the feasibility of showing a T to T type of suppression there are some problems with their interpretation. One is the question of how good were the methods used for eliminating B cells? They surely were good enough to prevent any detectable antibody formation. Diehards may insist that this is still not adequate, but the technicological limitations we face in achieving purity of cell populations reduce the argument to a immunological solipsism and at present only semi-religious answers can be found.

A more serious objection to these types of studies is that neither of the two cell populations that were mixed together were from tolerant animals. It therefore still remains important to demonstrate that isolated T cells from tolerant animals can effect specific suppression directly and in the absence of B cells so that a T to B to T mechanism can be ruled out. One should mention parenthetically because of the numerous demonstrations of suppressor activity effected by macrophages, (reviewed in 1 and 2) that one must always keep in mind the possibility that one is looking at a T to M to B or T type of suppression. However, if the suppression turns out to be specific, one can fairly reasonably

assign a secondary role at best to the macrophage as it is fairly
certain that antigen specific recognition is not an inherent property of macrophages.

A potentially excellent way for demonstrating a purer T type
of suppression is to look at the situation in mice suppressed with
anti-gamma M antibody from birth. Such mice are severely hypo-
gammaglobulinemic and have few if any immunoglobulin positive cells
in their lymphoid tissues. Using such mice in experiments we performed together with Max Cooper and Sandy Lawton, (unpublished
observations) we found that excess antigen severely inhibited the
delayed type hypersensitivity (DTH) response to sheep RBC. The
suppressed DTH response could be markedly augmented by pretreating
the mice with cyclophosphamide, suggesting that the poor response
in the mice given the excess antigen was due to some form of suppression. The cyclophosphamide treated mice (and untreated as well)
remained markedly agammaglobulinemic, deficient in circulating immunoglobulin positive cells and made no antibody to the sheep cells.
These results are quite preliminary and specificity controls as
well as adoptive transfers must be done before the suggested interpretation can be put on a firm basis.

Even after the appropriate experiments are done and a T to T
suppression is put on a firm basis it still will require a slight
to moderate leap in faith to think that the T dependent B cell suppression is similarly mediated. However, those that think that
"Occams razor" should be applied to immunology will feel that it
would be up to non-believers to prove an alternate mechanism and
only at that time will I personally feel that one can uncategori-
cally say that a T cell makes an immunosuppressive substance which
plays a significant role in the induction and/or maintenance of
immunological tolerance. Having said this I can add that at this
stage I would happily give better than ten to one odds that this
point will be firmly established within the next year or two.

SUPPRESSOR B CELLS

Several of the papers in this session deal with suppressor B
cells. Surely we all know that the B cell product antibody can be
highly immunosuppressive and our co-chairman has made a strong case
that antibody plays a significant role in the suppression seen in
immunological tolerance (10). However it would seem that some
forms of B cell suppression lack specificity and at the present
time I know of no demonstrated way by which antibody can be non-
specifically suppressive, at least directly. In this regard,
I have several speculative thoughts to offer. We have found that
there are subpopulations of mouse B cells which can be rendered directly tolerant by antigen without the need for participation of T
cells in any detectable form (1,2,11) and several other workers
have found that all the B cells of nude mice can be rendered tol-

erant directly by antigen (12,13). There is as far as I know no
evidence that this form of tolerance induction involves cell interactions. There are several discordant bits of information however
which should at least alert us to this possibility. One is the
recent finding of Cohen, Mosier and Scher in CBA/N mice, which have
a sex-linked recessive defect that prevents male F_1 mice from making
any type of thymus independent antibody response although their
thymus dependent response is fairly normal (14). Interestingly,
these male F_1 mice cannot be rendered tolerant to DNP with DNP-
conjugates which are supposed to be direct B cell tolerogens (15).
F_1 female littermates, which do not have a defect in their ability
to make responses to thymus independent antigens, are rendered
tolerant quite easily (even when tested with DNP on a thymus dependent carrier). A possible explanation for this type of result
is that appropriately stimulated thymus independent B cells shut
off thymus dependent B cells and thus mice which lack thymus independent B cells (male F_1) do not become tolerant. Cohen et al
have looked for suppressive interactions and have not been able to
find any. However, I think that they agree that further studies
are required before this possibility can be ruled out.

Carl Grumet and I (unpublished observations) have found that
C3H mice which make no thymus dependent response to the antigen
TGAL but which make a normal thymus independent response to that
antigen have cells in their spleens which can suppress the thymus
independent response of other C3H mice to TGAL. The suppressor
cells in this instance are generated in mice that have undergone
thymectomy, lethal irradiation and bone marrow grafting and act on
similarly treated mice, suggesting a total thymus independence of
the suppressive event. Therefore a B to B type of suppression
probably can exist. The mechanism is probably effected through IgM
antibody.

We have described another interesting form of B cell suppression; in this instance it seems to be a B to T to T type of suppression (16). We noted that sheep RBC immune B cells could cooperate quite nicely with immune T cells in Mishell-Dutton cultures.
However when normal T cells were added to the cultures, the response
was markedly suppressed. Non-immune B cells and immune T cells
could also cooperate quite nicely, in fact better than did immune
B cells and immune T cells. In this instance however, the addition
of normal T cells to the culture was not suppressive. These results suggest that immune B cells have a way of signaling normal T
cells to act as suppressors. They also suggest that immune T cells
are qualitatively different than normal T cells in the sense that
they are not equally influenced by the signals they receive from
the immune B cells. Again it would seem most likely that the product the immune B cell makes which signals the normal T cell is
antibody, although we were able to demonstrate this type of suppres-

sion in cases where precious little antibody, if any, could be detected. These types of results should alert us to the fact that
B cells and their products are intimately involved in some of the
feedback loops which result in suppression and must always be kept
in mind when analyzing experiments dealing with suppressor effects.

SUPPRESSION BY T CELL SUBSETS

Some of the papers being presented here will deal with the
effect of adult thymectomy on the activity of suppressor T cells.
These, as well as others (see 1-5) have suggested that the "suppressor T cell" may be a short - lived cell which depends on an
intact thymus to function properly. If this turns out to be true,
it would seem to me that one could dismiss the "suppressor T cell"
as an important factor in most forms of tolerance; this because
adult thymectomy has very little gross effect on most forms of
immunoregulation or on the ability to induce tolerance. However,
since we have shown the importance of interactions between cells
in the generation of suppressor activity, as in the examples given
above and in numerous others, (reviewed in 1,2,9 and 17) I am dis-
inclined to dismiss the importance of the suppressor T cell on the
basis of these results. I think it more likely that short - lived
T cells play a role in the interactions which lead to suppression
but are not themselves the suppressors, nor is their presence obligatory for suppression to occur. This point however is far from
firm at the present moment.

HORMONES AND SUPPRESSION

Two other interesting points will be considered in the papers
being presented here. One deals with the effects of hormones and
also peripherally with the well known reciprocal relationship between delayed hypersensitivity and antibody formation. We have
shown that this reciprocity is not necessarily causatively related
i.e.: that it is not the antibody production per se which suppresses the delayed hypersensitivity in all instances (18).

The role of hormones in regulating the immune response is a
very important underinvestigated area of immunology. It is clear
that lymphocytes have receptors for epinepherine (19) histamine (20)
and cortisone (21) and that these substances can affect the behavior of the lymphocytes. The histamine effect is one that is particularly interesting as it has been shown that depletion of cells
which stick to histamine columns leads to a significant augmentation
of the immune response of the remaining cells, suggesting that
"suppressor T cells" may have histamine receptors on them (22).
We (S. Fuchs and C. Metzler) have been able to identify a subpopulation of T cells which have histamine receptors and which synthesize cyclic AMP in response to histamine (unpublished observations).
In addition, we (A. Schwartz) have shown that intraperitoneal in-

jection of histamine into a mouse is a highly immunosuppressive
event. It should be remembered that histamine has very little effects on vascular pemeability in mice as these animals lack receptors for histamine on their blood vessels (23). It seems most
likely that histamine is acting directly on the lymphocytes which
do have H2 receptors in the mouse. The importance of the effect
of sex hormones, which will be discussed, is emphasized by the fact
that most autoimmune diseases have a predilection for affecting
females. Perhaps the paper by Fabris and Piantanelli will shed
some light on the mechanisms behind this.

Lastly, there will be a paper on the T cell dependence of
antibody heterogeneity. The connection between this observation
and suppression is tenuous at best but it is atribute to the wide
spread recognition suppression is attaining that the authors should
have considered it at all. Previous demonstrations of similar
findings, even though made by workers intimately involved in the
suppression field, have never had suppression invoked as a causative mechanism (24-26).

ACKNOWLEDGEMENTS
My research was supported by U.S.P.H.S. CA-08593 and AI-10497
and a contract, CB-43994, from the National Cancer Institute.

I am deeply indebted to my colleagues, students and technical
assistants who participated in the studies reported.

REFERENCES

1. Gershon, R.K. Contemporary Topics in Immunobiology, M. Cooper &
   N. Warner, eds., 3:1, Plenum Press, New York, 1974.
2. Gershon, R.K. Proceedings of 7th Miami Winter Symposium (in
   press).
3. Katz, D.H. and Benacerraf B. eds. Immunological Tolerance:
   Mechanisms and Potential Therapeutic Applications. Academic
   Press, N.Y., 1974.
4. Singhal, S.K. and Sinclair, N.R., eds. Suppressor cells in
   immunity. The University of Western Ontario Press, London,
   Ontario, (in press).
5. Möller, G. ed. Transpl. Rev. 26: (in press).
6. Gershon, R.K., Cohen, P., Hencin, R. and Liebhaber, S.A. J.
   Immunol. 108:586, 1972.
7. Gershon, R.K., Lance, E.M. and Kondo, K. J. Immunol. 112:546,
   1974.
8. Gershon, R.K., Liebhaber, S. and Ryu, S. Immunology 26:909,
   1974.
9. Gershon, R.K. The Immune System: genes, receptors, signals,
   E. Sercarz, A. Williamson and C. F. Fox, eds., p. 471,
   Academic Press, New York, 1974.

10. Voisin, G.A., Progr. Allergy 15:328, 1971.
11. Gershon, R.K. and Kondo, K. Immunology 18:723, 1970.
12. Mitchell, G.F. Immunological Tolerance: Mechanisms and Potential Therapeutic Applications, D.H. Katz and B. Benacerraf, eds., p. 283, Academic Press, New York, 1974.
13. Schrader, J.W. J. Exp. Med. 141:962, 1975.
14. Scher, I., Ahmed, A., Strong, D.M., Steinberg, A.D. and Paul, W.E. J. Exp. Med. 141:788, 1975.
15. Cohen, P.L., Mosier, D.E. and Scher, I. Science, (in press).
16. Gershon, R.K., Orbach-Arbouys, S. and Calkins, C. Progress in Immunology II, L. Brent and J. Holborow, eds., Vol. 2, p. 123, North Holland Publishing Co., Amsterdam, 1974.
17. Gershon, R.K. Immunological Tolerance: Mechanisms and Potential Therapeutic Applications. D.H. Katz and B. Benacerraf, eds., p. 413, Academic Press, New York, 1974.
18. Askenase, P.W., Hayden, B.J. and Gershon, R.K. J. Exp. Med. 141:697, 1975.
19. Bach, M.A. J. Clin. Investigation 55:1074, 1975.
20. Bourne, H.R., Melmon, K.L. and Lichtenstein, L.M. Science 173:743, 1971.
21. Dougherty, T.F. Physiol. Rev. 32:379, 1952.
22. Shearer, G.M., Melmon, K.L., Weinstein, Y., and Sela, M., J. Exp. Med. 136:1302, 1972.
23. Gershon, M.D., and Ross, L.L. J. Exp. Med. 115:367, 1962.
24. Gershon, R.K. and Paul, W.E. J. Immunol. 106:872, 1971.
25. Gershon, R.K. and Kondo, K. Immunology, 23:321, 1972.
26. Gershon, R.K. and Kondo, K. Immunology, 23:335, 1972.

IMMUNOSUPPRESSION BY FETAL LIVER AS A MODEL FOR TOLERANCE TO SELF

Tehila Umiel

Department of Cell Biology

The Weizmann Institute of Science, Rehovot, Israel

The nature of self tolerance is a complex phenomenon which as yet is poorly understood. Two major hypotheses have been formulated to explain the establishment of natural tolerance. The original hypothesis suggests that natural tolerance is acquired by elimination of specifically reactive cells (1). The alternative hypothesis suggests a mechanism whereby immunocompetent cells with potential to react against "self" exists, but are prevented from reactivity by inhibitory systems (2-7).

The embryonic liver chimera system in which lethally irradiated mice are reconstituted with allogeneic liver cells (8) may serve for studying the nature of tolerance. A permanent state of tolerance is induced in the embryonic liver cells and thus this model can be used for understanding the ontogenic development of tolerance to self antigens in the embryo.

Materials & Methods

Mice: Adult C57BL/6, C3H/eb and (C3H/eb x C57BL/6)F_1 hybrids and fetal C57BL, (C3H/eb x C57BL/6)F_1 or (C3H/eb x Balb/c)F_1 hybrids were used throughout these experiments.

Thymectomy and irradiation: Thymectomy was performed on 6-8 week old (C3H/eb x C57BL/6)F_1 mice under nembutal anesthesia and thymuses were removed by suction. Mice were exposed to 850 R and 450 R total body irradiation from a ^{60}Co source (Gamma beam 150A, Atomic Energy of Canada) 60R/min, focal skin distance 34 inches.

Preparation of liver cells: Liver cells from embryos were dissected in phosphate buffered saline supplemented with 10% Fetal calf serum

(Difco Laboratories, Detroit, Mich.) cell suspensions were prepared by gentle pipetation of the cells with a 5 ml pipete, the cells were filtered through a fine stainless steel mesh. Cells were washed 3 times and nucleated cells were counted. A dose of $3-5 \times 10^7$ liver cells was injected into irradiated mice 1-3 h after exposure.

Mixed lymphocyte culture (MLC): Responder cells were mixed with mitomycin-C treated (C3H/eb x C57BL/6)F_1 spleen cells 10^6 of each. Incorporation of ^{3}H thymidine was measured, according to the procedure described in detail elsewhere (9).

Experimental & Discussion

Allogeneic fetal liver cells can reconstitute lethally irradiated mice without development of secondary disease, thus a permanent state of tolerance was assumed to be established in these chimeras. The assumption was that if liver cells develop a state of tolerance because they lack reactive cells then subsequent inoculation of immunocompetent cells syngeneic with liver donors will induce a response against the host. On the other hand, if tolerance of liver cells in the host is due to suppressive mechanisms which prevent reactivity of liver cells, then inoculation of immunocompetent cells syngeneic with the liver will also be suppressed and no activity against host antigens will be manifested.

An experiment was designed to distinguish between these two possibilities. (C3H/eb x C57BL/6)F_1 mice were irradiated with 850 R and reconstituted with either syngeneic or C57BL fetal liver cells. Two months later, mice were irradiated with 450 R and challenged with 10^7 adult spleen cells either syngeneic or allogeneic with the donor liver cells. The rate of mortality was recorded as an indication of lethal graft versus host diseased produced by donor cells (10). It was found (table 1) that mice which received C57BL liver cells followed by a challenge of C57BL spleen cells showed no signs of GVH reaction. (Only 20% mortality was detected in this group after 100 days.) In contrast mice injected with spleen cells allo-

TABLE 1. Percent of mortality in (C3H/eb x C57BL/6)F_1 liver radiation chimeras following challenge with spleen cells

origin of liver cell inoculum	origin of spleen cells	No. mice	% mortality at days:				
			20	40	60	80	100
(C3H/ebxC57BL/6)F_1	C3H/eb	70	0	10	100		
(C3H/ebxC57BL/6)F_1	C57BL	70	0	10	100		
C57BL/6	C3H/eb	70	0	20	100		
C57BL/6	C57BL	70	0	10	20	20	20

TABLE 2. Effect of embryonic liver cells on lymphocyte response to mitomycin-C treated (C3H/eb x C57BL/6)F_1 spleen cells measured by incorporation of ^{3}H-thymidine

Liver cell source[1]	Age	Cell mixture[2]	cpm $\pm$ SE[3]	S.I.[4]
-	-	ab/abm	4518 $\pm$ 171	8.3
-	-	a/abm	37562 $\pm$ 3419	
a	15	ab/abm	6619 $\pm$ 1317	3.16
a	15	a/abm	20981 $\pm$ 609	
a	17	ab/abm	6293 $\pm$ 683	2.2
a	17	a/abm	13871 $\pm$ 252	
-	-	ab/abm	5630 $\pm$ 223	6.4
-	-	a/abm	36371 $\pm$ 2559	
b	15	ab/abm	12905 $\pm$ 334	1.4
b	15	a/abm	18538 $\pm$ 1072	
b	17	ab/abm	16144 $\pm$ 464	1.57
b	17	a/abm	25452 $\pm$ 1023	
bc	17	ab/abm	12860 $\pm$ 93	1.98
bc	17	a/abm	25543 $\pm$ 397	
bc	19	ab/abm	16570 $\pm$ 372	1.64
bc	19	a/abm	27222 $\pm$ 230	

1) 10^6 liver cells were added to the MLC of 10^6 responder and 10^6 stimulator spleen cells.
2) a: C57BL; b: C3H; ab: C3H/eb x C57BL; bc: (C3H/eb x Balb/c)F_1 m: mitomycin-C treated.
3) SE: standard error
4) S.I.: stimulation index = $\dfrac{\text{cpm experimental}}{\text{cpm syngeneic control}}$

geneic to donor liver cells died within 60 days after inoculation of immunocompetent cells.

The present data suggest that suppressor cells may differentiate within the liver cells which subsequently can specifically interfere with the reactivity of syngeneic immune reactive cells. Consequently, we decided to test whether differentiation of suppressor cells within the liver is experimentally induced by exposure to the host environment or whether liver cells contain a priori suppressor cells which may interfere with immune responses of competent cells. We tested whether embryonic liver cells can interfere with mixed lymphocyte reaction (MLC) of syngeneic responder spleen cells against allogeneic target cells. A remarkable reduction in MLC was found in cultures containing liver cells as compared

TABLE 3. Mortality rate of C57BL liver chimeras (C3H/eb x C57BL/6)F[1] intact or thymectomized mice following challenge with parental C57BL[1] spleen cells

# of mice	Treatment	% Mortality at days:				
		20	40	60	80	100
20	-	0	0	0	0	0
20	thymectomy	0	28	30	74	80

to control cultures (Table 2), this effect was noticed with embryonic cells at different stages of the gestation period. Liver cells interfered with the reactivity of cells possessing syngeneic or allogeneic antigens to embryonic liver cells. Thus it can be concluded that embryonic liver cells contain suppressor cells able to interfere with reactivity of competent cells. It seems that at this stage of development suppression is not specific to self nor is directed preferentially to any particular antigen. Similar results of liver suppressive activity have been recently reported using the cell mediated lysis assay (11). It thus appears that tolerance in the liver chimera system is maintained by embryonic liver suppressor cells. However, a period of "education" of these cells within the irradiated host is required for the development of specific discrimination between self and nonself.

In an attempt to find out how specificity in this system is acquired, intact and thymectomized mice were irradiated and reconstituted with allogeneic liver cells and then challenged with competent spleen cells syngeneic to the donor liver cells. It was found (Table 3) that while intact mice did not develop a GVH mortality, 80% of thymectomized mice died within 100 days after the challenge. These results suggest that the thymus plays a role in the differentiation of "naive" suppressor cells into suppressors which can specifically discriminate self from nonself (12).

Summary

The embryonic liver chimera system was used as a model to study the development of tolerance to self antigens. It was found that the permanent tolerant state which was induced in (C3H/eb x C57BL/6)F[1] irradiated hosts following reconstitution with parental C57BL liver cells could be due to the development of suppressor cells within the liver cell inoculum, which specifically prevent reactivity of immunocompetent cells. General suppressor activity could be found in embryonic liver cells at early stages of gestation. However, the differentiation of such cells into specific suppressor of "self" antigens is dependent on the presence of the thymus.

Acknowledgment. - These studies were supported by the National Institute of Health, Contract number NO1-CB-23890.

References

1. Burnet, M. 1959. 'The clonal selection theory of acquired immunity'. Vanderbilt University Press, Nashville, Tennessee
2. Hildemann, W.H. and Walford, R.L. 1966. Proc. Soc. Exp. Biol. Med. 123: 417.
3. Micklem, H.S. and Asfi, C. 1970. Advan. Exp. Med. Biol. 12: 57.
4. Cohen, I.R., Globerson, A. and Feldman, M. 1971. J. Exp. Med. 133: 834.
5. Wekerle, H., Cohen, I.R. and Feldman, M. 1973. Nature New Biol. 241: 25.
6. Wegman, T.G., Hellström, I., Hellström, K.E. 1971. Proc. Nat. Acad. Sci. 68: 1644.
7. Hellström, I., Hellström, K.E. and Allison, A.C. 1971. Nature 230: 49.
8. Uphoff, P.E. 1959. J. Nat. Cancer Inst. 20: 625.
9. Umiel, T. and Trainin, N. 1974. Eur. J. Immunol. 5: 85.
10. Trentin, J.J. 1956. Proc. Soc. Exp. Biol. Med. 92: 688.
11. Globerson, A., Zinkernagel, R.M. and Umiel, T. Submitted.
12. Umiel, T. 1975. Transplantation, June.

SUPPRESSOR CELLS IN THE EMBRYONIC THYMUS MEDIATE ALLOGRAFT TOLERANCE

Wulf Droege and Margaretha Tuneskog

Basel Institute for Immunology

Grenzacherstrasse 487, CH-4058 Basel, Switzerland

ABSTRACT. Thymus cells from non-immunized young chickens suppress the allograft rejection in lightly irradiated syngeneic or allogeneic recipients and mediate longlasting skingraft survival in a significant proportion of recipients across a strong histocompatibility difference. Suppressive activity of this kind is already found in the embryonic thymus and is therefore believed to mediate also self tolerance and neonatal allograft tolerance.

INTRODUCTION AND DESCRIPTION OF THE EXPERIMENTAL SYSTEM

Thymic suppressor cells from unprimed donors have been found to suppress the antibody formation in chickens (1,2). More recently, they were also found to significantly prolong the allograft rejection time of syngeneic recipients and to mediate long lasting skingraft survival (>200 days) across strong histocompatibility differences in a significant proportion of recipients (3,4).

The experimental system has essentially been described previously (4). Chickens of the WC line with the major histocompatibility alleles B2/B2 received an irradiation of 360R at 16 days of age, a transfer of syngeneic or allogeneic thymus cells from unprimed donors 2 days later, and allogeneic skin grafts one day after the transfer (Fig. 1). The skin graft donors (FS line) carried the major histocompatibility alleles B15/B21. Control animals that did not receive suppressive thymus cell preparation rejected usually the allograft with acute necrosis within 15 days.

The experimental groups that received thymus cells from syngene-

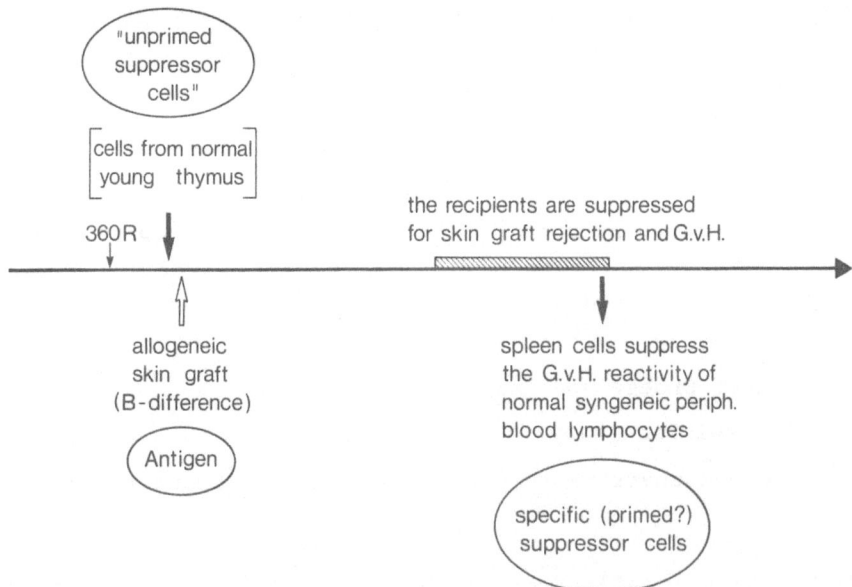

Fig. 1; Schematic illustration of the experimental system

ic or allogeneic young donors showed a significant increase in the
mean rejection time (harmonic means) (see Table 1), and contained a
significant proportion of animals with long surviving (>200 days)
healthy grafts (4). The healthy grafts grew feathers and contained
still antigenically intact donor tissue five months after grafting
as shown by regrafting on normal WC and FS recipients (4). The
animals with intact grafts showed a state of specific suppression:
a third party graft, when grafted 3 weeks after the first graft, was
always rejected with acute necrosis, while a second FS graft usually
did not develop necrosis and was retained significantly longer than
the third party graft, and also much longer than FS grafts on non-
suppressed control animals (4).

   Spleen cells from some of the suppressed animals also showed a
specifically decreased G.v.H. reactivity against FS embryos. Spleen
cells with suppressed G.v.H. reactivity were also able to inhibit the
G.v.H. reactivity of normal WC blood lymphocytes in FS embryos without affecting the reactivity of the normal WC-cells in third party
embryos (manuscript in preparation). It is believed, but not yet
proven, that the specific suppressor cells in the spleen were derived from the unprimed thymic suppressor cells after antigenic stimulus while the non-stimulated suppressor cells are believed to die
in the recipient. The specific suppressor cells are apparently analogous to the suppressor cells described in 1971 by Gershon (5). They
were found in high dose tolerance (6) and low dose tolerance (7). The

Table 1; The Suppressive Effect of 2×10^8 Syngeneic or Allogeneic Thymus Cells on the Skin Graft Rejection (FS Grafts on WC Recipients)

Thymus cells donors		Rejection Completed		Graft Survival beyond 100d
		days	P	%
No cells		15.4		3
9d	WC	23.3	(<.05)	33
18d	WC	24.6	(<.005)	27
9d	Ra	20.8	(<.12)	25
14d	Ra	22.1	(<.02)	25
9d	FS	28.4	(<.01)	50
14d	FS	26.0	(<.02)	50

unprimed suppressor cells were first described in 1971 by Droege (1). They are probably analogous to the suppressor cells that are found in the young mouse thymus (8). The present report deals mainly with the nature and identity of the "unprimed" thymic suppressor cell.

The choice of the chicken for the present experiments was based on two major advantages: 1) prenatal and early postnatal chickens yield relatively more thymus cells than newborn mice or mouse embryos, and 2) the early postnatal chicken contains one relatively well defined thymocyte subpopulation (9,10) and no G.v.H. reactivity (unpublished observation), while the early postnatal mouse contains already G. v.H. reactivity and a heterogenous mixture of subpopulations (11).

SYNGENEIC AND ALLOGENEIC THYMUS CELLS ARE SUPPRESSIVE

The response of WC-chickens against FS skingrafts is significantly suppressed by thymus cells from WC donors as well as allogeneic thymus cells from third party donors (random bred white leghorn) or from the skingraft donors (Table 1). Cells from third party donors were as effective as syngeneic thymus cells, while thymus cells from the skingraft donor strain produced by far the best suppressive effects. Thymus cells syngeneic to the skingrafts cannot necessarily be considered unprimed; but the following experiments will show that the suppressor cells from FS donors are by several criteria similar to the suppressor cells from WC donors, and represent probably the same cellular subpopulation.

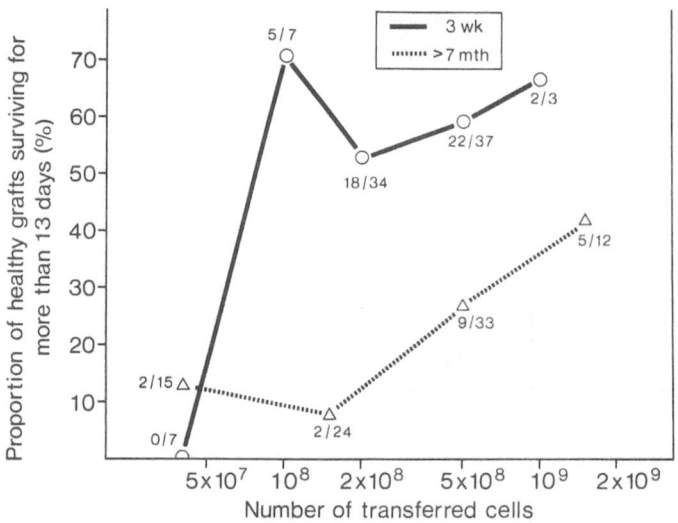

Fig. 2: Effect of thymus cells from adult and from 3 week old donors
on the skin graft survival

Table 2: Effect of 2-5 x 10^8 FS-thymus Cells from Donors of Different Ages (pooled results)

	Age of the Donor	Proportion of Healthy Grafts Surviving for more than 13 days
I	No cells	7/186 4%
II	19d Embryo	10/18 56%
III	9d	7/13 54%
IV	3wk	40/71 56%
V	6-11wk	18/41 44%
VI	>7mth (Adult)	11/57 19%

P <.001 for group VI different from group IV (χ^2 Test)

Table 3: Cell types and Reactivities in the Chicken Thymus

Age	Cell Types	Reactivities
0-2 wks	I	poor GvH, Suppr.
8-16 wks	I,II,III	GvH, Suppr.
8 mths	III	GvH, poor Suppr.

THE IDENTITY OF THE SUPPRESSOR CELL

Bursal cells, spleen cells, peripheral blood lymphocytes and ery-throcytes were not suppressive in this experimental system, irrespect-ive of whether obtained from WC or FS donors. Poor suppressive acti-vity is also found in thymus cells from syngeneic adult donors (data not shown) or adult FS donors (Fig. 2 and Table 2). On the other hand suppressive activity is found already in embryonic thymus cells both from syngeneic (data not shown) or allogeneic donors (Table 2).

The analysis of the cellular composition of the chicken thymus with a combination of density gradient centrifugation, cell electro-phoresis and size distribution analysis revealed 3 major subpopula-tions of small lymphocytes (9,10,12). Table 3 shows the sequential appearance and disappearance of the three cell types in the chicken thymus. The perinatal thymus contains only cells of type I (9), and carries also suppressive activity (see Table 2) but no G.v.H. react-ivity (unpublished observation). Between 8 and 16 weeks after hat-ching, the thymus contains all three cell types, and carries both G.v.H. and suppressive activity; and the adult chicken thymus, after strong involution particularly of the cortex (13), contains only cell type III, and carries G.v.H. reactivity but poor suppressive activity.

DISCUSSION

The present experiments show that transfer of syngeneic or allo-geneic thymus cells from young donors in combination with a light whole body irradiation can significantly suppress the allograft rej-ection and can lead to longlasting skin graft survival across a strong histocompatibility barrier in a proportion of recipients. Thymus cells syngeneic to the skin graft donors were most effective and resulted in long surviving healthy skin grafts in 50-80% of the recipients. The suppressive effect on the allograft rejection may find an application in medical problems like organ transplantation. For technical reasons, it is particularly relevant in this connection that the effect is given by cells from unprimed donors and from allo-geneic donors.

The suppressive effect of the allogeneic thymus cells is appa-rently not a result of G.v.H. reactivity, since thymus cells from adult donors have relatively high G.v.H. reactivity (13) and poor suppressive activity, while embryonic thymus cells were found to be suppressive in the absence of any G.v.H. reactivity. Chicken thymus cells before three weeks of age carry also no detectable B-cell act-ivity (14) or B cell precursors (15), indicating that the suppressor cell is different from B-cells or G.v.H. reactive T-cells. Since

the involuted adult thymus carries little suppressive activity, and
contains practically only medulla and little cortex (13), it is
reasonable to assume that the suppressor cell resides predominantly
in the thymus cortex.

The biologically most interesting observation is the suppressive
activity in the embryonic thymus. This may explain the immunological
nonreactivity to self antigens or antigens that are administered to
the embryo. At the time when the self antigens have their first
contact with the immune system, these antigens are facing a system
which consists largely if not only of the thymus. The thymus is at
this time readily penetrated by all kinds of antigens (16-18) and
contains at this time no immunocompetent elements except suppressor
cells. By analogy to our experiments, we expect this first encounter to lead to specific suppression, even for such strong antigens
as the major histocompatibility antigens. We expect this to be at
least one of the mechanisms of self tolerance and of the neonatally
induced allograft tolerance.

REFERENCES

1.   W. Droege, Nature 234,549 (1971)
2.   W. Droege, Eur. J. Immunol. 3,804 (1973)
3.   W. Droege, Z. Immun. Forsch., 147,294 (1974)
4.   W. Droege, Proc. Natl. Acad. Sci. U.S. 72, No. 6 (1975) in press
5.   R.K. Gershon and K. Kondo, Immunology, 21,903 (1971)
6.   A. Basten, J.F.A.P. Miller, J. Sprent, and C. Cheers, J. Exp.
     Med. 140,199 (1974)
7.   G. Weber and E. Kölsch, Eur. J. Immunol. 3,767 (1973)
8.   D.E. Mosier and B.M. Johnson, J. Exp. Med. 141,216 (1975)
9.   W. Droege, R. Zucker and K. Hannig, Cell. Immunol. 12,186 (1974)
10. W. Droege and R. Zucker, Transplant. Rev. 25,3 (1975)
11. W. Droege, R. Zucker and U. Jauker, Cell. Immunol. 12,173 (1974)
12. R. Zucker, U. Jauker, and W. Droege, Eur. J. Immunol. 3,812
     (1973)
13. N.L. Warner, Aust. J. Exp. Biol. Med. Sci. 42,401 (1964)
14. P. Toivanen, A. Toivanen, and R.A. Good, J. Exp. Med. 136,816
     (1972)
15. P. Toivanen, A. Toivanen, and P. Tamminen, Eur. J. Immunol. 4,
     405 (1974)
16. I. Green and K. Bloch, Nature 200,1099 (1963)
17. J. Mitchell and G.J.V. Nossal, Aust. J. Exp. Biol. Med. Sci.
     44,211 (1966)
18. A. Horiuchi, J. Gery, and B.H. Waksman, Yale J. of Biol. and
     Med. 41,13 (1968).

TOLERANCE IN TETRAPARENTAL MOUSE CHIMAERAS

R. D. Barnes

Clinical Research Centre

Harrow

The concept of tolerance in early embryo aggregation derived mouse chimaeras has recently been questioned.

Upon the basis of the persistence of parental strain skin grafts, Mintz and Silvers proposed that such chimaeras were an example of both 'permanent and intrinsic tolerance' (1). Both views have since been disputed. Whilst Wegmann and his colleagues have shown that lymphoid cells from such chimaeras can react against parental antigens in vitro (2,3) we have shown that such an interaction can also occur in vivo and result in a form of graft-versus-host like disease (4,5) leading to the rejection of a parental strain skin graft (6). In vitro it appears that a serum factor in the chimaeras 'blocks' both cytotoxicity (2) and mixed lymphocyte reactivity (3). This led to the suggestion that tolerance in such chimaeras is dependent upon the in vivo activity of the same serum blocking factor (2,3). Here we have re-examined the situation of tolerance in the chimaeras using a local graft-versus-host (GVH) assay in an attempt to learn whether their lymphoid cells are capable of reacting against corresponding Fl recipients in vivo.

Chimaeras were derived by aggregation of early embryos obtained from inbred AKR, CBA/H-T6, C57/Bl, colony bred PO and naturally derived hybrids. Naturally derived hybrids were used as recipients in the GVH assay.

The local popliteal lymph node weight gain assay originally described by Ford and his colleagues (7) modified for use in the mouse (8) was employed here. Natural hybrids were used as recipients.

In the assay, varying numbers of lymphoid cells from the chimaeras were injected into one rear footpad of a corresponding FI recipient. Controls in this assay included FI mice injected with lymphoid cells from one or other parental strain, but also on occasions mixtures of <u>both</u> parental strain cells. In each case cell suspensions were prepared from lymph nodes, washed (x3) in 199 standardised upon viability (trypan blue) and doses adjusted in 199 to unit volume (50 μl).

Controls for the assay included determining the cell-dose response curve for the injection of parental strain cells into corresponding FI recipients. All the recipients used in the GVH assay were aged between 6-12 weeks and in each case were killed and examined seven days after injection - the peak of popliteal lymph node weight gain enlargement in the GVH assay (8). In both the test and also the dose response controls enlargement was expressed as a ratio of injected (I): non-injected (N) popliteal lymph node weights (8).

The number and composition of the various chimaeras examined here together with a summary of results in the popliteal lymph node weight gain assay following the injection of chimaera lymphoid cells are shown in Fig. I. As can be seen in comparison with the results in the controls shown in Fig 2 lymph node enlargement was seen following the injection of lymphoid cells from the chimaeras was minimal and furthermore was totally unrelated to the number of cells injected. Clearly the chimaeras lymphoid cells appear unreactive compared with the parental strain ➤FI controls.

Earlier findings using the popliteal lymph node weight gain assay noted that injection of various groups of <u>non-reactive cells</u> normally caused some slight enlargement in the popliteal lymph node weight gain GVH assay (8). Injecting 5.0×10^6 X-irradiated, heat killed and syngeneic (FI) cells into parental strain recipients resulted in I/U ratios of 1.167, 1.375 and 1.239 respectively (8), ratios that are remarkably similar to the findings here following the injection of the same number of viable chimaera lymphoid cells. Again in contrast to our earlier findings using normally reactive cells (8) (and also the controls here) enlargement following injection of chimaera lymphoid cells appeared totally unrelated to the number of cells injected. Both features point to the fact that in this assay lymphoid cells from chimaeras appear immunologically inert within the concept of basic immunological tolerance. This perhaps is not surprising since such chimaeras are commonly obtained by aggregation of very early eight-cell embryos - a perfect situation for immunological self-tolerance to be induced.

In contrast to our findings, Wegmann and his associates

CHIMAERA - DONOR (NO.)	RECIPIENT - HOST (NO.)	NO. OF CELLS INJECTED ($\times 10^6$)	ENLARGEMENT INDEX INJECTED/NON-INJECTED		
			Range	Mean	S.D.
AKR ↔ CBA (10)	(AKR × CBA)FI (26)	2.5	0.909 – 1.640	1.274	0.091
	(21)	5.0	1.008 – 1.640	1.313	0.141
	(20)	10.0	1.173 – 1.568	1.382	0.093
CBA ↔ C57/Bl (2)	(CBA × C57/Bf)FI (5)	2.5	0.808 – 1.473	1.141	0.071
	(5)	5.0	0.980 – 1.492	1.288	0.114
	(6)	10.0	1.123 – 1.578	1.394	0.137
CBA ↔ PO (2)	(CBA × PO)FI (3)	2.5	0.972 – 1.420	1.178	0.291
	(5)	5.0	1.100 – 1.473	1.314	0.211
	(4)	10.0	1.123 – 1.472	1.300	0.214
C57/Bl × PO↔PO (2)	(C57/Bl × PO)FI (4)	2.5	1.323 – 1.498	1.429	0.081
	(4)	5.0	1.201 – 1.537	1.415	0.070
	(4)	10.0	1.229 – 1.620	1.441	0.221

FIG I. POPLITEAL LYMPH NODE WEIGHT GAIN ASSAY FOLLOWING INJECTION OF CHIMAERA CELLS INTO FI HYBRIDS.

DONOR	RECIPIENT (NO. OF MICE)	NO. OF CELLS INJECTED ($\times 10^6$)	ENLARGEMENT INDEX INJECTED/NON-INJECTED
AKR	(AKR x CBA/H–T6)F1 (27)	2.5	2.12 ($\pm$ 0.63)
		5.0	4.17 ($\pm$ 0.72)
		10.0	6.23 ($\pm$ 0.72)
CBA/H–T6	(32)	2.5	1.97 ($\pm$ 0.32)
		5.0	4.03 ($\pm$ 0.46)
		10.0	6.03 ($\pm$ 0.91)
CBA/H–T6	(CBA/H–T6 x C57/Bl)F1 (21)	2.5	2.73 ($\pm$ 0.98)
		5.0	5.17 ($\pm$ 0.73)
		10.0	7.07 ($\pm$ 1.23)
C57/Bl	(19)	2.5	2.90 ($\pm$ 0.68)
		5.0	4.95 ($\pm$ 0.84)
		10.0	5.75 ($\pm$ 2.32)
CBA/H–T6	(CBA/H–T6 x PO)F1 (14)	2.5	1.74 ($\pm$ 0.24)
		5.0	3.04 ($\pm$ 0.61)
		10.0	5.12 ($\pm$ 0.73)
PO	(17)	2.5	1.63 ($\pm$ 0.27)
		5.0	1.98 ($\pm$ 1.47)
		10.0	5.23 ($\pm$ 1.07)

FIG. 2. POPLITEAL LYMPH NODE WEIGHT GAIN ASSAY FOLLOWING INJECTION OF PARENTAL CELLS INTO F1 HYBRIDS

demonstrated that lymphoid cells from the chimaeras react in vitro
in cytotoxicity against cells with the corresponding parental strain
antigens (2). Again and also in vitro Phillips and his co-workers
showed similar reactivity in mixed lymphocyte culture (3). In both
cases the reaction could be blocked by a factor present in the sera
of the corresponding chimaera. Our results here clearly conflict
with the earlier findings. One obvious explanation is that, whereas
the earlier work was done in vitro our assays were performed
in vivo. Although this is one obvious explanation other factors
need to be considered.

     Although we do not dispute the findings of Wegmann and his
colleagues (2) we have failed to confirm their findings but in
perhaps an atypical situation. Using the same Hellström
microcytotoxicity assay (9) we were unable to demonstrate 'blocking'
activity in the sera of any of four NZB↔CFW chimaeras (10).
There were obvious limitations in considering this finding in
general in a potentially autoimmune (NZB) situation particularly
since evidence suggested the presence of a GVH-like-disease in
these chimaeras (4,5,6,11,12,13,14). Conceivably, absence of
serum blocking activity and GVH-like-disease might have been
related. It was interesting to note that whereas a hyperactive
response in the popliteal lymph node assay was seen in these
NZB↔CFW chimaeras at a time when there was GVH-like activity (6)
a hypoactive response was recorded when GVH-like activity had
ceased (13).

     From the results here one is lead to conclude that lymphoid
cells from the chimaeras are in general unresponsive against Fl
recipients, in the local popliteal lymph node weight gain assay -
the exception being when GVH-like activity occurs. In this
context it would seem that the potential for reactivity is
present but generally suppressed, a hypothesis that has some support.
Phillips recently showed that in spite of his earlier findings (14)
lymphoid cells from the chimaeras do not respond to parental cells
in vitro. Intriguing is the fact that these same cells are also
capable of preventing an interaction between the two corresponding
parental strain cell lines. From this work has emerged the
possibility of the existence of a suppressor cell population.
Presumably inactive in the earlier in vitro studies of Wegmann (1)
and Phillips (2) it is this cell population that is manifest in the
most recent in vitro studies and also is a likely explanation for
the results here. It remains to identify the cell population
involved and also the factors that influence its activity -
including the possibility of serum mediated blocking activity. In
this respect recent evidence has provided a vital clue. A group
of seven tetraparental BALB/c ↔ C57/Bl chimaeras have been
investigated in collaboration with Dr. Hilliard Festenstein and
other colleagues. In each case in spite of chimaerism being

confirmed in mixed coat colour composition, red cells (glucose
phosphate isomerase) and serum allotype only one parental strain
peripheal blood lymphocyte could be identified by H-2
cytotoxicity. Absence of the antigenicity of one or other
lymphoid cell population was also confirmed in uni-directional
mixed lymphocyte reactivity (M.R.L.). The fact that XX:XY
lymphoid mosaicism was shown in the peripheral blood of at
least one chimaera confirms that both parental strain cell
populations are present, in spite of this only one was
identified antigenically.

In M.L.R. using artificial mixtures of corresponding A → AB
cells no suppression of reactivity could be demonstrated in the
presence of either sera or spleen cells from the chimaeras. This
was in contrast to the earlier findings of Phillips (2,15). One
is left to explain absence of one or other H-2 defined
lymphocyte population in the chimaeras. Although we have failed
to demonstrate either humoral and cellular suppression, at this
stage cannot with certainty be excluded. It seems possible
that an alternative mechanism such as antigenic modulation
might be effective or that what we have seen is evidence of the
elimination of one or other 'forbidden' clue of potentially
auto-reactive cells - auto-reactive in the context of the
two parental strain cells populations in the chimaeras being
potentially self-reactive against the other cell populations.
Either hypothesis remains is feasible but remain to be
confirmed.

REFERENCES

 1. Mintz, B., Science, 1967, 158, 1484.
 2. Phillips, S.M., Martin, W.J., Shaw, A.R., and Wegmann, T.G.,
       Nature, 1971, 234, 146.
 3. Wegmann, T.G., Hellstrom, and Hellstrom, K.E., Proc. Nat. Acad.
       Sci. U.S.A., 1971, 68, 1644.
 4. Barnes, R.D., and Tuffrey, M., Microenvironmental Aspects of
       Immunity (B.D. Jankovic and K. Isakovic Eds.) Plenum Pub.
       Corp. N.Y., 1972, 427.
 5. Barnes, R.D., and Tuffrey, M., Scand. J. Immunol., 1972, I, 284.
 6. Barnes, R.D., Tuffrey, M., Kingman, J., Thornton, C.,
       Turner, M.W., Clin. exp. Immunol., 1972, II 605.
 7. Ford, W.L., Burr, W., and Simonsen, M., Transplantation, 1970,
       10, 258.
 8. Twist, V., and Barnes, R.D., Transplantation 1973 15, 183.
 9. Hellstrom, K.E., and Hellstrom, I., Annu. Rev. Microbiol., 1970,
       24, 373.
10. Barnes, R.D., and Tuffrey, M., Europ. J. Immunol. 1973 3, 60.

11. Barnes, R.D., Holliday, J., and Tuffrey, M., Immunol., 1974, 26, 1195.
12. Barnes, R.D., Tuffrey, M., Graham, C.F., Holliday, J., and Thornton, C., Scand. J. Immunol., 1974, 3, 789.
13. Barnes, R.D., Tuffrey, M., and Wills E.J.,J.,Immunogenetics, 1974 ,(In press)
14. Tuffrey, M., Holliday, J., and Barnes, R.D.,Path., 1974, 113, 61.
15. Phillips, S.M., and Wegmann, T.G., J. exp Med., 1973, 137, 291.

STUDIES ON SUPPRESSOR T CELLS IN TOLERANCE

I. Zan-Bar, D. Nachtigal and M. Feldman

Department of Cell Biology, The Weizmann Institute of
Science, Rehovot, Israel

The study of the cellular mechanisms which determine the establishment of a state of specific immune unresponsiveness is one of the most
controversial areas of immunological research. The interpretations proposed to explain this phenomenon center around a genetically oriented
clonal elimination hypothesis on the one hand and around several suppressive hypotheses on the other. Our studies on immune tolerance to protein
antigens in mice (1) yielded information which is relevant to this controversy. The following report summarizes the pertinent observations concerning the role of suppressor T lymphocytes in the mechanism of tolerance, as well as some of the characteristics of these cells.

MATERIALS AND METHODS

Either inbred mice or F1 crosses of these were employed for induction
of unresponsiveness to human serum albumin (HSA). This was done in
either one of two ways without affecting the basic results: Adult mice (2—
3 months old) were made tolerant by administering 8—10 weekly intraperitoneal injections of 10 mg HSA each. Young mice, 18—19 days old, were
given to this end a single i. p. injection of 10 mg aggregate-free protein.
The mice were tested for their responsiveness after challenging them with
a mixture of the test antigen (HSA) and a control antigen (RSA), 0.5 mg of
each one incorporated in complete Freund's adjuvant. The antibody response was assayed by means of the Farr technique in terms of micrograms
protein bound per milliliter of serum.

585

Cell interactions were tested in adoptive transfer experiments into lethally irradiated syngeneic recipients. The cell grafts constituted 60 x 10^6 viable cells from each donor.

RESULTS

Analysis of the model of immune unresponsiveness to HSA in mice demonstrated clearly that unresponsiveness in this case did not result from a specific loss of a competent clone, since it could be shown that the tolerant mice carried a distinctive memory for the tolerizing antigen. This memory persisted after tolerance induction in a mode of specific suppression which was demonstrated to be basically reversible. The suppressive mechanism involved proved to be relatively radiosensitive and could therefore be abrogated by differential irradiation of the tolerant animals, whereby the suppressed priming of tolerant mice could be reactivated. This was done by irradiating the animals and reconstituting their T cell systems with normal syngeneic lymphocytes. Upon challenge with the tolerizing antigen a specific anamnestic response was elicited in tolerant mice, as compared with nontolerant animals treated identically (Fig. 1). Evidence suggested that this specific suppression of response of tolerant mice was effected by suppressor T cells which exhibited strict specificity for the tolerogen. The cells in question could be demonstrated in the spleens, lymph nodes and thymuses of tolerant animals, but were conspicuously absent from their bone marrow.

Technically suppressor cells in tolerance could be demonstrated in adoptive transfer experiments when lymphoid cells from tolerant donors were mixed with spleen cells of normal syngeneic donors and the mixtures grafted into lethally irradiated recipients. It was invariably demonstrated that the cells from tolerant origin suppressed specifically the responsiveness of the normal spleen cells in the mixture. In this system, the characteristics of the suppressor cells could be, therefore, investigated. Evidence was provided that the phenomenon in question represented actual specific suppression and could not be interpreted as competition, neither for space nor for the antigen (1). Moreover, Segal and his associates have recently demonstrated that suppressor T cells in tolerance constitute a separate subpopulation of T lymphocytes which carry characteristic surface receptors capable of binding to histamine and which can, therefore, be selectively retained by histamine-conjugated substrates (2).

These cells were found to be present exclusively in T cell tolerance (3). Evidence for this was provided by the following experiment: Specific unresponsiveness could be induced in T deprived 'B' mice as well as in intact

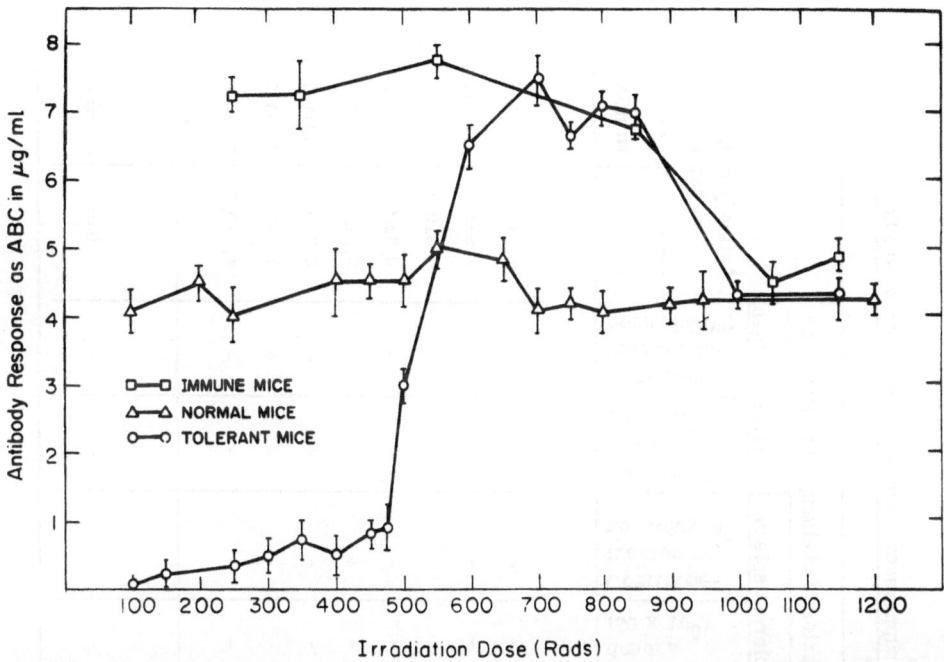

Figure 1. Response to HSA of mice irradiated with various doses of gamma rays and subsequently restored with 6×10^7 normal syngeneic spleen cells each. The animals, either tolerant to HSA or primed with HSA or normal controls, were challenged with the test antigen (HSA). No differences were found in response to a control antigen between tolerant and normal mice.

mice, employing identical techniques. The resulting tolerance, however, exhibited characteristics which differed from those of unresponsiveness induced in intact animals. It was of a shorter duration (4), it could be abrogated by supplementing nonirradiated tolerant mice with syngeneic normal spleen cells and, most significant, no suppressor cells could be demonstrated in the lymphoid tissues of these unresponsive animals.

It was found that the suppressors were relatively radiosensitive, θ-positive and cortisone-resistant lymphocytes (3). Evidence was available, however, that suppressor lymphocytes, although cortisone-resistant, are the progeny of cortisone-sensitive precursors. This conclusion was deduced from the observation that cortisone-sensitive thymic lymphocytes are essential for the induction of 'T-type' tolerance. In the relevant experiment tolerance was induced in T-deprived 'B' mice which had been restored by grafts of syngeneic normal thymocytes in addition to normal bone marrow cells (Table 1). Such mice could be made tolerant to HSA even

TABLE 1

Resistance to hydrocortisone acetate of specific suppressor T cells in mice tolerant to HSA

Group of mice	Irradiation (750 R)	Cell supplements administered to mice prior to challenge with HSA+RSA								Antibody response on day 14	
		Normal spleen		Normal thymus		Tolerant spleen		Tolerant thymus			
		Untreated donors (60 x 10^6)	Cortisone-treated donors (50x10^6)	Untreated donors (50 x 10^6)	Cortisone-treated donors (5x10^6)	Untreated donors (50 x 10^6)	Cortisone-treated donors (50x10^6)	Untreated donors (50 x 10^6)	Cortisone-treated donors (5x10^6)	to HSA	to RSA
Normal recipient mice											
1	+	+	+	−	−	−	−	−	−	3.4±1.1	4.7±0.5
2	+	+	−	+	−	−	−	−	−	2.9±1.2	3.2±1.2
3	+	+	−	−	+	−	−	−	−	4.0±0.9	7.2±1.2
4	+	+	−	−	−	+	−	−	−	0.5±0.6	3.1±1.3
5	+	+	−	−	−	−	+	−	−	0.0±0	4.0±0.6
6	+	+	−	−	−	−	−	+	−	0.2±0.3	3.3±0.7
7	+	+	−	−	−	−	−	−	+	1.9±0.7	7.1±1.2
8	+	−	−	−	−	−	−	−	−	4.1±0.8	7.0±0.8
Tolerant mice											
9	−	−	−	−	−	−	−	−	−	0±0	6.5±0.8

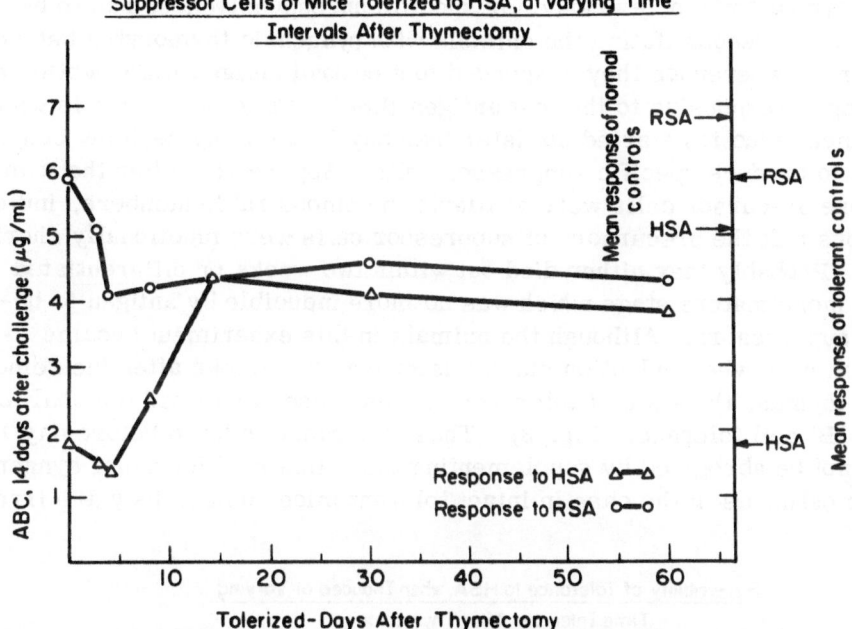

Figure 2. Tolerance was induced in mice at various time intervals after thymectomy and when tolerance was verified the spleens were removed and tested for suppressor cells. The antibod response of the adoptively transferred mice is reported.

when the bone marrow originated from cortisone-treated donors. However, when the thymus donors had been pretreated with cortisone, the recipients became refractory to tolerance induction. That corticosteroids can interfere with the induction of unresponsiveness has been demonstrated in other experimental models as well (5, 6). Since cortisone-sensitive thymic lymphocytes are believed to represent the immature T cell population (7), it was suggested that these precursors are the target cells which, on receipt of a signal transmitted from the antigen, differentiate into mature cortisone-resistant suppressor cells. Assuming, thus, that the induction of suppressor T cells depended on the availability of appropriate precursor lymphocytes, it was of interest to investigate the life history of these precursors. Initially, we approached the problem of the functional life span of the precursor cells (8). The experiment was based on the premise that the origin of the immature T cells is the thymus. Adult mice were therefore thymectomized so that they would be unable to replenish their pool of peripheral cortisone-sensitive lymphocytes. These animals were divided into several groups which were made tolerant to HSA each starting at a different time after thymectomy (Fig. 2). Since the mice had

been thymectomized, evidence for specific unresponsiveness had to be obtained after reconstituting the animals with syngeneic thymocytes before
challenge, whereupon they responded to a control antigen (RSA) while remaining unresponsive to the test antigen (HSA). Only those mice in which
tolerance induction started not later than day 14 after thymectomy could be
shown to produce specific suppressor cells. Apparently, after that time
no more precursor cells were available in demonstrable numbers, indicating thus that the precursors of suppressor cells were functionally short-
lived. Probably they either died out within two weeks or differentiated
into a more mature stage which was no more inducible by antigen to become suppressors. Although the animals in this experiment became
tolerant even when induction started later than two weeks after the removal
of the thymus, the state of tolerance in these cases exhibited the character-
ics of 'B' cell tolerance (Fig. 3). Thus, tolerance induced before day 14
could not be abrogated by supplementing the animals with normal syngeneic
spleen cells, as in the case in intact tolerant mice, unless they are irradi-

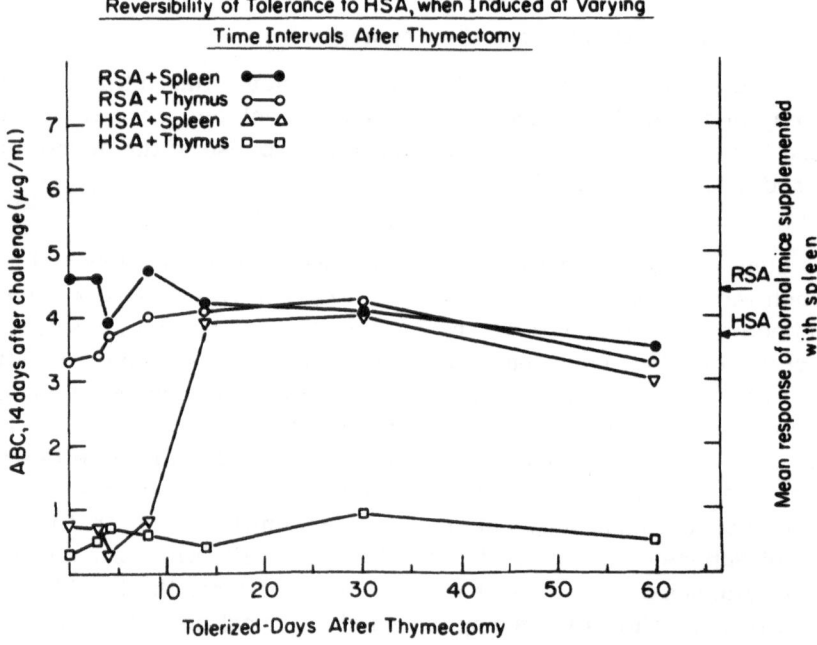

Figure 3. Mice made tolerant at various time intervals after thymectomy
were restored either with normal syngeneic thymus or with normal syngeneic spleen cells. Thymus cells failed to restore specific reactivity, while
spleen cells did so, but only in those animals which were made tolerant
from day 14 and later after thymectomy.

ated before cell grafting. Those mice, however, which were made tolerant later than 14 days after thymectomy and which were shown to lack
suppressor cells, could be made competent to the tolerizing antigen by
reconstitution with normal spleen. Apparently they did not require prior
irradiation, since they did not harbor suppressor cells which suppress the
responsiveness of the normal cell graft. Subsequently we studied for comparison the functional life span of the mature suppressor cells as well.
This was done by rendering first the mice tolerant to HSA and afterwards
thymectomizing the tolerant animals, thus ensuring that the pool of preformed suppressor cells would remain cut off from possible replenishment.
The mice were tested for the presence of suppressor lymphocytes at increasing time intervals after thymectomy and the suppressive activity of
their spleens could be demonstrated as late as 63 days. It appears, thus,
that the short-lived precursors differentiate as a result of antigen stimulation into comparatively long-functioning suppressor cells.

SUMMARY

(1) Evidence is provided that tolerance induced in mice to HSA depends
on a suppressive mechanism which inhibits the responsiveness of potentially competent cells.

(2) The suppression is apparently the function of suppressor T cells
which are comparatively radiosensitive and are resistant to cortisone.

(3) The cortisone resistant suppressor cells are apparently the progeny of cortisone-sensitive precursors, the differentiation of which into
mature suppressors seems to be signalled by antigen.

(4) The precursor lymphocytes are comparatively short functioning
cells (about 14 days), while the mature suppressor T cells function for at
least two months.

REFERENCES

1. Zan-Bar, I., Nachtigal, D., and Feldman, M. (1974) Cell. Immunol.
   10:19
2. Segal, S., Weinstein, Y., Melmon, K. L., and McDevitt, H. O., J.
   Exp. Med., in press
3. Zan-Bar, I., Nachtigal, D., and Feldman, M. (1975) Cell. Immunol.
   17:202

4. Chiller, J. M. , Habicht, G. S. , and Weigle, W. O. (1971) Science 17:
    813
5. Zan-Bar, I. , Nachtigal, D. , and Feldman, M. (1975) Cell. Immunol.
    17:215
6. Dukor, P. and Dietrich, F. M. (1970) Proc. Soc. Exp. Biol. Med.
    133:280
7. Weissman, I. L. (1973) J. Exp. Med. 137:504
8. Nachtigal, D. , Zan-Bar, I. , and Feldman, M. , (1975) Transplant.
    Rev. 26 (in press)

DEPLETION OF SUPPRESSOR T-CELLS IN SYNGENEIC CHIMERIC MICE

Varda Rotter and Nathan Trainin

Department of Cell Biology, The Weizmann Institute of

Science, Rehovot, Israel

T-cells are known to play an important role in the expression of the immune response. Data accumulated recently suggest that T-cells are in addition involved in the suppression and regulation of the immune response to certain antigens (1). It was observed that depletion of suppressor T-cells by means such as ALS treatment (2-4) adult thymectomy (5,6) or induction of a mild graft vs host reaction (7,8) causes an increased immune reactivity to antigens such as III pneumococcal polysaccharide or polyvinylpyrrolidone. The regulatory mechanism of Lewis Lung (3LL) carcinoma growth in mice also involves suppressor T-cell activity. Indeed reduction of the suppressor T-cell population by different means resulted in an increased resistance of the host to the growth of this tumor (9-11).

We present here results suggesting that lethally irradiated mice reconstituted with syngeneic bone marrow cells are deficient in a suppressor T-cell population. This was expressed by increased resistance to 3LL growth and augmentation of the response to PVP. In addition when other aspects of T-cell activity were studied we found that while the mixed lymphocyte culture (MLC) reactivity was intact the capacity to elicit a cell mediated lysis (CML) reaction was impaired in these mice.

MATERIALS AND METHODS

<u>Mice</u>: 2-6 month old female (C3H/eb x C57BL/6)F$_1$ hybrids were used throughout these experiments.
<u>Irradiation and bone marrow reconstitution</u>: (C3H/eb x C57BL/6)F$_1$ mice were submitted to a single 800 R dose of total body irradiation from a ^{60}Co gamma source (Atomic Energy of Canada Ltd. Gamma beam

150 A dose rate 1000 R per min). Within 2 h after irradiation mice
were injected 5-8 x 10^6 syngeneic bone marrow cells each.
Lewis Lung (3LL) Carcinoma: This is a malignant metastasizing tumor
which arose spontaneously in C57BL/6 mice (12) and is maintained in
our laboratory by subcutaneous transfer into C57BL/6 male mice.
12-20 days after s.c. injection of 2 x 10^5 tumor cells into (C3H/eb
x C57BL/6)F_1 mice a solid tumor appears at the site of injection.
Mice injected with tumor cells were checked daily and tumor takes
were considered positive when a visible solid tumor appeared. Mice
died 4-6 weeks later from lung metastases.
Preparation of cell suspensions: Spleen cells were prepared by pressing the organ through a fine stainless steel mesh into cold RPMI-
1640 medium (Gibco USA). Bone marrow cells were prepared by flush-
ing out the marrow from the bones with a stream of Eagle's medium
using a syringe. 3LL tumor cell suspension was prepared from a
local tumor mass removed from a mouse, minced and treated for 30 min
in a 0.3% trypsin solution. Cells were washed several times counted and injected into the mice.
Immunization and assay: The immune response to sheep red blood
cells (SRBC) and polyvinylpyrrolidone (PVP) was measured by determining the number of specific plaque forming cells (PFC) by means
of the Jerne technique (13) and modifications (6).
Mixed lymphocyte culture (MLC) reaction: The capacity of lymphoid
cells from (C3H/eb x C57BL/6)F_1 mice to elicit a MLC reaction (14)
was tested against stimulator spleen cells of Balb/c origin. Balb/c
spleen cells as well as control (C3H/eb x C57BL/6)F_1 cells were
treated with mitomycin-C 20 µg/ml for 30 min in 37°C. 10^6 effector
spleen or lymph node cells were mixed with 10^6 stimulator cells in
each test tube culture and cell cultures were incubated in humidified air with 5% CO_2 for 72 h. At the end of this incubation period
2 µCi of ^{3}H-thymidine (Negev, Israel) were added for another 16 h
incubation period and radioactive content was measured.
Cell mediated lysis (CML): The capacity of lymphoid cells from
(C3H/eb x C57BL/6)F_1 mice to lyse blast target cells of a Balb/c
origin was tested as described (15). Spleen or lymph node cells
were mixed with irradiated (1000 R) Balb/c spleen cells for 4-5
days. These sensitized cells were mixed with blast cells (by Con A
stimulation) of Balb/c origin labeled with ^{51}Cr, and ^{51}Cr release
evaluated.

EXPERIMENTAL AND DISCUSSION

We observed previously that lethally irradiated mice reconstituted with syngeneic bone marrow cells manifest 2 month later an
increased response to PVP (6,16). In the present study we followed
the kinetics of the immune response to PVP of these chimeric mice
and in parallel we studied their response to SRBC, an antigen known
to be dependent on T-helper activity (17). As seen in Fig. 1 the
response to PVP raises above normal early after irradiation and
bone marrow reconstitution, reaching a plateau around 70 days later.

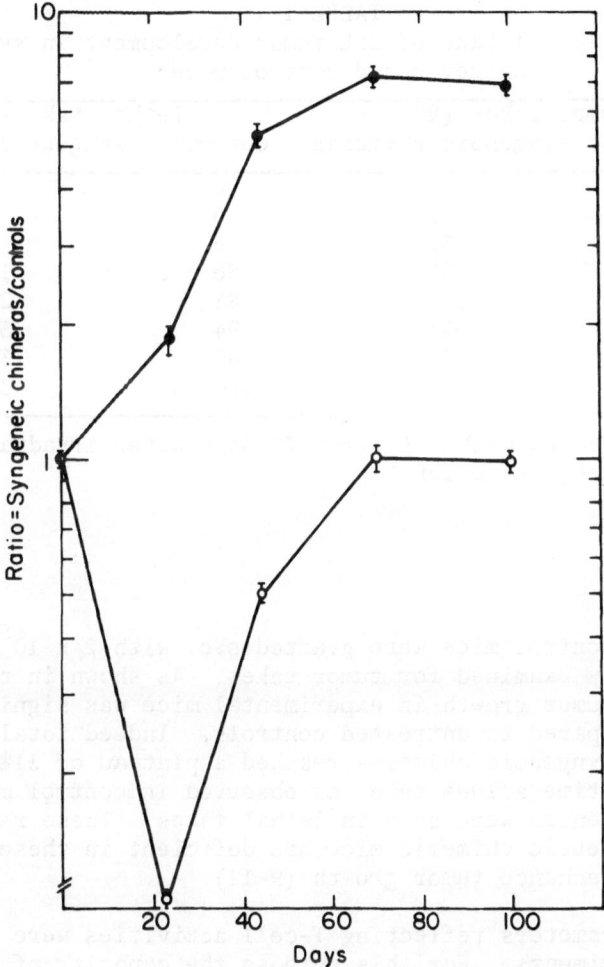

<u>Fig. 1</u>: Antigenic response to PVP (●——●) and SRBC (o——o) in syn-
geneic chimeric mice. Each point represent the ratio of the mean
response of experimental mice and controls.

The response to SRBC on the other hand, was strongly damaged, but
returned to normal 70 days after irradiation and remained constant.
Altogether these results suggest that suppressor T-cells are a distinct T-cell population which is remaining impaired in chimeric
mice. Another system regulated by suppressor T-cells is that related to the development of 3LL tumors in mice. Indeed the incidence
of 3LL tumors was shown to be reduced under some experimental conditions which lead to a rise in the response to PVP. It was therefore of interest to study 3LL tumor growth in syngeneic chimeras as
another model for evaluating suppressor T-cell activity. Syngeneic

TABLE 1

Incidence and lethal take of 3LL tumor development in syngeneic
chimeric and control mice*

Days	Tumor takes (%)		Lethal take (%)	
	Control	syngeneic chimeras	Control	syngeneic chimeras
11	56	6	0	0
16	87	16	0	0
19	100	31	6	0
29	100	31	56	16
35	100	31	81	26
40	100	31	94	31
46	100	31	100	31
50	100	31	100	31

*
Mice were injected with 3LL tumor 70 days after irradiation and
bone marrow reconstitution.

chimeras and control mice were grafted s.c. with 2×10^5 tumor
cells and daily examined for tumor takes. As shown in table 1 the
incidence of tumor growth in experimental mice was significantly
reduced as compared to untreated controls. Indeed total tumor
takes in the syngeneic chimeras reached a plateau of 31% at 19 days
while at that time a 100% take was observed in control mice.
Similar differences were seen in lethal takes. These results indicate that syngeneic chimeric mice are deficient in these suppressor
T-cells which enhance tumor growth (9-11).

Other parameters reflecting T-cell activities were studied in
the next experiments. For this purpose the capacity of lymphoid
cells of syngeneic chimeric and control mice to elicit MLC and CML
reactions was studied. As shown in table 2 a similar MLC reaction
was observed when lymphoid cells of either chimeric or intact
(C3H/eb x C57BL/6)F_1 mice were tested against same Balb/c stimulating cells, thus suggesting that T-cells involved in this reaction
are in syngeneic chimeric mice as active as in control mice. On the
other hand when CML was assayed a significant reduction in the capacity of chimeric spleen cells to lyze Balb/c target cells was
observed as compared to normals (Table 3). This impaired CML reaction was also observed when lymph node cells from syngeneic chimeras
were tested (Table 3). These findings are in line with the concept
that different T-cell populations are involved in MLC and CML reactions (18,19).

TABLE 2

MLC response of lymphoid cells obtained from (C3H/eb x C57BL/6)F_1 chimeric mice and controls*

Mice	Effector cells	Stimulating cells**	CPM $\pm$ SE
Normal mice	F_1 sp. cells	F_1 sp. cells	3114 + 365
	F_1 sp. cells	Balb/c sp. cells	10141 + 980
	F_1 LN cells	F_1 LN cells	3895 + 405
	F_1 LN cells	Balb/c sp. cells	19383 + 585
Chimeric mice	F_1 sp. cells	F_1 sp. cells	4965 + 1196
	F_1 sp. cells	Balb/c sp. cells	10585 + 465
	F_1 LN cells	F_1 LN cells	2827 + 734
	F_1 LN cells	Balb/c sp. cells	21348 + 660

*   MLC response was measured 70 days after irradiation and bone marrow reconstitution.

** Stimulating cells were incubated for 30 min with mitomycin-C 20 μg/ml at 37°C.

TABLE 3

Reduced CML response of lymphoid cells obtained from (C3H/eb x C57BL/6)F_1 chimeric mice as compared to controls*

Exp. #	% of ^{51}Cr release from target cells	
	controls	syngeneic chimeras
Spleen cells		
1	29.8 + 7.1	-3.0 + 3.2
2	28.0 + 1.7	-0.4 + 1.0
3	19.6 + 4.8	-4.5 + 2.6
LN cells		
1	30.2 + 5.6	5.7 + 0.7
2	18.2 + 1.4	0.5 + 1.2
3	11.8 + 1.8	5.7 + 1.8

*   CML response was measured 70 days after irradiation and bone marrow reconstitution.

SUMMARY

The present results suggest that some T-cell activities of
syngeneic chimeric mice such as T-cells involved in the antibody
response to SRBC and MLC reaction are intact. On the other hand,
suppressor T-cells involved in the regulation of the immune response to PVP and enhancement of 3LL tumor growth, and cells
mediating CML reaction are damaged.

Acknowledgement: Supported by a grant from the National Institutes
of Health, under Agreement NCI-G-72-3890

REFERENCES

1.   Gerson, R.K. Contemporary Topics in Immunobiology. M.C.Cooper
         & N.L. Warner, eds., Vol. 3, p. 1, Plenum Press, 1974.
2.   Baker, P.J., Barth, R.F., Stashak, P.W. and Amsbaugh, D.F.
         J. Immunol. 104, 1313, 1970.
3.   Baker, P.J., Stashak, P.W., Amsbaugh, D.F., Prescott, B. and
         Marth, R.F., J. Immunol. 105, 1581, 1970.
4.   Kerbel, R.S. and Eidinger, D., J. Immunol. 106, 917, 1971.
5.   Kerbel, R.S. and Eidinger, D., Eur. J. Immunol. 2, 114, 1972.
6.   Rotter, V. and Trainin, N., Cell. Immunol. 13, 76, 1974.
7.   Rotter, V. and Trainin, N., Cell. Immunol., in press.
8.   Byfield, P., Christie, G.H.,and Howard, J.G., J. Immunol. 111,
         72, 1973.
9.   Umiel, T. and Trainin, N., Transplantation 18, 244, 1974.
10.   Treves, A.J., Carnaud, C., Trainin, N., Cohen, I.R., Feldman,
         M., Eur. J. Immunol. 4, 722, 1974.
11.   Carnaud, C., Markowicz, O. and Trainin, N., Cell. Immunol. 14,
         87, 1974.
12.   Sugiura, K. and Stock, C.C., Cancer Res. 15, 38, 1955.
13.   Jerne, N.K., Nordin, A.A., Henry, C. in B. Amos and H. Koprowski
         eds., Cell Bound Antibodies, The Wistar Institute Press
         Inc., Philadelphia, Pa. 1963, p. 109.
14.   Hayry, P., Andersson, L.C., Nording, S. and Virolainen, M.,
         Transplant. Rev. 12, 91, 1972.
15.   Feldman, M., Cohen, I.R. and Wekerle, H., Transplant. Rev.
         12, 57, 1972.
16.   Rotter, V. and Trainin, N., Transplantation, in press.
17.   Claman, H.N., Chaperon, E.A., Triplett, R.F., Proc. Soc. Biol.
         Med. 122, 1167, 1966.
18.   Bach, F.H., Segall, M., Stouber-Zier, K., Sondel, P.M., Alter,
         B.J. and Bach, M.L., Science 180, 403, 1973.
19.   Stobo, J.D., Paul, W.E. and Henney, C., J. Immunol. 110, 652,
         1973.

REGULATORY CELLS IN THE BONE MARROW

S. Adler[*], S. K. Singhal[+], and E. E. Sercarz[*]

[*]Department of Bacteriology, University of California,
Los Angeles, California 90024 USA
[+]Department of Bacteriology and Immunology, University
of Western Ontario, London, Ontario, Canada

INTRODUCTION

Regulation of the immune system has been attributed primarily
to thymus-derived T cells (1,2). Here we present evidence that
suppression can be mediated by another cell type, found in the bone
marrow, that is neither a T cell nor a macrophage. Others have also
shown that bone marrow-derived (B) cell suppression can inhibit both
humoral and cell-mediated immunity (3-6).

As a main source of progenitor and mature cells, the bone marrow
is the most complex hemopoietic organ in the adult animal, and is a
likely candidate to play an influential regulatory role on the immune
response. Initially, the bone marrow suppression observed by Singhal
was measured on a primary sheep red cell (SRC) response in DBA/2J
spleen cell cultures (7,8). The experiments reported here have been
carried out with the lysozyme antigen system in C57BL/6 mice. The
similar nature of the results in these systems supports the gener-
ality of this non-T cell regulatory phenomenon.

EXPERIMENTAL

The Assay System

Two days prior to use, C57BL/6 mice were primed i.v. with
4×10^7 burro red cells conjugated with hen egg white lysozyme
(BRC-HEL). Spleen cell suspensions were prepared from these primed

animals and 10×10^6 cells/ml were cultured with BRC-HEL (10×10^6 red cells/ml) in a standard Mishell-Dutton culture (9). On day five the cultures were assayed for direct HEL specific plaque forming cells (PFC) on a target of HEL-coated, goat red cells by the Cunningham slide technique(10). The number of PFC's observed in these control cultures represents the normal anti-HEL PFC response (control response = 100%). Graded numbers of bone marrow cells, from normal or BRC-HEL primed animals, were compared and the results are expressed as % of the HEL control response.

The Suppressive Effect of Bone Marrow Cells

The suppressive effect of normal and primed bone marrow cells on primed spleen cell cultures is shown in Fig. 1. When increasing concentrations of bone marrow cells (from 10^4 to 5×10^6 cells/ml) were added to the responding spleen cell cultures, the PFC response was suppressed to as low as 1% of the control culture. It is interesting to note that when low concentrations of bone marrow cells ($< 10^4$/ml) were added to cultures, an augmentation of the HEL response was often observed (data not shown). This happened more frequently when the bone marrow cells were added to cultures of spleen cells primed for 1-2 weeks rather than for 2 days.

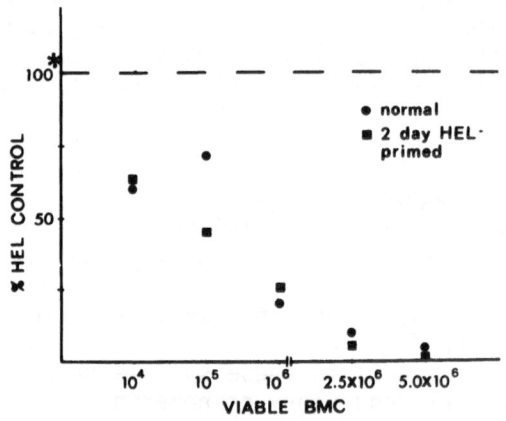

*100 % = 41,220 direct PFC's/culture

Fig. 1. Increasing Concentrations of Normal or Primed Bone Marrow Cells (BMC) Suppress the IgM PFC Response by HEL-primed Spleen Cells In Vitro. Viable BMC were added to 2 day HEL-primed spleen cells (10×10^6 cells/ml). The cultures were assayed for PFC's on day 5.

Lack of Specificity of the Suppression

The fact that normal and primed bone marrow cells suppressed the response to approximately the same extent suggested that the suppression was immunologically nonspecific. This lack of specificity is shown by the results presented in Fig. 2. Spleen and bone marrow cells were taken from animals primed with unrelated antigens. When bone marrow cells from GRC-primed animals were added to GRC-primed spleen cell cultures, the GRC response was suppressed.

Suppression by Early Addition of Bone Marrow Cells

Studies have shown that for an immune response to occur, various cell interactions or products of cell interactions are needed early in the response. If bone marrow cells were exerting a general toxic effect, it would be expected that they would interfere with the response whenever they were added. However, the bone marrow cells in our studies appear to act on the inductive process of antibody formation (Fig. 3). Bone marrow cells which were added at the onset of culture or up to 24 hours strongly suppressed the antibody response of the spleen cell cultures. The later addition of bone marrow cells had little effect on the response.

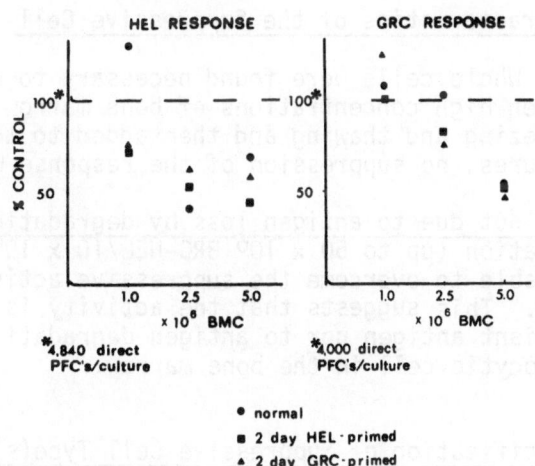

Fig. 2. Lack of Specificity in BMC Suppression. For the HEL response, the BMC were added to 2 day HEL-primed spleen cells (10 x 10^6/ml). For the GRC response, the BMC were added to 2 day GRC-primed spleen cells (10 x 10^6/ml). The cultures were assayed, respectively, for HEL and GRC PFC's on day 5.

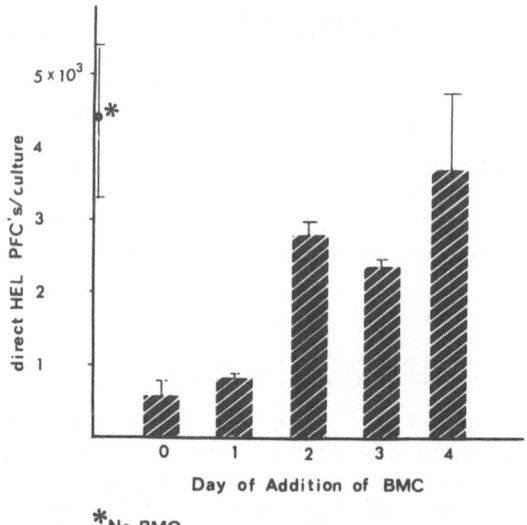

*No BMC

Fig. 3. Suppression by BMC Added Early in the Response.
Day of addition of 4 x 10⁶ viable BMC to 2 day HEL-primed spleen
cells (10 x 10⁶/ml). Triplicate cultures were individually
assayed for PFC's on day 5. The bars represent average PFC's
± standard deviation.

Characteristics of the Suppressive Cell

Viability. Whole cells were found necessary to elicit this
suppression. When high concentrations of bone marrow cells were
submitted to freezing and thawing and then added to the responding
spleen cell cultures, no suppression of the response was observed.

Suppression not due to antigen loss by degradation. High
antigen concentration (up to 50 x 10⁶ BRC-HEL/10 x 10⁶ spleen cells
cultured) was unable to overcome the suppressive activity of the
bone marrow cell. This suggests that the activity is neither due to
a lack of sufficient antigen nor to antigen degradation or elimination by a phagocytic cell in the bone marrow.

Identification of Suppressive Cell Type(s)

The cell types present in the adult bone marrow of mice can
be roughly divided as follows: one-half granulocytes, one-fourth
lymphocytes, and one-fourth erythrocytes. Small percentages of
platelets, eosinophils, basophils, mast cells, monocytes and macrophages can also be found along with immature cells of each cell

type. Some of the lymphocytic bone marrow cells are Ig⁺ while there
are few, if any, θ⁺ cells (11).

In order to assess whether the small population of T cells or
the larger population of macrophages might be responsible for the
suppression observed, the bone marrow cells were treated with specific antisera. The data in Fig. 4 show that the treatment of bone
marrow cells with either anti-θ or anti-macrophage sera plus complement had no effect on their suppressive activity.

DISCUSSION

Our results show that normal or primed, intact bone marrow
cells can nonspecifically inhibit an early step in antibody formation in vitro. This suppressive activity is neither due to antigen
degradation by phagocytic cells nor to unfavorable cell densities
in culture. The addition of increasing numbers of primed spleen
cells (data not shown) or normal thymus cells to spleen cell cultures
does not significantly reduce the PFC response (7). The suppressor
cell is not sensitive to anti-θ or anti-macrophage treatment.
Further evidence for the non-macrophage nature of this cell is based
on the fact that the suppressor activity is associated with the nonadherent bone marrow cell population (8). Furthermore, the suppressor activity is not removed when cells were treated with iron

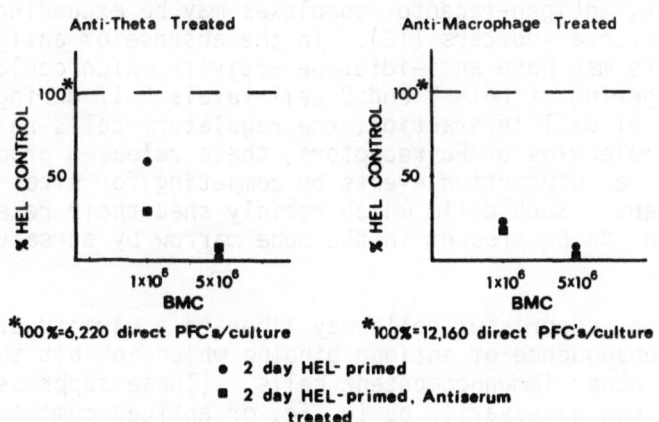

*100%=6,220 direct PFC's/culture   *100%=12,160 direct PFC's/culture

● 2 day HEL-primed
■ 2 day HEL-primed, Antiserum
   treated

*Fig. 4. Lack of Effect of BMC Treatment with Anti-Theta
or Anti-Macrophage Sera on Suppression.* 2 Day HEL-primed BMC
were pretreated with anti-θ or anti-macrophage sera before addition to cultures as indicated. Control and serum-treated BMC
were added to 2 day HEL-primed spleen cells (10 x 10⁶ cells/ml).
The cultures were assayed for PFC's on day 5.

filings and placed in a magnetic field (A.K. Duwe and S.K. Singhal, unpublished).

Although we have shown that an intact cell is necessary for suppression, the cell need not be dividing. When mitomycin C-treated bone marrow cells were mixed with the responding spleen cells, they were still suppressive. This preliminary experiment suggests that DNA synthesis is not necessary for suppression, and that marked expansion of the bone marrow cells to inhibitory densities is not a relevant factor.

These observations and others implicating an Ig^+ suppressor cell population suggest that a bone marrow-derived cell or another cell type with Ig-like receptor, either synthesized by that cell or passively acquired, may act as an important regulator in humoral immunity (3,5,6). In addition, B cell suppression has been implicated in cell-mediated immunity of tumor bearing mice (4,5) and delayed hypersensitivity in guinea pigs (6).

A generalized mechanism involving regulation of T cell activity by B cell products would be expected late in the response (2). However, it is necessary to explain the interference with immune functions very early in this response (3,4,7,8). During this inductive process, a complex set of interactions among T cells, macrophages, B cells, and factors derived from these cells usually results in antigen presentation at the appropriate site. The target cell(s) of the inhibition may be affected in a number of ways. With antigen present, antigen-receptor complexes may be exceedingly effective as tolerance inducers (12). In the absense of antigen, some or all receptors may have anti-idiotype activity which could interfere with triggering at both T and B cell levels. If during the crucial period of cell interaction, the regulatory cells release their receptors, Ig molecules or Fc receptors, these released products might subvert the interaction events by competing for sites of receptor attachment. Such cells which rapidly shed their receptors have been shown to be present in the bone marrow by ourselves and others (13,14).

In addition, suppressor cells may liberate a variety of substances as a consequence of antigen binding which inhibit the functioning of other immunocompetent cells. (These suppressor cell products would not necessarily be Ig, Fc, or antigen complexes.) Now there is evidence for (5,6) and against (3,4) the release of such material from these suppressor B cells. The evidence for a soluble factor mediating the B cell suppression of the bone marrow will be presented in the following paper by Duwe and Singhal.

ACKNOWLEDGMENTS

This work was supported by NATO Grant 606, NIH Grant AI-08198, and Contract NIH NCI CB-43972.

REFERENCES

1. Gershon, R.K. In: Contemporary Topics in Immunobiology, v. 3, eds. M.D. Cooper and N. Warner (Plenum Press, New York) p. 1 (1974).
2. Gershon, R.K., Orbach-Arbouys, S., and C. Calkins. In: Progress in Immunology, v. II, eds. L. Brent and J. Holborow (North-Holland Publishing Co., Amsterdam) p. 123 (1974).
3. Okumura, K. and M. Kern. Cellular Immunol. 17:19-29 (1975).
4. Eggers, A. and J. Wunderlich. J. Immunol. 114:1554-1556 (1975).
5. Gorczynski, R. J. Immunol. 112:1826-1838 (1974).
6. Katz, S.I., Parker, D., and J.L. Turk. Nature. 251:550-551 (1974).
7. Singhal, S.K., King, S., and P.J. Drury. Int. Arch. Allergy. 43:934-951 (1972).
8. Drury, P.J., and S.K. Singhal. Int. Arch. Allergy. 46:707-724 (1974).
9. Mishell, R., and R. Dutton. J. Exp. Med. 126:423 (1967).
10. Cunningham, A.J., and A. Szenberg. Immunol. 14:599-600 (1968).
11. Raff, M. Transplant. Rev. 6:52 (1971).
12. Diener, E., and M. Feldman. Transplant. Rev. 8:76 (1972).
13. DeLuca, D., Miller A., and E. Sercarz. Cellular Immunol. 18 (1975) in press.
14. Melchers, F., vonBoehmer, H., and R. Phillips. J. Exp. Med. (1975) in press.

SUPPRESSION BY SOLUBLE FACTOR RELEASED FROM B CELLS

A. K. Duwe and S. K. Singhal

Department of Bacteriology and Immunology
University of Western Ontario
London, Ontario, Canada N6a 5C1

INTRODUCTION

Whereas suppression of immune responses by T cells has been well documented (1), the role played by B cells in the regulation of the immune response is less well known. The mouse bone marrow contains a radiosensitive, non-T, non-macrophage cell population which dramatically suppresses the primary and secondary IgM PFC response of spleen cells both in vivo and in vitro (2-4). In this communication we will present evidence for the release of suppressive and augmenting materials from cells in the bone marrow and attempt to clarify the target and mechanism of action of the suppressor cell.

METHODS AND RESULTS

Culture conditions and reagents used were essentially those described by Mishell and Dutton (5). Briefly, 20 x 10^6 DBA/2J spleen cells and SRBC were cultured in 1 ml of medium for 5 days, after which they were harvested and assayed for PFC.

The Effect of ATC on Suppression by Bone Marrow Cells

Kinetic studies revealed that the bone marrow cells (BMC) must be added during the first 24-48 hours of culture to be suppressive (2), suggesting that the suppressor might be preventing induction at the level of either a B or a T cell. We therefore added a population of pre-activated T cells (ATC) and BMC to cultures of

spleen cells. Lethally irradiated (850R) recipients were injected
with 50 x 10⁶ syngeneic thymocytes plus SRBC and their spleens
removed 6-8 days later as a source of ATC.

While the addition of 10⁶ ATC alone to spleen cells in the
presence of antigen resulted in a marked augmentation of the
response, this dose of ATC failed to abrogate the suppression
mediated by 2 x 10⁶ BMC (Fig. 1). This suggested that the BMC were
not preventing induction of T cells, although the possibility remained that release of T-cell factor(s) was inhibited or that
suppression might act via a T cell.

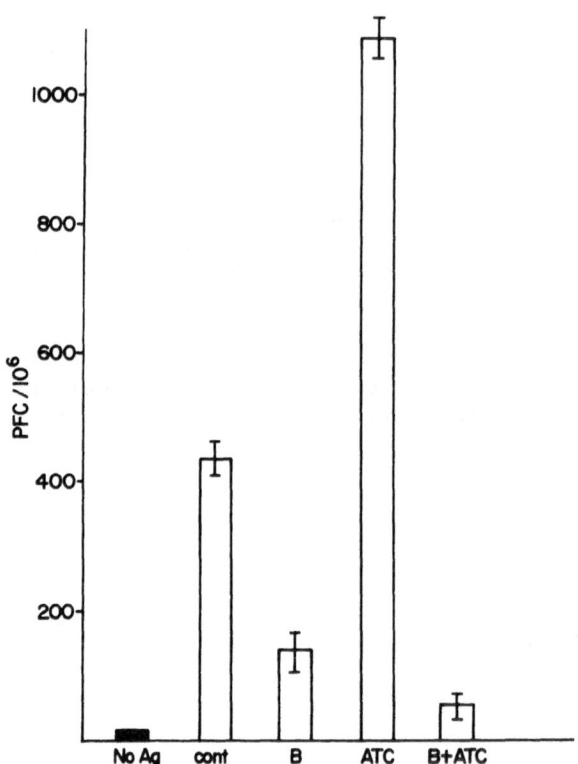

Fig. 1 The effect of addition of ATC on the suppressive activity
of BMC. Spleen cells were cultured with or without SRBC (controls)
or with 10⁶ ATC and 2 x 10⁶ BMC added either together or separately
on day 0. PFC/10⁶ values represent the mean of duplicate
determinations.

BMC Suppression does not Act Via a T Cell

It is possible to replace T-cell function with factors obtained from cultures of allogeneic spleen cells (6). Supernatants were obtained by culturing DBA/2J and C57Bl spleen cells for 24 hrs either alone as controls or together as a source of allogeneic factors, and added in 0.5 ml volumes to normal or anti-θ treated spleen cells. As presented in Fig. 2, control supernatants did not restore the response, whereas cultures receiving allogeneic supernatants responded normally. Addition of 10^6 or 2×10^6 BMC to these cultures resulted in suppression comparable to that observed with normal spleen cells. Similar results were obtained with allogeneic supernatants added at day 0. Thus presence of a T cell was not required for expression of suppressor activity, suggesting the target cell to be a B cell.

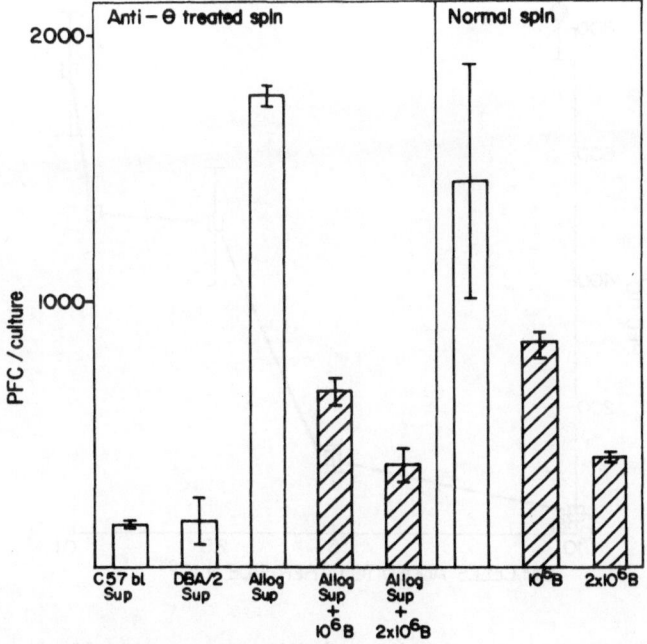

Fig. 2. Suppression of the SRBC response of anti-θ treated spleen cells reconstituted with allogeneic supernatant. Spleen cells were cultured at $8 \times 10^6/0.5$ ml for 2 days. Anti-θ treated spleen cells then received 0.5 ml of control or allogeneic supernatants while normal spleen cells received 0.5 ml of medium. PFC/10^6 values represent the mean of duplicate determinations.

Suppressor Factor Released by BMC

As our attempts to demonstrate a soluble suppressor in cell-
free BMC supernatants failed and instead resulted in a slight but
consistent augmentation of the response similar to that observed
upon addition of small numbers of BMC (10^5), we considered it a
possibility that small quantities of a soluble suppressor material
might be responsible for this stimulation or that more than one
factor was being released. In order to test this, a double-chamber
system was constructed wherein 10^7 spleen cells plus SRBC were
cultured across a 0.2 u nuclepore membrane from varying numbers of
BMC. These experiments showed that the suppression was indeed
mediated by a soluble factor (Fig. 3), and that the degree of
suppression was dependent on the number of BMC cultured across
the membrane. Spleen or thymus cells showed no suppressive
activity when cultured across the membrane.

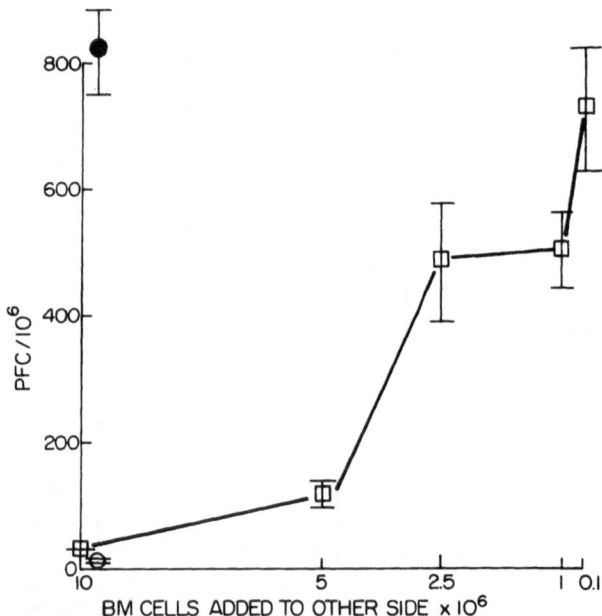

Fig. 3. Ab-suppressive activity of BMC across a cell-impermeable
membrane. 10^7 spleen cells were cultured without SRBC (O); with
SRBC (●); or with SRBC plus graded numbers of BMC across a 0.2 u
nuclepore membrane (□). PFC/10^6 values represent the mean of
duplicate cultures.

Separation of an Augmenting Factor by Dialysis

In an attempt to isolate this soluble suppressor by concentration,the supernatants were extensively dialyzed against 10 times
diluted phosphate buffered saline before lyophylization. A dose-
dependent augmentation of the response was obtained upon addition
of this material. In addition, subsequent experiments showed that
the BMC could also suppress the Ab-response across a dialysis
membrane, indicating that the suppressor material has a molecular
weight of less than 10,000.

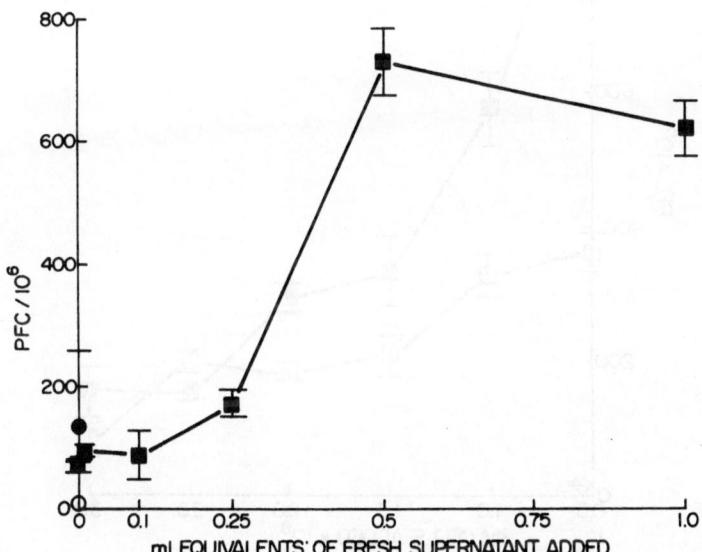

Fig. 4. Ab-augmenting activity of dialyzed, lyophylized super-
natant from BMC. Spleen cells were cultured without SRBC (0); with
SRBC (●); or with SRBC plus increasing amounts of supernatant
(■). The supernatant was obtained from 3 x 10^6 BMC/ml cultured
for 24 hrs in serum-free medium, dialyzed, and lyophylized.
PFC/10^6 values represent the mean of duplicate cultures.

BMC Supernatants Compete with the Suppressive Activity of BMC

The preceding experiments led us to conclude that BMC may release both a stimulatory and a suppressive factor, and that these factors are antagonistic. Spleen cells and SRBC were therefore cultured together with both 0.1 ml of fresh, whole BMC supernatant plus increasingly suppressive doses of BMC. Fig. 5 illustrates that a definite competition was observed between the suppressive activity of BMC and the augmenting activity of supernatant.

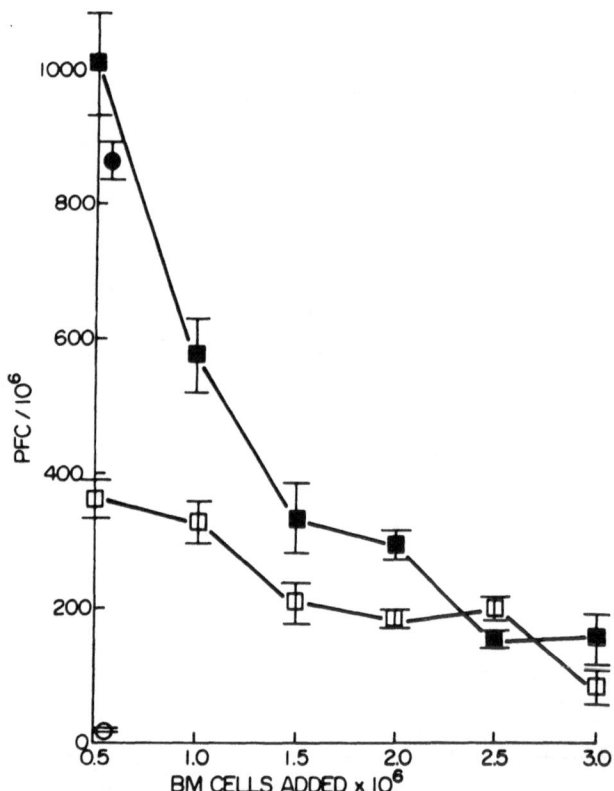

Fig. 5 Competition between Ab-suppressive activity of BMC and Ab-augmenting activity of their supernatants. Spleen cells were cultured for 5 days without SRBC (0); with SRBC (●); with SRBC plus increasing numbers of BMC (□); or with SRBC, increasing numbers of BMC plus 0.1 ml of supernatant from 3×10^6 BMC/ml precultured for 24 hrs in standard medium (■). PFC/10^6 values represent the mean of duplicate determinations.

DISCUSSION

Small numbers of BMC non-specifically suppress the Ab-response of spleen cells. This suppression is mediated by a non-adherent cell which is resistant to anti-θ and anti-macrophage serum but sensitive to radiation and anti-Ig treatments (2-4). In addition, this suppression cannot be removed with carbonyl iron (unpublished observation). Okumura and Kern (7) have recently confirmed our findings in the rabbit. They found that the suppressor cell in rabbit bone marrow is also resistant to anti-T cell serum, sensitive to anti-Ig serum, and could not be removed with glass wool.

Kinetic studies indicated that the BMC suppressor was acting on an early event in the immune response, possibly by preventing induction of Ag-reactive B or T cells (2). The inability of ATC to overcome BMC-induced suppression indicated that the BMC suppressor may act directly on the B cell. Another possibility was that the suppressor prevented release of soluble mediator(s) of T-cell function, or alternatively that suppressor T cells were being generated. This was studied using a T-cell free system in which T-cell function was replaced by allogeneic spleen cell supernatants (6). It was found that no T cells were needed for expression of suppressor activity since the BMC suppressed the response of T-depleted spleens equally as well as that of normal spleen cells.

The ability of BMC to suppress across a cell-impermeable membrane and our inability (2) and that of others (7) to detect suppressor activity in whole BMC supernatants was reconciled by the finding that BMC release an augmenting factor that competes with the soluble suppressor material. Preliminary results indicate that the suppressor released by BMC and that released by macrophages (8, 9) are different. The BMC suppressor has a molecular weight greater than 1,000, as compared to 600-800 for the macrophage factor. Furthermore, unlike the macrophage supernatant, the BMC factor does not suppress DNA synthesis in bone marrow, spleen or thymus cells (unpublished observations).

The antagonism between suppressor and stimulator factors could constitute a mechanism of dynamic regulation of the immune response if these two factors were secreted into the serum. The molecular weight of the BMC suppressor (1-10,000) is in the same range as the active component of immunoregulatory alpha-globulin (10) found in normal serum. Veit and Michael (11) have also reported enriched suppressive activity in the serum of irradiated mice reconstituted with BMC, but not thymocytes.

It is also apparent that a suppressor mechanism is required in the bone marrow component of the intact animal to prevent activation

of immature B cells. If adult BMC are incubated with specific Ag
in vitro and transferred to an irradiated host, they are incapable
of synthesizing Ab specific for that Ag (12), and it was suggested
that this is due to elimination of the specific Ag-reactive clone
of cells. Strayer et al (13) obtained analogous results by injection of specific anti-receptor Ab which produced long-term
unresponsiveness in neonatal but not adult animals. Thus the
activation of immature B cells must be avoided in order to prevent
elimination of specifically reactive clones, and a suppressor
produced in the bone marrow and acting directly on B cells would
fulfill this requirement.

Suppressor B cells have been described in a number of other
systems. Gorczynski has reported participation of a soluble factor
released by θ-negative, B-derived cells in an immunosuppressed
state of MSV-induced tumour-bearing mice (14), and B cells have
been implicated in the suppression of delayed hypersensitivity in
guinea pigs (15) as well as a cell-mediated auto-immune response
in NZB mice (16). Thus there is increasing evidence that B cells
play an important role as regulators in a variety of immune systems.

ACKNOWLEDGEMENTS

The authors wish to thank Ulla Kallstrom and Ann Levstek for
their technical assistance and Judy Verge and Phyllis Hobson for
the preparation of the manuscript. This work was supported by
the Medical Research Council of Canada.

REFERENCES

1.   Gershon, R.K., Orbach-Arbouys, S., and Calkins, C. Prog.
       Immunology 2: 122, 1974.

2.   Singhal, S.K., King, S., and Drury, P.J. Int. Arch. Allergy
       App. Immunol. 43: 934, 1972.

3.   Drury, P.J. and Singhal, S.K. Int. Arch. Allergy App.
       Immunol. 46: 707, 1974.

4.   Singhal, S.K. and Duwe, A.K. In Suppressor Cells In Immunity,
       edited by S.K. Singhal and N.R. Sinclair, University of
       Western Ontario Press, London, Canada, 1975.

5.   Mishell, R.I. and Dutton, R.W. J. Exp. Med. 126: 423, 1967.

6.   Schimpl A., and Wecker E. Nature 226: 1258, 1970.

7.   Okumura K., and Kern M.   Cell. Immunol. 17: 19, 1975.

8.   Waldman, S.R. and Gottlieb, A.A.   Cell Immunol. 9: 142, 1973.

9.   Calderon, J., Williams, R.T., and Unanue, E.R.   Proc. Nat.
     Acad. Sci. 71: 4273, 1974.

10. Occhino, J.C., Galsgow, A.H., Cooperband, S.R., Mannick, J.A.,
     and Schmid, K.   J. Immunol., 110: 685, 1973.

11. Veit, B., and Michael, J.G.   J. Immunol. 111: 341, 1973.

12. Nossal, G.J.V. and Pike, B.L.   J. Exp. Med. 141: 904, 1975.

13. Strayer, D.S., Cozenza, H., Lee, W.M.F., Rowley, D.A., and
     Kohler, H.   Science 186: 640, 1974.

14. Gorczynski, R.   J. Immunol. 112: 1826, 1974.

15. Katz, S.I., Parker, D. and Turk, J.L.   Nature 251: 550, 1974.

16. Russell, A.J., Liburd, E.M., and Diener, E.   Nature 249:
     43, 1974.

THE REGULATORY INFLUENCE OF THE THYMUS-DEPENDENT IMMUNE SYSTEM ON THE HETEROGENEITY OF IMMUNOGLOBULINS IN IRRADIATED AND RECONSTITUTED MICE

W.B. van Muiswinkel, J. Radl[*] and D.J. van der Wal

Department of Cell Biology and Genetics
Erasmus University, Rotterdam and [*]Institute for
Experimental Gerontology, TNO, Rijswijk,
The Netherlands

The transient appearance of homogeneous immunoglobulins (H-Ig), "paraproteins", in serum is a frequent finding during the reconstitution of the immune system after bone marrow transplantation in children with severe combined immunodeficiency (1) or in patients with aplastic anaemia or leukemia pretreated with an immuno-suppressive regimen (unpublished observation). Similar findings were obtained in lethally irradiated and bone marrow-reconstituted animals (2). Moreover, it was shown in rhesus monkeys that these H-Ig represent a specific antibody response towards antigenic stimulation (3).

In the present work the role played by the T-system in the regulation of the heterogeneity of serum immunoglobulins was investigated in thymectomized or sham-thymectomized mice. The animals were lethally irradiated and reconstituted with bone marrow cells or foetal liver cells. It was observed that a delay in maturation of the T cell population or the absence of the T-system contributed substantially to the appearance of H-Ig during the reconstitution period.

EXPERIMENTAL DESIGN AND METHODS

(DBA/2 x C57BL/Rij)F1 male and female mice were thymectomized (Tx) or sham-thymectomized (STx) at 5-6 weeks of age (4).

In the first experiment (exp. A, table I) the animals were lethally irradiated (825 rad of X-rays, 250 kV, 1 mm Cu filter) and injected intraveneously (i.v.) with 3×10^6 anti-Θ serum treated syngeneic bone marrow cells 2-4 weeks after surgery (4). The STx mice were subdivided: one group of STx mice received 3 intraperitoneal (i.p.) injections of 10^7 corticosteroid-resistant thymocytes (CRT) during the first week after transplantation (STx + T). The CRT were obtained from 6 weeks old mice 48 hours after i.p. injection with 30 mg/kg dexamethasone-21-phosphate (Merck & Comp. Inc., U.S.A.). The other group of STx mice received no extra CRT. Blood samples were obtained by heart puncture under nembutal anesthesia in the period between 3 and 13 weeks after transplantation. The criterion for a designation of H-Ig in the serum sample was the occurrence of a narrow, homogeneous extra band in the β-γ region when tested by agar electrophoresis according to Wieme (5) and/or of a symmetric deviation of a precipitin line in the same region by immunoelectrophoretic examination using polyvalent and monospecific antisera for mouse immuno-globulin classes and subclasses.

In the second experiment (exp. B, table I) the STx and Tx mice were reconstituted with 1.5×10^6 foetal liver cells. These liver cells were derived from embryos at 14-15 days gestation. At that time foetal liver does not contain B lymphocytes (6,7).

As a control the sera of 50 normal mice of comparable age were investigated in the same way.

RESULTS

No H-Ig were found in any of the serum samples from 50 normal untreated mice aged 5-6 months.

However, a number of H-Ig were detected in the sera of irradiated and bone marrow reconstituted mice. The frequency at which the H-Ig appeared in the various groups of mice is given in table I, experiment A. Only 3-7% of the STx + T mice developed H-Ig during the period of 3 months after transplantation. The STx mice showed a higher frequency of H-Ig (15-19%). Even higher numbers of H-Ig were detected in the sera of Tx mice (33-45%). Most of the animals could be followed during the whole period of 3 months or even longer (details of this follow-up study will be published elsewhere). The H-Ig were usually transient, but they persisted in the sera of some animals for one or even two months. On several

TABLE I

Homogeneous immunoglobulins (H-Ig) in the sera of irradiated and reconstituted mice.

Exp.	Group	Age in months	Percentage of mice with H-Ig		
			3-5	7-9	12-13
			weeks after transplantation		
A	STx + T*	3-6	7 (28)**	3 (32)	3 (28)
	STx	3-6	16 (25)	19 (36)	15 (27)
	Tx	3-6	33 (60)	45 (60)	37 (57)
B	STx	4-6	9 (23)	13 (31)	23 (30)
	Tx	4-6	20 (25)	28 (32)	33 (30)

* STx + T = sham-thymectomized mice that received 3×10^7 corticosteroid-resistant thymocytes after bone marrow transplantation; STx = sham-thymectomized mice; Tx = thymectomized mice. All mice were irradiated and injected with 3×10^6 anti-Θ serum treated bone marrow cells (Exp. A) or 1.5×10^6 foetal liver cells (Exp. B).
** Number of animals tested in parentheses.

occasions, they gradually changed into a more heterogeneous population of immunoglobulins. One homogeneous component usually appeared at a time, but two or more H-Ig were observed in some cases. Practically all immunoglobulin classes and subclasses were represented among the H-Ig observed in the immunoelectrophoresis.

In the second experiment, where STx and Tx mice were reconstituted with foetal liver cells, a similar picture was seen (Table I, Exp. B), with one exception where the maximum changes appeared later. The agreement of the results of the two experiments indicates that the H-Ig observed in the first experiment were also produced by B cell clones newly developed from hemopoietic stem cells and not from committed B cells present in the bone marrow graft.

DISCUSSION

Radl and co-workers have shown that transient H-Ig appear frequently in the serum of man (1) and monkeys (2) during reconstitution of the immune system after bone marrow transplantation. The simplest explanation of this finding is that a limited number of B cells will first arise during the development of the immune system. Later, more B cell clones will develop and a gradual transition

from homogeneous to heterogeneous responses will occur.
However, the question arises whether cell populations
other than B cells are also important in the regulation
of antibody heterogeneity. It was shown that B cells in
mice reach their normal values 3-4 weeks after irradiation and reconstitution (4,6,7). It is interesting,
therefore, that in our experiments, H-Ig were observed
in the period between 7 and 13 weeks after transplantation. The greatest numbers of H-Ig were observed in
Tx mice, but they were also frequently observed in STx
mice. It is important in this respect to realize that
the recovery rate of the T cells in normal or STx mice
after irradiation and reconstitution is slower than that
of the B cells. It has been shown that the T cell population is still below its normal level at 15 or even 30
weeks after reconstitution. (7,8). The difference in development of the T and B cells is schematically presented
in figure 1. These data, together with the observation
that the addition of T cells during the recovery period
(STx + T mice) favours a heterogeneous immunoglobulin

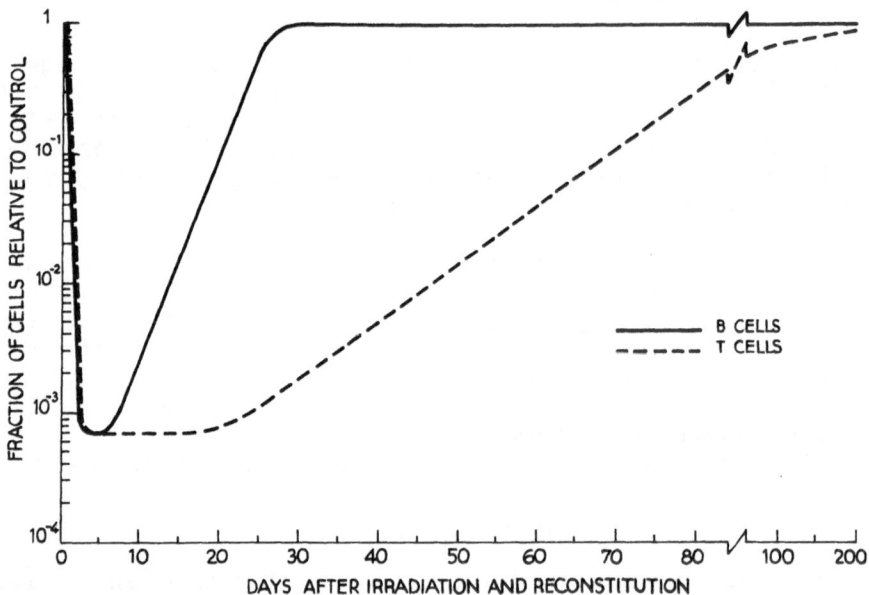

Fig. 1. A schematic diagram of the development of the B
        and T cell population in the spleen of normal
        mice after irradiation and reconstitution with
        hemopoietic stem cells.

spectrum, strongly suggest an important role of the T-system in the regulation of immunoglobulin heterogeneity. The role of the T cells may be twofold: (a) as helper cells, they can promote a response of multiple B cell clones towards thymus-dependent antigens; (b) as suppressor cells, they may prevent an overshoot reaction of a restricted number of B cell clones towards thymus-dependent (9) or "thymus-independent" antigens (10).

ACKNOWLEDGMENT

The excellent technical assistance of Miss P. van den Berg, Miss E. van der Veer and Mr. P.L. van Soest is gratefully acknowledged.

REFERENCES

1. J. Radl and P. van den Berg, p. 263, in "Protides of the Biological Fluids", Vol. 20, 1973.

2. J. Radl, P. van den Berg, M. Voormolen, U.W. Schaefer, and W.D.H. Hendriks, Clin. exp. Immunol., 16, 259, 1974.

3. P. van den Berg, J. Radl, B. Löwenberg and A.C.W. Swart (in preparation).

4. W.B. van Muiswinkel, J.J. van Beek and P.L. van Soest, Immunology, 29, (in press, 1975).

5. R.J. Wieme, Studies on agar gel electrophoresis, Arscia, Bruxelles, 1959.

6. G.J.V. Nossal and B.L. Pike, p. 11, in "Microenvironmental aspects of immunity", Plenum Press, N.Y., 1973.

7. J. Rozing and R. Benner (in these proceedings).

8. O. Vos, p. 149, in "Effects of radiation on cellular proliferation and differentiation", I.A.E.A., Vienna, 1968.

9. R.K. Gershon, p. 1, in "Contemporary topics in immunobiology", Vol. 3, Ed. by M.D. Cooper and N.L. Warner, Plenum Press, N.Y., 1974.

10. D.R. Barthold, S. Kysela and A.D. Steinberg, J. Immunol., 112, 9, 1974.

INTERFERENCE WITH ANTIBODY-FEEDBACK BY IRRADIATION, THYMUS CELLS,

THE ALLOGENEIC EFFECT, AND SERUM FACTORS

N.R.StC. Sinclair, R.K. Lees and P.L. Chan

Department of Bacteriology and Immunology
Faculty of Medicine
University of Western Ontario
London, Ontario, Canada, N6A 5C1

INTRODUCTION

Many experimental approaches have been used to analyze the mechanisms by which antibody controls various forms of immune responses. These approaches include an analysis of the structural requirements for antibody, the conditions under which antibody-mediated suppression is optimal, the determinants on antigen to which antibody must be directed and bound to attain feedback suppression, and the effects of antibody-feedback suppression on the various cellular components involved in immune responses. Another approach to the study of antibody feedback is to ask the question, "What interferes with immunosuppression by antibody?" This communication reports on four forms of interference in four different immune responses and attempts to explain these interference phenomena in terms of a single mechanism for antibody control of immune responses.

METHODS AND RESULTS

Radiosensitivity of Fc-Dependent Suppression

Many aspects of the immune response are suppressed by ionizing radiation. However, low doses of radiation have, under certain conditions, increased immune responses (1). Because of the possibility that antibody-feedback may depend upon some radiosensitive cellular activity, we compared suppression by antibody in animals which had or had not received low doses of radiation. Fig. 1 indicates the results of one such experiment in which 300 rad

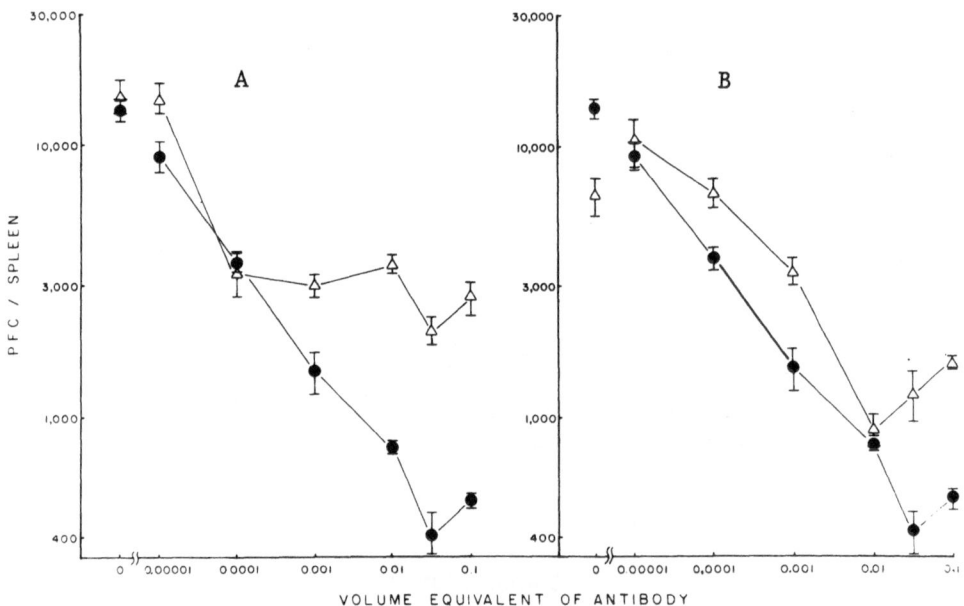

Figure 1.   Three month old male C57B1/6J mice were unirradiated
($\bullet$) or γ-irradiated with 300 rad ($\triangle$) just prior to (A) or 3 days
after (B) the intravenous injection of 10^8 sheep erythrocytes.
Varying quantities of intact IgG antibody were injected intravenously into all 4 groups of mice 3 days after the administration of
antigen.   The numbers of direct plaque-forming cells (PFC) in the
spleens were assessed by the Jerne assay 7 days after injection of
antigen.   Each point represents the mean response of 6 mice and
the vertical lines represent standard errors.

γ-irradiation decreased the sensitivity of mice to the suppressive
effects of antibody.   This radiation-induced change in sensitivity
to antibody was more noticeable when the animals were irradiated
at the time of antigen administration.   The dose of irradiation
employed altered slightly control responses (in the absense of
antibody).   Therefore, a dose of irradiation, which was ineffective
in altering the PFC response to sheep erythrocytes, conferred on
this response a degree of resistance to the immunosuppressive
effects of anti-sheep erythrocyte antibodies.

We have shown over the past number of years that there is a
structural requirement for the Fc portion of antibody for the
inhibition of anti-sheep erythrocyte immune responses (2-5).
Pepsin-digested F(ab)$_2$ antibody is suppressive but only minimumly
so and only when given at the beginning of an immune response.   To
help understand the relationship between immunosuppression

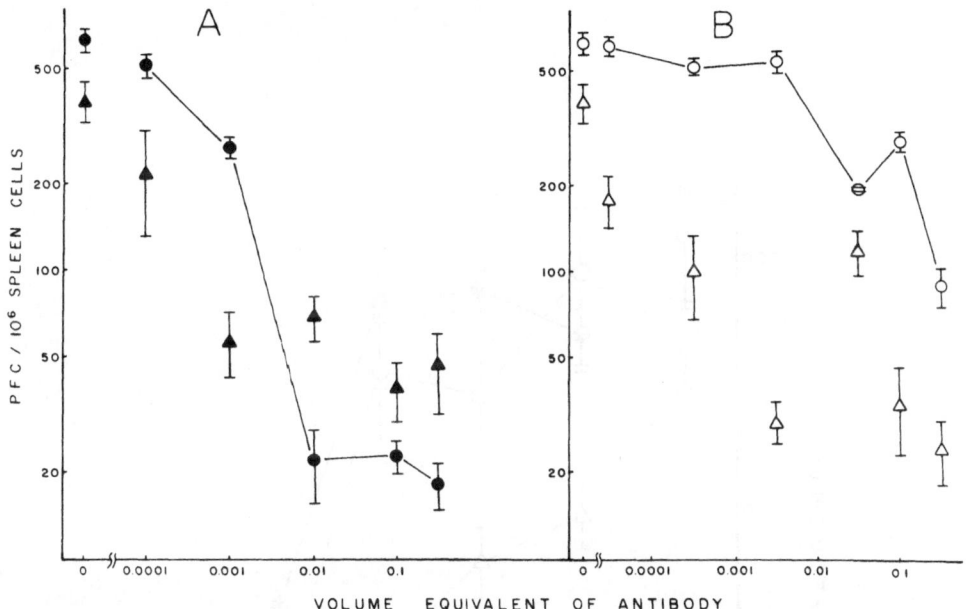

Figure 2. C57B1/6J mice, not irradiated (circles) or γ-irradiated with 300 rad (triangles) just prior to the injection of 10^8 sheeperythrocytes, were given varying quantities of intact IgG (A) or F(ab')$_2$ (B) anti-sheep erythrocyte antibody intravenously one day after the injection of antigen. The direct PFC numbers at 5 days after injection of antigen were determined, and each point represents the mean response of 6 mice with the standard errors indicated.

by antibody and irradiation, we carried out experiments to determine if irradiation-induced resistance was seen in both Fc-dependent and Fc-independent forms of immunosuppression by antibody. Non-irradiated or irradiated (300 rad) C57B1/6J mice were given varying quantities of intact IgG or F(ab')$_2$ anti-sheep erythrocyte antibody. Irradiation increased somewhat inhibition by intact IgG antibody at low doses of antibody but interfered with inhibition at high doses of antibody. The maximum depression obtained in the irradiated group was 10% of the non-antibody treated group, whereas, in non-irradiated animals, antibody reduced the PFC response to 5% or lower (Fig. 2A). This was in marked contrast to the effect of irradiation on the rather poor suppression by F(ab')$_2$ anti-sheep erythrocyte antibody (Fig. 2B). Here, 300 rad γ-irradiation potentiated the suppression of immune responses by F(ab')$_2$ antibody to an extent that the degree of suppression was similar to that obtained by intact IgG antibody in irradiated mice. These experiments

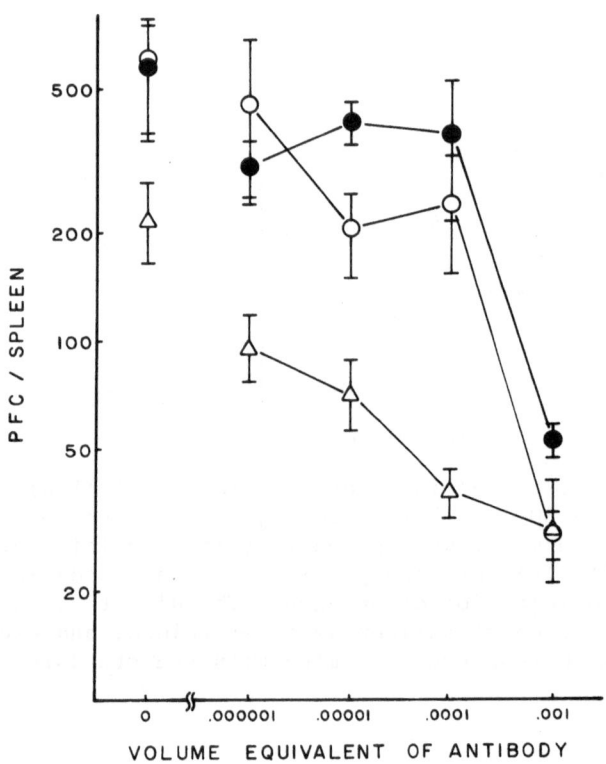

Figure 3.   Inbred Swiss mice were irradiated with 850 rad and injected with 2×10^8 sheep erythrocytes mixed with 10^7 bone marrow cells ($\triangle$), 10^7 bone marrow cells and 2×10^6 thymus cells ($\bigcirc$) or 10^7 bone marrow cells and 6×10^7 thymus cells ($\bullet$).   Three days later, varying quantities of intact IgG antibody were injected.   The numbers of antibody-forming cells in the spleen, 7 days after cell transfer and antigen injection are expressed as PFC/spleen.   Each point represents the mean of 12 mice and the vertical lines indicate standard errors.

indicate that the $F(ab')_2$ derivative of intact antibody is rather poor in causing feedback inhibition, and that low doses of irradiation interfere with feedback suppression by intact IgG antibody while potentiating feedback suppression by $F(ab')_2$ antibody.

Thymus Cell Concentration and Sensitivity to Suppression by Antibody

It has long been a contention of ours that the thymus-dependency of IgG responses (6,7) and the marked feedback potentialities of IgG antibodies (8) were somehow related (4). One possibility worth considering was that thymus cells interfere with feedback suppression by IgG antibodies, generated by activated B cells, and allow the switch from IgM to IgG synthesis to occur. An adoptive transfer experiment was carried out using inbred mice in which additional quantities of thymus cells could be transferred with a constant number of bone marrow cells. Addition of thymus cells to a bone marrow adoptive transfer gave only a modest increase in the immune response but increased resistance to antibody feedback by a factor of 10 - 100 - fold (Fig. 3). Statistically significant increases in resistance to antibody feedback were obtained in the absence of a helper augmentation of immune responses under two conditions, delaying the transfer of thymus cells until 3 days in an adoptive transfer system and adding thymus cells to a suboptimal number of spleen cells in the Marbrook culture system for an in vitro immune response (unpublished observation).

It appears then that an increase in the thymus cell concentration decreased the sensitivity of the system to immunosuppression by antibody, and that this increased resistance may occur in the absence of any augmentation of the immune response due to the presence of additional T cells.

Interference with Antibody Feedback by an Allogeneic Reaction

The above experiments indicated that thymus cells interfered with feedback suppression by antibody. One well known function of of thymus cells is the ability to induce nonspecific stimulatory factors in allogeneic reactions. This immunostimulation has been called the allogeneic effect. We carried out experiments to investigate the influence that an allogeneic reaction had on immunosuppression by antibody (Table 1). In these experiments, antibody was added either at the initiation of the cultures or one day later. The presence of an allogeneic reaction induced resistance to the feedback suppressive effect of anti-sheep erythrocyte antibody, but only when the antibody was added 1 day after the initiation of the cultures in the presence of allogeneic cells. Suppression by $F(ab')_2$ antibody was not affected by the presence of an allogeneic effect (unpublished observations).

TABLE 1

Allogeneic Effect - Interference with Antibody-Immunosuppression

	PFC/CULTURE[1]			
Antibody ml equivalent /culture	Antibody Added at Day 1		Antibody Added at Day 0	
	Without Allogeneic Cells	With Allogeneic Cells	Without Allogeneic Cells	With Allogeneic Cells
None	185 ± 37^{2}	1253 ± 46	488 ± 71	1564 ± 108
0.1	14 ± 3	598 ± 46	42 ± 4	160 ± 27

[1]
10^{7} CBA/H spleen cells were incubated in Marbrook cultures with
4×10^{6} sheep erythrocytes in the presence or absence of 10^{7}
irradiated Swiss spleen cells. The exact culture conditions
have been previously described (5).

[2]
Average of 5 cultures ± standard error.

Interference by Fetal Calf Serum with Antibody-Suppression of an In Vitro Cell-Mediated Immune Response

We have recently published data indicating that immunosuppression of an in vitro cell-mediated immune response by antibody was difficult to obtain, dependent upon limiting doses of
stimulating antigen and not dependent upon an Fc-mediated mechanism
(9). One possible explanation for these results is that an in vitro
cell mediated immune response has incorporated into it an allogeneic
effect which induces resistence to immunosuppression by antibody.
In an attempt to circumvent this inbuilt allogeneic effect, we
omitted the fetal calf serum (FCS) from the culture medium for the
first 6 hours of culture. Antibody was added at the initiation of
the cultures, and we reasoned that there may be insufficient time
for antibody to induce immunosuppression prior to the development
of an allogeneic effect. In this in vitro system for cell-mediated
immunity, 10^{7} CBA/H spleen cells were cultured with 10^{6} irradiated
(2,500 rad) DBA$_2$ spleen cells with the addition of FCS to bring the
concentration to 20% either at 0 time or at 6 hours. Anti-
stimulator cell antibody was added at the initiation of the cultures.
The absence of FCS for the first 6 hours did not effect the production of cytotoxic cells, when assayed against ^{51}chromium-labelled

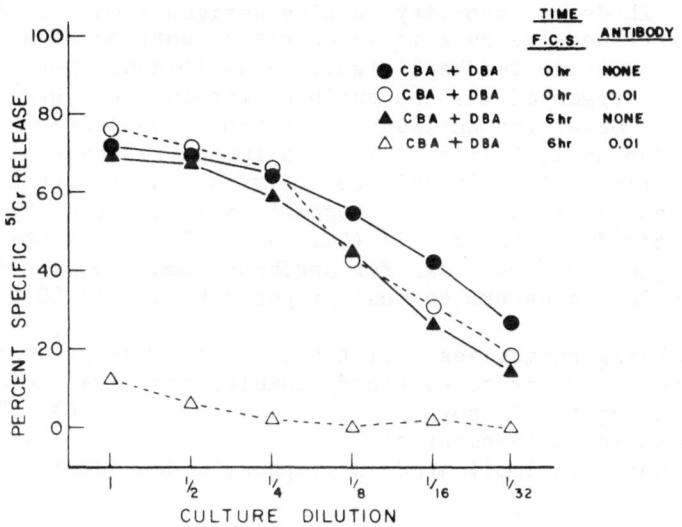

Figure 4. Ten million CBA spleen cells were incubated in CMRL 1066 at 37°C for 5 days with 10^6 DBA$_2$ spleen cells. Cultures were given FCS (20% final concentration) either at 0 time (closed symbols) or 6 hours later (open symbols) and were (triangles) or were not (circles) given anti-DBA$_2$ antibody (0.01 ml volume equivalent). The cultures were serially diluted and assessed for specific cytotoxicity against ^{51}Cr-labelled DBA$_2$ mastocytoma.

P815X DBA$_2$ mastocytoma as targets (10), in the experimental groups not receiving antibody (Fig. 4). If FCS was omitted from the culture medium for a period of 6 hours, this normally resistant in vitro cell-mediated system was made sensitive to the immuno-suppressive effects of antibody (Fig. 4).

DISCUSSION

The Fc portion of antibody is required for strong antibody-feedback (2-5). Other laboratories have confirmed this finding in various systems (11-13), but still other investigations have not revealed a significant role for the Fc portion of antibody in systems employing soluble antigens (14) or allogeneic responses (9, 15). Therefore, there appear to be differences in the requirement for the Fc portion of antibody in antibody-immunosuppression depending upon the immune response under study, and, indeed, T cell responses appear to be resistant to Fc-mediated feedback (9, 24)

Having established that the requirement for the Fc portion of antibody was not a product of some artifactual consideration, such

as loss of antibody or inability to bind antigen (3-5), we developed
a model for antibody-feedback in which the Fc portion of antibody
transmitted a negative feedback signal to an immunocompetent cell
(16), which we suggested was the antibody-forming cell precursor, a
B cell (4). In order for antibody to be immunosuppressive, antibody
must bind to the antigen stimulating the immune response. By binding
to antigen, antibody is able to interact with, and suppress, B cells
binding the same antigen, via a cytophilic attachment of the Fc
portion of antibody to the B cell (Fig. 5A). Other investigators
have since suggested mechanisms for antibody-immunosuppression
which are similar in nature to that proposed by us (17-20).

Besides being themselves resistant, T cells may prevent these
forms of Fc-mediated antigen-antibody complex inactivation of
B cells by binding the Fc portions of antibody (Fig. 5B). This
prevents the direct attachment of Fc portions to the B cells. Since
T cells have not been implicated in lymphocyte-dependent antibody

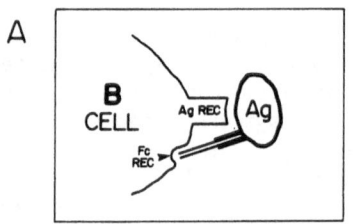

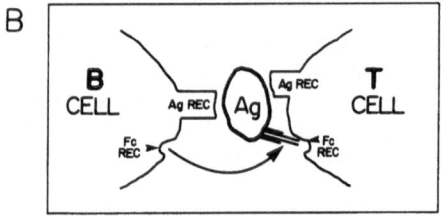

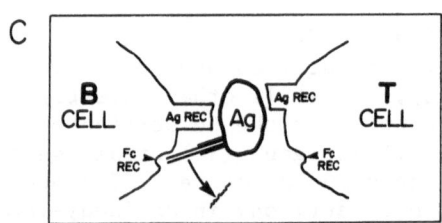

Figure 5. Fc-dependent models for (A) B cell inactivation (B)
T cell prevention of B cell inactivation and (C) T cell accentuation
of B cell inactivation by antigen-antibody complexes.

cytotoxicity, this form of interaction would not lead to a cytotoxic attack by T cells on B cells. Activation of T cells involves an increase in Fc receptor density (21), and this increase may prevent Fc-dependent antibody-feedback. However, one reason to suspect that this increase may not relate to T cell prevention of antibody-feedback, comes from experiments performed in Herzenberg's laboratory (22) which may indicate that, in the activation of T helper cells, little in the way of Fc receptors can be found either prior to or after activation, whereas Fc receptors do appear on T cells which become cytotoxic in cell-mediated immune responses.

In the process of allogeneic activation of T cells, either the Fc receptor density on T cells may increase or nonspecific factors, produced by T cells undergoing allogeneic activation, may bind to the Fc portion of antibody and prevent their binding to B cells.

The resistance of the _in vitro_ cell-mediated immune response to antibody immunosuppression in the presence of FCS and its sensitivity in the absence of FCS could be explained in a number of ways. The absence of FCS may prevent T cell activation which may not occur until the addition of FCS to the culture system. During this time, anti-stimulator cell antibody may bind to stimulator cell antigen and induce an antigen-antibody complex inhibition of T cells. Another possibility is that factors present in FCS can bind to the Fc portion of antibody such that antibody does not interact with T cells in a way necessary to cause T cell suppression. FCS does not possess factors inhibiting the Fc-mediated inactivation of B cells since inactivation can be demonstrated in the presence of FCS (5). We are in the process of determining whether or not suppression by antibody in the absence of FCS is dependent upon the Fc portion of antibody.

In mounting an adequate helper cell effect, T cells may present antigen-antibody complexes to the surface of B cells in such a way that the B cells can interact with antigenic determinants on the immunogen without interacting with Fc portions of attached antibody (Fig. 5B). However, if T cells are unable to pre-empt the Fc portions of antibody, B cells will receive concomitant signals from antigenic determinants and the Fc portions of antibody to become inactivated (Fig. 5C). This may happen when the T cells are present in insufficient numbers (4), when the Fc receptors on T cells are not adequate for binding Fc portions, when the initial B cell product overwhelms T cell activities such that T cells cannot handle these feedback suppressive products (23) and when exogenous antibody enters the system in amounts which exhaust the ability of T cells to bind Fc portions. In such situations, T cells would function as suppressor cells (23).

Low doses of irradiation may impair the ability of T cells to respond to antigen. The limited number of T cells may be fully occupied in cooperating with B cells in response to the earlier injection of antigen. With the administration of antibody at some time following the stimulation of the immune response, there may be too few circulating T cells which could recognize the antigen–antibody complexes and bring these complexes to responding B cells. Another possibility is that 300 rad γ-irradiation is not high enough to reduce the T cell numbers below the functional reserve and the T cell system is activated to replace the loss due to irradiation; hence, low doses of irradiation may increase resistance to antibody-immunosuppression by increasing T cell activity as in other experimental systems described in this paper. Irradiation augmented the immunosuppression by $F(ab')_2$ antibody, given 1 day after antigen and irradiation. Irradiation may impair the ability of the lymphoid system to sequester antigen in a form which is resistant to the suppressive effect of $F(ab')_2$ antibody; and $F(ab')_2$ antibody given with antigen is more immunosuppressive than that given 1 day after antigen (4).

SUMMARY

Low doses of irradiation, increased number of T cells, increased T cell activity as in the allogeneic effect, or early activation of an _in vitro_ cell-mediated immune response all confer resistance to antibody feedback. In some of these systems, the resistance is directed against immunosuppression by intact IgG antibody whereas suppression by $F(ab')_2$ antibody is either not changed or increased. These forms of interference with immunosuppression by antibody, are explained in terms of an Fc-dependent model for antibody-feedback regulation.

ACKNOWLEDGEMENTS

This work has been supported by grants from the Medical Research Council of Canada and the National cancer Institute of Canada.

REFERENCES

1. Taliaferro, W.H., Taliaferro, L.G., and Janssen, E.F., J. Infect. Diseases, 91: 105, 1952.

2. Sinclair, N.R.StC., J. Exp. Med., 129: 1183, 1969.

3. Sinclair, N.R.StC., Lees, R.K., Chan, P.L., and Khan, R.H., Immunology, 19: 105, 1970.

4. Chan, P.L., and Sinclair, N.R.StC., Immunology, 21: 967, 1971.

5. Lees, R.K., and Sinclair, N.R.StC., Immunology, 24: 735, 1973.

6. Sinclair, N.R.StC., Clin. Exp. Immunol., 2: 701, 1967.

7. Mitchell, G.F., Grumet, F.C., and McDevitt, H.O., J. Exp. Med., 135: 136, 1972.

8. Uhr, J.W., and Moller, G., Adv. Immunol., 8: 81, 1968.

9. Sinclair, N.R.StC., Lees, R.K., Fagan, G., and Birnbaum, A., Cell. Immunol., 16: 330, 1975.

10. Cerottini, J.C., and Brunner, K.T., Adv. Immunol., 18: 67, 1974.

11. Abrahams, S., Phillips, R.A., and Miller, R.G., J. Immunol., 137: 870, 1972.

12. Kappler, J.W., van der Hoven, A., Dharmarajan, U., and Hoffman, M., J. Immunol., 111: 1228, 1973.

13. Wason, W.M., and Fitch, F.W., J. Immunol., 110: 1427, 1973.

14. Feldmann, M., and Diener, E., J. Immunol., 108: 93, 1972

15. Kaliss, N., Sinclair, N.R.StC., and Cantrell, J.L., in preparation.

16. Sinclair, N.R.StC., and Chan, P.L., Adv. Exp. Biol. Med., 12: 609, 1971.

17. Gorczynski, R., Kontiainen, S., Mitchison, N.A., and Tigelaair, R.E., in Cellular Selection and Regulation in the Immune Response, edit. by Edelman, G.M., p. 143, Raven Press, New York, 1974.

18. Gordon, J., and Murgita, R.A., Cell. Immunol., 15: 392, 1975.

19. Sachs, D.H., and Dickler, H.B., Transplant. Rev., 23: 159, 1975.

20. Waldmann, H., and Lachmann, P.J., Europ. J. Immunol., 5: 185, 1975.

21. Yoshida, T.O., and Anersson, B., Scand. J. Immunol., 1: 401, 1972.

22. Herzenberg, L., in General Discussion, Suppressor Cells in Immunity, edit. by Singhal, S.K., and Sinclair, N.R.StC., The University of Western Ontario Press, 1975.

23. Gershon, R.K., Contempt. Topics Immunobiol., 3: 1, 1974.

24. Hoffmann, M.K., Kappler, J.W., Hirst, J.A., Oettgen, H.F., Eur. J. Immunol., 4: 282, 1974.

EFFECT OF CHORIONIC GONADOTROPINS ON HUMORAL AND CELL-MEDIATED IMMUNITY

Fabris N. and Piantanelli L.

Exp. Geront. Ctr - Research Dept. - I.N.R.C.A.

Via Birarelli, 8 - 60100 A N C O N A - Italy

In order to explain the depression of cell-mediated immunity observed during pregnancy, serum bloking antibody, as well as, known hormones, such as corticosteroids, progesterone, oestrogens and chorionic gonadotropins have been taken into consideration (for review see Fabris, Piantanelli and Muzzioli, submitted). That immune responses may be influenced by some female hormones is proven by the observation that in numerous species females outperform the males in terms of antibody production and that males may be turned off to female pattern by castration (Eidinger and Garrett, 1972). Moreover, the possibility that some female hormones may, in particular, depress cell-mediated immunity is supported by the observation that women taking oral contraceptives show a reduced "in vitro" blastic trasformation to P.H.A. (Barnes et al, 1974) and that the menstrual cycle itself may modulate P.H.A. responses (Fabris, Ghislieri and Bevilacqua, submitted).

The assumption, how ever, that the peculiar hormonal balance of pregnancy is responsible for the immunological disturbances observed in that period, needs further experimental evidence, which avoids the oversimplification to consider pregnancy in different species as characterized by identical hormonal patterns (for review see Davies and Ryan, 1973). In mice we have shown that contact allergic reactions to picryl chloride are depressed during pregnancy, while plaque-forming-cell (PFC) responses are increased, the positive effect of pregnancy on PFC capacity being more indicative of possibile hormonal influences than the simple depression of cell-mediated immunity (Fabris, 1973).

In order to prove whether a unique hormonal mechanism is responsible for the opposite effect of pregnancy on humoral and

cell-mediated immunity, we have compared the PFC capacity against sheep erythrocytes and the mixed unidirectional leucocytes
reaction (UMLR) of spleen cells from pregnant mice with those of
spleen cells from mice daily treated with hormones, such as human
chorionic gonadotropins (HCG), human luteotropic hormone (LTH)
and progesterone, whose synthesis is physiologically increased
during pregnancy. Pregnant Charles River mice at different stages of gestation and virgin female mice treated for 15 days with
HCG, LTH or progesterone were used. These hormones were kindly supplied in highly purified form by Richter, through the cour-
tesy of Prof. Matscher. The results given by pregnant or hormones treated mice were compared to those observed in control mice,
the difference being expressed as index of variation : the unit (1)
indicates no variation, higher values enhancement, lower values
inhibition. Details will be published else were (Fabris, Piantanelli and Muzzioli, submitted).

PFC capacity, as measured by the 4th day peak response, is
significantly increased during pregnancy whereas UML reactions
are strongly depressed (see table). Both depression of UML reactivity and increased PFC capacity are observable at mid-pregnancy.

Daily treatment of virgin female mice with HCG, but not with
LTH or progesterone, induces immunological alterations, which
are strikingly similar to those observed at mid-pregnancy.

Days of pregnancy		UML reaction index of variation		Haemolitic plaques index of variation	
8		0.60	P< 0.05	1.90	–
12		0.51	P< 0.05	2.45	P < 0.05
15		0.98	–	3.07	P < 0.001
18		1.20	–	1.19	–
Horm. treatment					
HCG	20 μg	0.22	P< 0.001	0.92	–
HCG	100 μg	0.25	P< 0.001	3.10	P < 0.001
HCG	500 μg	0.41	P< 0.05	2.18	P < 0.05
LTH	20 μg	0.79	–	1.17	–
LTH	100 μg	1.11	–	1.16	–
LTH	500 μg	1.22	–	1.5	–
Prog.	20 μg	0.75	P< 0.05	not done	
Prog.	100 μg	1.10	–	1.42	–
Prog.	500 μg	0.96	–	1.37	–

Effect of pregnancy or of 15 daily injections with HCG, LTH
or progesterone, at the daily dose indicated above, on humoral
(PFC response) or cell-mediated (UMLR) immunity.
Index = 1, no variation   Index = 0, complete inhibition
Index   1, enhancement

Moreover the total number of nucleated cells in the slpeen is not significantly modified by hormonal treatment, thus suggesting that dilution effects are not main cause of the observed alterations. An incidental observation is that the spontaneous "in vitro" blastic trasformation by spleen cells increases either at mid-pregnancy or after HCG or progesterone treatments.

The similarity between the immunological behaviour of HCG treated mice and that observed during pregnancy favours the assumption that HCG may be factor playing, directly or undirectly, the major role on the immunological disturbances of gestation, at least in the mouse. Other hormones, which are also synthetized in higher amounts during pregnancy in the mouse, such as oestrogens or corticosteroids, have been discarded in our investigation, because the progressive increase of their synthesis until delivery does not correlate with the mid-pregnancy patterns of immunological alterations.

With regard to the specificity of the action of HCG on the UML reactivity it seems to us not casual the fact that the depression of PHA response observed in women lymphocytes at mid-menstrual cycle (Fabris, Ghislieri and Bevilacqua, submitted) correlates well only with the cyclic pattern of luteinizing hormone, which shares with HCG the majority of its functions.

The opposite effect of HCG on humoral and cell-mediated immune response, besides representing a factor for the safety of the foetus either by depressing transplantation immunity or by favouring enhancing antibody production, may help to understand a number of related problems, such as the increased frequency of autoantibody in women, the shorter life-expectancy recorded in suffering from tumors arisen during pregnancy and, may be, the extremely high invasiveness of HCG producing molar carcinomas.

Moreover the different effect of HCG on humoral and cell-mediated immunity, together with the findings on hormones other than HCG gives evidence to the existence of an "Hormonal-dependent" compartimentation of the lymphoid system (Fabris and Piantanelli, submitted).

REFERENCES

Barnes E.W., Loudon N.B., MacCuish A.C., Jordan J. and Irvine W.J. - Lancet, i, 898, 1974
Davies J. and Ryan K.J., Vitam. Horm. 30, 223, 1972
Eidinger D. and Garrett T.J.-J. exp. Med. 136, 1098, 1972.
Fabris N., Experientia, 29, 610, 1973
Fabris N., Piantanelli L. and Muzzioli M., Clin. exp. Immunol. (submitted for pubblication)

Fabris N., Ghislieri L. and Bevilacqua P., The Lancet (submitted for pubblication)

Fabris N. and Piantanelli L., J. exp. Med. (submitted for publication)

AUGMENTATION OF CELL MEDIATED LYSIS (CML) BY THF

Tehila Umiel, Amnon Altman and Nathan Trainin

Department of Cell Biology

The Weizmann Institute of Science, Rehovot, Israel

Cell-mediated immunity can be studied in detail in the in-vitro mixed lymphocyte culture (MLC) system which consists of two sequential phases: A proliferative phase which is believed to represent the recognition phase of the homograft response (1,2) and cell mediated immune lysis which is considered to represent the effector phase of this response (3). Experimental data suggest that T-cells proliferating in MLC may be distinct from those T-cells which differentiate into killer cells and cause cell mediated lysis (CML) (4,5,6). We have found that THF, a thymic hormone, increases the reactivity of T-cells responding in the proliferative phase of MLC (7). In the present study we attempted to analyze the effect of THF on the reactivity of effector cells involved in CML.

MATERIALS AND METHODS

Mice: Two-3 month old male C57BL/6, C3H/eb and (C3H/eb x C57BL/6)F_1 hybrids were supplied by the Animal Breeding Center of the Weizmann Institute of Science, Rehovot.

Thymectomy: Thymectomy was performed on 6-8 week old C57BL/6 mice under nembutal anesthesia and thymuses were removed by suction. Mice later found to contain thymus remnants were discarded from the experiments.

Preparation of cells: Spleens were removed aseptically. The organs were gently dispersed through a stainless steel mesh and the cells were suspended in RPMI-1640 medium (Grand Island Biological Co., N.Y., N.Y.) buffered with sodium bicarbonate, and supplemented with penicillin (100 units/ml) and streptomycin (10 µg/ml) and 15% heat inactivated fetal bovine serum (FBS) (Rehatuin, Reheis Chemical Co., Chicago, Ill.), cells were washed twice in RPMI-1640 medium and counted in Turk's solution in a hemocytometer.

Mixed lymphocyte culture (MLC): C57BL/6 spleen cell suspensions (10×10^7 cells) prepared in RPMI-1640 supplemented with 15% FBS were incubated with an equal number of mitomycin-C treated (C3H/eb x C57/6)F_1 spleen cells in a volume of 10 ml in 100 mm plastic petri dishes. The cell mixtures were incubated for 6 days at 37^oC in a humidified atmosphere of 5% CO_2 in air.

Exposure of cells to THF: Partially purified calf thymus extract (THF) prepared as previously described (8) was used at a concentration of 1 mg protein/ml of 0.005 M Na phosphate buffer pH 7.4. THF (20 µg/ml) was supplemented to culture medium for the entire experimental period or added to the effector phase only.

CML assay: Effector cells were harvested from the cultures 6 days after sensitization. Cells were counted and resuspended to a cell concentration of 4×10^6/ml in Dulbecco's modified Eagle's medium supplemented with 10% FBS. Target cells were prepared by culturing the cells with 4 µg/ml of Concanavalin A for 48 hrs. Blast cells obtained by this procedure were labeled in 0.6 ml of medium containing 150 µCi Na_2 $^{51}CrO_4$ for 90 min. Cells were then washed and resuspended to a cell concentration of 4×10^4/ml in Eagle's medium. Effector and target cells in a ratio of 100:1 were incubated for 4 hrs in plastic tubes and then 1.5 ml cold PBS was added to each tube. The tubes were centrifugated for 10 min and samples of 1 ml of supernatant from each tube were removed into counting tube and counted. CML was calculated according to the following formula:

$$\% \text{ CML} = \frac{\text{CPM in 1 ml samples of sup x 2}}{\text{total CPM}}$$

EXPERIMENTAL AND DISCUSSION

It has been suggested that the presence of the thymus is a prerequisit for the generation of effector T cells in the MLC system (9). We have shown that THF, a hormone produced by the thymus can augment the reactivity of T lymphocytes in the recognition phase of MLC when cell proliferation was measured (7). It was of interest to find out whether THF can also participate in the processes which lead to the generation of effector cells in MLC. Thus, responder C57BL spleen cells were incubated for 6 days in a MLC system together with mitomycin-C treated stimulator (C3H/eb x C57BL/6)F_1 spleen cells with or without THF. The cells were then harvested and tested for their lytic effect (CML) on ^{51}Cr labeled target cells with or without THF. It was found (Table 1) that THF stimulated generation of killer cells when present in the culture

TABLE 1

Increase of cell mediated lysis (CML) by effector C57BL/6 spleen cells following their sensitization against mitomycin-C treated (C3H/eb x C57BL/6)F_1 spleen cells in the presence of THF during MLC period

THF[a] during sensitization phase (MLC)	THF[a] during effector phase (CML)	% cytolysis $\pm$ SE[b,c]	P
-	-	29.3 $\pm$ 1.3	
-	+	32.2 $\pm$ 0.9	N.S.[d]
+	-	40.5 $\pm$ 2.5	< 0.01
+	+	37.6 $\pm$ 2.7	< 0.05

a) 20 µg protein/ml
b) CML was assayed against C3H/eb ^{51}Cr labeled target cells.
c) SE = standard error
d) N.S. = non significant difference

medium during the MLC. When THF was added only to the effector phase no stimulatory effect by THF could be observed. This may suggest that THF affects the process of generation of effector cells responding to allogeneic stimulus but does not influence cytolysis itself.

Since the effect of THF on CML was established by these experiments, we attempted to find out whether THF also functions in a MLC system in which responder cells were derived from thymectomized mice. It was found (Table 2) that a marked reduction in the CML activity was apparent 2 months after thymectomy, this reduction being even more severe 5 months following thymus deprivation. When THF was present in the culture medium during the MLC period, an increase in the cytolytic activity of spleen cells of such mice by THF to the level of spleen cells of intact donors was observed. This suggests that THF could compensate for the defect caused by adult thymectomy to the population of cells differentiating into effector cells in the MLC system. Thus, it was concluded that THF can increase the activity of cells participating in the MLC proliferative phase (7) as well as the cells participating in the effector phase of such assay.

Whether THF affects a cell population which first proliferate as a result of antigenic stimulation and then further differentiate into effector cells or whether THF can activate a different cell population, those participating in MLC and others in the CML, cannot be resolved as yet. More data is needed to define the source of T cells participating in the different phases of the MLC.

TABLE 2

The activity of THF on generation of effector C57BL/6 spleen cells
from thymectomized mice stimulated with mitomycin-C treated (C3H/eb
x C57BL/6)F_1 spleen cells.

Responder cells	THF[a]	% cytolysis $\pm$ SE[b,c]	P
spleen of intact mice	-	42.1 $\pm$ 1.00	
spleen of thymectomized mice 2 months after	-	29.1 $\pm$ 0.55	<< 0.001
thymectomy	+	43.8 $\pm$ 2.35	N.S.[d]
spleen of thymectomized mice 5 months after	-	19.0 $\pm$ 2.30	<< 0.001
thymectomy	+	38.8 $\pm$ 1.39	N.S.

a) THF was present in the culture medium for 6 days at 20 µg protein/ ml.
b) CML was assayed against C3H/eb ^{51}Cr labeled target cells.
c) SE = standard error.
d) N.S. = non significant difference.

SUMMARY

The in-vitro model of cell mediated lysis (CML) was used to
study whether a thymic hormone (THF) participates in the processes
which lead to generation of effector cells. It was found that THF
increases the capacity of effector cells from spleens of intact
mice in the CML assay. This effect of THF on generation of effect-
or cells was manifested when THF was present during the mixed
lymphocyte culture. On the other hand, addition of THF to the
effector (CML) phase did not elevate the lytic capacity of killer
cells. Moreover, THF compensated the impaired lytic capacity of
effector cells from adult thymectomized mice and raised it to the
level of intact mice.

These results are compatible with the hypothesis that THF
acts on the generation of CML effector cells of both intact and
adult thymectomized mice.

ACKNOWLEDGMENT

This work was supported by the National Institutes of Health, under agreement NC1-G-721-3890.

REFERENCES

1. Wilson, D.B., Bluth, J.L. and Nowell,P.C.   J. Exp. Med. 1968. 128: 1157.
2. Bach, F.H., Back, H., Graunper, K., Day, E. and Klosterma, H. Proc. Natl. Acad. Sci. USA 1969. 62: 374.
3. Hayry, P., Andersson, L.C., Nordling, S. and Viralainen, M. Transplant. Rev. 1972. 12: 91.
4. Bach, F.H., Segall, M., Stanberizer, K., Sondel, P.M. and Alter, B.J. Science 1973. 180: 403.
5. Stobo, J.D., Paul, W.E. and Henney, C. J. Immunol. 1973. 110: 652.
6. Kono, S., Bloom, B.R. and Howe, M.L. Proc. Natl. Acad. Sci. USA 1973. 70: 2299.
7. Umiel, T. and Trainin, N. Eur. J. Immunol. 1975. 5: 85.
8. Trainin, N. and Small, M. J. Exp. Med. 1970. 132: 885.
9. Andersson, L.C., Hayry, P., Bach, M.A. and Bach, J.F. Nature 1974. 252: 252.

CONCLUDING REMARKS TO SESSION EIGHT:

SUPPRESSOR CELLS AND ENHANCING ANTIBODIES: IMMUNE AGENTS

OF THE FACILITATION REACTION

G. A. Voisin

Centre d'Immuno-Pathologie et d'Immunologie Experimentale
de l'INSERM et de l'Association Claude-Bernard, Hopital
Saint-Antoine, 75102 Paris, France)

Suppressor cells and enhancing antibodies can be understood as the
cellular and humoral agents of what I have called the facilitation reaction
(FR). Under physiological conditions, this active, specific immune reaction does always take place in front of a (at least potential) rejection
reaction (RR), so that one is led to write the equation IR = RR + FR,
indicating that the immune reaction is the result of a rejection reaction
interfered with by a facilitation reaction.

The role of the FR is to insure an active homeostasis of the RR. It
prevents the latter from reaching an exaggerated and dangerous level.
Its highest degree culminates in immunological tolerance (the physiologically most meaningful form of immunological tolerance), as already proposed -- but rejected -- in 1961 and demonstrated further since that time.
This very process of active tolerance appears necessary for both individual
and species survival.

Among the two types of immune agents are the following:

(1) The suppressor cells. These have been mostly studied in this session.
Among the many very interesting facts that we have learnt (and that were
very adequately summarized at the beginning of the session) I shall take a
few home with my luggage. In particular:

(a) The multiplication of the types of suppressive cells — T, B and
others—as well as of the types of suppressive activities and targets for

645

suppression -- antigen-specific and nonspecific activities; suppression of activities of B-, T-helpers, T-killers, GVH, MLC, CLM, etc. Still no one has spoken of mast cells yet.

(b)   New data on ontogeny of suppressor T cells from different laboratories seem to indicate that cortisone resistant suppressor cells stem from cortisone-sensitive precursors, themselves originating from non-T cells.

(c)   Even discrepancies between several groups of results may eventually bring some light on significant factors of variation such as different proportions of different cell populations of lymphocytes (especially of antagonistically acting cells) in different strains, during reactions to different antigens, at different steps of the evolution of an essentially dynamic process.

But rather than trying to influence your own choice, I should try to re-establish the balance of the session by saying a few words on the humoral factors of suppression.

(2) Enhancing antibodies. Although they are on the program they have not been dwelt upon this morning. Still it would have been of interest to learn -- or to be reminded of -- the following.

Enhancing antibodies have usually been mainly considered for their peripheral action (the easiest to be studied), that is one of competition for antigen leading both to a decreased immune stimulation and to a protection of the antigen-bearing target against the immune agents of the rejection reaction.

Still more interesting is their central action on the immune system, although not clearly understood yet.

Two aspects seem to be of particular interest: the class of the responsible antibodies and their form of action.

A.   Their class: non complement fixing, anaphylactic antibodies (especially of mouse IgG_1 class) have consistently been found in our hands to be linked with enhancing and facilitating properties in several situations. Let me mention, for instance:

(i)   In transplantation sera raised in different ways, the enhancing properties were found to be linked to the presence of anaphylactic activity, not to that of C'-fixing one (Transplantation, 1972, 13:452).

(ii) In DEAE-cellulose fractions of transplantation sera, the enhancing activity was found most intense in the fractions most anaphylactic, without respect to the C'-fixing activity. The latter, on the contrary, was not usually found linked to an inhibitory activity of IgG_2 fraction (idem).

(iii) In the case of experimental allergic encephalomyelitis induced in the guinea pig by encephalitogenic basic protein in complete adjuvants, a negative correlation was also found between the incidence of specific anaphylactic antibodies in the serum (Int. Arch. Allergy 1974, 46:82).

(iv) Finally, studying the active production of anti-DNP classes of antibodies in the guinea pig it was found, among other things, that the production of anti-DNP IgG_1 antibodies was decreased by passive injections of anti-carrier IgG_1 antibodies, while it was eventually increased by anti-hapten IgG_1 (Eur. J. Immunol. 1973, 3:90; J. exp. Med. 1973, 137:265).

These experiments stress the importance of IgG_1 as immunoregulatory agents.

In view of the discrepancies between the preceding results of those who found IgG_2a antibodies to be the agents of immune enhancement, new experiments were performed in our laboratory. During these, IgG_2 antibodies could be rendered enhancing in two ways: by dilution and by complexing to the corresponding antigens.

B. The form of action of enhancing antibodies is actually important. It is now clear that at least some types of antibodies are active under the form of of circulating immune complexes. This has been shown in simple experiments where specific transplantation immune sera were mixed with various proportions of corresponding antigens. Only the specific immune complexes in antibody excess, or at equivalence, were found to be active. Antibody alone and antigen alone were inactive (Ann. Immunol. Inst. Pasteur 1973, 124:567).

C. The importance of the role of enhancing antibodies under physiological circumstances is attested by in vivo experiments. For instance, immunoglobulins (mainly of the IgG_1 type) are found to stay fixed on mouse placentae even after washing. They can be eluted (acid elution) and studied. They can be fixed on thymocytes of the father's (not the mother's) strain, and, when injected to normal mice of the mother's strain, they can render them unable to reject a tumor graft of the father's strain (J. Reprod. Fertil. 1974, suppl. 21:89).

A last and most important chapter, a chapter for the future (but the future begins today), is the next chapter.

(3) The functional relation between suppressor cells and enhancing anti-bodies. If these two immune agents are really part of a common physio-logical process, namely, the facilitation reaction, they must have some functional relation.

Two attractive possibilities are explored in our laboratory, related to the roles of immune complexes and anaphylactic antibodies, respectively.

(a) Immune complexes are expected to be retained by cells having the specific receptors for the antigen and to react on these cells through their activated Fc portion. This may require a Fc receptor at the cell surface. One may imagine that such immune complexes (possibly of a given class) inactivate potentially reactive cells (T or B) or, alternatively, activate suppressor cells.

(b) Anaphylactic antibodies are known to be able to fix on mast cell Fc receptors and to degranulate these mast cells upon contact with the cor-responding antigen. This leads to the release of active amines (histamine, serotonine) and other substances. The regulatory role of anaphylactic antibodies might conceivably be exerted by mast cells and their degranula-tion products.

That this is possible was shown by experiments showing that the pro-duct of mast cell degranulation is able to depress a primary in vitro re-sponse as measured in a Mishell and Dutton system. The response can be re-established by anti-histamin. The depressive effect can be obtained also by adding to the culture either mast cells sensitized to the immunizing anti-gen (sheep or horse RBC), histamine or serotonine.

Here again the phenomenon appears to have some physiological rel-evanace since it has also proved to be effective in vivo.

This concept of "suppressor mast cells" might enlighten the meaning of histamine receptors at the surface of T suppressor cells. It might also bring the beginning of an answer to the long-asting riddle: What is the biological significance of anaphylaxis ?

Immunophathology

IMMUNOPATHOLOGY

J.D. Feldman

Scripps Clinic and Research Foundation

La Jolla, California, 92037, U. S. A.

This session of immunopathology covers the subject from A to T, i.e., from amyloidosis to tumorigenesis. We shall hear about T and B lymphocytes dysfunction in amyloidosis and systemic lupus erythematosus; about autoimmune disease and a suggestion for its cure by use of a biological factor that induces differentiation of T lymphocytes; about association of cellular disorders with a genetic disability and with neoplastic states; and we shall hear about certain morphological changes in diseased tissues that are related to immunologic processes, as in certain forms of chronic liver disease and amyloidosis.

The session of immunopathology reflects the state of the art and science in immunopathology. Although there is considerable activity in immunopathology and clinical immunology, there is still a lag in transferring and translating the mass of information that constitutes the infrastructure of immunology to diseases and tissue injuries that occur in the living host as a result of immunologic phenomena. To achieve its full potential, I perceive three goals that should be attained so that immunopathology may be considered a discipline of biomedicine in its own right.

First, a supply of reliable standard reagents should be developed, especially for human patients, for examination and detection of immunologic reactants in the tissues of living animals. Such reagents should be capable of measuring antibodies of different classes and antibodies of different specificities both in the circulation, in diseased tissues and in single cells. It is no longer sufficient to report antibody titers of 1:256 or 1:10,000. Rather the presence and amount of IgG_1, IgG_2, IgM etc. in microgram or nanogram quantities can be recorded. Even more important, it would be desirable to know the antigens to which antibody is

being made. In diseased states, the crucial unknown component of
immunologic processes is usually tissue antigen; it is therefore
difficult to ascertain which antigens are eliciting an antibody
response.

A second category of reagents should be available to distinguish
unequivocally, in situ, T and B lymphocytes, macrophages, K cells,
blast elements and other effector cells still unidentified. Imagine
the immunopathologist examining a biopsy with immunologic reagents
and being able to determine a deficiency or excess of T cells, or
macrophages or whatever elements compose the injured area.

After suitable and sensitive reagents are available, immunopathologists should learn if the many immunologic reactions that
occur in vitro, also occur in vivo. Is there biologic reality to
a microcytotoxicity test? Do mitogenic stimulations with lectins
have their counterparts in the living host?

A third and most important goal for immunopathology is to determine if the immunologic reactants in damaged tissues and organs
are the cause or the result of disease. Since immunopathology is
in a pivotal position that connects it with basic research and with
disease in animals and humans, immunopathologists have the advantage of being able to discover etiology, trace the course of
disease, and establish the markers of immunologic disorders.

Let us proceed now with our session on Immunopathology. I
hope we may enjoy a lively interchange of ideas and knowledge and
that we make some progress in determining what is cause and what
is effect in immune disorders.

LYMPHOCYTE SURFACE-ATTACHED IMMUNOGLOBULINS IN SOME CLINICAL

CONDITIONS

Judith Warren

Department of Immunology, University of Leeds

The General Infirmary, Leeds U.K.

In the past five years much interest has been shown in the detection of lymphocyte sub-populations using tests which appear to group cells on the basis of their surface characteristics. As far as is known, these groupings correlate broadly with the main divisions of lymphocytes into thymus-dependent and thymus-independent cells.

In some clinical conditions of relatively rare occurrence, such as systemic L.E., immune complexes are extensively implicated as the mediators or catalysts of tissue disruption. Depressed T-cell function is almost invariably associated with SLE whereas absolute lymphopenia is not. This has led to various theories as to the probable blocking of lymphocytes by immunoglobulins[1,2,3].

Depressed T-cell function is common to many cancer states and the presence of blocking immune complexes has been given as a reason for the apparent inability of sensitised cells to mount a clinically measurable destruction of tumour tissue.

In an attempt to test these explanations for depressed CMI, a rosette test was devised using washed human 'O' red blood cells which were tanned and coated with a precipitated globulin fraction of a rabbit antiserum to normal human globulin. Incubation of these TEAG (tanned, erythrocyte anti-globulin) cells with separated lymphocytes was performed in the hope that a specific interaction between the anti-globulin coating of the red cells and elements of globulin which may exist in some form on the surface of lymphocytes could be detected as stable rosettes.

MATERIALS AND METHODS

Normal subjects were 12 males and females aged between 20-50 years of age, tested on at least one and up to 9 occasions over a period of approximately 12 months. Patients were as follows (a) 6 with diagnosed and active systemic lupus erythematosus (SLE), (b) 10 with liver disease diagnosed as active chronic hepatitis (ACH), some with established cirrhosis (c) 7 diagnosed as carcinoma of lung (samples taken prior to surgical resection). Patients were always tested in conjunction with normal controls. All patients included in these groups were between 20-55 years.

Treatment of blood for separation of lymphocytes

Venous blood, heparinised at 10 i.u./ml was diluted 1:2 in saline and layered 7 ml onto 3 ml of Ficoll-Metrizoate prepared after the method of Böyum[4]. After centrifuging at 1200 r.p.m. ($\simeq$ 400g) for 15 mins, at 20°C, the white cell layer was removed into Hanks balanced salt solution (HBSS) and washed 3 times at 1100 r.p.m. for 10 mins. Cells were then resuspended in HBSS and counted.

In accordance with procedures recommended by the IUIS/WHO Workshop[5] no attempt was made at physical elimination of blood mono-cytes from Ficoll-separated preparations. Instead, differential counts and a standard peroxidase stain[6] were used to estimate mono-cytes. Table 1 shows that the average monocyte contamination was $<5\%$. In some cases it has been found useful to include 1μ polystyrene beads in TEAG rosette tests to give an indication of actively phagocytosing cells.

TABLE 1

Mean Percentages of Mononuclear Cells (not Lymphocytes) in Ficoll/Metrizoate Separations from Peripheral Blood

Group	Peroxidase Stain	Differential Count	Phagocytosing* TEAG Rosettes
Normal	4.2 (90)	<5 (20)	1.5 (15)
Active Chronic Hepatitis	5.9 (60)	<5 (20)	5.5 (10)
Carcinoma Lung	8.3 (50)	<5 (10)	
Systemic L.E.	3.2 (50)	<5 (6)	

Figures in brackets represent number of observations.

* TEAG rosette forming cells phagocytosing 1μ polystyrene beads.

E-rosette test

This test was performed after the method of Jondal[7] using 0.05% washed sheep RBC in HBSS. All tests were performed in triplicate. Criteria for counting were 100 white cells per aliquot.

EAC-rosette test

Preparation of EAC (erythrocyte-antibody-complement) was after the method of Bianco[8] using human complement. Counts were made on 300 lymphocytes per sample. Lymphocytes with 3 or more RBC adhering were counted as rosettes. No effort was made to exclude monocytes from EAC counts unless they had phagocytosed SRBC. This preparation of EAC would be expected to include in the results lymphocytes with Fc receptors.

Tanned erythrocytes with antiglobulin (TEAG)

A high-titred precipitating antiserum to normal human globulin (NHG) (Lister Institute, Elstree) was prepared in N.Z. White Rabbits. After bleeding, a crude globulin fraction was prepared by ammonium sulphate precipitation. This fraction, which was shown to be directed predominantly against IgG and which had a precipitin titre of >1:100,000 was absorbed with the washed cells from human 'O' blood before use.

A 2.5% suspension of washed group 'O' human red cells were tanned and coated with rabbit anti-NHG (globulin fraction)[9,10]. 0.4 ml of anti-NHG containing 10-12 mg protein was used in the coating process for every 10 ml of the original red cell suspension. The washed, coated red cells were resuspended to a 1.25% suspension in a stabiliser medium of 0.05% w/v crystalline bovine albumen in saline[11].

Test system for TEAG-rosettes

Duplicate samples of 0.25 ml TEAG + 0.25 ml human lymphocyte suspension containing 10^6 cells, were incubated in 4" x $\frac{1}{2}$" screw-top glass tubes in a shaking water bath at 37°C for $\frac{1}{2}$-1 hour. The cells were spun down at 1,000 r.p.m. for 5 mins, left overnight at 4°C and then counted. The following controls were included in each test:-

1. TEAG in 0.5 ml volume alone

2. 0.25 ml of 1.25% suspension of washed human RBC (in 0.05% BSA) plus 0.25 ml human lymphocyte suspension (10^6 cells)

3. 0.25 ml of 1.25% suspension of tanned HRBC (in 0.05% BSA) plus 0.25 ml human lymphocyte suspension (10^6 cells)

These controls were uniformly <7% "false rosettes".

Other routine tests

Plasma samples from all subjects were subjected to fluorescent testing for antibody to a range of cell and tissue antigens. In addition IgM, G and A were estimated in samples, and levels of DNA-binding antibody were estimated in patients with positive anti-nuclear factor antibody. A total and differential white blood cell count was performed on whole blood and separated cells.

RESULTS

The reproducibility of the results of three rosette tests over a period of one year in a typical normal control is illustrated in Table 2 (see Table 3 for normal mean and S.D.). In order to obtain an overall picture of the behaviour of lymphocytes in the clinical conditions being investigated by the rosette methods, results from patients were grouped and compared with the means for the normal controls (Table 3). There were large increases in mean TEAG rosettes in all clinical groups and also a highly significant difference between mean percentage EAC and TEAG rosettes. E-rosettes are mostly not significantly different from normal in any group though there is considerable variability in E-rosettes of SLE patients and the unavoidable inclusion of steroid treated patients may have a contributory effect in this group.

Lymphopenia was not severe in any group included here and only 2/9 SLE and 2/20 ACH had lymphocyte counts of less than 10^9/litre whole blood.

TABLE 2

Variation with time of the percentage of rosette-forming cells in the peripheral blood of a normal female aged 32

Date	Percentage Rosettes		
	E	EAC	TEAG
22.5.74	60	36	21
3.6.74	52	36	31
9.9.74	52	32	25
25.9.74	64	33	25
20.1.75	61	25	25
29.1.75	57	32	26
21.2.75	65	25	25
19.5.75	71	25	20
2.6.75	70	25	26
Mean	61.33	29.88	24.88
S.D.	±6.53	±4.58	±2.96

TABLE 3

Mean percentage of E, EAC and TEAG rosette tests in patients and normal subjects

Diagnosis	No. of Samples	Rosette Test	Mean	S.D.	Patient Rosettes v Normals (P) (by 't' test)
NORMAL	40	E	64.18	+8.8	
		EAC	27.42	7.2	
		TEAG	25.28	5.5	
ACTIVE CHRONIC HEPATITIS	20	E	59.19	4.71	<.01
		EAC	35.63	6.71	<.001
		TEAG	47.00	11.08	<.001** <.001
SYSTEMIC L.E.	9	E	56.75	7.93	<.05
		EAC	19.77	8.82	<.02
		TEAG	60.85	7.08	<.001** <.001
CARCINOMA LUNG	7	E	63.52	6.5	ns
		EAC	33.33	9.04	ns
		TEAG	51.00	8.1	<.001** <.001

** = TEAG rosettes v EAC rosettes

SLE is classed as an autoimmune condition and as an immune complex disease. There is a common association with anti-lymphocyte antibodies. High percentages of TEAG rosettes were found in all active cases of SLE. Table 4 shows the results of tests on a typical case (JG) on three occasions over 9 months, together with a normal control.

TABLE 4

Mean percentages of E, EAC and TEAG rosettes tested on three occasions in a patient (J.G.) with active SLE, and a normal control. Blood lymphocyte counts and C3 levels are included

Date	Patient/ Control	Mean % of rosette tests			Lymphocytes x 10^9/litre blood	C3 mg%
		E	EAC	TEAG		
3. 6.74	J.G.	56	22	60	1.2	56
	Control	60	36	31	2.5	*
8.10.74	J.G.	50	16	48	0.75	82
	Control	61	26	25	2.0	*
3. 3.75	J.G.	72	22	64	0.75	76
	Control	64	35	36	2.2	*

* Normal range 104 - 161.

It is possible to draw the conclusion from the above results that a higher proportion of blood mononuclear cells than can be accounted for by lymphocytes with C' and Fc receptors, or monocytes, interact with antiglobulin coated HRBC, not only in SLE but also in ACH and the group of patients with lung cancer.

SUMMARY

The TEAG rosette test was not devised as an immediate diagnostic indicator, but in order to detect gross differences over a period of time between the lymphocytes of patients with conditions where immune complexes may be formed, and those of normal people. In summary these results indicate that:-

1. Percentage TEAG rosettes were highly significantly increased in patients with SLE, active chronic hepatitis and carcinoma of lung compared with normal controls, when the tests were performed on suspensions, containing over 90% lymphocytes, separated from peripheral blood.
2. Estimates of mean B lymphocytes plus blood monocytes in the separated suspensions, as measured by EAC rosettes (and peroxidase and differential counts for monocytes) are exceeded by TEAG-rosetting cells in the patients tested.
3. Tests on patients with chronic autoimmune conditions (e.g. ACH and SLE) do not show a highly significant difference from normal controls with respect to mean total cells forming E-rosettes.
4. It may be speculated that some TEAG rosettes are formed by T-cells which could have immune complexes or autologous anti-lymphocyte globulin on their surface and that such a condition may account for the depressed T-cell function found in these conditions.

REFERENCES

1. Mellbye, O.J., Messner, R.P., De Bord, J.R. and Williams, R.C. (1972) Arthritis Rheum. 15, 371.
2. Messner, R.P., Lindstrom, F.D. and Williams, R.C. (1973) J. clin. Invest. 32, 3046.
3. Wernet, P., Fotius, M., Thorburn, R., Moore, A. and Kunkel, H.G. (1972) Arthritis Rheum. 16, 137.
4. Böyum, A. (1968) Scand. J. clin. lab. Invest. 21, suppl. 97, 31.
5. Aiuti, F. et al. (1975) Clin. Immunol. and Immunopathology, 3, 584.
6. Hayhoe, F.G.J., Quaglino, D. and Doll, R. (1964) The Cytology and Cytochemistry of Acute Leukaemias, H.M.S.O., London. pp.19.
7. Jondal, M. Holm, G. and Wigzell, H. (1972) J. exp. Med. 136, 207.
8. Bianco, C., Patrick, R. and Nussensweig, V. (1970) J. exp. Med. 132, 702.
9. Gowland, G. (1958) Ph.D. Thesis, University of Leeds.
10.Boyden, S.V. (1951) J. exp. Med. 93, 107.
11.Stein, B. and Desowitz, R.S. (1964) Bull. Wld. Hlth. Org. 30, 45.

CONTROL OF AUTOIMMUNE PROCESSES BY A THYMIC HUMORAL FACTOR (THF)

Myra Small and Nathan Trainin

Department of Cell Biology

The Weizmann Institute of Science, Rehovot, Israel

The demonstration that lymphocytes with the potential for anti-self reactivity exist in adult rodents (1,2) leads us to ask what control mechanisms prevent such reactivity under normal conditions. Although the thymus has been implicated in discrimination between self and non-self (3,4) control of autoreactivity by the thymus still requires experimental evaluation. THF, a noncellular agent of thymic function, has been found previously to confer immunoreactivity against allogeneic tissues by regulating the maturation of developing lymphocytes (5,6). We here present evidence that THF can inhibit anti-self reactivity of lymphocytes and that this function also involves processing of immature lymphocyte populations. Details of the experimental procedures are given elsewhere (7).

TABLE 1. Cytotoxicity against syngeneic fibroblasts by C57BL spleen cells sensitized on C57BL fibroblast monolayers with or without THF

Spleen cells assayed	THF present	replicates tested	surviving fibroblasts at 48 hrs$\pm$ SE	% cytoto-xicity
sensitized	-	24	45.6 $\pm$ 2.3	44
sensitized	+	24	70.0 $\pm$ 3.8	13
nonsensitized		23	78.7 $\pm$ 3.0	3
-		22	80.9 $\pm$ 5.1	

The first experiments were performed with spleen cells sensitized on syngeneic monolayers of embryonic fibroblasts, with or
without addition of THF. After four days these lymphoid cells were
added to microcultures of the same fibroblasts and the number of
surviving fibroblast cells evaluated 48 hrs later by phase contrast
microscopy. In table 1, it can be seen that spleen cells manifest-
ing an inhibitory effect on the growth of syngeneic fibroblasts after
in vitro sensitization against these fibroblasts were less cytotoxic against self when THF had been added to the sensitizing cultures.

In order to evaluate anti-self reactivity against non-embryonic
tissue we measured the capacity of auto-sensitized lymphocytes to
induce a graft-versus-host response against syngeneic spleens. For
this purpose we modified the in vitro GVH assay of Auerbach and
Globerson (8) usually used to detect allogeneic reactivity. Here
we measured the splenomegaly induced in newborn spleen explants by
syngeneic lymphocytes autosensitized on syngeneic fibroblast monolayers with or without addition of THF. We can see in table 2 that
spleen cells sensitized on syngeneic (but not allogeneic) monolayers
for either 4 days (upper portion) or 1 day (lower position) induced
a GVH reaction against syngeneic tissue which was clearly inhibited
by addition of THF to the sensitizing cultures. Incubation of the
spleen cells in THF before sensitization inhibited their subsequent
anti-self reactivity as well.

In the next experiments, the spleen cells submitted to autosensitization were obtained from neonatally thymectomized mice.
This enabled simultaneous evaluation of the effect of THF on autoreactivity and on alloreactivity, which we had shown previously to

TABLE 2. In vitro GVH response against syngeneic tissue by spleen
cells sensitized on syngeneic fibroblasts with or without THF

Donor of graft cells	Sensitizing monolayer	Extract tested	Incidence of reactive cultures			% response
Intact C57BL	C57BL	-	5/6	7/8		86
	C57BL	THF	1/6	1/8		14
	Balb/c	-	1/6			17
Intact C57BL	C57BL	-	5/6	4/6	4/4	81
	C57BL	THF	1/6	1/5	1/5	19
	C57BL	THF before sensiti-ation	1/7	2/6		23
	C57BL	Spleen			4/5	80
	Balb/c	-	0/5			0

be conferred by THF treatment (5,6). Thus, as shown in table 3,
C57BL spleen cells sensitized for 24 hrs on syngeneic fibroblast
monolayers with or without addition of THF were tested in parallel
against syngeneic or allogeneic tissue in the GVH assay.

It can be seen that the same cell suspensions which lost anti-
self reactivity after interaction with THF gained reactivity against
allogeneic tissue after processing by THF. This suggested that the
process of T-cell maturation involves acquisition of immunocompetence against allogeneic tissue and concomitant loss of autoreactivity
as a result of THF directed maturation of lymphocytes.

Since the thymus is the source of developing T-cells, we then
looked at the GVH response induced in vitro by autosensitized
thymocytes. As shown in table 4, while more mature cortisone-resistant thymocytes failed to induce a syngeneic GVH response after
autosensitization, autoreactivity was apparent when the total thymocyte population was sensitized and assayed against self. Again,
this anti-self reactivity was inhibited by addition of THF to the
sensitizing cultures.

At this point we wished to determine the effect of THF on the
autosensitized lymphocytes themselves and so measured the uptake
of tritiated thymidine in a syngeneic MLC of spleen cells sensitized on syngeneic fibroblast monolayers with or without addition of
THF. Autosensitized cells showed an uptake of ^{3}H-thymidine which
was four fold that of control nonsensitized syngeneic cells and the
reaction was significantly reduced when the cells were autosensitized with the addition of THF (7).

The results described indicate that within the spleen and the
thymus there are cells which, when cultured on syngeneic fibroblasts
in the absence of the controlling influence of the thymus,developed
anti-self reactivity as reflected in cytotoxicity, MLC or GVH react-

TABLE 3. In vitro GVH responses of spleen cells from neonatally
thymectomized mice sensitized on syngeneic fibroblasts with or
without THF

Donor of graft cells	THF during sensitiz-ation	Host spleen explants	Incidence of reactive cultures		% response
Neona-	-	C57BL	5/6	4/7	69
tally	+	C57BL	2/6	0/7	15
Tx	-	Balb/c	1/6	0/7	8
C57BL	+	Balb/c	4/7	6/7	70

TABLE 4. In vitro GVH response against syngeneic tissue by thymocytes sensitized on syngeneic fibroblast with or without THF

Graft cells (C57BL)	Extract tested	Incidence of reactive cultures		% response
sensitized cortisone-resistant thymocytes	-	1/4	0/4	13
sensitized thymocytes	-	5/6	3/4	80
sensitized thymocytes	THF	1/5	0/4	11
sensitized thymocytes	spleen	4/5		80

ivity against syngeneic tissue. Interaction of these lymphocytes
with THF inhibited the anti-self reactivity of these cells. The
evidence so far suggests that autoreactivity is a characteristic
of immature T-cells and is lost as these cells mature under the
influence of THF.

Since it was shown here that spleen cells from neonatally thymectomized mice are potentially autoreactive, and shown previously
that serum of thymectomized animals failed to prevent anti-self
reactivity (9) we then tested the activity of spleen cells from
neonatally thymectomized mice in a syngeneic GVH assay without in
vitro sensitization. The results shown in table 5 indicate that
spleen cells from mice deprived of the thymus had undergone in vivo
sensitization against components of self, and their autoreactivity
was prevented by exposure of the cells to THF (after the sensitization had occurred).

Finally, we wished to reproduce the entire process of self-
sensitization, administration of THF, and testing of syngeneic GVH
reactivity in vivo. For this purpose spleen cells from intact, or

TABLE 5. Effect of THF on the in vitro GVH response against syngeneic tissue by spleen cells from neonatally thymectomized mice

Donor of graft cells	Extract tested	Incidence of reactive cultures				% response
Neona-tally Tx C57BL	none	6/6	3/5		3/6	71
	spleen		4/5	4/5		80
	THF	2/6	0/5	0/5	0/5	10

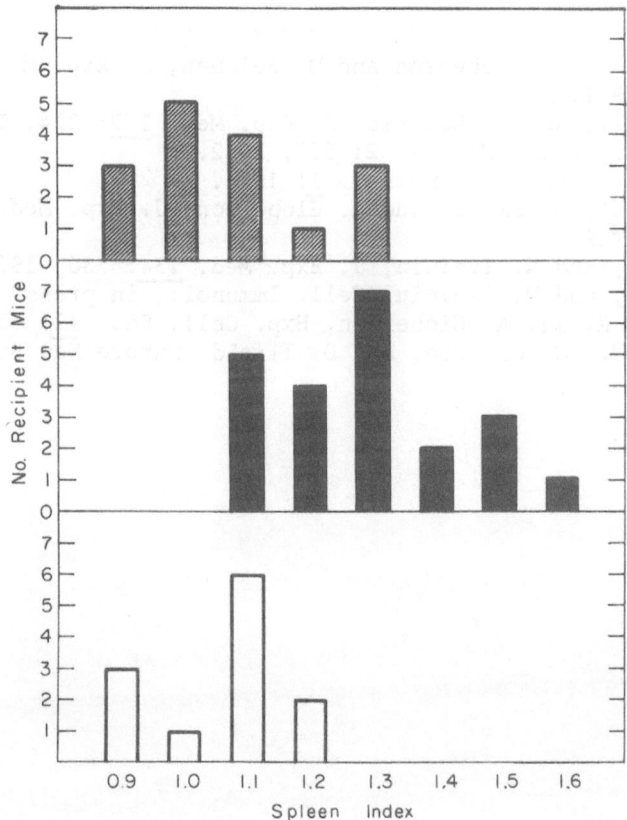

Fig. 1. In vivo GVH response induced in 10 day old C57BL recipients by 20 x 10⁶ syngeneic spleen cells from a) intact mice (bottom panel) b) neonatally thymectomized mice (middle panel) or c) neonatally thymectomized mice injected with THF for 5 successive days before GVH assay (top panel).

neonatally thymectomized mice, or neonatally thymectomized mice injected with THF were injected into syngeneic 10 day old recipients and splenomegaly measured in these recipients 10 days later. As can be seen in fig. 1, a moderate but definite syngeneic GVH response was caused in vivo by cells from thymectomized donors and was clearly reduced by injection of THF to the donor mice.

These experiments demonstrate a role of the thymus in the processes controlling autoreactivity which is mediated by THF.

REFERENCES

1. Cohen, I.R., A. Globerson and M. Feldman, J. Exp. Med. 133: 834, 1971.
2. Cohen, I.R., and H. Wekerle, J. Exp. Med. 137: 224, 1973.
3. Burnet, M., Brit. Med. J. 2: 807, 1962.
4. Jerne, N.K., Eur. J. Immunol. 1: 1971.
5. Trainin, N., M. Small, and A. Globerson, J. Exp. Med. 130: 765, 1969.
6. Small, M., and N. Trainin, J. Exp. Med. 134: 786, 1971.
7. Small, M., and N. Trainin, Cell. Immunol., in press.
8. Auerbach, R. and A. Globerson, Exp. Cell. Res. 42: 31, 1966.
9. Trainin, N., C. Carnaud, and D. Ilfeld, Nature New Biol. 245: 253, 1973.

CLINICAL, IMMUNOLOGICAL AND HISTOPATHOLOGICAL EVIDENCE FOR THYMIC DEFICIENCY IN DOWN'S SYNDROME (MONGOLISM)

M. Schlesinger*, S. Levin*, Z. Handzel*, T. Hahn*,
Y. Altman*, B. Chernobilski** and J. Bos***

The Pediatric Research Dept.* and Pathology Dept.**,
Kaplan Hospital, Rehovot and Pathology Dept.***, Hebrew
University - Hadassa Medical School Jerusalem, Israel

Down's syndrome (DS) is a chromosomal disorder leading to genetic malformations of various systems, the most marked giving rise to mental retardation and skeletal and heart abnormalities. The incidence of this disorder ranges from 1 per 1000 births in young mothers, to 1 per 50 births in mothers over 40 years of age. Certain clinical observations have recently lead investigators to study the immune system in DS.

It is known that these children suffer an inordinate number of infections in childhood (1), and no adequate explanation for this observation has been forthcoming. The incidence of leukemia is about 18 times higher in DS than in non-DS children, and this increase is due to a higher incidence of the lymphocytic form of the neoplasm (2). A high incidence of a chronic carrier state of Australian antigen has been linked to a possible defect in the immune system of DS (3), as has been the finding of increased auto-antibodies to thyroid in these cases (4).

Studies of the B system have shown non-consistent "minor" abnormalities of immunoglobulin production, none in themselves being sufficient to explain the above clinical observations. These include increased levels of IgG and IgA with diminished IgM, depending on age of the DS patients and whether they are institutionalised or not (5) (6). IgD levels were lower too (7), and present evidence is that this is probably related to the lower values of IgM in these cases (8). It is likely that these variations are the result of infections in DS rather than the cause of them. Minor variations in Gm antigenic titres have also been reported in DS adults. The finding of defective antibody response to bacteriophage

does not in itself implicate the B system (9). Studies of leucocyte
function have shown that phagocytic activity in DS is reduced (10).

The evidence for T-system dysfunction is much stronger. Using
the mixed leucocyte reaction a qualitative deficiency of T-cells
has been found (11), and the response of DS lymphocytes to PHA in
culture has been shown to be impaired (12) (13). Our own studies
using a cytotoxic test with anti-human-T-cell serum (ATS) has
shown consistently that DS patients of all ages including newborns
have less peripheral lymphocytes than normal and this deficit
is due to a significantly diminished number of peripheral T lymphocytes (14). This has been confirmed using the T-rosette test. More
significantly we have shown a defect in T-cell function in these
patients, who have marked deficiency of leucocyte migration inhibitory factor (LIF) production following stimulation of their
lymphocytes with PHA, although response to PPD is only slightly
diminished (15). However we have shown by means of the Stimulation
of Protein Synthesis test (SPS) that DS lymphocytes react to PHA
normally in the early production of protein (16).

It became therefore of interest to study the histopathology of
the thymus gland in these patients shown to have a partial T-system
deficiency. In a previous study (17) in which we analysed the
occurence of lymphocyte depletion (LD) in the thymus, lymph-glands
and spleen of infants coming to autopsy at the Kaplan Hospital over
a 10 year period, we found that in two groups of children matched
for age and cause of death, but differing in the presence or
absence of LD, all 13 cases of DS fell into the group with genera-
lised lymphocyte depletion, and none were in the group without
lymphocyte depletion. Numerous clinical and therapeutic parameters
evaluated showed no significant differences between the groups. The
present report analyses the histopathological preparations of the
thymuses of 13 DS patients aged 1 day to 15 months and compares
them with 13 non-DS children matched for age, cause of death and
length of terminal illness.

A major finding was that in DS thymuses, lymphocyte depletion
was severe in 9 cases, mild in 3 cases, and absent in a single case.
In the non-DS thymuses, moderate LD was found in 1 case, mild
changes in 6 cases and none was found in the rest.

The lobules were usually smaller than normal, some distorted
with blurring of the cortico-medullary junction due to LD of the
cortex, with increase of reticular epithelial cells. The main
changes were noted in the cortex where the majority of lymphocytes
are found, whilst in severe cases, LD was pronounced in the medulla
as well (Fig. 1 and 2).

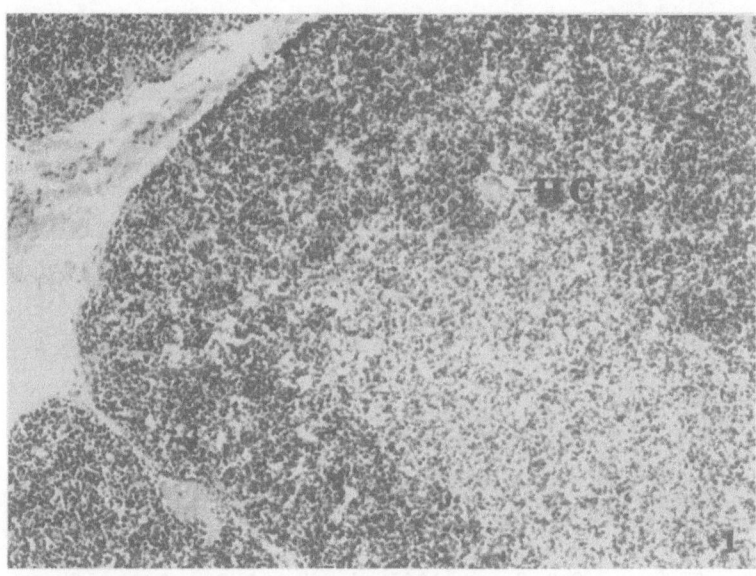

Figure 1. Normal thymus (x 100), with lymphocytes mainly in cortex, and a single H.C. in medulla.

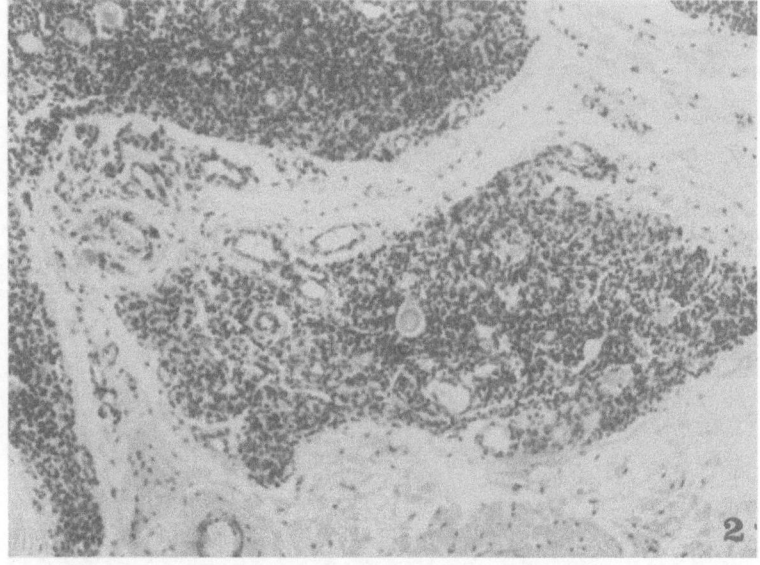

Figure 2. Involuted thymus (x 100) with lymphocyte depletion (L.D.), loss of corticomedullary demarcation, and increased number of H.C.

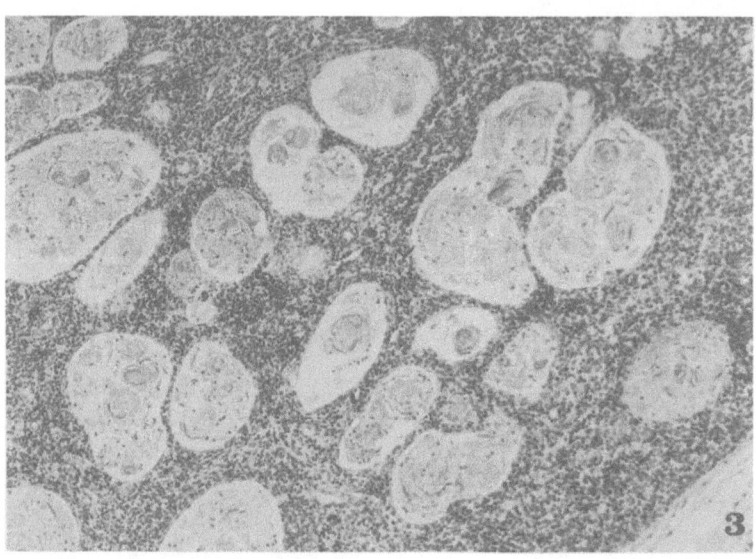

Figure 3. Thymus of D.S. (x 100) showing L.D., loss of demarcation between cortex and medulla, and increased number and size of H.C.

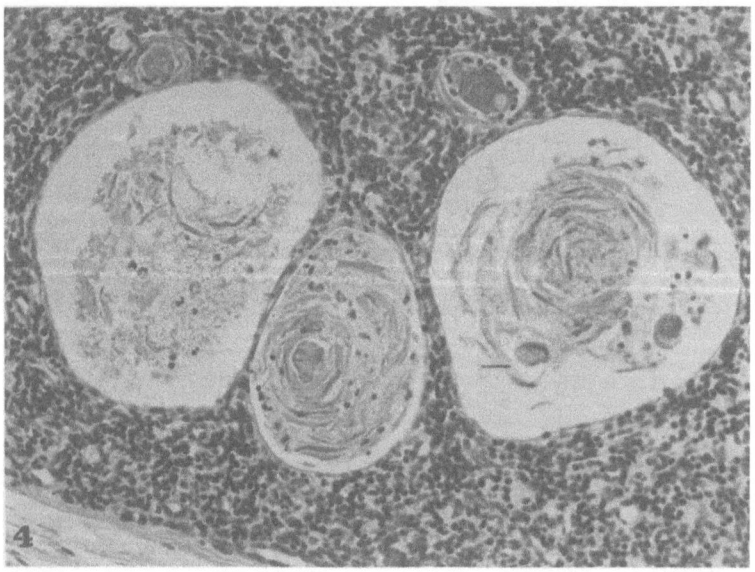

Figure 4. Thymus of D.S. (x 250) showing large cystic H.C. containing debris.

A remarkable finding was the tremendous enlargement of the epithelial cords or so-called Hassal's corpuscles (HC) in the medulla, most having tubular or cystic appearances (Fig. 3 and 4). These represent nests of epithelial cells which develope by folding of "villae" or "buds" of the epithelial anlage into the mesenchymal tissue. A normal HC is about 25-75μm in diameter, with peripheral epithelial cells showing evidence of high metabolic enzyme activity, with some resemblance to the epidermis of human skin. In DS the enlarged degenerative centers contained much cellular and nuclear debris, and often calcified. This appearance was compatible with accelerated involution at the stage of advanced atrophy.

Our study showed that of the 13 DS cases, the size of HC reached 1200 x 800μm, with many larger than 800μm in diameter. The mean area of HC measured in five microscopic fields (x 128) was 48,000 sq.microns (131 corpuscles), whereas in the matched control group, the largest HC was 250 x 200μm, and the mean area of a single body was 6800 sq.microns (106 corpuscles). Individually 11 of 13 DS cases the HC were also cystic, filled with amorphous material and degenerated cells, whilst mild cystic changes were seen only in 2 control cases. The number of HC per field was slightly higher in DS than in the control groups. Interestingly the 4 cases of DS with mild or no LD all had large HC, in three of them with cystic changes. Thus every case of DS examined had abnormal findings in the thymus.

An examination of spleens from these cases showed extreme depletion of lymphocytes in the white pulp, although the number of lobules appeared normal. The thymic-dependent periarteriolar sheath was almost non-existent. The red-pulp was less involved and in some cases germinal follicles were diminished or absent.

Examination of the clinical parameters in these two groups showed that 8 out of 13 DS cases suffered from gastro-enteritis in their final illness, the rest mainly from respiratory and other infections. In the control groups 5 children died with respiratory illness, and the rest mainly with severe infections. Dystrophia or malnutrition was found in 6 cases of DS and only in 2 control cases. The length of the last illness or "stress" situation in both groups was similar. No significant differences in treatment was found between the two groups.

DISCUSSION

Benda and Strassman (18) were the first to note the marked abnormalities of the HC in DS, although neither they nor Kouvalainin (19) analysed these findings in relation to concurrent diseases, age or other "stress" situations. Our study could not demonstrate any extrinsic factor which could account for the marked difference in thymus pathology between DS and non-DS patients.

The exact function of the HC is still in doubt. In the development of the thymus, the epithelial cells are first to appear beginning in the fetus as an epithelial tube, which folds and refolds with the lumen becoming narrower, and only subsequently is this organ infiltrated with lymphocytes (20). The epithelial and reticulum cells are known to secrete substances, one of them probably being a thymic humoral factor (THF) (21). This factor is known to be involved in the induction of immune-competency of T-cells. It is possible therefore that diminished numbers of T cells and abnormal function in DS could be due to defective secretion of thymic humoral factor from these abnormal HC. Our preliminary observations in vitro and in vivo indicate that THF can correct these deficiencies. As phagocytic activity has been demonstrated in HC, a suggestion has been made that these are graveyards for thymocytes (19), and possibly some subpopulations of T cells are more actively eliminated in the large HC of DS, leading to T-cell deficiency. As far as we are aware these large HC are not seen in other T-cell deficiency syndromes, although HC tend to become larger and filled with amorphous material as the gland involutes. We are unaware of a direct relationship between LD and enlargement of HC. In measles, where there is an acquired T-system deficiency, there is LD of the thymus with diminished number of small HC (22). Also diminution in size and number of HC has been found after experimental viral infections (23). The higher incidence of leukemia in DS may have a relationship to the finding of LD and hyperplasia of the epithelial reticular elements (HC) in pre-leukemic mice (24).

SPECULATION

The finding of marked LD of the thymus with giant, often cystic HC, in cases of DS, even as young as 1 day old is compatible with accelerated involution and atrophy of the thymus, and is an unusual and specific observation not seen regularly in any other condition. These children suffer increased numbers of infections and have T-system deficiency characterized by diminished number of peripheral T-cells and some T-cell functional deficiency. It is speculated that there is a primary defect in the epithelial anlage of the thymus, with diminished secretion of THF necessary for the maturation of T-cells. Alternatively, abnormal overactivity of the phagocytic function of the HC, or premature involution, may lead to increased destruction of T-cells in these patients.

REFERENCES

1. Oster, J., Mikkelson, M. and Nielson, A., Internat.Copenhagen Cong.Sci.Study Ment.Retard., 1, 231, 1964.
2. Miller, R.W., Ann.N.Y. Acad.Sci., 171 (ii), 637, 1970.
3. Sutnick, A.I., London, W.T., Blumberg, B.S. and Gerstley, B. J.S., Am.J.Clin.Path., 57, 2, 1972.
4. Fialkow, P.J., Blumberg, B.S., London, W.T., Sutnick, A.I. and Thuline, H.C., J.Ment.Def.Res., 15, 177, 1971.
5. Stiehm, E.R. and Fudenberg, H.H., Pediatrics, 37, 715, 1966.
6. Sutnick, A.I., London, T. and Blumberg, B.S., Arch,Int.Med., 124, 722, 1969.
7. Rundle, A.T., Clothier, B. and Sudell, B., Clin.Chem.Acta., 35, 389, 1971.
8. Rowe, D.S., Hug, K., Forni, L. and Pernis, B., J.Exp.Med., 138, 965, 1973.
9. Lopez, V., Ochs, H.D., Thuline, H.C. Davis, S.D. and Wedgwood, R.J., Jnl.Ped., 86, 207, 1975.
10. Rosner, F., Kosinn, P.J. and Jervis, G.A., N.Y. State J.Med., 675, 1973.
11. Sasaki, M. and Yoshitaka, O., Nature 222, 596, 1969.
12. Hyakawa, H., Matsui, I., Higurashi, M. and Kobayashi, N., Lancet, 1, 95, 1968.
13. Agarwal, S.S., Blumberg, B.S., Gerstley, B.J.S., London, W.Y., Sutnick, A.I. and Loeb, L.A., J.Clin.Invest., 49, 161, 1970.
14. Levin, S., Nir, E. and Mogilner, B.M., Pediatrics, 1975 (in press).
15. Hahn, T., Levin, S. and Handsel, Z., J.Clin.Exp.Immun., 1975 (submitted).
16. Schecter, B., Nir, E. and Levin, S., Isr.J.Med.Sci., 10, 1170, 1974.
17. Schlesinger, M., Doctorate thesis, Hebrew University - Hadassah Medical School, Jerusalem, 1973.
18. Benda, C.E. and Strassman, G.S., J.Ment.Deficiency Res., 9 (2), 109, 1965.
19. Kouvalainen, H., International Congress of Pediatrics (Wien), 4 September, 1971.
20. Shier, K.J., Lab.Invest., 12, 316, 1963.
21. Trainin, N., Cook, A.I., Umiel, T. and Albala, M., Ann.N.Y. Acad.Sci., 249, 349, 1975.
22. White, R.G. and Boyd, J.F., Clin.Exp.Immun., 13, 343, 1973.
23. McCollough, B., Krakowke, S. and Koestner, A., Am.J.Path., 74, 155, 1974.
24. Sutnick, A.J., London, W.T., Blumberg, B.S. and Gerstley, B.J., J.Nat.Cancer.Inst., 47, 923, 1972.

IMMUNOMORPHOLOGICAL LYMPH NODE PROCESSES
IN SOME CIRRHOGENIC LIVER DISEASES

Mariana Laky and D. Laky

Victor Babeş Institute

Spl.Independenţei 99,Bucureşti 35,Romania

Summary

Dynamics of the lymph node modifications as well as hepatic and immunoserological in various cirrhogenic hepatopathies have been studied on human and experimental material. Lymph nodes showed early and progressively immunomorphological reactions with maximum intensity in evolutive stades of certain cirrhoses. Such reactions as well as in other areas of reticulo-endothelial system are decreasing during the immunosuppressive treatment and in advanced stades of cirrhosis.

The lymph nodes participation in the pathogenic mechanism of some cirrhogenic hepatopathies has been very little studied, whereas that of the liver and of the spleen has been more approached. Our previous investigations (1) have disclosed the existence of some chronic lymphadenites as well as reactional reticuloses on necroptic material from young cirrhotics. Equally, during some preliminary experimental studies (7) we remarked intense lymph node reactions even in incipient phases of cirrhoses, which fact stirred us up to examine them thoroughly.

Material and Methods

Experimental Material.   Various cirrhogenic hepa-

topathies have been reproduced at 3oo Lewis and Wistar
rats and at AKR mice. Chronic intoxication with CC14 has
been performed by inhaling or by subcutaneous via. At some lots there have been effected splenectomies which were
sometimes associated with immunosuppressive treatment
(corticoids, imuran), during which was continued the treatment with CC14. At other lots were effected incomplete cho-
ledoc or portal vein ligatures. The experiments lasted 2-
45o days, the animals were periodically sacrified by bleeding. Cervical, thoracal, abdominal, subcutaneous lymph nodes as well as fragments from all the organs have been taken. Such fragments have been fixed in Carnoy and in neu-
tral formalin lo%. The next staining methods were used on
sections : hematoxiline-eosine, Van Gieson, Gömöri, Bra-
chet, Hotchis-Mc′Manus and certain techniques for distin-
guishing certain enzymes : acid and alkalin phosphatases,
, ATP-ases, in some cases have been employed electrono-
microscopical investigations. Electrophoresis and immunoelectrophoresis have also been performed.

    Human material.   For the present study there have
been selected 25o cases of chronic hepatopathies and cirrhoses from young people and children. The etiological factor was chiefly viral hepatitis and in the other cases the
chronic alcoholism and colostases. Hilar hepatic and splenic lymph nodes (obtained intraoperatively), those from
supraclavicular, cervical axilar and inguinal areas (obtained bioptically) and from other areas on necroptic material have also been studied. In all the cases there have been performed hepatic biopsies and in some cases were
examined also bone marrow and spleen. Besides, all the
organs obtained from necropsies were treated as above.
The immunoglobulins value has also been investigated.

                            Results

    In all experimental models the histological lymph
node statement showed immunomorphological features. Thus,
during the first week of experiment we remarked the presence of numerous macrophages, containing acid phosphatases and PAS positive material, at the level of follicular centers, of marginal sinus and in the surrounding
areas. The germinal centers grow larger progressively
and we observed numerous mitoses and frequent intense
pyroninophilic blast cells. The immunoblast cells appeared
in paracortical zone and showed frequent contacts with
cytoplasmic prolongations of macrophages. Tumefaction and
hyperplasia of reticuloendothelial elements and their

presence as well as of macrophages in sinusoidal lumen
are generating pictures of catharral sinusitis. The frequency of mitoses at immunoblast cells level in the paracortical zones determines their extension in medullar
cords, setting up contacts with macrophages and rising
up plasmocytoid and plasma cell differentiation. To their
intense pyroninophily corresponds in electronomicroscopy
the marked hyperplasia of ribosomes and of endoplasmic
reticulum with the dilatation of ergastoplasmic structures. Plasma cells are grouped in clums and cords surrounding the sinusoids and reaching an important percentage even at the end of the first decade. Compared with
the hepatic histologic statement, there was observed the
fact that in early stades of experiments the immunomorphological lymph nodes processes highly exceed in intensity those of the liver. During the experiments we observed the appearance and successive enlargements of new
pyroninophilic germinal centers followed by cell differentiation processes, similar to those as above mentioned. The cellular elements of lymph nodes appeared pyroninophilic, nearly completely, forming compact plasmocytoid and plasma cell cords in medulla and cortex, and
decreasing the lymphoid follicles. This histologic picture persists for a period during which we assist to extensive immunomorphological reactions at the liver, these
reactions lead to hepatic cirrhosis. Watching simultaneously the dynamics of cytodifferentiations in other areas
of R.E.S., we notice important reactional similitudes at
certain visceral lymphoid structures, at the spleen, at
the bone marrow and at the stroma of parenchymal organs.

The immunoglobulin level reaches important values,
IgG and IgM are predominant in evolutive stade of cirrhosis. We have obtained interesting results on lots of
animals at which we performed splenectomies during the
CC14 intoxication. In some of these cases was associated
the immunosuppressive treatment. At animals at which only
splenectomies were effected, the immunomorphological
lymph node reactions were accentuated unlike to the other
lots to which was associated also an immunosuppressive
treatment. In advanced stades of predominant fibrosis
and sclerosis processus in cirrhoses, we observed at the
lymph node level the decrease of the immunomorphological
reactions. We observe inequal thickness, colagenisation
of reticulinic trama as well as of capsular and septal
structures and also a tendency to sclerosis. The decrease-
ment of immunomorphological processes takes place also
in the other R.E.S. areas, being accompanied by the diminution of the seric immunoglobulins.

The human material in spite of not having been studied chronologically, allowed the reconstitution of some links of the reactional dynamics from the obtained pictures. In evolutive phases of some chronic hepatites, in incipient stades of hepatic cirrhosis as well as in bantian syndroma, the statement of the reactional lymph node shows similar features to those described in the experimental material. Thus we often found numerous pyroninophilic elements, especially plasma cells on the background of a diffuse reactional reticulosis with catharral sinusitis. Numerous germinal centers rendered themselves evident. We would draw the attention to the minimal intensity of immunomorphological processes in case of alcoholic and nutritional cirrhosis.

At advanced stades of cirrhosis, the pyroninophilic elements are appreciably decreasing up to disappearing, at the lymph node as well as in liver, spleen and other R.E.S. areas, although macrophages and germinal centers are seen at some levels. The fibrillo-forming processes are setting out chronic lymphadenitis process. Similar reactions are taking place also in other areas of the immune system which accounts for the decrease of the immunoglobulin values.

Discussion

The purpose of our investigations was to get the immunomorphological bases of pathogenetic processes enlarged within some chronic cirrhogene hepatopathies, specifying the modalities and the degree of lymph node participation in the given context. The references studied did not offer sufficient information, being limited often to some studies on hilar hepatic lymph nodes (8). The said reference gave estimations with respect to the possibility of lymph node reactions determining immunoserological disturbances (3) as well as limiting the efficiency of splenectomies in certain bantian syndroma and in cirrhogenic hepatopathies (6). This situation is due to the difficulties in approaching some lymph node areas on human material and in interpreting the obtained morphological pictures. Inguinal lymph nodes are not recommanded in the histopathological study, they are often suffering sclerogene lesions. The systematic study of lymph nodes on necroptic material can offer interesting data only on the condition that the study should be limited with young people and that the respective patients sould be unharmed by other chronical disease or by secondary infectious complications which might render the interpretation of lesional and reactional pictures more difficult. From this material there had to be especially investigated the patients having incipient stades of cirrhosis, for the lesions of chronic sclerogenic lymphadenitis in advanced stade are predominant, particularly in the abdominal region, such modification being partially generated by circulatory troubles within the portal hypertension. In order to avoid such difficulties we seized the occasion of some surgical interventions when we deducted hilar hepatic and splenic lymph nodes concomitently with hepatic biopsy and surprised some reactional aspects. The results obtained from biopsies of lymph nodes in supraclavicular and cervical regions which were effected concomitently with hepatic biopunctures and immunoserological investigation seemed to be encouraging. Immunological features of the lymph node reactions chiefly represented by the abundance of pyroninophilic plasma cells correlated with the intensity of hepatic mesenchymal reaction and with the increase of IgG and IgM supply an exact appreciation on the pathogenetic frame, on the indication and efficieney of immunosuppressive treatments. Not all cirrhogenic hepatopathies are presenting such immunological disturbances. Thus in nutritional, alcoholic cirhhosis the immunomorphological reactions appear minimal at lymph and in serum predominates IgA.

The experimental researches remain, of course, the most accessible way to study of lymph nodes dynamic in these affections, they show the development of an immunomorphological reactional range similar to the human ones (2, 3, 4). Lymph node reactions appear early, in initial stades (7), they depass in intensity the hepatic mesenchymal reactions. They often take place in the condition of a progressive hyperreactivity of various R.E.S. areas (2, 3, 4, 5) reaching the maximum intensity when the hepatic cirrhosis was settled in and corresponds to a hypergammaglobulinemia with an increase of IgG and IgM. The performance of the splenectomy at some animals intoxicated chronically with CC14 only can lead to an intensification of the immune system and of the remaining R.E.S.(3). Such pictures have been found also after splenectomies at normal rats. In human pathology the failures of splenectomies effected in some bantian syndroma and chronic evolutive hepatites have been explained by the compensatory hyperreactivity and by functional disturbance of immune system (6). The restrain of the immunomorphological lymph node reactions concomitently with hepatic lesions at animals at which it was associated splenectomy and the

immunosuppressive treatment in conditions of continuing
CC14 intoxication, seemed to us interesting. These data
are equivalent with those found after the complexe immu-
nosuppresive therapy of the human pathology and demonstrate the role of lymph nodes within the pathogenic process.

REFERENCES

1. Laky (D), Gălеşanu (M.R.): Aspecte morfofiziopatolo-
   gice în cadrul cirozelor hepatice. Viaţa Medicală
   (Bucureşti) 1956, 1, 86
2. Laky (D), Golgoţiu (L), Quintesco (M): Modèles expé-
   rimentaux pour l'étude des hépatopathies chroniques.
   Les modifications du S.R.E. hépatique et général au
   cours de l'évolution des hépatopathies cirrhogènes.
   Virchows Arch.Abt.A.Path.Anat.1971, 353, 45-59
3. Laky (D): Corelaţii între sistemul reticuloendotelio-
   histiocitar hepatic şi cel general în hepatopatii cro-
   nice. Teza de doctorat I.M.F. Iaşi, 1971
4. Laky (D), Quintesco (M), Bratianu (Ş): Changes of
   R.E.S. during cirrhosis. IX.Intern.Congr.on Intern.
   Acad.Path. 1972, Jerusalem. Abstracts p.89
5. Laky (D): Les réactions immunomorphologiques pulmo-
   naires au cours des hépatopathies cirrhogènes. Acta
   morphol.Acad.Scient.Hung. 1973, Suplim.Abstr.of Fourth
   Congress of Europ.Soc.Path., p.125
6. Mantz (M.J.), Mantz-Le Correler (J): Hypersplénisme
   et système réticulo-endothélial. La Presse méd.(Paris)
   1955, 63, 1345-1348
7. Quintesco (M), Laky (D), Gălеşanu (M.R.): Leziuni inci-
   piente în cadrul cirozelor hepatice. Spitalul (Bucureşti) 1957, 2, 156-164
8. Velican (D): Morfopatologia şi histiochimia ganglio-
   nilor limfatici din hilul ficatului în forma cronică
   a hepatitei epidemice. Studii şi cerc.med.int.(Bucureşti) 1962, 3, 755

CASEIN-INDUCED MURINE AMYLOIDOSIS: AMYLOID AND IMMUNOGLOBULIN

PRODUCTION AND PROLIFERATIVE CAPACITY OF SPLENOCYTES

Reuben Baumal, Ester Pass and Bill Wilson

The Departments of Immunology and Pathology

The Hospital for Sick Children, Toronto, Canada

A study of the chemical composition and immunological reactivity of amyloid fibrils in human amyloidosis has revealed 2
classes of amyloid (1, 2). The amyloid derived from primary amyloidosis and multiple myeloma consists of immunoglobulin (Ig) light
(L) chains or the variable region fragments of L chains. The amyloid obtained from secondary amyloidosis consists of a non-Ig
protein. Soluble circulating components which cross-react with
amyloid may represent precursors of the tissue deposits (3, 4).
These observations suggest possibilities as to the pathogenesis of
amyloid formation. The present studies seek to determine how murine
amyloidosis can serve to elucidate the pathogenesis of human amyloidosis. Attention will focus on lymphocytes and reticuloendothelial
cells since they are the probable producers of amyloid.

Experimental models for amyloidosis. Amyloid deposition was
induced in mice by the daily administration of casein. This system
is considered analogous to secondary human amyloidosis because
repetetive antigenic stimulation is common to both. In our hands,
amyloid began to appear after 10 to 15 injections of casein, accumulated gradually and after 30 or more injections, massive amounts
were present. The chemical composition of this amyloid has shown
it to consist of a protein ressembling the non-Ig form of human amyloid. A model analogous to myeloma-associated human amyloidosis
was sought using transplantable mouse myeloma tumors. The organs
and tumor masses of mice with 19 different Balb/C and C_3H tumors
were surveyed. The group included tumors producing IgG, IgA, IgM,
L chains and non-producers. Amyloid deposits were found only in
mice bearing the IgG_{2a} producing MOPC 173 tumor. The identification
of this murine amyloid as Ig is necessary if the model is truly
analogous to human myeloma-associated amyloidosis.

We have raised antisera against extracted, denatured casein-
induced and myeloma-associated murine amyloid and have used them
in immunofluorescent tissue studies. Casein-induced amyloid deposits reacted intensely with anti-casein amyloid antiserum and
cross-reacted with anti-MOPC 173 amyloid antiserum. Myeloma associated MOPC 173 amyloid cross-reacted with the anti-casein antiserum but failed to react with the anti-MOPC 173 antiserum, possibly because the latter was too weak. These studies indicated that
either casein induced and myeloma-associated murine amyloid were
the same substance, they were different but had common antigenic
determinants or they were distinct but occurred together. Studies
on the chemical composition of myeloma-associated amyloid will
distinguish these possibilities.

Immunoglobulin production in experimental amyloidosis. The Ig
form of human amyloid may arise because of disordered Ig biosynthesis. Amyloidosis might be characterized by the production of excess L chains or of N-terminal fragments, both of which occur in
mouse myeloma tumors (5, 6). Spleen lymphocytes and tumor cells
from casein-induced and tumor bearing amyloidotic mice were examined. In the first study, the intracellular ratio of L and H
chains was determined. Normal non-amyloidotic mice immunized with
sheep RBC or hemocyanin produced a 1.5 fold molar excess of L
chains. Casein injected amyloidotic mice produced a similar molar
ratio, indicating that this form of amyloidosis was not associated
with excess L chains. Myeloma tumor bearing mice produced L chains
in amounts equivalent to or in moderate to vast excess over H
chains. However, since the MOPC 173 mice produced only a 1.5 fold
molar excess of L chains, the presence of amyloidosis in this model
was also not correlated with excess L chain production.

In a second study, spleen lymphocytes and tumor cells of amyloidotic mice were labelled with ^{14}C amino acids and aliquots of
the intracellular and secreted proteins were immunologically precipitated with anti-Ig antiserum. The immunoprecipitates were
analyzed on sodium dodecyl sulfate containing polyacrylamide gels,
which separates the various species on the basis of size. Figure
1 shows the gel electropherograms observed using spleen lymphocytes
of casein-injected amyloidotic mice. The top 2 panels show the
intracellular proteins, non-precipitated and precipitated with
anti-Ig antiserum. In the former there is a peak of radioactivity
in the low mol. wt. region while the latter shows the Ig intermed-
iaries μH_2L_2, μHL, γH_2L_2, free L chains but no L chain fragments.
The low mol. wt. component was also observed in non-amyloidotic
mice, was not precipitated by anti-Ig antiserum and was not considered unique to amyloidosis or related to Ig. The bottom 2 panels
show the proteins secreted, again non-precipitated and precipitated,
namely, IgM, IgG, free L chains, the low mol. wt. non-Ig constituent,
but no L chain fragments. Amyloidotic MOPC 173 mice also lacked L
chain fragments. Therefore, these studies showed that there was no

disorder of Ig biosynthesis in murine amyloidosis and imply that
the Ig type of human anyloidosis arises from post-synthetic degradation of L chains.

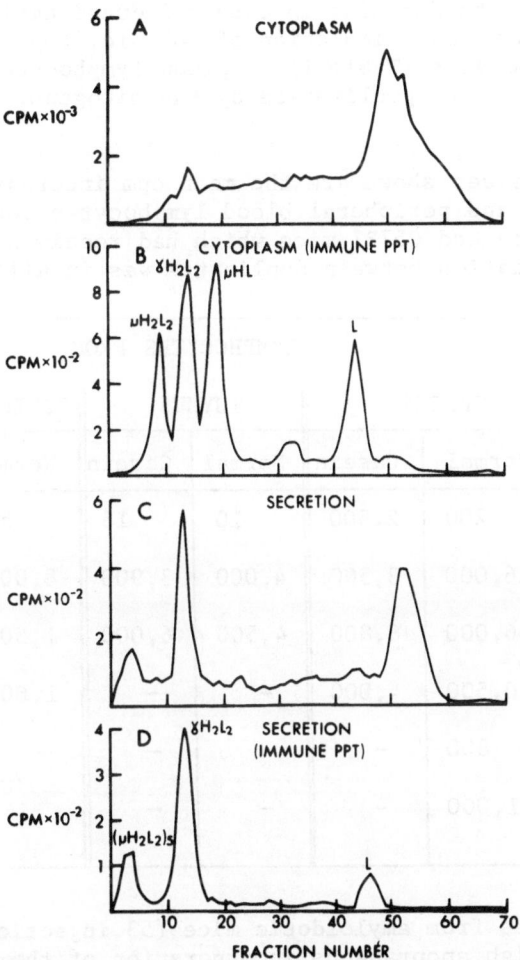

Figure 1. Sodium dodecyl sulfate polyacrylamide gel electropherograms of spleen lymphocytes from casein-induced amyloidotic mice.
Cytoplasmic lysates (A and B), secretions (C and D), non-immunologic-
ally precipitated (A and C), and precipitated with anti-Ig antiserum.
(B and D). Direction of migration is from left to right.

Cellular immunity in casein-induced murine amyloidosis. Thymus-
derived (T) lymphocytes play a central role in cellular immunologic
responses and may become depleted during induction of murine amyloidosis (7). As a consequence, amyloidotic animals demonstrate decreased PHA responsiveness and decreased migration inhibitory
factor production. In addition, amyloid deposition is enhanced by

measures which deplete T lymphocytes such as neonatal thymectomy.
These observations suggest that diminished cellular immunologic
reactivity is important in the pathogenesis of amyloidosis. We
studied T lymphocyte function in casein-induced amyloidotic mice,
as assessed by mitogen stimulation of splenic, thymic and peripheral blood lymphocytes (Table I). Spleen lymphocytes from normal
mice are stimulated to proliferate by the mitogens. PHA, Con A, and
PWM.

Table 1. The values shown are the mean cpm incorporated by the
spleen, thymus, and peripheral blood lymphocytes obtained from
normal C57Bl mice and C57Bl mice which had received 53 injections
of casein. Variation between duplicates was in all cases less
than 20%.

MITOGEN	LYMPHOCYTES FROM					
	SPLEEN		THYMUS		PERIPHERAL BLOOD	
	Normal	Casein	Normal	Casein	Normal	Casein
Nil	200	2,500	10	15	50	150
PHA-P	26,000	3,500	4,000	3,900	8,000	9,000
Con-A	36,000	8,800	4,500	6,000	1,500	1,800
PWM	20,500	4,000	-	-	1,600	7,000
Amyloid	800	-	-	-	-	-
Amyloid & PHA	1,000	-	-	-	-	-

Spleen lymphocytes from amyloidotic mice (53 injections of casein)
demonstrated a high spontaneous incorporation of thymidine and a
diminished response to PHA, Con A and PWM. Thymus and peripheral
blood lymphocytes showed normal mitogenic responses. These studies
showed that the impaired lymphocyte transformation of amyloidotic
mice was localized to the spleen. Since the spleens were infiltrated with amyloid, the possibility was considered that it played a
role in decreasing lymphocyte responses. This was tested by incubating amyloid extracts with normal lymphocytes. A weak mitogenic response was observed but the amyloid inhibited PHA induced
lymphocyte transformation. Therefore, the decreased response of
spleen lymphocytes to T cell mitogens may have been caused by an
inhibitory effect of the in vivo splenic amyloid deposits. Spleen
lymphocytes have been widely used in studies which show diminished
cellular immunologic responses in experimental amyloidosis. Our

results suggest that they may not truly reflect cellular immunologic integrity.

Cellular aspects of casein-induced murine amyloidosis. Light
and electron microscopic examination of organs from amyloidotic
mice and patients with secondary amyloidosis indicate that reticular, endothelial or reticuloendothelial cells (i.e. macrophages) are
the source of amyloid (8, 9). Macrophages are involved in processing of antigens and a subpopulation of these cells may be adversely
affected by repeated amyloidogen injections so that instead of
performing their normal function, they begin producing amyloid.
We have been studying the properties of amyloid producing cells in
casein-injected mice. At various times during induction, spleens
were removed and sections were stained with Congo red to detect extracellular amyloid deposits. The cut edge of the spleens were
also touched to glass slides, stained with Congo red and examined
for the presence of intra-and extracellular amyloid deposits. Isolated cell suspensions were prepared from a third aliquot of the
spleens and they were placed in dishes containing coverslips. After
various intervals in culture, the coverslips were removed, stained
with Congo red and examined for intra-and extracellular amyloid.

Extracellular amyloid appeared after 15 injections of casein
and progressively accumulated. Cells staining with Congo red
appeared in the touch preparations 4 days prior to the extracellular amyloid. Further proof for intracellular amyloid was provided
by staining with fluorescent labelled anti-casein amyloid antibody
and by electron microscopic examination of the spleens. The number
of amyloid containing cells in the touch preparations was small
and did not increase as more amyloid was deposited. This may indicate that these cells were not important in amyloid formation
and that cells containing soluble amyloid precursors, not detected
by the methods used, were involved. On the other hand, if the
amyloid containing cells detected do play a role in amyloid formation, the fact that they do not increase in number suggests that
amplification of synthesis rather than recruitment of new cells
was responsible for progressive amyloid deposition. The amyloid
containing cells adhered to tissue culture dishes and presumably
represented a subpopulation committed to amyloid synthesis. This
latter conclusion was supported by examination of the cultured
cells which adhered to the coverslips. Again, amyloid containing
cells appeared prior to amyloid deposits in the spleen. At one
time point examined in detail (10 injections of casein), the proportion of amyloid containing cells increased to 50% at 4 weeks and
then it fell to 10%. Such a high percentage of cells, in contrast
to the low proportion observed in the touch preparations, suggests
that cells acquire the property of amyloid synthesis in vitro due
to loss of control when put into culture. This culture system may
provide a means for obtaining large numbers of cells to study the
regulation of amyloid synthesis.

Summary. We have examined some aspects of lymphocyte and macrophage function in experimental murine amyloidosis. Casein-induced murine amyloidosis is a good model for studying secondary human amyloidosis while myeloma-associated murine amyloidosis is a poor model for human myeloma-associated amyloidosis. The amyloid of casein-induced and myeloma-associated murine amyloidosis cross-reacted immunologically. Neither form of amyloidosis was associated with L chain fragments or excess L chain production. Cellular immunologic reactivity of casein-induced amyloidotic mice, as assessed by lymphocyte transformation with mitogens, was abnormal using spleen lymphocytes but completely normal when thymus and peripheral blood lymphocytes were examined. The depressed activity could be attributed to splenic amyloid deposits. Intracellular amyloid was detected in the spleens of casein-injected mice prior to extracellular amyloid deposits. Amyloid containing cells could also be cultured from the spleen in a much higher proportion than that found in vivo. These cells may represent a subpopulation committed to amyloid synthesis.

REFERENCES

1. Glenner, C. G., Terry, W. D. and Isersky, C., Seminars in Hemat. 10: 65, 1973.
2. Husby, G., Sletten, K. Michaelsen, T. E. and Natvig, J. B., Scand. J. Immunol., 1: 393, 1972.
3. Husby, G. and Natvig, J. B., J. Clin. Invest., 53: 1054, 1973.
4. Levin, M., Pras, M. and Franklin, E. C., J. Exp. Med. 138: 373, 1973.
5. Baumal, R. and Scharff, M. D., J. Immunol., 111: 448, 1973.
6. Schubert, D. and Cohn, M., J. Mol. Biol., 53: 305, 1970.
7. Hardt, F. and Claessen, M. H., Immunol., 22: 677, 1972.
8. Heefner, W. A. and Sorenson, G.D., Lab. Invest. 11: 585, 1962.
9. Zucker-Franklin, D. and Franklin, E. C., Amer. J. Path., 59: 23, 1970.

T AND B BLOCKING FACTORS IN HODGKIN'S DISEASE

Z. Bentwich, R. Cohen and C. Brautbar

Department of Medicine A. and Immunology, Hebrew
University-Hadassah Medical School, Jerusalem, Israel

INTRODUCTION

Considerable evidence has been brought forward to show that patients with Hodgkin's disease (H.D.) have an impaired immune response (1,2). Since antibody production is relatively preserved, these findings seem to indicate that H.D. patients have a selective deficit in their cell mediated immunity. A number of studies have tried to correlate this deficit to a quantitative and/or qualitative deficit of peripheral T lymphocytes. The results of some of these studies are, however, conflicting. Decreased (3) as well as normal (4) percentage of peripheral T lymphocytes, has been found by some investigators, while normal (5) as well as impaired (6) reaction of H.D. lymphocytes to mitogens and allogeneic cells, have been reported by others. In other studies, decreased (7), normal (8), or elevated (9) number of peripheral B cells, have also been observed.

In the present study, we report on lymphocyte "blocking" factors in the sera of H.D. patients, which may possibly account for these as well as other observations in this disease.

SUBJECTS AND METHODS

Subjects. Thirty six patients with Hodgkin's disease referred to 3 central hospitals in Israel between April and October 1974, were studied. Their ages varied between 15 and 64 years; nineteen were males and seventeen were females. Fourteen were untreated, thirteen had received a course of radiotherapy 1-5 years prior to the study and nine had received either radiotherapy or chemotherapy

during the last 6 months. All patients were staged according to
the Ann Arbor classification (11) after thorough diagnostic
evaluation. There were 5 patients in stage I, 13 in stage II, 8 in
stage III and 10 in stage IV.

Healthy persons were used in each set of experiments and the
results supplied the normal range for each test.

Methods. Cell were isolated from heparinized or defibrinated
venous blood by the Ficoll-hypaque technique. Serum samples were
heat inactivated and then stored at -20°C until used. Identification
of phagocytic cells was routinely made by latex ingestion.

Spontaneous sheep erythrocyte (E) rosettes (12) served as a
T cell marker, while complement coated erythrocyte (EAC) rosette (13)
and binding of fluorescinated aggregated human gamma globulin (14)
were used as B cell markers. To study inhibition of rosette
formation and/or aggregate binding by sera of patients, 0.1 ml of
cell suspension were incubated overnight at room temperature with
0.1 ml serum previously absorbed with sheep red blood cells. The
cells were then washed three times in HBSS and rosette formation
and/or aggregate binding determined. The presence of surface Ig on
lymphocytes was measured by direct immunofluorescence(15).

The fluorochromatic cytotoxicity assay (16) was used for HL-A
typing, as well as for determining the presence of lymphocytotoxic
antibodies in the sera of the patients.

RESULTS

E-rosettes. E-rosette formation by peripheral blood lymphocytes (PBL) was determined in 23 H.D. patients and ten normal
controls, in parallel. In 9 patients, the assay was performed
immediately after cell separation, while in 14 other patients, it
was performed after overnight incubation of the separated cells in
culture medium (HBSS with 10% FCS). The mean percentage of rosette
forming lymphocytes in the two groups of patients was 16.5+ 12.6
and 38.0 + 13.2, respectively, and was significantly lower (p< 0.001),
than that of the respective normal controls (66.0 + 7.0 and
70.0+ 6.0). A significant increase in rosette formation by the cells
obtained from the same patient was observed after short term culture
of the cells.

EAC-rosette. EAC rosette formation by PBL was determined in
9 H.D. patients and ten normal controls, immediately after cell
separation. The mean percentage of rosettes in the patients was
3.3 + 3.0 which was significantly lower (p< 0.001)than in normal
controls 12.6 + 2.1. With the EAC rosettes, too, a significant

increase in rosette formation was observed after the same cells
were incubated overnight in HBSS with 10% FCS.

   Blood monocytes. The mean percentage of monocytes found in
the Ficoll purified blood cell suspensions obtained from 14 patients
was 38.0+ 8.2, and was significantly higher (p< 0.001) than that
found in 18 normal controls 13.0+ 2.1. The conditions under which
the assay is performed were found to be very important. When Ficoll
separation of blood samples was not performed shortly after the blood
was taken, no such differences between patients and normal controls
were observed.

   The proportions of T and B rosette forming lymphocytes and of
monocytes in the H.D. peripheral blood, did not seem to have any
correlation with clinical stage or anatomical extent of the disease,
despite the significant differences observed between all patients and
controls.

   Inhibition of rosette and aggregate binding by H.D. sera. Several
H.D. sera were found to inhibit both E and EAC rosettes formation and
the binding of fluorescinated gamma globulin, by normal lymphocytes.
This was seen either when normal cells from one donor were preincubated with the sera of several patients(Table I), or when normal
cells obtained from a number of donors were preincubated with 2-3
H.D. sera. Marked differences in the rosette inhibiting capacity of
the various H.D. sera can be seen, some sera causing none or only
negligible inhibition. The inhibition of EAC rosette formation was
generally greater than that of E rosettes. Inhibition of the
aggregate binding was generally much stronger, though variations in
the inhibition among the various H.D. sera can be seen. The degree
of rosette and/or aggregate binding inhibition, did not seem to show
any correlation with the clinical stage of the disease nor with
previous or present therapy. Normal human sera (other than AB serum)
showed no or only slight inhibition of rosette formation or aggregate
binding.

   Antilymphocyte antibodies. Using the microcytotoxicity assay,
nine of the H.D. sera were studied for the presence of lymphocytotoxic antibodies against a panel of normal and H.D. lymphocytes. In
only three sera were such antibodies found. The specificity of these
antibodies is not yet clear. Preliminary studies have not yet
disclosed specific anti HL-A or anti H.D. lymphocyte activity, and
no clear correlation with rosette and/or aggregate binding inhibition,
was observed.

   In another series of experiments, HL-A phenotype of several H.D.
lymphocytes was not found to vary when it was determined immediately
after cell separation and after short term culture.

Preliminary immunofluorescent studies also revealed the presence of antilymphocytic antibodies in a number of H.D. sera.

TABLE I

INHIBITION OF NORMAL ROSETTE AND AGGREGATE BINDING BY H.D. SERA[*]

H.D. serum no.	%E	%EAC	% aggregated γ-globulin
1	55(9.3)[+]	9(30.7)	5(61.5)
2	41(31.6)	4.5(65.3)	5(61.5)
3	36(40.0)	4.5(65.3)	7(46.1)
4	44(26.6)	3(76.9)	5(61.5)
5	45(25.0)	6(53.8)	6(53.8)
6	60(0)	13(0)	5(61.5)
Normal AB serum	60	13	13

[*]Representative experiment using lymphocytes from one normal donor.

[+]Number in brackets express inhibition as percent of the values obtained after preincubation with the reference normal AB serum.

DISCUSSION

These findings suggest that the low proportion of rosette forming lymphocytes in the peripheral blood of patients with Hodgkin's disease cannot be ascribed to the low number of T and B cells, but rather to some alteration in their function, caused at least in part, by some extracellular factor present in the serum of these patients. Varied results have been reported for the proportions of T and B lymphocytes in the peripheral blood of H.D. patients (3,4,7,8,9). Variations in the procedure used for preparing rosettes, may account for some of the differences observed (17). It is apparent from our study however, that E and EAC rosette formation may be inadequate to identify all peripheral blood T and B cells in Hodgkin's disease (and possibly in other diseases as well), unless the cells are left in a short term culture prior to

the test. Similar findings have only very recently been reported
also by Kaplan et al., who however studied only T and not B
rosettes (18).

One of the surprising features of current investigation of T
and B cells in disease is the widespread occurrence of antibodies,
particularly against T cells. We have also found anti-lymphocyte
antibodies in some of the H.D. sera, both by microcytotoxicity and
immunofluorescent assays. It has been shown, however, that there
are many antibodies that are not readily detected by the cytotoxic
and fluorescence assays and can be detected only by their inhibitory
effect on the mixed lymphocyte reaction (MLR). Such antibodies have
also been shown to coat the cells in vivo and shed from the surface
during short term culture (19). Whether such antibodies are indeed
present in H.D. sera, and if so can account for all the rosette and
aggregate blocking activity of these sera is not yet clear. It is
also possible that other non-antibody factors like serum ferritin(20)
or serum migration inhibitory activity (21) that are increased in
H.D. patients can be implicated in the blocking activity.

It has been recently shown that the Fc receptor on murine
cells (also detected by the binding of aggregated human globulin),
may be specifically blocked by antisera directed against the immune
response associated (Ia)gene products (22). This would indicate that
this receptor and the cell on which it is located are crucial for
the normal immune response, probably both cellular and humoral.
The blocking of this receptor by the H.D. sera that we have observed
may probably hold considerable promise for gaining an understanding
of the character of the equivalent human Ia gene product.

There are probably various mechanisms by which tumor cells can
escape from immunological destruction by the host's lymphocytes.
Most notably is the one involving blocking factors present in the
serum (23). Little is known however about the molecular nature,
mode of action and effects of these factors on various functions
of T and B lymphocytes and of macrophages. The results of the
present study may shed light on some of these effects by serum
factors present in Hodgkin's patients. Further study of these
factors in other malignancies and diseases and their correlation
with clinical stage and/or manifestation of the disease is fully
warranted, and will be the subject of subsequent reports.

REFERENCES

1. Aisenberg, A.C. Cancer, 1966, 19, 385.
2. Eltringham, J.R., Kaplan, H.S. Natn. Cancer Inst. Monograph, 1973, 36, 107.
3. Cohnen, G., Augener, W., Brittinger, G., Douglas, S.D. New Engl. J. Med. 1973, 289, 863.
4. Kaur, J., Spiers, A.S.D., Catovsky, D., Galton, D.A.G. Lancet, 1974, II, 800.
5. Lang, J.M., Tongio, M.M., Oberling, F., Mayer, S., Waitz, R. Lancet, 1972, I, 1261.
6. Levy, R., Kaplan, H.S. New Engl. J. Med. 1974, 290, 181.
7. Gajl-Peczalska, K.J., Hansen, J.A., Bloomfield, C.D., Good, R.A. J. Clin. Invest. 1973, 52, 3064.
8. Cohnen, G., Augener, W., König, E., Brittinger, G., Douglas, S.D. New Engl. J. Med. 1973, 288, 161.
9. Grifoni, V., DelGiaco, G.S., Manconi, P.E., Tognella, S. Lancet, 1972, I, 848.
10. Lukes, R.J., Craver, L.F., Hall, T.C., Rappaport, H., Rubin, P. Cancer Res. 1966, 26, 1311.
11. Carbone, P.P., Kaplan, H.S., Musshof, K., Smithers, D.W., Tubiana, M. Cancer Res. 1971, 31, 1860.
12. Bentwich, Z., Douglas, S.D., Siegal, F.P., Kunkel, H.G. Clin. Immunol. Immunopath. 1973, 1, 511.
13. Shevach, E.M., Jaffe, E.S., Green, I. Transplantation Rev. 1973, 16, 3.
14. Dickler, H.B., Kunkel, H.G. J. exp. Med. 1972, 136, 191.
15. Siegal, F.P., Pernis, B., Kunkel, H.G. Europ. J. Immunol. 1971, 1, 482.
16. Bodmer, W., Tripp, M., Bodmer, J. In "Histocompatibility Testing" (E.S. Curtoni, P.L. Mattinz, R.M. Tosi. eds.) p. 341, Munksgaard, Copenhagen.
17. Bentwich, Z., Kunkel, H.G. Transplantation Rev. 1973, 16, 29.
18. Kaplan, H.S., Bobrove, A.M., Fuks, Z., Strober, S. New Engl. J. Med. 1974, 290, 971.
19. Wernet, P., Kunkel, H.G. J. exp. Med. 1973, 138, 1021.
20. Jones, P.A.E., Miller, F.M., Worwood, M., Jacobs, A. Br. J. Cancer 1973, 27, 212.
21. Cohen, S., Fisher, B., Yoshida, T., Bettigole, R. New Engl. J. Med. 1974, 290, 882.
22. Dickler, H.B., Sachs, D.H. J. exp. Med. 1974, 140, 779.
23. Hellström, K.E., Hellström, I. Adv. Immunol. 1974, 18, 209.

PROPERTIES OF TRANSPLANTABLE RETICULUM CELL SARCOMAS IN SJL/J MICE

S.P. Lerman, N.M. Ponzio, E.A. Carswell and G.J. Thorbecke

Dept. of Pathology, New York University School of Medicine, New York, N.Y. and Sloan-Kettering Institute for Cancer Research, Walker Lab., Rye, N.Y.

The transplantable reticulum cell sarcomas (RCS-5 and RCS-19 of SJL/J mice, derived in the Sloan-Kettering Institute for Cancer Research by Drs. Carswell and Old from spontaneous tumors in this strain, have two very unusual properties. Firstly, these tumor cells induce an extremely high proliferative response in syngeneic cells from normal, non-tumorous mice (1) and secondly, while they are readily transplantable in normal syngeneic hosts, they fail to grow if the mice have been irradiated prior to tumor cell injection (Carswell and Old, unpublished observations; 2,3). We are reporting here on studies aimed at elucidating: 1) The nature of the antigen which induces the strong T cell proliferation in both thymus and peripheral T cells (1); 2) The basis for the relatively limited but definite immunity which the SJL/J mice exhibit upon immunization (4); 3) That property of irradiated mice which prevents RCS growth; and 4) The nature and characteristics of the tumor cells themselves.

The studies on the proliferative response represented in Table 1 show that the antigen involved is resistant to treatment with 25 U/ml neuraminidase and to 1 mg/ml of pronase. Other preliminary observations suggest that the antigen(s) may be trypsin sensitive. Pretreatment of the stimulating tumor cells with various antisera and control sera in the presence of C shows no cytotoxic effect of anti-Ig or anti-Thy 1.2 and also no significant inhibition of the stimulatory property. In contrast anti-Ia (kindly donated by Dr. D.C. Shreffler, University of Michigan) + C kills >50% of the tumor cells and greatly reduces their capacity to induce proliferation (Table 1). The tumor cells thus appear to lack Thy 1.2 and Ig, while a large percentage possess Ia antigens.

In spite of the strong proliferation induced in syngeneic cells

Table 1

CHARACTERIZATION OF THE STIMULATING CELL IN THE
PROLIFERATIVE RESPONSE OF NORMAL SJL/J LYMPH NODE
(LN) CELLS TO SYNGENEIC IRRADIATED RCS CELLS

Responding LN cells (2×10^5)[1]	Stimulating X-RCS-5 (10^5)[1]	cpm/culture[2]	
		Expt 1	Expt 2
+	None	163	466
+	Untreated	11,863	13,365
+	Neuraminidase (25 U/ml)[3]	12,255	
+	Pronase (1 mg/ml)[3]	9,472	
+	anti-Ig + gp C[4]	6,938	
+	NRS + gp C[4]	8,286	
+	anti-Thy 1.2 + RC[4]		13,067
+	NMS + RC[4]		11,996
+	anti-Ia + RC[4]		3,219
-	Untreated	328	578

[1] Cells cultured in Linbro microplates (#15-FB-96-TC), RCS-5 cells received 6000 R γ-irradiation. Medium-modified MEM + 10% Fetal calf serum. [2] H[3]-thymidine added on day 3, cultures terminated 24 hours later. [3] 20 min. at 37°C, neuraminidase (Vibrio cholera). [4] NRS and anti-Ig diluted 1:30; gpC diluted 1:15; anti-Thy 1.2 and NMS diluted 1:45; anti-Ia diluted 1:100; RC 1:45.

which, as other studies in this laboratory show, also occurs in vivo, induction of cytotoxic activity in host cells is not readily obtained. The results in Table 2 illustrate that immunization with irradiated RCS leads to the generation of a cytotoxic effect in cells of allogeneic mice, both in vivo and in vitro, whereas neither procedure results in cytotoxic activity with syngeneic cells. In fact, in vitro, there appears to be an inverse relationship between the proliferative and cytotoxic responses (Table 2). However, cytotoxic effector cells may not be totally absent from this syngeneic system, since preliminary results suggest that challenge in vitro of cells from in vivo immunized SJL/J mice may lead to a low degree of cytotoxicity (Ponzio, unpublished observations). Other attempts to facilitate a primary cytotoxic response in vitro have all failed. Trinitriphenylated (TNP) RCS cells induce a good cytotoxic response in SJL/J LN cells to TNP-RCS without eliciting any effect on the unconjugated RCS cells (5). Neither does the addition of mitomycin-treated allogeneic (BALB/c) cells to mixtures of SJL/J LN and RCS lead to any cytotoxicity towards RCS cells (5). Thus, the situation here is clearly different from those where a weak cytotoxic effect is the result of limited H_2 differences (6). The most comparable results in the literature concern the M locus differences which also lead to strong proliferation without detectable cytotoxicity (7).

The lack of growth of RCS in irradiated syngeneic mice is illustrated in Fig. 1. This figure also shows a similar effect on the

Table 2
FAILURE OF RCS TO INDUCE CYTOTOXIC ACTIVITY IN SYNGENEIC CELLS AFTER EITHER IN VIVO OR IN VITRO "IMMUNIZATION"

EXPOSED TO RCS	EFFECTOR CELLS	RATIO E/T[1]	% CYTOTOXICITY[2]		STIMULATION[3] INDEX MLR
			51Cr-RCS	51Cr-PU5	
In Vivo[4]	SJL/J,PE	50	1.0		
		100	8.4	-1.2	
	LAF₁,PE	25	47.3	4.3	
		50	68.1		
	SBF₁,Spl	100	3.1	0.0	
	SJL/J,Spl	200	0.4	-0.5	
	LAF₁,Spl	100	23.2	3.4	
In Vitro[5]	SJL/J,LN	100	1.1	1.2	29.8x
	BALB/c,LN	100	39.5	13.3	6.3x
	SJL/J,LN	50	2.6	6.9	246.5x
	BALB/c,LN	50	26.3	14.3	45.4x

[1] E/T = effector to target cell ratio in cytotoxic tests; 4 hrs at 37°C. [2] (specific-spontaneous) release x 100/(maximal-spontaneous) release ^{51}Cr-target cells were RCS of SJL/J and PU-5 of BALB/c origin. [3] Stimulation indices were determined from 0.2 ml microplate cultures containing 2 x 10⁵ responding and 5 x 10⁴ stimulating cells (table 1) and calculated as cpm in mixed cells/sum of cpm of each cell alone. [4] Immunized by 3 biweekly injections of 10⁷ γ-irradiated (10,000R) RCS cells. [5] LN cells (4 x 10⁷) of the strain indicated were cultured for 5 days with 10⁷ irradiated RCS cells in Falcon flasks (#3013).

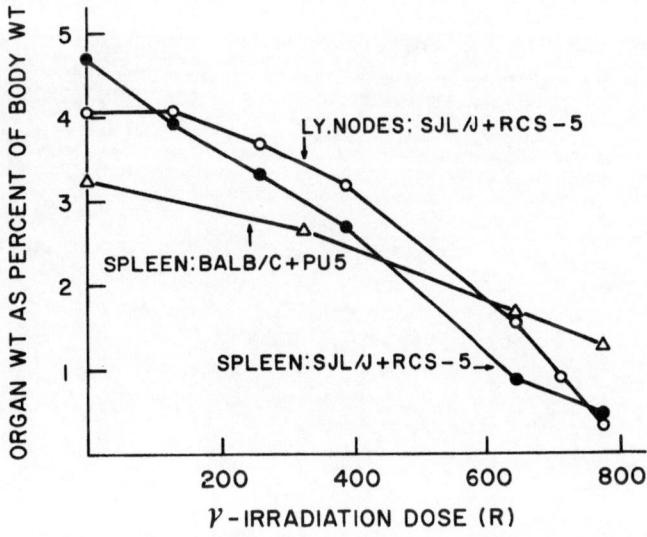

Fig. 1. Growth (see table 3) on day 6 after iv injection of 10⁷ tumor cells into syngeneic mice, irradiated on day -1.

Table 3
ROLE OF T CELLS AND MACROPHAGES IN PROMOTING
RCS GROWTH IN IRRADIATED SYNGENEIC MICE

TREATMENT OF RECIPIENTS			$(LN + SPLEEN\ WT/BODY\ WT)^3 \times 100$	
Day -2 γ-ray[1]	Day -1 Ly Node Cells[2]	Day 0 RCS-5[3]	Expt 1	Expt 2
-	None	+	5.23 ± 0.01	6.41 ± 0.38
+	None	+	1.32 ± 0.05	1.34 ± 0.18
+	Untreated	+	2.82 ± 0.22	2.73 ± 0.51
+	Macr. Depleted	+	1.02 ± 0.11	1.60 ± 0.21
+	NMS + C	+	3.27 ± 0.52	2.70 ± 0.12
+	Anti-Thy 1.2 + C	+	2.70 ± 0.18	2.01 ± 0.17

[1] 650 R γ-irradiation. [2] 4×10^7 viable cells i.v. in all cases except after anti-Thy 1.2 + C treatment (3×10^7); macrophage depletion was by incubation with carbonyl iron and passage over magnet.
[3] 10^7 tumor cells i.v.; Axillary + mesenteric LN + spleen of recipients were weighed on day 5 or 6 as a measure of tumor growth.

growth of another lymphoid tumor (PU-5) in syngeneic mice. This BALB/c tumor has been characterized as of B cell origin (8) and grows primarily in spleen or locally. For both tumors a progressively greater inhibition of growth is obtained as the dose of whole body γ-irradiation of prospective recipients is increased.

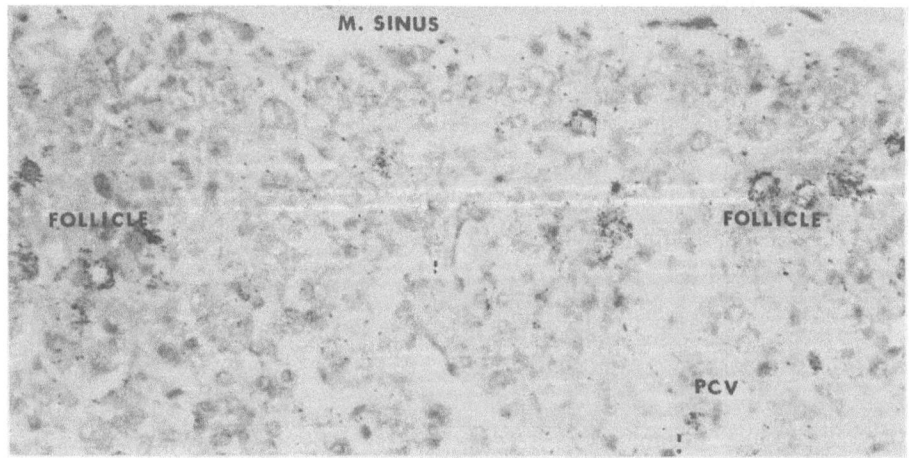

Fig. 2. Autoradiograph of lymph node from irradiated SJL/J mouse 24 hours after iv injection of 2×10^7 ^{3}H-uridine labeled RCS cells. (120x). M. sinus = marginal sinus, PCV = postcapillary venule.

Table 4
ABILITY OF MACROPHAGE INHIBITORY AGENTS TO DEPRESS
RCS-5 GROWTH IN LYMPH NODES OF SYNGENEIC HOSTS

	% OF CONTROL GROWTH[1]	
TREATMENT OF RECIPIENTS	Expt 1	Expt 2
Untreated	100	100
	(2.05 ± 0.17)	(1.47 ± 0.06)
Trypan blue, daily[2]	45	
Trypan blue, pretreatment[3]	62	
Silica, pretreatment[4]		63
450 R[5]	52	75
450 R[5] Trypan blue, pretreatment	27	
450 R[5] Silica[6]		52

[1] 10^7 RCS-5 cells injected i.v. on day 0; growth determined on day
5 or 6 and expressed as (Ax + Mes. LN wt/Body wt) x 100. [2] Trypan
blue, 4 mg i.v. on day 0, 1 mg i.p. every day thereafter. [3] Trypan
blue, 4 mg i.v. on day -2, 4 mg i.p. on day -1. [4] Silica, 5 mg i.v.,
2 Hrs prior to tumor. [5] 450 R on day -2. [6] Silica, 5 mg i.v. on day -1.

Studies which are described in detail elsewhere (9) have shown
that ^{3}H-uridine labeled RCS cells localize effectively in spleen
and lymph nodes of both irradiated and normal SJL/J mice upon intravenous injection. Neither histological localization nor overall distribution of the radioactivity indicate a failure of the cells to
reach specific areas of the lymphoid tissue or to survive injection.
In irradiated and normal recipients, these tumor cells localize within 24 hours after injection primarily in follicular areas (Fig. 2).
In normal recipients, the amount of radioactivity per cell rapidly
diminishes over the next 2-3 days and marked enlargement of typical
tumor areas is noted in all the lymphoid tissues. In irradiated
recipients the dilution of the label per cell is much less rapid, as
is seen not only in the lymphoid tissue itself but also in the peri-
portal areas of the liver and in the lung (Fig. 3A and B). The persistence of labeled cells in irradiated recipients indicates a marked
inability to proliferate and also the absence of a destructive effect
of the host on these cells. Thus, the failure to grow in irradiated
hosts appears due to a defect of the milieu rather than to an inability of the cells to home to proper areas. Neither does a cytotoxic
effect appear to be the reason for the lack of growth. In addition,
the homing of these tumor cells to follicles in a manner similar to
normal bone marrow or spleen B cells (9,10) suggests a B cell origin
for the RCS tumors. This contention is also supported by the presence of Ia antigen on their surfaces (11) and by the supposed origin
of the primary tumors in germinal centers (12).

In further studies on the defect in irradiated hosts it has
been found that the growth of RCS in 650 R irradiated mice can be
enhanced by the intravenous injection of normal lymphoid cells 1 day

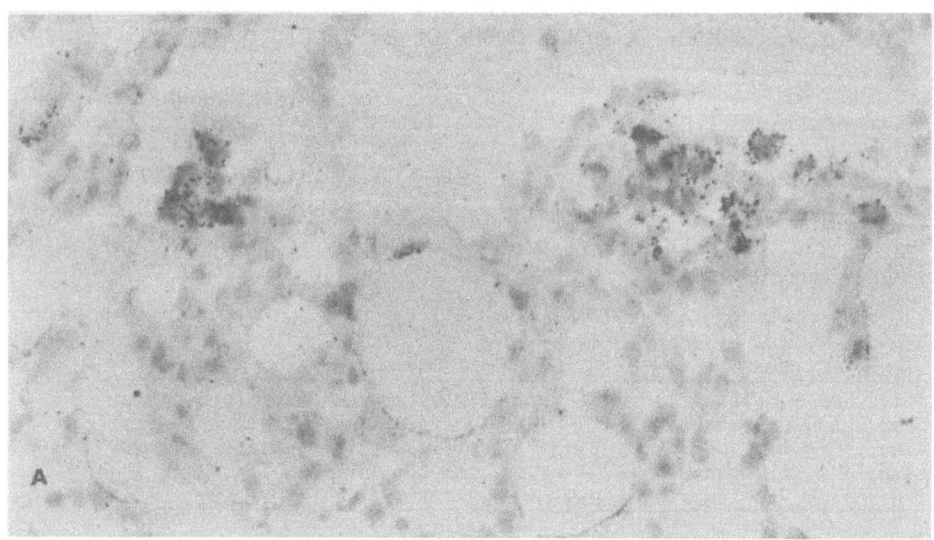

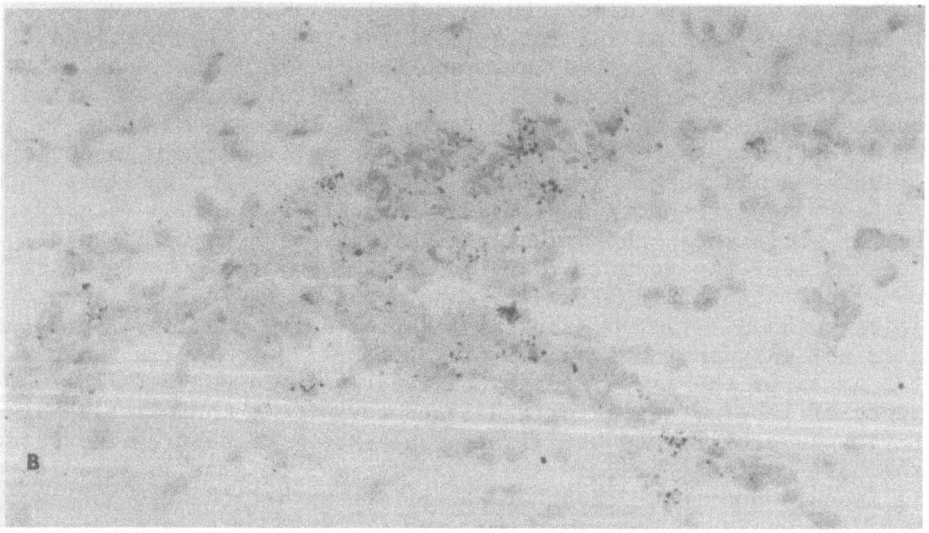

Fig. 3. Autoradiographs of lung from irradiated (A) and unirradiated
(B) SJL/J mice taken 48 hours after iv injection of 2 x 10^7 ^{3}H-uri-
dine labeled RCS cells. Note the contrast between small areas of
heavily labeled cells in A and larger tumor area with far fewer grains
per cell in B, suggesting a much more marked dilution of the label
through the better proliferation of tumor cells in the normal than
in the irradiated host (120 x, methyl green pyronin).

prior to tumor cells (3). Initial findings suggest that a cooperation between thymus and bone marrow derived cells might be operative
here. Table 3 shows the results of our efforts to identify the
cells which promote growth of RCS in the irradiated environment.
While the removal of T cells from the normal lymph node suspensions
does not much diminish their ability to help tumor growth, depletion
of macrophages greatly reduces this property. Other findings also
suggest that macrophages are important for the growth promotion of
RCS in both normal and 450 R irradiated mice (Table 4). Pretreatment
with two agents, silica and trypan blue, known to be inhibitory to
macrophage function (13,14) decreases growth of RCS in normal mice
and significantly aggravates the effect of the relatively low dose
of irradiation used in these experiments. Thus, it appears that
macrophages, perhaps in conjunction with T cells, facilitate RCS
growth, possibly through elaboration of a factor which promotes
tumor cell division. A definitive answer as to the role of T cells
must await results of studies with thymusless mice of SJL/J genetic
background (3).

Bibliography

1. Lerman, S.P., Chapman, J.M., Carswell, E.A., and Thorbecke, G.J.,
   Int. J. Cancer 14:808, 1974.
2. Lerman, S.P., Chapman, J.M., Carswell, E.A., and Thorbecke, G.J.,
   Fed. Proc. 33:616, 1974.
3. Lerman, S.P., Jacobson, E.B., Carswell, E.A., and Thorbecke, G.J.,
   Fed. Proc. 34:852, 1975.
4. Carswell, E.A., Wanebo, H.J., Old, L.J., and Boyse, E.A., J. Natl.
   Cancer Inst. 44:1281, 1970.
5. Ponzio, N.M., Lerman, S.P., and Thorbecke, G.J., submitted.
6. Alter, B.J. and Bach, F.H., J. Exp. Med. 140:1440, 1974.
7. Abbasi, J., Festenstein, H., Eur. J. Immunol. 3:430, 1973.
8. Green, I., Shevach, E.M., Stobe, J., Frank, M., and Herberman, R.,
   Adv. Exp. Med. 29:491, 1972.
9. Carswell, E.A., Lerman, S.P., and Thorbecke, G.J., submitted.
10. Howard, J.C., Hunt, S.V., and Gowans, J.L., J. Exp. Med. 135:
    200, 1972.
11. Shreffler, D.C. and David, C.S., Adv. in Immunol. 20:125, 1975.
12. Siegler, R. and Rich, M.A., J. Natl. Cancer Inst. 41:125, 1968.
13. Allison, A.C., Harington, J.S., and Birbeck, M., J. Exp. Med.
    124:141, 1966.
14. Hibbs, J.B., Transplantation 19:77, 1975.

Acknowledgments
    We thank Dr. K. Roback, Essen-Krey, Germany for a gift of silica
particles and Ms. J. Chapman for competent assistance. Supported by
USPHS grant CA 14462 and by the New York Cancer Research Institute, Inc.
N.M. Ponzio is a postdoctoral trainee on USPHS Training Grant GM 00127.

SKIN AS A VEHICLE FOR HORIZONTAL TRANSMISSION OF GROSS PASSAGE A LEUKEMIA IN ADULT MICE. A UNIQUE MICROENVIRONMENT?[1]

T. Mariani[2]

Department of Laboratory Medicine and Pathology

University of Minnesota, Minneapolis, Minnesota U.S.A.

In malignancy in vivo studies, skin is one of the frequently manipulated organs. It has been painted or injected subcutaneously with carcinogens in order to induce tumor growth. Attempts to induce immunity to tumor growth have included intradermal injection and scarification techniques. But in all these manipulations, the skin is used only as an "experimental medium" through which some other element of the oncogenic process is studied - either the tumor itself or the immune response to the challenge of the tumor. A recent discovery in my laboratory, however, has strongly suggested that the skin microenvironment itself may play a role in the oncogenic process.

It is well established that mice injected as neonates with leukemic virus regularly develop malignancy. In contrast, when they are injected as weanling or adults, the mice regularly develop immunity. This pattern is the rule in my Gross passage A (GPA) virus-mouse system.

Because of this high degree of age-related immunologic resistance, attempts to induce virus-related malignancy in adult animals have in the past met with limited success. For example, Dr. Ludwik Gross injected C3H mice (51 days, average age) with GPA virus intracranially and intraperitoneally. These manipulations induced leukemia in only 37% of the animals with a mean latent period (MLP) of 8.8 months.

[1]Aided by grants from USPHS CA-12929 from the National Cancer Institute, Leukemia Society of America, Inc., Minnesota Medical Fdn.

[2]Scholar of the Leukemia Society of America, Inc.

Despite this extensive immunologic barrier, I have recently induced leukemia in 100% of the treated animals - regardless of age.
The method I used is unique. It involved grafting normal weanling
or adult mice with skin taken from animals which had been exposed
to GPA virus. All the animals treated in this way ultimately died
of disseminated lymphoma.

The discovery of this method itself was not the product of a
single experiment. It has evolved from a series of studies (1-6).

MATERIALS AND METHODS

C3H/Bi, DBA/2,and F_1 hybrids of these inbred mice were used in
these investigations. The mice were initially foster-nursed on C57B1
females to eliminate the milk-borne mammary carcinoma agent and have
been maintained by rigorous inbreeding procedures.

The GPA virus, originally obtained from Dr. Ludwik Gross, has
been maintained by serial passage in newborn C3H/Bi mice. My method
for growing the GPA lymphoma in the ascites form in C3H/Bi and
(C3H/Bi x DBA/2)F_1 strains was reported in (7).

Skin grafting was always female to female and male to male.
The method was described in (1). Routinely grafts were observed
daily and measured weekly. Graft acceptance was characterized by
luxuriant hair growth. Complete sloughing of the graft or little or
no hair growth indicated rejection. Each grafted animal was housed
in an individual plastic cage, and given Purina Laboratory Chow
pellets and water ad libitum.

In Table 1 the various virus-skin transplantation protocols are
illustrated. For the initial skin-grafting series (Group I, 2-3
months old), syngeneic (C3H/Bi x DBA/2)F_1 mice (47 total) were
grafted with skin taken from 2 groups of leukemic donors: 1) with
ascites-form lymphoma 10-15 days after IP tumor transfer; and 2) with
lymphoma 3-4 months after neonate virus injection intrathymically
(IT, 0.05 ml) or intraperitoneally (IP, 0.1 ml). In these experiments, the implication was that the leukemic skin would contain tumor
cells and virus (endogeneous) that had migrated to the site as a result of the malignant process.

In the next series (Group II, 2-3 months old), GPA virus was
exogenously introduced into the skin. C3H/Bi mice (34 total) were
grafted with normal syngeneic skin. Twenty-four hours post-trans-
plantation, the newly placed grafts were directly injected subder-
mally (ID) with purified GPA virus (0.1 ml) either in a cell-free
filtrate from leukemic tissue preparation (25 animals) or in an irradiated (in vitro, 5000 R) cell-free ascites form (25 animals).

Between 1 and 1½ years after virus injection, these 50 animals were further divided for additional treatment: 1) Seven mice from each of the two virus preparation groups received no further treatment; 2) An exchange of skin was performed between treated animals and normal syngeneic recipients. 20 graft-beds (10 from each of the two virus preparation groups) were transplanted onto the normal recipients, and the normal skin was grafted onto the treated animals at the original graft site; 3) Eight mice from each virus preparation group (16 in all) were sacrificed. Their graft beds and abdominal skin were transplanted onto normal syngeneic recipients. The 68 recipients of this treated skin, C3H/Bi mice (2-11 month old), are designated as Group III.

The third series involved preleukemic skin transplantation. The assumption was made that this preleukemic skin did not contain tumor cells. It was also assumed that if virus was present in pre-leukemic skin, it would be endogenous in nature since the donors had been virus-injected as neonates. Preleukemic skin was routinely taken from 4-5 week old donors neonatally injected IT with GPA virus (0.05 ml) but not yet showing malignant signs. Two groups of normal C3H/Bi mice were grafted with preleukemic skin (Group IV, 1 month old, 49 total; Group V, 2-18 months old, 119 total).

To verify the presence of typical disseminated GPA lymphoma, lymphoid organs (thymus, spleen, inguinal, axillary, mesenteric nodes) were excised from all mice (killed or spontaneous death) and processed by routine histologic methods for light microscopy examination. Donors' skin taken at the time of grafting was similarly processed.

RESULTS

The successful horizontal transmission of GPA lymphoma to over 300 animals using skin transplantation protocols is illustrated in Table 1. The latent periods and percentages of thymus (primary target site) enlargement are also indicated. Though not presented in tabular form, autopsy revealed that other lymphoid tissues (spleen, lymph nodes) were extensively involved in all experimental groups (60-100%). All of the experimental animals eventually died of typical disseminated GPA lymphoma as verified by gross and microscopic examination.

In the initial study, 47 (C3H/Bi x DBA/2)F$_1$ mice (Group I) were grafted with syngeneic skin taken from leukemic donors with ascites form lymphoma (1). All these recipients died within 21 days. 62% showed thymus enlargement. Similar pathologic findings (not shown in Table 1) were observed in C3H/Bi recipients of syngeneic skin taken from leukemic donors that had been virus injected (IT) as neonates.

TABLE 1

SUCCESSFUL HORIZONTAL TRANSMISSION OF GPA LEUKEMIA IN ADULT INBRED
MICE: A VIRUS-SKIN INTERACTION

Group*	Age (months)	Route of Virus Introduction	Thymus Enlargement Total No. Animals	%	Latent Period (days) Range	Mean
I	2-3	leukemic skin graft	29/47	62	16-31	21
II	2-3	normal skin graft + GPA virus ID	26/34	76	211-739	558
			5/16+	31	sacrificed	
III	2-11	skin graft from ID virus-injected group	49/68	72	120-545	422
IV	1	preleukemic skin graft	41/49	84	95-319	174
V	2-18	preleukemic skin graft	84/119	71	13-644	363

* C3H/Bi - Groups I, II, IV, V; (C3H/Bi x DBA/2)F$_1$ - Group III.

+ Sixteen mice were sacrificed 390 days after virus injection.

In Group II, 50 C3H/Bi mice were grafted with normal syngeneic skin which was directly injected ID with GPA virus preparation 24 hours after grafting (5). Sixteen of these animals were sacrificed approximately 390 days after treatment. The other 34 animals showed a MLP of 558 days with a 76% incidence of thymus enlargement. The lower incidence of thymus enlargement (31%) in the sacrificed group probably results from the significantly shorter latent period (168 days less) at time of sacrifice.The Group III normal recipients of treated skin taken from the Group II animals showed a MLP of 422 days with a 72% occurrence of thymus enlargement.

The two groups which were grafted with preleukemic skin both showed high thymus involvement rates: Group IV, 84%; Group V, 71% (8,9). However, significant differences in the length of the latent period were observed. The one month old recipients of preleukemic skin grafts showed a MLP of 174 days in contrast to 363 days for the 2-18 month old recipients. A general trend emerged: The latent periods were inversely related to the age of the recipients at time of grafting. A second general pattern was the rate of thymus involvement: As the age of the recipient at grafting increased, the incidence of thymus involvement decreased.

All the skin grafts taken from leukemic donors were regularly rejected with graft-site tumor development (Group I). In contrast, the preleukemic skin grafts were accepted, and no tumor developed at the graft-site (Groups IV, V). All grafts were accepted by both the skin-virus-injected recipients (Group II) and the normal recipients (Group III) that were grafted with skin taken from Group II mice. No graft-site tumors developed. Histologic examination revealed the presence of tumor cells in all grafts that were rejected. In contrast, no tumor cells were found in any accepted graft.

DISCUSSION

The most exciting aspect of this discovery is that I can now regularly induce GPA lymphoma in weanling and adult mice. Horizontal transmission of a leukemic virus malignancy is not only possible, it is now a reality.

Several provocative findings have emerged from these studies. First and foremost, of course, is the fact that skin or the "virus-skin microenvironment" can play a role in the transmission of a malignancy. Other observations pertain to age-related differences in the interaction between the malignancy and the host's immune system during leukemogenesis. The inverse relationship between the duration of the latent period and the age of the animal when virus was presented by preleukemic skin grafts suggests the possibility of an age-related decline in immunocompetence. Further, as the age of the animal at time of virus presentation increased, the incidence of thymus involvement decreased reflecting perhaps the current postulate that thymic function declines with age. This hypothesis is strengthened by the observation that no decline in involvement patterns occurred with any other lymphoid organs. These differences may also reflect subtle variations in the responses to GPA virus between neonate and adult animals. In a larger sense, they may be indicative of subtle immunologic differences between the neonate and adult animals.

Though several different manipulations were involved in the evolution of this new method, preleukemic skin grafting proved to be the most effective of the procedures. The extraordinary success of this method - compared with all other routes of virus introduction - compels analysis of the special microenvironment of this preleukemic skin. Undoubtedly it is the key to understanding the mechanism underlying this unusual phenomenon.

At this initial phase of exploration, several hypotheses should be considered and eventually tested. Apparently, the virus contained in the environment of the skin graft escapes immunologic surveillance and can therefore induce leukemia rather than immunity. An immuno-deviation, e.g., tolerance or enhancement, may exist in which antibody produced would be ineffective in viral neutralization. Or, possibly, virus in skin is in a special or processed form - a form that when in the environment of the skin escapes immunologic surveillance but eventually disseminates to the primary target sites - the lymphoid organs.

Thorough investigation will reveal which mechanisms are operant in this horizontal malignancy transmission phenomenon. Discovery of this unique skin-graft model to induce malignancy in adult mice provides a powerful tool for investigating basic aspects of oncogenesis and immune system dynamics.

REFERENCES

1. Mariani, T., Dent, P.B. and Good, R.A., J. Nat. Cancer Inst. 44: 319-328, 1970.

2. Mariani, T., Maruyama, Y. and Good, R.A., J. Nat. Cancer Inst. 47:361-366, 1971.

3. Mariani, T., Maruyama, Y. and Good, R.A., J. Nat. Cancer Inst. 48:363-366, 1972.

4. Mariani, T., Maruyama, Y. and Good, R.A., J. Nat. Cancer Inst. 49:879-885, 1972.

5. Mariani, T., Maruyama, Y. and Good, R.A., Nat. Cancer Inst. Monogr. 35:309-320, 1972.

6. Mariani, T. and Maruyama, Y., J. Nat. Cancer Inst. 53:1661-1664, 1974.

7. Mariani, T., Dent, P.B. and Good, R.A., Proc. Soc. Exp. Biol. Med. 138:889-892, 1971.

8. Mariani, T., Maruyama, Y. and Good, R.A., Proc. Soc. Exp. Biol. Med. 137 (No. 2):513-515, 1971.

9. Mariani, T., J. Nat. Cancer Inst. (submitted).

THE RELATIONSHIP BETWEEN PHAGOCYTOSIS, RELEASE OF LYSOSOMAL ENZYMES

AND 3', 5' CYCLIC ADENOSINE MONOPHOSPHATE IN MOUSE MACROPHAGES 1)

H. Dieter WELSCHER and André CRUCHAUD

Division of Immunology and Allergy

Hôpital cantonal, 1211 Geneva 4, Switzerland

Polymorphonuclear leukocytes (PMNL) selectively release lyso-somal enzymes when exposed to immune reactants (1-4). The same phe-nomenon has been demonstrated for mouse peritoneal (PM) and alveo-lar macrophages following phagocytosis of zymosan (5), latex parti-cles (6), immune complexes (7) and asbestos (8). Excretion of enzy-mes by PMNL is controlled by cyclic nucleotides (9, and reviewed in Ref. 10). The data presented here show that the rate of lysosomal enzyme release by macrophages depends upon the nature of the endo-cytosed material. The role of 3',5' cyclic adenosine monophosphate (cAMP) in this process seems to be much less important than has been shown for PMNL.

MATERIALS AND METHODS

Particles : Zymosan was obtained from Sigma (St. Louis, Mo., USA); heat-aggregated human IgG (ΔHGG) and immune complexes made of ΔHGG and rheumatoid factor (ΔHGG-RF) were prepared as described by Weissmann et al. (1). Peritoneal macrophages (PM) were obtained from the peritoneal cavity of Swiss mice 3 days following injection of proteose peptone. In enzyme release studies PM were suspended in Eagle's medium (MEM) supplemented with 10% inactivated foetal calf serum (FCS). One-ml aliquots containing $8-10.10^6$ PM were cultured in the presence and in the absence of particles and drugs at 37°C in 95% air and 5% CO_2, using 35x10 mm Falcon dishes. Supernatants were carefully removed after 0-180 min incubation and cells were

1) This work was supported by grant No. 3.768.72 of the Swiss National Foundation for Scientific Research.

lysed with 2 ml of 0.2% Triton X-100. For <u>determination of cAMP</u>
<u>levels</u>, one-ml aliquots containing 5.10^6 cells were cultured in
Falcon tubes and incubations stopped after 0-10 min by heat inactivation. <u>β-D-glucuronidase</u> and <u>β-D-galactosidase</u> were determined as
described by Kato et al. (11) and Conchie et al. (12) respectively,
and the activity expressed as nmoles p-nitrophenol/10^7 macrophages/
min. <u>LDH</u> activity was assessed using the Boehringer UV test combination and expressed as mU/10^7 macrophages. The amount of enzyme
released into the medium was expressed as the percentage of total
enzyme activity for 10^7 cells. <u>cAMP</u> was assayed as described by
Gilman (13); cAMP levels were expressed as pmoles/10^7 cells. For
<u>evaluation of phagocytosis</u> 5.10^6 PM in 0.5 ml MEM plus FCS were in-
cubated with various concentrations of either dibutyryl-cAMP (DBcAMP)
or theophylline for 10 min at 37°C. Sheep red blood cells (SRBC)
labelled with ^{51}Cr and opsonized with rabbit anti-SRBC serum were
then added and phagocytosis was estimated after 1 hr as previously
described (14).

                          RESULTS AND DISCUSSION

     Fig. 1 A and B illustrates that during the entire incubation
time of 180 min there was an increase in β-glucuronidase and β-galactosidase activity in the culture medium. In most experiments
this increase, as compared to 0 min incubation, became already statistically significant (p<0.05) after 10 min and represented 1.5 to
4 times the control value after 180 min. The enzyme release was not
a consequence of cell death as proved by the low increase of LDH, a
non-lysosomal enzyme. Zymosan and ΔHGG-RF both appeared to be more
potent than ΔHGG in inducing enzyme release. Control cells also released enzymes though to a lesser extent than phagocytizing cells
and probably as a consequence of activation induced by adherence to
culture dishes. When macrophages were exposed to identical amounts
of aggregated protein particles (i.e. 640 µg of either ΔHGG or ΔHGG-
RF per 8.10^6 PM), the difference between ΔHGG and ΔHGG-RF became
statistically significant for β-galactosidase after 30 min of incubation (+29%; p<0.05), and for β-glucuronidase after 60 min (+48%;
p<0.01). It should be pointed out that the total amount of lysosomal
enzymes (intracellular and released; see legend to Fig. 1) remained
constant for the duration of the experiments as already noted by
others (8) and was not influenced by the nature of the phagocytized
material. This makes it likely that released enzymes were not replaced by newly synthesized molecules at least during the period of
time studied in our experiments, although <u>de novo</u> synthesis of proteins was not investigated.

     When an attempt was made to raise the cellular level of cAMP
by adding either DBcAMP or theophylline (an inhibitor of phospho-
diesterase) to macrophage preparations, a decrease of the rate of
enzyme release was observed with theophylline at 10^{-3} M, but with

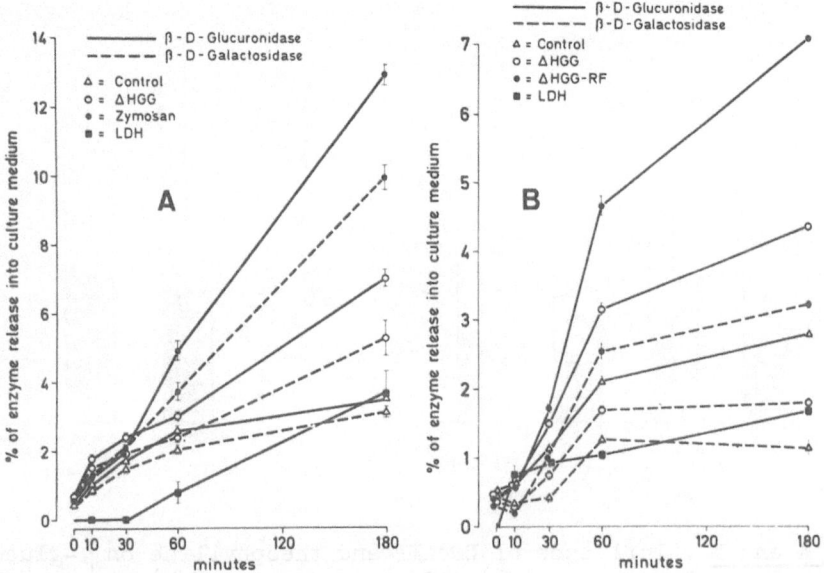

Fig. 1 A and B : Release of lysosomal enzymes by resting and phagocytizing macrophages. A: ΔHGG, 130 μg/8.10^6 cells: Zymosan,
3 mg/8.10^6 cells; B: ΔHGG, 640 μg/8.10^6 cells; ΔHGG-RF, 640 μg/8.10^6
cells. Each value represents the mean ± S.E.M. of 2-4 cultures.
Mean total amounts of enzymes + S.E.M. (intracellular + released)
per 10^7 cells were : β-D-glucuronidase 21.90 + 0.34 units, β-D-ga-
lactosidase 11.77 + 0.27 units and LDH 1764 + 27 mU.

DBcAMP only at the concentration of 10^{-2} M (i.e. 10^{-6} and 10^{-5}
moles per 8.10^6 cells respectively) as examplified for glucuronidase in Fig. 2. This decrease could not be ascribed to cell toxicity.
Theophylline inhibited the release of glucuronidase and galactosidase by 33 and 29% respectively and DBcAMP (10^{-2} M) by 16 and 22%
respectively. These changes although very modest were all statistically significant (p<0.005). DBcAMP at a concentration of 10^{-3} M
slightly increased the release of both enzymes (by 20 and 12% respectively). Adding both substances at a concentration of 10^{-3} M to
the same preparation did not result in a synergistic effect. The
rate of enzyme release of control cells remained unchanged.

When both substances were tested for their effect on phagocytosis, it appeared that theophylline (5.10^{-3} and 5.10^{-4} M) induced
a dramatic reduction in the uptake of SRBC by PM whereas only the
highest concentration (10^{-2} M) of DBcAMP had a similar effect
(Table 1). It is therefore not unlikely that the decreased rate
of enzyme release in the presence of DBcAMP and theophylline is

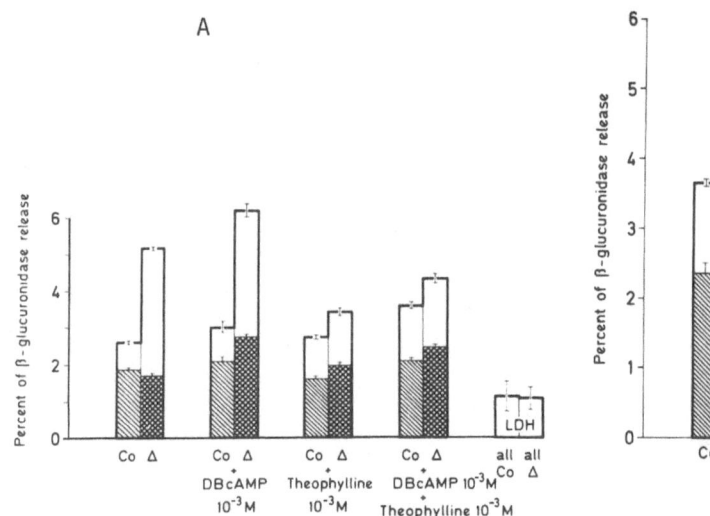
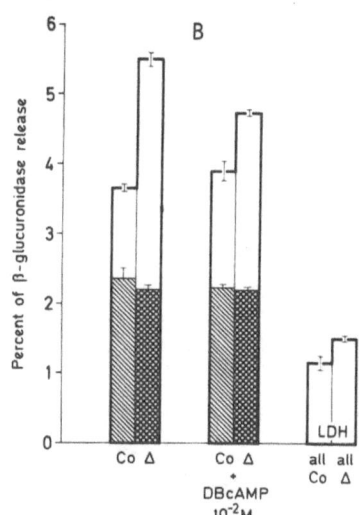

Fig. 2 A and B : Influence of DBcAMP and theophylline on β-glucuronidase release by resting (Co) and phagocytizing (△) macrophages
(640 μg ΔHGG/8.10⁶ cells). DBcAMP (10⁻³ and 10⁻² M) and theophylline
(10⁻³ M) were added 10 min prior to particulate material. Cross-
hatched bars, cells at 0 min; open bars, cells at 60 min incubation;
vertical lines, ± S.E.M.

related to reduced phagocytosis as is also suggested for PMNL by
the observations of Ignarro et al. (9).

   Isoproterenol (a stimulator of β-receptors) added to PM at the
concentration of 10⁻³ M 10 min prior to zymosan induced a moderate
increase of total cAMP after 10 min incubation. However, the cAMP
level was much higher in cells exposed to zymosan than in control
cells exposed to either zymosan or isoproterenol alone (Table 2).
To be sure, these modifications were strikingly less important than
those observed with PMNL in comparable conditions (9).

   Our results agree with those of others (5, 6) showing that
macrophages may release lysosomal enzymes without losing their viability. The finding that more enzymes were released by cells exposed to zymosan and ΔHGG-RF than by cells exposed to ΔHGG suggests
that the rate of enzyme excretion is related to the nature of phagocytized particles (9).

   In view of our observations, the regulator role of cAMP on
lysosomal enzyme release by mouse macrophages seems rather weak :
1) the decrease of enzyme release in the presence of substances
known to increase cellular cAMP was quite moderate;

Table 1 : Effect of DBcAMP and theophylline on phagocytosis
         (in % of control)

Agents	Concentration			
	$10^{-2}M$	$5.10^{-3}M$	$5.10^{-4}M$	O
None	−	−	−	100
DBcAMP	−41.6*	−11.9	+0.3	−
Theophylline	−	−86.3*	−47.0*	−

* p < 0.001, all other changes N.S. Cell viability as determined by
the trypan blue dye exclusion test ranged from 81-96%.

Table 2 : cAMP (pmoles/10^7 cells) in mouse peritoneal macrophages.
         Effect of phagocytosis and β-adrenergic stimulation.

Incubation time	Control		Isoproterenol $10^{-3}M$ *)	
	−	zymosan	−	zymosan
O min	69 + 1	80 + 5	83 + 10	111 + 8
10 min	89 + 6	87 + 8	85 + 8	136 + 8

*) Isoproterenol was added to cell suspensions 10 min prior to
zymosan. Figures represent means of 3 separate experiments + S.E.M.

2) DBcAMP and theophylline modified the rate of enzyme release in phagocytizing but not in resting cells, and they did so only at concentrations that also inhibit phagocytosis. By itself, decreased phagocytosis may well be responsible of reducing the rate of enzyme release; 3) even with a potent β-stimulator such as isoproterenol, it was markedly more difficult to raise cAMP level in macrophages than it appears to be for PMNL.

ACKNOWLEDGMENTS

We wish to acknowledge the valuable technical assistance of Monika Berney.

REFERENCES

1) Weissmann, G., Zurier, R.B., Spieler, P.J. and Goldstein, I.M., J. exp. Med., 134, 149s, 1971.
2) Hawkins, D., J. Immunol., 108, 310, 1972.
3) Henson, P.M., Johnson, H.B. and Spiegelberg, H.L., J. Immunol., 109, 1182, 1972.
4) Wright, D.G. and Malawista, S.E., J. Cell. Biol., 53, 788, 1972.
5) Weissmann, G., Dukor, P. and Zurier, R.B., Nature (New Biol.), 231, 131, 1971.
6) Ackerman, N.R. and Beebe, J.R., Nature, 247, 475, 1974.
7) Cardella, C.J., Davies, P. and Allison, A.C., Nature, 247, 46, 1974.
8) Davies, P., Allison, A.C., Ackerman, J., Butterfield, A. and Williams, S., Nature, 251, 423, 1974.
9) Ignarro, L.J., Lint, T.F. and George, W.J., J. exp. Med., 139, 1395, 1974.
10) Weissmann, G., Zurier, R.B. and Hoffstein, S., in Cyclic AMP, Cell Growth and the Immune Response, Edited by Braun, W., Lichtenstein, L.M. and Parker, C.W., p. 176, Springer-Verlag, Berlin, 1974.
11) Kato, K., Yoshida, K., Tsukamoto, H., Nobunaga, M., Masuya, T. and Sawada, T., Chem. Pharm. Bull. (Tokyo), 8, 239, 1960.
12) Conchie, J., Findlay, J. and Levy, G.A., Biochem. J., 71, 318, 1959.
13) Gilman, A.G., Proc. Natl. Acad. Sci., 67, 305, 1970.
14) Cruchaud, A. and Unanue, E.R., J. Immunol., 107, 1329, 1971.

THE STILL UNSOLVED GERMINAL CENTRE MYSTERY

(INVITED LECTURE)

J.H.Humphrey

National Institute for Medical Research, Mill Hill
London NW7 1AA, UK

When I was invited to give a lecture at this Conference I
looked through the list of titles of the other contributions, and
saw that Germinal Centres figured very little, despite the fact that
the 5th Conference includes them in its main title. In the event
we have heard a few very interesting papers on germinal centres,
but I decided that these structures had been unduly neglected and
that it would be opportune to try to restore to them something of
their earlier status.

No one who spends much time examining the histology of lymphoid
tissues can fail to conclude that their functional anatomy must be
important. They possess a remarkably complex, delicate and flex-
ible architecture which is similar in general design in very many
species. It seems clear that such an architecture would not have
evolved if it did not have important survival value for these species
in an environment full of microbes and other parasites ready to
colonize them the moment their protective external barriers were
breached. It seems to me that the fine control of the immune response must be regulated in real life, as opposed to tissue culture
vessels, by the interaction between antigens and cells, and of
cells with one another, constrained by the topographical relationships and the humoral influences which obtain within the complex
lymphoid tissues where they meet.

Of course in vitro studies of B cells, T cells and macrophages
have yielded a great deal of information, which could have been
obtained in no other way, about how B cells are stimulated to make
and secrete antibody. We have heard at this Conference about surface receptors for antigens, for Fc, for C3, for Ir gene products

and about soluble specific and nonspecific T cell factors which
can stimulate or inhibit B cells. Even though these soluble factors
can be shown to act when added to dispersed cells in tissue culture
vessels, there is strong evidence that in vivo interaction must
take place between cells which are in direct contact or very close
to one another. For example Rajewsky, Roëlants and Askonas (1)
showed that mouse spleen cells primed with a hapten-carrier could
not efficiently be stimulated to make anti-hapten antibody by
injection of the carrier alone or together with the hapten on an
unrelated carrier, and later (2) that when stimulation was by
hapten-carrier already taken up by macrophages - which was very
effective in triggering B memory cells - the hapten and the carrier
had to be associated with the same macrophages. Furthermore even
when T cell help was elicited by an allogeneic interaction (such
that soluble nonspecific T cell factors able to cause B cell differentiation would be produced in vitro), anti-hapten antibody production was only stimulated when the hapten-primed B memory cells
were targets for the allogeneic aggressor cells. They could find
no evidence that other B cells, as innocent bystanders, were involved and concluded that any active factor could only act over a
very short range.

    This is only part of the evidence that in vivo the outcome of
antigenic stimulation is determined by intimate contact between
antigen and all the cells concerned. Furthermore in vivo other
local factors are likely to modify the outcome, such as prosta-
glandins, histamine, noradrenaline, lymphocyte activation products,
and the stimulatory and inhibitory products of activated macrophages
recently described by Calderon and Unanue (3). We cannot dismiss,
either, thymin of which we have heard earlier, or even ubiquitin (4),
or other more conventional hormones such as insulin, somatotropin
and corticosteroids for which lymphocytes are known to have receptors.
Perhaps glutathione is the equivalent of the magic 2×10^{-5} M
2-mercaptoethanol which has so improved the performance of our
tissue cultures in vitro? At present we do not know which, if any,
of such factors are of primary importance, and their interplay may
be too complex to analyze in detail - but we should nevertheless be
aware of them.

    Let me return now to my theme, the Germinal Centre mystery.
The scenario is set in the lymph nodes and the spleen. I will not
describe it in detail but point out only the main features relevant
to the story. The traffic of T and B lymphocytes requires separate
descriptions in respect of lymph nodes (e.g. 5, 6) at which cells
arrive both via the afferent lymphatics and the arteries,and the
spleen (e.g. 7,8) which has no afferent lymphatic vessels. Van
Ewijk and Brons have shown at this Conference their striking scanning electron micrographs demonstrating the passage of T and B
lymphocytes between the lining endothelium of postcapillary venules
in the lymph node,and in the marginal sinus of the splenic white

pulp where the penicillary arteries arborize and end. So far as primary follicles (9) germinal centres are concerned, the important feature is that they contain only B cells,except for scanty T cells in primary follicles (6) and the T cells at the cortical poles of active germinal centres now described by Weissman, Gutman and Friedberg at this meeting. The distribution of antigens has also to be considered. This has been followed both by immunofluorescence, or by the much more sensitive technique of using ^{125}I labelled materials, to which I shall largely refer. Where and for how long antigens are retained depends upon a number of factors:- the route of administration (e.g. via the afferent lymphatic or via the blood stream), the nature of the antigen, its speed of degradation within macrophages, whether it is particulate, and whether there is pre-existing antibody (as there very often is). Soluble protein anti-gens or polysaccharides such as linear 1:3 dextrans in the absence of antibody sweep through lymphoid tissues, but small amounts are retained (until degraded) in or on macrophages of the subcapsular and marginal zones and in the medulla of lymph nodes and the red pulp of the spleen. Some other indigestible antigens, such as poly D-TGL (10), D-(TG) poly-ProL (11) or type 3 pneumococcal polysaccharide (12) are retained in large amounts and for long periods undegraded mainly in macrophages of the medulla and red pulp. Others still, such as ficoll or branched chain dextrans become predominantly and lastingly localized in the subcapsular sinus and marginal zones, although they also are present to some extent in macrophages elsewhere (12). Antigens generally are retained only to a small extent in scattered macrophages in the thymus dependent areas, unless the lymphoid tissues have been disorganized by complete Freund's adjuvant. When antibody is present, or when the antigen is an aggregated Ig, a further pattern of retention is superposed. More is retained in macrophages generally, though degradable mat-erials are largely broken down within a day or so, apart from a small proportion retained at the surface (13), but now there is prominent and lasting localization in germinal centres. I shall return to this later.

The last part of the scenario concerns the sites of antibody formation. Both in primary and secondary responses antibody form-ation first occurs in the medulla of lymph nodes (after 4-6 days and 2-4 days respectively) and/or at the margin of the white and red pulp of the spleen (after 2-4 days). Although preexisting germinal centres may be present, new germinal centres, induced by the antigen, do not appear until after 5-7 days in primary and 4-6 days in secondary responses. This implies that germinal centres cannot be involved in the initiation of antibody production. However when no antibody is produced, new germinal centres are not formed.

The Origin of Germinal Centres

Workers at the Hall Institute (9) have distinguished primary

follicles, consisting of small spherical aggregates of lymphocytes
in the B cell area interspersed with scattered dendritic reticular
cells, present in lymph nodes and spleen of animals subject to
minimal antigenic stimulation. After antigenic stimulation the
dendritic reticular cells appear to migrate towards one another,
and an increasing number of large pyroninophilic dividing cells
become present at the site, surrounded by a sphere of medium sized
lymphocytes and outside these a cuff of small lymphocytes. Among
the large pyroninophilic cells are "tingible body" macrophages -
i.e. macrophages containing dead cell debris, notably pyknotic
nuclei. Evidently considerable cell destruction goes on simultaneously with cell division, but the identity of the dying cells and
the reason for their death are unknown. These are the corpses of
the germinal centre mystery - and I fear that this part of the
mystery remains unsolved. It is not certain either what becomes
of the offspring of the dividing cells. They do not usually contain Ig (although antibody containing cells can be found in germinal centres in vigorous secondary responses and late in the response
in the spleens of chickens (14)). Presumably they contribute to the
mantle of surrounding cells, and must leave the area in the spleen
either into the red pulp by the bridging channels described by
Mitchell (15) or by the lymphatics (16), and in the lymph nodes by
retrograde passage through post-capillary venules and/or by passing
into the medulla. Sometimes in lymph nodes there appears to be a
continuous progression of cells from blast cells in the germinal
centre to mature plasma cells in the medulla, as though the blast
cells had burst out from the germinal centre and had acquired the
capacity to secrete Ig as a result of further stimulation en route.

It is a matter of interest, that germinal centres are not
formed in nu nu mice, although they are present in neonatally thymectomized or irradiated and foetal liver reconstituted animals,
and are restored when nu nu mice are reconstituted with thymus cells
(17); nevertheless the capacity of dendritic reticular cells in nu
nu mice to capture antigen antibody complexes is unimpaired (18).
Whether the requirement for some T cells reflects a need for the
synthesis of enough of the right sort of antibody to allow follicular localization of antigen, or whether T cell help is required
for the B cells to become blasts is uncertain.

The Dendritic Reticular Cells

The dendritic reticular cells have been aptly described as the
immunologists' Cinderella. Their origin is uncertain, and they are
not included in the proposed Mononuclear Phagocyte System (19).
Nossal and his colleagues have shown that they are present early in
phylogeny, for example in the juxtaglomerular organ of Buffo
marinus (9). They have the striking property of binding aggregated
Ig and antigen-antibody complexes, which are retained at the surface

of the cells for long periods of time - except insofar as they may
be gradually be broken down by enzymes in the surrounding fluid
(20). Binding depends upon the presence of the Fc portion of Ig
(9). The presence of C3 as well as of IgG and IgM has been shown
in germinal centres of human lymph nodes (21), and indeed none of
the experiments of Ada and his colleagues (9) excludes the possibility that binding may be via C3. Hanna, who showed that dendritic
reticular cells in germinal centres gradually lose the fine in-
folding of their plasma membranes, suggested that this might be due
to damage by fixed complement; however they also showed that these
cells are damaged by moderate doses (400-600r) of irradiation and
could not exclude the possibility that the changes might be due
to the radioactive antigen which was employed (22).

The follicular dendritic reticular cells are quite unselective
in localizing antigen-antibody complexes, and the same cells can
pick up two different complexes administered 2 weeks apart (23).
How such complexes reach these cells, particularly in the spleen,
is not perfectly clear. Within a few minutes of injection into
the blood stream in mice complexes are found in the marginal zone
of the white pulp, and only reach germinal centres after 4-6 hours.
Brown and his colleagues have argued that the complexes become
bound via Fc receptors to B lymphocytes in the marginal zone and
are transported by them to the dendritic cells (24). Their evidence is not fully convincing to me, and such a process does not
seem to occur in the chicken where dendritic cells have been shown
by White themselves to carry the complexes into splenic germinal
centres (14).

Steinman and Cohn recently reported the presence in peripheral
lymphoid organs of mice of a novel cell type which they named
dendritic cells, because of their morphological appearance (25).
I would like to think that these are the same as dendritic reticular cells, but they evidently are not. Although they are distinct
from normal macrophages, are very sensitive to hydrocortisone and
to ionizing radiation and do not ingest antibody coated sheep
erythrocytes, they lack the cardinal property of retaining immune
complexes at their surface (26). It seems to me more probable that
they correspond to the "frilly cells" which occur in afferent lymph,
and which may represent migrating Langerhans cells of the dermis
(27 and B.M.Balfour, personal communication).

C3 and the Localization of Antigen-Antibody Complexes

Dukor and his colleagues (28) last year presented preliminary
evidence that mice deprived of C3 by treatment with cobra venom
factor (CVF) failed to trap ^{125}I-labelled aggregated HGG in their
splenic follicles. Dr.Pryjma and I have confirmed this (29).

We have also shown that CVF is a strictly thymus dependent immunogen, and that thymus deprived (TxB) mice can be maintained depleted
of circulating C3 by repeated injections of CVF for several weeks.
This enabled us to compare the antibody response in mice to T-indep-
endent immunogens in the continued presence or absence of C3. We
have used various polysaccharides or their DNP derivatives trace-
labelled with ^{125}I by means of a small number of tyramine groups
(conjugated via CNBr). The outcome of our experiments has been
to show that once antibody is present (largely IgM) a variety of
antigens (DNP-Ficoll, DNP-S3, DNP-dextrans) become localized in
germinal centres, in addition to localization in macrophages in
other sites. Such localization occurs equally in TxB or sham Tx
control mice. Deprivation of C3 prevents localization in germinal
centres, but not in other sites, and has no or only a small effect
on the antibody response to these immunogens. These findings
indicate that C3 activation is necessary for attachment of immune
complexes to dendritic reticular cells. They also rule out any
role for antigen bound in germinal centres in the primary antibody
response - a not very surprising conclusion, in view of the time
course of the immune response discussed earlier.

We also observed that levan or DNP-levan became extensively
localized in germinal centres within a few hours after injection,
long before antibody formation, measured by plaque forming cells,
could be detected. This also was abolished by C3 deprivation.
Levan is a large molecule forming semi-colloidal solutions and,
alone among the antigens which we tested, is a potent activator of
C3 via the alternate pathway. The implication is that C3 activation
is not only a necessary but also a sufficient condition for localization in germinal centres.

Changes in the Functional Anatomy of Lymph Nodes following Antigen Administration

Lymph nodes draining the site of administration of an immunogen
swell. Some recent work analyzing what changes occur in them is
relevant to my theme. One concerns the vascular circulation, which
can be visualized by microangiography (32). Two days after injecting
typhoid 'O' antigen into the foot pad of rabbits there is an extraordinary redistribution of the capillary circulation in the draining
lymph nodes. The relatively avascular paracortical (T-dependent) areas
become uniformly and highly vascularized, and the subcapsular and medullary cord capillaries also enlarge and the number patent increases.
The changes reach a peak at 5 days and have subsided by 15 days.
The number of post-capillary venules with high endothelium is also
increased, but not proportionately.

The second concerns the effect of lymphocyte activation products formed at the site of antigen deposition, and travelling up

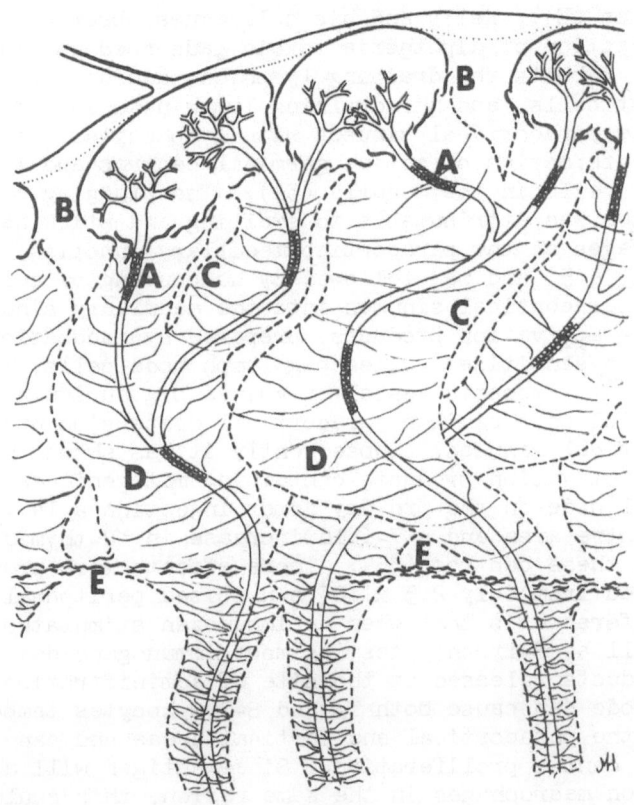

Figure 1. Anatomical drawing showing lymphocyte migratory routes
through the lymph node paracortex. Blood-borne cells enter at the
high endothelial segments of the post-capillary venules (A). Three
different migratory routes may be followed from this point: the
perifollicular route (B), the paracortical sinus route (C), and
the paracortical cord route (D). Most recirculatory lymphocytes
which pass through the paracortical cords leave these structures
at the paracortico-medullary border (E) to enter the medullary
sinuses (F) and eventually reach the efferent lymphatic.
(From Kelly, R.H.(33)).

the afferent lymphatic vessels. Kelly has described (33) three
migratory routes whereby lymphocytes, which enter the paracortical
area of a lymph node via high endothelial segments of post-capillary venules, can migrate into the medulla. These are illustrated
in the accompanying diagram. The main pathway is along the paracortical cords (D in the drawing) and across the paracortico-

medullary border (E). Kelly and his colleagues observed that 2-3
days after injection of diphtheria toxoid (adsorbed on alum) into
the footpad of rabbits the draining lymph contained a substantial
number of blast cells, and the draining lymph node showed extensive
plugging of the paracortical sinuses with lymphocytes, followed
shortly by the formation of active germinal centres and the appearance of plasma cells in the medulla (34). The plugging of the paracortical sinuses was attributable to swelling and stickiness of the
lining macrophages at the paracortico-medullary junction; this ended
abruptly at day 4-5, and was followed by outpouring of cells from
the congested paracortical sinuses into the medullary sinuses.
When lymphocyte activation products, prepared by incubation with
antigen in vitro/sensitized guinea pig lymph node cells, were infused
into the afferent lymphatic vessel of guinea pig auricular lymph
nodes there resulted a similar paracortical distension and plugging
of the paracortical sinuses. Subsequently it was shown that infusion
of lymphocyte activation products containing mitogenic factor caused
in the regional node on the 3rd day after injection a 14-fold increase
in germinal centre area and a 7-fold increase in ^{3}H-thymidine labelled cells in these centres (35). These effects were produced by
material derived from only 2.5 x 10^4 sensitized peritoneal exudate
cells. The inference is that when an immunogen stimulates T-lymphocytes as well as B-lymphocytes (as most immunogens do), lymphocyte
activation products released at the site of administration or within
the draining node can cause both T- and B-lymphocytes temporarily to
accumulate in the paracortical and cortical areas and can also stimulate germinal centre proliferation. Since antigen will also be
present in or on macrophages in the same region, this could provide
the ideal microenvironment for interaction at close quarters between
the three cell types. That this inference is not merely fanciful
is indicated by the demonstration by Hay et al.(36) of MIF and mitogenic activity in the lymph of sheep draining sites into which
bacteriophage ØX 174 or tuberculin had been injected.

Are Germinal Centres Sites of Generation of B-memory Cells?

It has been proposed by Cottier, Nossal, Thorbecke and other
workers that germinal centres could be the sites where antigen,
attached to dendritic reticular cells and in intimate contact with
B cells, acts to stimulate B cell memory. If T-cells are also
required for this (which I doubt), they also have been shown by
Weissman to be present very nearby in the cortical poles. This
would be an attractive solution of at least a major part of the
germinal centre mystery, but there has been to my mind the following major difficulty in accepting it. As already pointed out,
antibody production precedes germinal centre formation. Consequently antigen attached to the dendritic follicular cells will be
coated with excess antibody, and its epitopes unavailable to the
receptors on B-cells. However recent work by my colleagues

Dr.B.A.Askonas and M.E.Roux may have resolved these doubts. They
have been studying the mechanism of "clonal dominance"(37), which
is observed when clones of potential antibody forming cells are
serially transferred in irradiated mice. Such clones contain both
T- and B-memory cells. The question was how the clone persists -
i.e. memory cells remain available - even after antigenic stimulation, which elicits a clonal antibody product which can inhibit its
own B-memory cells. They selected anti-DNP clones which could be
stimulated by T-cell help induced by DNP on another carrier. The
DNP specific B-memory cells in such clones, treated with DNP-
carrier in vitro before transfer, could be stimulated, with the
help of T-cells responding to the separate carrier, even in the
presence of their own clonal anti-DNP antibody product. This means
that the epitope in an antigen antibody complex can be recognized
by receptors on B-cells. Since B-cells in a germinal centre would
be capable of interacting with complexes at the surface of dendritic
cells via C3 and Fc receptors as well as by specific receptors for
a suitable epitope, the interaction could presumably be sufficient
to trigger them to multiply as B-memory cells.

What seems to me the clearest evidence that germinal centres
are a site, and perhaps the main or even the only site of generation of B-memory cells in vivo, comes from an elegant experiment
by Cottier and his colleagues (38). They studied the response of
mice primed against tetanus toxoid (TT) to secondary stimulation by
fluid TT injected into the foot pad. This elicited the transient
appearance of very many plasma cells in the medulla of the regional
nodes, maximal at 3 days and largely subsided by 5 days after boosting.
Germinal centre enlargement began a little later, reached a maximum
at 5 days followed by a second increase at 12 days. When the mice
were irradiated (600r) 4 days after the boost, the germinal centres
disappeared within one day and did not reappear. Nevertheless the
time course of synthesis and release of antibody against TT was
almost unaffected by irradiation at this time, and was attributable
to the radio-resistant mature plasma cells. When mice which had
received no irradiation were given a third injection of TT they
gave a vigorous tertiary antibody response, but those irradiated
as described showed no evidence of immunological memory. Although
other explanations are possible, the most obvious is that germinal
centres are required for generating new B-memory cells.

Since C3 is required for localization of antigen in germinal
centres, it should be possible to test whether B memory cells can
be generated in response to an immunogen administered to mice chronically deprived of C3 by means of CVF and consequently without antigen on the dendritic reticular cell web. Since B cell memory can
be generated in Txb mice my colleague G.G.B.Klaus and I have compared the B-memory generated in TxB mice, with and without C3, by
DNP-KLH administered 3 weeks earlier. The presence of B-memory

cells for DNP was tested by transfer of spleen cells together with
ovalbumin-primed helper cells to irradiated syngeneic mice, which
were challenged with DNP-ovalbumin and assayed for anti-DNP plaque
forming cells. We have only completed one experiment, but I mention
it because it showed no generation of memory in the absence of C3,
and again provides support, though not proof, for the proposition
that germinal centres are the site of generation of B-cell memory.

In mice infected with malaria due to Plasmodium berghei yoellii,
during the phase of parasitaemia germinal centres are disorganized
and fail to localize aggregated HGG (39). According to the present
hypothesis such mice should fail to generate memory cells against
a non persistent antigen administered during this period, and it is
of some interest that mice primed with sheep erythrocytes during
the parasitaemic phase show greatly impaired IgG memory when re-
challenged later (40).

The Strange Story of Germinal Centres in the Chicken

R.G.White and his colleagues have made an extensive study of
the development of germinal centres in the spleen of chickens,
especially in response to the intravenous injection of moderate
doses (1-10 mg) of the soluble protein antigen human serum albumin
(HSA). The sequence of events which they describe is as follows:-
HSA continues to circulate in the bloodstream for about 30 hours.
Antibody (initially IgM) is then produced by cells in the red pulp
near the margin of the white pulp, and antigen-antibody complexes
are formed. Some of the complexes enter the white pulp through the
walls of the Schweigger-Seidel sheaths and become attached to the
surface of preexisting scattered dendritic reticular cells. These
antigen-bearing cells migrate through the white pulp alongside the
penicillary vessels to the point of their bifurcation from the
central arterioles of the white pulp. From 72 hours onwards germinal centres appear as aggregations of dendritic cells and B-
lymphocytes at this site; this process continues until by about
6 days all the antigen bearing cells have become enclosed within
the boundaries of newly formed germinal centres. If preformed HSA-
anti HSA complexes are injected instead of soluble HSA,the whole
process is accelerated . Correspondingly, in bursectomized irradiated birds, which fail to make antibody, localization on dendritic
cells and germinal centre formation does not take place. Heat
aggregated HGG (but not material treated with pepsin to remove the
Fc protein) becomes very rapidly attached to dendritic reticular
cells, and this is followed by their migration to form germinal
centres as described above. In bursectomized irradiated chickens,
lacking B-cells, aggregated HGG attaches equally well to dendritic
cells but no germinal centres are subsequently formed. The description so far is in accord with that already given for the mouse. So
also is the effect of 3 injections of CVF given within 24 hours,

before injecting HSA, which prevented the usual localization of
antigen on dendritic cells and subsequent germinal centre formation.   Interestingly, if passive hyperimmune chicken anti-HSA
antibody was administered to CVF treated birds 1 hour before HSA
was injected, the dendritic cells picked up HSA-anti-HSA complexes
in the usual way and migrated to form germinal centres - but these
were relatively few and poorly outlined compared to those in controls
(41).

The strange part of the story is that which follows.

The antibody response of normal chickens to soluble HSA or to
sheep erythrocytes consists of an early rise of IgM followed shortly
by IgG antibody.   Antibody levels, both IgM and IgG, reach a peak
at 6-8 days after which IgM production abruptly ceases.   IgG production also declines, but more slowly (42).   White and his colleagues
(14) have shown that late in the response, from the 13th day onwards
(by which time all antibody producing cells have disappeared from
the spleen) antibody containing cells appear in some of the germinal
centres, and probably account for the 'tail' of IgG production.   This
is not inconsistent with germinal centres being the sites of production of B-memory cells.   White has postulated that both IgM and
IgG antibody synthesis are switched off by high affinity IgG, and that
the latter depends upon germinal centres.   This hypothesis is supported by some striking effects which occur when germinal centre formation is prevented or does not take place.

Intravenous administration of 10^9 Salmonella adelaide organisms
results in a rapid IgM antibody response which reaches a peak at
4-7 days and then declines.   This is followed by a further series of
at least four peaks of IgM antibody production at about 10 day
intervals; after about 40 days a small amount of IgG antibody begins
to appear, and the IgM peaks cease (42).   The picture is not unlike
that of the response to bacterial 'O' lipopolysaccharide in the
mouse (44).   Histological examination of the spleens of chickens
injected with S.adelaide showed that a massive development of plasma
cells occurred in the medulla by the 4th day, as expected, but that
from the 6th day onward germinal centres were not detectable, and
they did not re-appear until 3 or more weeks later.   Whether this
was due to C3 depletion owing to activation of the alternate pathway by the injected organisms was not tested.   However when 10^{10}
sheep erythrocytes were administered to chickens treated with CVF
(to prevent germinal centre formation), instead of the usual single
sharp peak of anti-erythrocyte antibody there occurred two or even
three well marked consecutive peaks of IgM antibody with virtually
no IgG (43).   To complete the picture White and Nielsen injected
chickens with 10^9 S.adelaide mixed with 10^{10} sheep erythrocytes,
and found that both the anti-erythrocyte and the anti S.adelaide
responses consisted of a series of peaks of IgM antibody.   Passive

administration on day 9 of IgG antibody from birds hyperimmunized
against sheep erythrocytes promptly cut short the response to
that antigen, so that only a single peak occurred; IgG from birds
hyperimmunized against S.adelaide,however, cut short the response
to both antigens. Following administration of IgG antibody against
S.adelaide there was a prompt and massive development of germinal
centres, much greater than the late recovery which took place in
chickens injected with S.adelaide only.

White has argued (45) that the effect of Freund's adjuvant,
which disorganizes lymphoid tissues in mammals and birds, and in
the chicken causes abnormal germinal centres in which dendritic
cells are clumped and not interspersed with B-lymphocytes, is
to interfere with the normal germinal centre dependent feed-back
 mechanism which switches off antibody production. This argument
requires that B-cells able to respond to the antigen should be
suppressed by contact with antigen on the dendritic cells. I know
of no direct evidence that this occurs, and there are alternative
explanations which lie outside the scope of this lecture.

I hope that I have convinced you that germinal centres are not
only intriguing but important, and were rightly included in the
title of our Conference. Although it has been possible to report
progress in unravelling the mystery of their origin and function,
I suspect that we shall need to understand much more about the
ecology of lymphocytes in the micro-environment of lymphoid tissues
before the mystery is finally revealed.

REFERENCES

1.   Rajewsky, K., Roelants, G.E. and Askonas, B.A., Eur.J.Immunol.
        2,592 (1972).
2.   Askonas, B.A. and Roelants, G.E., Eur.J.Immunol. 4, 1 (1974).
3.   Calderon, J. and Unanue, E.R., Nature (Lond.) 253, 359 (1975).
4.   Schlesinger, D.H. and Goldstein,G., Nature (Lond.) 255, 423,
        (1975).
5.   Parrott, D.M.V. and de Sousa, M.A.B., Clin.Exp.Immunol. 8,
        663 (1971).
6.   Gutman, G.A. and Weissman, I.L. Immunology, 23, 465 (1972).
7.   Mitchell, J., Immunology 22, 231 (1972).
8.   Nieuwenhuis, P. and Ford, W.L., in preparation.
9.   Nossal, G.J.V. and Ada, G.L."Antigens, Lymphoid Cells and the
        Immune Response". Academic Press Inc., New York and London
        (1971).
10. Janeway, C.A.,Jr., and Humphrey, J.H., Immunology 14, 225 (1968)
11. Medlin, J., Humphrey, J.H. and Sela, M., Folia Biologica 16,
        156 (1970).
12. Humphrey, J.H.,(unpublished.)
13. Unanue, E.R. and Askonas, B.A., J.exp.Med., 127, 915 (1968).
14. White, R.G., French, V.I. and Stark, J.M., J.Med.Microbiol.
        3, 65 (1970).

15. Mitchell, J., Immunology 24, 93 (1973).
16. Veerman, A.J.P. and van Ewijk. Cell Tiss.Res. 156, 417 (1975).
17. de Sousa, M. and Pritchard, H., Immunology 26, 769 (1974).
18. Mitchell, J., Pye, J., Holmes, M.C. and Nossal, G.J.V.,
    Austral.J.exp.Biol.med.Sci. 50, 637 (1972).
19. "Mononuclear Phagocytes" ed.R.van Furth., Blackwell Scientific
    Publications, Oxford, 1970.
20. Humphrey, J.H., Askonas, B.A., Auzins, I., Schechter, I. and
    Sela, M., Immunology 13, 71 (1967).
21. Gail-Peczalska, K.J., Fish, A.J., Meuwissen, H.J., Frommel, D.
    and Good, R.A., J.exp.Med. 130, 1367 (1969).
22. Hanna, M.G. and Szakal, A.K., J.Immunol. 101, 949 (1969).
23. van Rooijen, N., Immunology 27, 617 (1974).
24. Brown, J.C., Harris, G., Papamichail, M., Slijvic, V.S. and
    Holborow, E.J., Immunology 24, 955 (1973).
25. Steinman, R.M. and Cohn, Z.A., J.exp.Med. 137, 1142 (1973).
26. Steinman, R.M. and Cohn, Z.A., J.exp.Med. 139, 380 (1974).
27. Kelly, R.H., Nature (Lond.) 227, 510 (1970).
28. Dukor, P., Dietrich, F.M., Gisler, R.H., Schumann, G. and
    Bitter-Suermann, D., Progress in Immunology 2. eds.L.Brent
    and J.Holborow. Vol.3., p.99. North-Holland, Amsterdam.
29. Humphrey, J.H. and Pryjma, J. (to be published).
30. Pryjma, J. and Humphrey, J.H., Immunology 28, 569 (1975).
31. Pryjma, J., Humphrey, J.H. and Klaus, G.G.B., Nature (Lond.)
    252, 505 (1974).
32. Herman, P.G., Yamamoto, I. and Mellins, H.Z., J.exp.Med. 136,
    697 (1972).
33. Kelly, R.H., Int.Archs.Allergy appl.Immunol. 48, 831 (1975).
34. Kelly, R.H., Wolstencroft, R.A., Dumonde, D.C. and Balfour,
    B.M., Clin.Exp.Immunol. 10, 49 (1972).
35. Kelly, R.H. and Wolstencroft, R.A., Clin.exp.Immunol. 18, 321
    (1974).
36. Hay, J.B., Lachmann, P.J. and Trnka, Z., Eur.J.Immunol. 3, 127
    (1973).
37. Askonas, B.A. and Williamson, A.R., Nature (Lond.) 238, 339
    (1972).
38. Grobler, P., Buerki, H., Cottier, H., Hess, M.W. and Stoner,
    R.D., J.Immunol.112, 2154 (1974).
39. Greenwood, B.M., Brown, J.C., de Jesus, D.G. and Holborow, E.J.
    Clin.exp.Immunol. 9, 345 (1971).
40. Greenwood,B.M., Playfair, J.H.L. and Torrigiani, G., Clin.exp.
    Immunol. 8, 467 (1971).
41. White, R.G., Henderson, D.C., Eslami, M.B. and Nielsen, K.H.,
    Immunology 28, 1 (1975).
42. White, R.G. and Nielsen, K.H., Immunology 28, 959 (1975).
43. Nielsen, K.H. and White, R.G., Nature (Lond.) 250, 234 (1974).
44. Britton, S. and Moller, G., J.Immunol. 100,1326 (1968).
45. White, R.G.. In:"Immunopotentiation". Ciba Foundation Symposium
    18. ASP, Amsterdam. 1973.